Your Pregnancy and Childbirth

SEVENTH EDITION

MONTH TO MONTH

From the Leading Experts in Women's Health Care

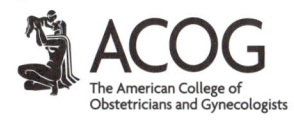

ACOG
The American College of
Obstetricians and Gynecologists

Your Pregnancy and Childbirth: Month to Month, Seventh Edition, was developed by a panel of experts working with staff of the American College of Obstetricians and Gynecologists (ACOG):

Editorial Task Force Members
Brian M. Mercer, MD, Chair
Dane M. Shipp, MD, Vice Chair
D. Ware Branch, MD
Lisa M. Foglia, MD
Manijeh Kamyar, MD
Gayle Olson Koutrouvelis, MD
Maria Mascola, MD
Barbara M. O'Brien, MD
T. Flint Porter, MD, MPH
Adrienne D. Zertuche, MD, MPH

ACOG Staff
Christopher Zahn, MD, Vice President, Practice Activities
Jennifer Walsh, Publisher and Product Officer
Jennifer Hicks, MS, Director, Patient Education
Olivia Bobrowsky, Product Manager, Patient Education
Sandra Patterson, Managing Editor, Clinical Content
Jeanette Smith, MPA, Editor
Elizabeth Frey, Production Manager
Hosnia N. Jami, Graphic Designer
Samantha Lee, Marketing and Graphics Manager

The contributions of the following people are gratefully acknowledged:
Robin Marwick, Writer
Debra Naylor, Naylor Design, Inc., Book Design
John Yanson, Illustration
Lightbox Visual Communications Inc., Illustration
Cade Martin Photography with Photogroup Inc./DC Studios

Library of Congress Cataloging-in-Publication Data

Names: American College of Obstetricians and Gynecologists.
Title: Your pregnancy and childbirth : month to month / from the leading experts in women's health care, ACOG, The American College of Obstetricians and Gynecologists.
Description: Seventh edition. | Washington, DC : American College of Obstetricians and Gynecologists, [2021] | Includes index.
Identifiers: LCCN 2019059300 (print) | LCCN 2019059301 (ebook) | ISBN 9781934984901 (paperback) | ISBN 9781948258029 (ebook)
Subjects: LCSH: Pregnancy--Popular works. | Childbirth--Popular works.
Classification: LCC RG525 .A26 2021 (print) | LCC RG525 (ebook) | DDC 618.2--dc23

LC record available at https://lccn.loc.gov/2019059300
LC ebook record available at https://lccn.loc.gov/2019059301

Copyright 2021 by the American College of Obstetricians and Gynecologists,
409 12th Street SW, Washington, DC 20024-2188.

All rights reserved. No part of this publication may be reproduced, stored in a retrieval system, posted on the internet, or transmitted, in any form or by any means, electronic, mechanical, photocopying, recording, or otherwise, without prior written permission from the publisher.

Designed as an informational resource for patients, *Your Pregnancy and Childbirth: Month to Month* sets forth current information and opinions on subjects related to women's health and reproduction. *Your Pregnancy and Childbirth: Month to Month* is a resource for informational purposes only. This resource does not constitute advice from your physician or health care professional and it is not intended to replace the advice or counsel of a physician or health care professional. You should consult with, and rely only on the advice of, physicians or health care professionals familiar with your particular condition. While *Your Pregnancy and Childbirth: Month to Month* makes every effort to provide information that is accurate and timely, the publisher cannot make any guarantees or warranties in that regard. The information does not dictate an exclusive course of treatment or procedure to be followed and should not be construed as excluding other acceptable methods of practice. Variations, taking into account the needs of the individual patient, resources, and limitations unique to the institution or type of practice, may be appropriate. The mention of a product, device, or drug in this publication does not constitute or guarantee endorsement of the quality or value of such product, device, or drug or of the claims made for it by the manufacturer.

12345/54321

Contents

Introduction xix

1 PREGNANCY MONTH BY MONTH 1

CHAPTER 1: Getting Ready for Pregnancy 3

The Prepregnancy Visit 3
Preexisting Health Conditions • Family Health History • Medications and Supplements • Past Pregnancies • Vaccinations • Protection Against Sexually Transmitted Infections • Prepregnancy Carrier Screening

A Healthy Lifestyle 9
Eating Right • Getting Regular Exercise • Taking Folic Acid • Reaching and Maintaining a Healthy Weight • Stopping Use of Unhealthy Substances • Keeping Your Environment Safe

Getting Pregnant 15
The Menstrual Cycle • When Are You Most Fertile? • Stopping Birth Control

RESOURCES 20

CHAPTER 2: Choosing Your Care Team 23

Types of Pregnancy Doctors 23
Obstetrician–Gynecologists • Maternal–Fetal Medicine Specialists • Family Medicine Doctors

Other Practitioners 24
Certified Nurse–Midwives and Certified Midwives • Certified Professional Midwives

Types of Practices 25

Questions to Ask 26

Prenatal Care Visits 26
What Happens During a Visit? • How Often Should You See Your Ob-Gyn?

Making Your Physical Exam More Comfortable 28
Special Concerns for Survivors of Sexual Abuse

RESOURCES 31

Illustrations of Fetal Development 32

III

CHAPTER 3: Months 1 and 2 (Weeks 1 to 8)   43

YOUR BABY   43

YOUR PREGNANCY   46

Your Changing Body   46
Signs and Symptoms of Pregnancy • Pregnancy Tests • Hormones • Your Estimated Due Date

Discomforts and How to Manage Them   50
Morning Sickness • Fatigue

Nutrition   52
Prenatal Vitamins • Weight Gain

Exercise   54

Healthy Decisions   55
Things to Avoid During Pregnancy • What Should I Do About Medications?

Other Considerations   60
A Safe Workplace • Tips for Working During Early Pregnancy

Prenatal Care Visits   61

Special Concerns   63
Miscarriage • Ectopic Pregnancy

When to Share the News   64

RESOURCES   65

CHAPTER 4: Month 3 (Weeks 9 to 12)   67

YOUR BABY   67

YOUR PREGNANCY   68

Your Changing Body   68

Discomforts and How to Manage Them   68
Nausea • Fatigue and Sleep Problems • Acne • Skin Color Changes • Breast Changes • Constipation • Emotional Changes

Nutrition   73
Weight Gain • Sugar and Sugar Substitutes

Prenatal Care Visits   75
Ultrasound Exam • Lab Tests • Screening for Birth Defects

Discussions With Your Ob-Gyn   80
Vaginal Birth After Cesarean Delivery • Prenatal Genetic Screening and Diagnosis

RESOURCES   82

CHAPTER 5: Month 4 (Weeks 13 to 16)   85

YOUR BABY   85

YOUR PREGNANCY   86

Your Changing Body   86

Discomforts and How to Manage Them   86
Lower Abdominal Pain • Mouth and Dental Changes • Excessive Salivation • Pregnancy-Related Stress • Spider Veins • Strange Dreams • Urinary Problems • Vaginal Discharge

Nutrition   90
Weight Gain • Food Cravings

Prenatal Care Visits   92
Discussions With Your Ob-Gyn   92
Birth Places • Home Birth
RESOURCES   93

CHAPTER 6: Month 5 (Weeks 17 to 20)   95

YOUR BABY   95

YOUR PREGNANCY   96

Your Changing Body   96
Your Baby's Movement

Discomforts and How to Manage Them   97
Congestion and Nosebleeds • Dizziness • Memory Changes • Sleeping Positions • Lower Back Pain

Nutrition   100
Healthy Snacking • Weight Gain

Prenatal Care Visits   101

Discussions With Your Ob-Gyn   103
Learning the Baby's Sex • Choosing Your Baby's Doctor

Special Concerns   104
Prenatal Lead Exposure

RESOURCES   107

CHAPTER 7: Month 6 (Weeks 21 to 24)   109

YOUR BABY   109

YOUR PREGNANCY   111

Your Changing Body   111
Body Image • Sexual Activity • Weight Gain

Discomforts and How to Manage Them   112
Heartburn • Hot Flashes • Aches and Pains • Fast or Racing Heartbeat

Exercise   114
Loss of Balance

Prenatal Care Visits   115

Discussions With Your Ob-Gyn   115
Labor and Delivery: Things to Start Thinking About

Special Concerns   116
Early Preterm Birth • Signs of Preterm Labor • Preeclampsia

Involving Your Other Children in Your Pregnancy   118

RESOURCES   118

CHAPTER 8: Month 7 (Weeks 25 to 28)   121

YOUR BABY   121

YOUR PREGNANCY   122

Your Changing Body   122
Body Image and Weight Gain

Discomforts and How to Manage Them   124
Lower Back Pain • Pelvic Bone Pain • Constipation • Braxton Hicks Contractions

Mental Health During Pregnancy   126
Depression • Anxiety and Stress

Prenatal Care Visits   130

Discussions With Your Ob-Gyn   131
Birth Plan • Cord Blood Banking • Birth Control After Pregnancy

Special Concerns   132
Preterm Labor • Vaginal Bleeding • Amniotic Fluid Problems

RESOURCES   134

CHAPTER 9: Month 8 (Weeks 29 to 32)   137

YOUR BABY   137

YOUR PREGNANCY   138

Your Changing Body   138

Discomforts and How to Manage Them   138
Shortness of Breath • Leg Cramps • Varicose Veins and Leg Swelling • Hemorrhoids • Itchy Skin

Nutrition   142

Exercise   142
Relaxation Techniques

Getting Ready for Delivery   142
Checklist for Delivery • Pain Relief During Labor • Childbirth Classes • Hospital Tour

Prenatal Care Visits   145

Special Concerns   145
Preterm Labor • Prelabor Rupture of Membranes • Activity Restriction and Bed Rest

RESOURCES   147

CHAPTER 10: Month 9 (Weeks 33 to 36)   149

YOUR BABY   149

YOUR PREGNANCY   150

Your Changing Body   150

Discomforts and How to Manage Them   150
Frequent Urination • Braxton Hicks Contractions • Trouble Sleeping • Leg Swelling and Pain • Pelvic Pressure • Numbness of Legs and Feet

Nutrition   153

Exercise   153

Getting Ready for Delivery   153
Packing for the Hospital • Preparing Your Home for the Baby • Buying a Car Seat

Prenatal Care Visits   155
Group B Streptococcus Screening • Other Screening Tests

Discussions With Your Ob-Gyn   157
Positions for Labor and Childbirth • Your Baby's Hospital Stay • Feeding Your Baby

CONTENTS • VII

Special Concerns 159
Preterm Labor • Preeclampsia • Breech Presentation
RESOURCES 161

CHAPTER 11: Month 10 (Weeks 37 to 40) 163
YOUR BABY 163
YOUR PREGNANCY 164
Your Changing Body 164
Having Sex • Nesting

Discomforts and How to Manage Them 166
Frequent Urination • Snoring • Nausea • Vaginal Spotting

Exercise 167

Preparing for Delivery 167
Knowing When You're in Labor • When to Go to the Hospital • Eating During Labor

Prenatal Care Visits 170

Discussions With Your Ob-Gyn 171
Elective Delivery • Cesarean Delivery on Request

Late Term and Postterm Pregnancy 174
Risks of Late Term and Postterm Pregnancy

Deciding to Induce Labor 175
RESOURCES 176

2 GETTING READY FOR LABOR AND DELIVERY 179

CHAPTER 12: Preparing for Birth 181
Your Birth Plan 182
Birth Places • Hospital Tour • Home Birth • Your Labor Partner • Doulas • Pain Management During Labor • Pain Medication • Other Pain-Relief Techniques • Labor and Delivery in Water • Other People in the Delivery Room

Childbirth Classes 186

Decisions About Your Baby's Health 187
Circumcision for Boys • Feeding Your Baby • Your Baby's Hospital Stay • Delayed Cord Clamping • Cord Blood Banking

Packing for the Hospital 191

Choosing Your Baby's Doctor 191

Preparing Your Home for the Baby 193
Car Seats • Safe Sleep

Child Care 197
RESOURCES 200

CHAPTER 13: Pain Relief During Childbirth 203
Medications for Pain Relief 204
Systemic Analgesics • Nitrous Oxide • Local Anesthesia • Regional Analgesia and Anesthesia • General Anesthesia

Opioid Use Disorder and Pain Relief During Labor   209

Pain Relief Techniques   210
Walking • Positions • Warm Showers • Sitting in Water • Music and Massage

Equipment for Labor and Delivery   212

Continuous Labor Support   212

Childbirth Classes   213

RESOURCES   217

CHAPTER 14: Labor Induction   219

Medical Reasons for Labor Induction   219
Late Term and Postterm Pregnancy

Elective Reasons for Labor Induction   220

When Is Labor Not Induced?   221

How Induction Is Done   222
Getting the Cervix Ready for Labor • Stripping or Sweeping the Amniotic Membranes • Oxytocin • Amniotomy

Risks of Labor Induction   225

If Your Labor Is Going to Be Induced   226

RESOURCES   227

CHAPTER 15: Labor and Delivery   229

Knowing When You're in Labor   229

Stages of Childbirth   232
Stage 1: Early Labor • Stage 1: Active Labor • Transition to Stage 2 • Stage 2: Pushing and Delivery • Stage 3: Delivery of the Placenta

After the Baby Is Born   241

RESOURCES   241

CHAPTER 16: Assisted Vaginal Delivery and Breech Presentation   243

Assisted Vaginal Delivery   243
Types of Assisted Vaginal Delivery • Risks of Assisted Vaginal Delivery

Breech Presentation   246
The Baby's Position • Turning the Baby • Options for Delivery

RESOURCES   251

CHAPTER 17: Cesarean Delivery and Vaginal Birth After Cesarean Delivery   253

Cesarean Delivery   253
Reasons for Cesarean Delivery • Cesarean Delivery on Request

What Happens During a Cesarean Delivery   256
Anesthesia • Preparing for Surgery • Making the Incisions • Delivering the Baby • Delivering the Placenta and Closing the Incisions

Risks of Cesarean Delivery   259

Recovery After Cesarean Delivery   259
Back at Home

CONTENTS • IX

Vaginal Birth After Cesarean Delivery   261
Factors to Consider • Benefits of a VBAC • Risks of a TOLAC • Be Prepared for Changes
RESOURCES   265

3 POSTPARTUM CARE   267

CHAPTER 18: After the Baby Is Born   269

The First Few Hours   269
Skin-to-Skin Care • Breastfeeding Your Baby

Your Baby's Health   270
Your Baby's First Breath • Your Baby's Apgar Score • Keeping the Baby Warm

Getting to Know Your Baby   272
Your Baby's Weight • How Your Baby Looks • How Your Baby Acts

What Happens Next for Your Baby   273
Medical Care • Newborn Screening Tests • Circumcision

Your Recovery After Delivery   275
Vaccinations • Pain Relief

Going Home With Your Baby   277

RESOURCES   279

CHAPTER 19: Your Postpartum Care   281

Planning Your Postpartum Care   281
Postpartum Visit Schedule • Postpartum Care Team

Physical Health After Childbirth   284
Postpartum Bleeding • Bladder Problems • Bowel Problems • Hemorrhoids • Vaginal Birth: Perineal Pain • Cesarean Birth: Incision Pain

Your Changing Body   288
Return of Periods • Swollen Breasts • Abdomen and Uterus

Your Feelings After Childbirth   289
Postpartum Mood Disorders

Lifestyle Habits   292
Sleep and Fatigue • Nutrition and Weight Loss • Exercise

Sex and Family Planning   293
Lack of Interest in Sex • Birth Control • Having Another Baby

Your Future Health   296
Health Problems During Pregnancy • Vaccinations • Ongoing Well-Woman Care

RESOURCES   299

CHAPTER 20: Feeding Your Baby   301

Benefits of Breastfeeding   301

When You Should Not Breastfeed   303
Infections • Prescription and Illegal Drug Use • Medications

Breastfeeding   304
Getting Started • Latching On • Baby's Breastfeeding Technique • How Long to Feed • Signs That Your Baby Wants to Feed • Vitamin D and Iron Supplements • Pacifiers

x • CONTENTS

Food, Drinks, and Medication While Breastfeeding 312
Nutrition • Medication • Tobacco • Alcohol

Breastfeeding Challenges 314
Sore Nipples • Engorgement • Delayed Milk Production • Low Milk Supply • Inverted or Flat Nipples • Breast Surgery • Blocked Ducts • Mastitis • Breastfeeding Twins

Feeding Expressed or Pumped Breast Milk 319
Expressing Milk by Hand • Using a Breast Pump • Storing and Using Breast Milk • Expressed Milk as Your Baby's Primary Feeding Method • Expressing Milk at Work

Feeding With Formula 325
Choosing a Formula • Using Formula Safely

How Long Should Breastfeeding Last? 327
Weaning

Final Thoughts on Feeding Your Baby 327

RESOURCES 328

CHAPTER 21: Birth Control After Pregnancy and Beyond   331

Choosing a Birth Control Method 331

Reversible Birth Control 332
Intrauterine Device • Implant • Injection • Combined Hormonal Methods • Progestin-Only Pills • Barrier Methods

Lactational Amenorrhea Method 341

Fertility Awareness Methods 342

Permanent Birth Control 343
Female Sterilization • Male Sterilization

Emergency Contraception 346

RESOURCES 347

4 HEALTH DURING PREGNANCY   349

CHAPTER 22: Nutrition During Pregnancy   351

Balancing Your Diet 351

Major Nutrients 352
Protein • Carbohydrates • Fats

Vitamins and Minerals 354
Calcium • Choline • Folic Acid • Iron • Omega-3 Fatty Acids • B Vitamins • Vitamin C • Vitamin D • Water

Planning Healthy Meals 359
The Five Food Groups • Tips for Healthy Eating • Healthy Eating on a Budget

Weight Gain During Pregnancy 363
Foods to Avoid or Limit During Pregnancy

Special Diets and Food Restrictions 366
Celiac Disease • Food Allergies • Lactose Intolerance • Vegetarian Diets

Food Safety 368
Common Types of Foodborne Illness • Foods to Avoid • Safe Food Preparation

RESOURCES 372

CONTENTS • XI

CHAPTER 23: Exercise During Pregnancy   375

Who Should Not Exercise During Pregnancy?   376

Guidelines for Physical Activity During Pregnancy   376
Tips for Safe and Healthy Exercise • Activities to Avoid • Pregnancy Changes That Can Affect Your Exercise Routine

Starting an Exercise Program During Pregnancy   379
Staying Motivated

Aerobic Activities   380

Activities for Balance, Strength, and Flexibility   381

Exercises You Can Do At Home   382
Kegel Exercises • 4-Point Kneeling • Seated Leg Raises • Seated Overhead Triceps Extension • Ball Wall Squat • Ball Shoulder Stretch • Seated Side Stretch • Kneeling Heel Touch • Standing Back Bend

Exercising After Childbirth   387
When to Start Exercising • Guidelines for Exercise After Childbirth

Postpartum Exercises   388
4-Point Kneeling • Leg Slides • Knee Raises • Heel Touches • Leg Extensions

RESOURCES   393

CHAPTER 24: Reducing Risks of Birth Defects   395

Teratogens and Pregnancy   395

What Is an Exposure History?   396

Medications   397
Prescription Medications • Over-the-Counter Medications

Alcohol   400

Environmental Toxins   401
Lead • Mercury • Pesticides

Infections   403

X-Rays and Other Radiation   403

Elevated Core Body Temperature   405

Hazards in the Workplace   405

RESOURCES   407

CHAPTER 25: Protecting Yourself From Infections   409

What Happens During an Infection   409

Vaccine Safety   410

How Vaccines Are Made   410

Vaccine-Preventable Diseases   412
Influenza (Flu) • Pertussis (Whooping Cough), Tetanus, and Diphtheria • Hepatitis • Human Papillomavirus • Measles, Mumps, and Rubella • Meningococcal Meningitis • Pneumococcal Pneumonia • Varicella (Chickenpox) and Herpes Zoster (Shingles)

Sexually Transmitted Infections   422
Genital Herpes • Gonorrhea and Chlamydia • Human Immunodeficiency Virus • Syphilis • Trichomoniasis

Other Infections   427
Yeast Infection • Bacterial Vaginosis • Urinary Tract Infection • Cytomegalovirus • Group B Streptococcus • Hepatitis C Infection • Listeriosis • Parvovirus • Toxoplasmosis • Tuberculosis • Zika Virus

RESOURCES   437

CHAPTER 26: Work and Travel During Pregnancy   439

Your Workplace Rights   439
Requesting Workplace Accommodations • Pregnancy Discrimination Act • Occupational Safety and Health Act • Family and Medical Leave Act • Break Time for Nursing Mothers Law

Health Insurance   443

Travel During Pregnancy   444
International Travel • By Plane • By Ship • By Car

RESOURCES   448

CHAPTER 27: Frequently Asked Questions   451

Personal Care   451
Is it safe to dye my hair during pregnancy? • Can I get a massage? • Can I get infections from pedicures? • Is there anything I can do about my varicose veins? • Is it safe to douche during pregnancy? • Can I use a sauna or hot tub early in pregnancy? • What causes stretch marks?

Health and Health Care   453
Where can I find information on coronavirus (COVID-19) and pregnancy? • Should I tell my ob-gyn that I have an eating disorder? • What if I need surgery while I'm pregnant? • Is it safe to see my dentist during pregnancy? • Can I have dental X-rays? • What medicine can I take for allergies? • Is it normal for my partner to be controlling and jealous?

Pregnancy and Technology   455
What should I know about pregnancy apps? • Can I trust the information I read in pregnancy chat rooms?

Your Pregnancy   456
How long does pregnancy last? • How much weight should I gain during pregnancy? • What causes nausea and vomiting during pregnancy? • How can I take care of my teeth after vomiting? • How can I tell if my sadness is normal or a sign of depression? • Does a positive ultrasound exam guarantee that my baby will be healthy? • What is expanded carrier screening? • What should I know about "keepsake" ultrasound pictures? • Will I need bed rest near the end of pregnancy? • Is it safe to have sex during pregnancy?

Nutrition and Exercise   458
How much exercise should I get early in my pregnancy? • How much caffeine can I have per day? • What can I do about the smell of my prenatal vitamins? • Can I eat sushi while I'm pregnant? • What is vitamin D deficiency? • How can I get all the calcium I need if I can't eat dairy products? • How much water should I be drinking each day? • Why is fiber important in the third trimester?

Potentially Harmful Substances   460
Why should I tell my ob-gyn about my medications and supplements? • What can I do to avoid secondhand smoke? • What do I need to know about Zika virus? • Is it safe to keep a cat during pregnancy? • What should I do if I've been exposed to chickenpox?

Labor and Delivery   461
Do I have to write a birth plan? • If coronavirus (COVID-19) is spreading as I get close to delivery, would it be safer to have a home birth? • How can I remember everything I need to do before I give birth? • Is there anything I can do to start labor? • What is "back labor"? • What is assisted vaginal delivery? • What is an episiotomy?

After the Baby Is Born   463
What is delayed cord clamping? • What are the benefits of breastfeeding? • How soon after delivery can I breastfeed? • What kind of birth control should I use after I have the baby?

RESOURCES   464

5 SPECIAL CONSIDERATIONS   467

CHAPTER 28: Multiples: When It's Twins, Triplets, or More   469

Making Multiples   469
Fraternal and Identical Twins • Three or More Babies

Signs That It's More Than One Baby   471

Terms to Know   472

Risks With Multiples   472
Preterm Birth • Problems With the Placenta and Umbilical Cords • Gestational Diabetes • High Blood Pressure and Preeclampsia • Growth Problems

Everyday Health   477
Nutrition • Weight Gain • Exercise

Health Care   478
Prenatal Genetic Screening and Diagnosis • Monitoring • Bed Rest and Hospitalization

Delivery   480

Getting Ready   480

RESOURCES   482

6 MEDICAL PROBLEMS DURING PREGNANCY   485

CHAPTER 29: Weight During Pregnancy: Obesity and Eating Disorders   487

Why Your Weight Is Important   487

Obesity and Pregnancy   489
Defining Obesity • Risks for You • Risks for the Baby • Risks for Childbirth • Exercise • Testing for Gestational Diabetes • Labor and Delivery • Losing Weight After Pregnancy • Future Health Risks

Pregnancy After Weight-Loss Surgery   494

Eating Disorders and Pregnancy   495
How Eating Disorders Can Affect You • How Eating Disorders Can Affect Your Baby • Types of Eating Disorders • Risk Factors and Warning Signs • Getting Help • If You Have a History of Eating Disorders

RESOURCES   499

CHAPTER 30: Hypertension and Preeclampsia 501

Blood Pressure 501

Hypertension 503

Chronic Hypertension 504
Risks • Treatment

Gestational Hypertension 506

Preeclampsia 507
Risks • Signs and Symptoms • Diagnosis

Treatment of Gestational Hypertension and Preeclampsia 509
Gestational Hypertension or Preeclampsia Without Severe Features • Preeclampsia With Severe Features

Prevention 510
Prepregnancy Care • Aspirin

RESOURCES 511

CHAPTER 31: Diabetes During Pregnancy 513

Gestational Diabetes Mellitus 514
Risk Factors • How Gestational Diabetes Can Affect You • How Gestational Diabetes Can Affect Your Baby • Testing for Gestational Diabetes • Controlling Gestational Diabetes • Tracking Blood Sugar Levels • Healthy Eating • Exercise • Medications • Specials Tests • Labor and Delivery • Care After Pregnancy

Pregestational Diabetes Mellitus 520
Risks to Your Pregnancy • Prepregnancy Care • Controlling Your Diabetes During Pregnancy • Tracking Blood Sugar Levels • Managing High and Low Blood Sugar • Healthy Eating • Exercise • Medications • Special Tests • Labor and Delivery • Care After Pregnancy

RESOURCES 526

CHAPTER 32: Other Chronic Conditions 529

Asthma 530

Autoimmune Disorders 532
Multiple Sclerosis • Rheumatoid Arthritis • Lupus

Blood Clotting and Bleeding Disorders 535
Inherited Thrombophilias • Antiphospholipid Syndrome • Von Willebrand Disease

Digestive Disorders 539
Celiac Disease • Inflammatory Bowel Disease • Irritable Bowel Syndrome

Epilepsy and Other Seizure Disorders 541

Heart Disease 542

Kidney Disease 543

Mental Illness 544

Physical Disabilities 545

Thyroid Disease 545

RESOURCES 547

7 TESTING   551

CHAPTER 33: Genetic Disorders, Screening, and Testing   553

Screening and Diagnostic Tests   553

Genes and Chromosomes   555

Inherited Disorders   557
Autosomal Dominant Disorders • Autosomal Recessive Disorders • Sex-Linked Disorders • Multifactorial Disorders

Chromosomal Disorders   560
Aneuploidy • Structural Chromosomal Disorders

Assessing Your Risk   562

Types of Tests for Genetic Disorders   564

Deciding Whether to Be Tested   564

Carrier Screening   566
Results and What to Do Next • Timing • If You or Your Partner Is a Carrier

Prenatal Screening Tests   569
First-Trimester Screening • Cell-Free DNA Testing • Second-Trimester Screening • Integrated and Sequential Screening • If Screening Test Results Show an Increased Risk

Diagnostic Tests   572
Amniocentesis • Chorionic Villus Sampling • Preimplantation Genetic Testing • How the Cells Are Analyzed

If Your Pregnancy Has a Disorder   575

RESOURCES   576

CHAPTER 34: Ultrasound Exams and Other Testing to Monitor Fetal Well-Being   579

Ultrasound Exams   579
How It Is Done • What the Results May Mean

Testing to Monitor Fetal Well-Being   581

Why Testing May Be Done   581

When Tests Are Available   583

Interpreting Test Results   583

Types of Special Tests   584
Kick Counts • Nonstress Test • Biophysical Profile • Modified Biophysical Profile • Contraction Stress Test • Doppler Ultrasound Exam

RESOURCES   589

8 COMPLICATIONS DURING PREGNANCY AND CHILDBIRTH 591

CHAPTER 35: When Labor Starts Too Soon: Preterm Labor, Prelabor Rupture of Membranes, and Preterm Birth 593

Preterm Labor 593
Risk Factors • Diagnosis • Management

Prelabor Rupture of Membranes 597
Risk Factors for PROM • Risk Factors for Preterm PROM • Diagnosis • Management

Cervical Insufficiency 599
Diagnosis • Evaluation • Management

Indicated Preterm Birth 600

Medications Before Preterm Birth 601
Corticosteroids • Magnesium Sulfate • Tocolytics

When Preterm Birth Happens 602
Breathing Support • Surfactant Replacement Therapy • Neonatal Intensive Care

What to Expect After Preterm Birth 603
Caring for a Preterm Baby

Preventing Another Preterm Birth 604

RESOURCES 604

CHAPTER 36: Blood Type Incompatibility 607

ABO Incompatibility 607
How It Affects the Baby • Treatment

Rh Incompatibility 608
What the Rh Factor Means for Pregnancy • How Rh Antibodies Can Cause Problems • Preventing Rh Problems During Pregnancy • Treatment if Antibodies Develop

Other Incompatibilities 612

RESOURCES 612

CHAPTER 37: Placenta Problems 615

Placenta Previa 615
Types • Signs and Symptoms • Diagnosis • Treatment

Placental Abruption 618
Types • Signs and Symptoms • Diagnosis • Treatment

Placenta Accreta 619
Types • Signs and Symptoms • Diagnosis • Treatment

RESOURCES 621

CHAPTER 38: Growth Problems 623

Fetal Growth Restriction 623
Causes • Diagnosis • Management • Prevention

Macrosomia 626
Diagnosis • Complications • Management • Prevention

RESOURCES 629

CHAPTER 39: Problems During Labor and Delivery   631

Abnormal Labor   631
Causes • Risks • Assessment • Management

Shoulder Dystocia   634
Risks • Management • Future Deliveries

Umbilical Cord Compression   635
Risk Factors • Signs and Symptoms • Management

Umbilical Cord Prolapse   636
Risk Factors • Signs and Symptoms • Management

Postpartum Hemorrhage   637
Causes • Signs and Symptoms • Risk Factors • Management

Endometritis   639
Risk Factors • Signs and Symptoms • Management

RESOURCES   640

9 PREGNANCY LOSS   643

CHAPTER 40: Early Pregnancy Loss: Miscarriage, Ectopic Pregnancy, and Gestational Trophoblastic Disease   645

Miscarriage   645
Causes • Signs and Symptoms • Diagnosis • Treatment • Recovery • Trying Again

Ectopic Pregnancy   648
Risk Factors • Signs and Symptoms • Diagnosis • Treatment • Medication • Surgery • Recovery and Trying Again

Gestational Trophoblastic Disease   653
Signs, Symptoms, and Diagnosis • Treatment • Trying Again

Coping With the Loss   654

RESOURCES   655

CHAPTER 41: Late Pregnancy Loss: Stillbirth   657

How Stillbirth Is Diagnosed   657

What Went Wrong?   658

Tests and Evaluations   658

Grieving   659

The Stages of Grief   660
Shock, Numbness, and Disbelief • Searching and Yearning • Anger or Rage • Depression and Loneliness • Acceptance

You and Your Partner   662

Seeking Support   662

The Future   663

Another Pregnancy   663

RESOURCES   664

10 LOOKING AHEAD 667

CHAPTER 42: Having Another Baby: What to Expect the Next Time Around 669

Timing for Another Baby 669
How Long Should You Wait? • Is Your Body Ready?

You're Pregnant Already 671
How Will It Be Different? • Possible Problems

Telling Your Other Children 673

RESOURCES 674

11 RESOURCES AND TOOLS 677

Terms You Should Know 679
Body Mass Index Chart 700
Medical History Form 702
Sample Birth Plan 708
My Postpartum Care Checklist 711
Environmental Exposure History Form 713
My Postpartum Care Team Chart 716

Index 717

Introduction

Pregnancy is a life-changing experience, and it's important that you have the best information from the start. This book, *Your Pregnancy and Childbirth: Month to Month,* comes from the experts at the American College of Obstetricians and Gynecologists (ACOG). For more than 60 years, ACOG has written the medical guidelines that obstetrician–gynecologists (ob-gyns) and other medical professionals use when taking care of women.

Why Use This Book?

First, because there's nothing like it on the market today. Since *Your Pregnancy and Childbirth* comes from ACOG, it offers the latest medical guidelines to help you make the best decisions for you and your pregnancy. You can trust that the information you read here is supported by medical research and the everyday experience of ob-gyns who have cared for millions of pregnant women.

Second, this book presents medical information in a straightforward, easy-to-understand way. *Your Pregnancy and Childbirth* encourages you to

- learn about prepregnancy health and planning, pregnancy, labor and delivery, and the postpartum period
- use the information you learn to talk with your ob-gyn and others who may care for you during pregnancy
- be an empowered, active decision-maker in your care

What's Different About This Edition?

This seventh edition of *Your Pregnancy and Childbirth* has been completely revised. Medical information has been updated, and new illustrations have been added. New content also has been added in response to reader feedback, including

- a new chapter on exercise during and after pregnancy
- updated information on when and how genetic testing is done
- an updated chapter on pain relief during labor
- a new chapter where you can find quick answers to frequently asked questions

Also, this book went to press during the coronavirus (COVID-19) health crisis. Check the index at the back of the book to find pages that talk about the impact of COVID-19 on telehealth, travel during pregnancy, breastfeeding, and more. Research about COVID-19 is ongoing, and you should talk with your ob-gyn about how to stay safe and healthy during pregnancy. You also can find up-to-date information at www.acog.org/COVID-Pregnancy.

How Is This Book Organized?

You'll notice that the first half of the book is a detailed prenatal guide. The chapters for each month of pregnancy talk about

- the development of your baby from week to week
- some of the changes taking place in your body
- how to manage some of the discomforts of pregnancy
- what may happen during that month's prenatal care visit

The second half of the book includes sections on labor, delivery, and the postpartum period, from right after your baby is born through the first 12 weeks and beyond. You'll also find chapters dedicated to

- nutrition during pregnancy
- work and travel during pregnancy
- common medical conditions that can affect pregnancy
- pregnancy complications and how they are managed

How Can You Use the Tools and Resources?

Also new for this edition are important tools that you can use when talking with your ob-gyn, including

- a medical history form to review before your first prenatal care visit
- a form to track possible exposure to toxic or harmful things at home or work
- a checklist for tracking symptoms or concerns during the postpartum period
- a chart to note contact information for friends, family, and health care practitioners who will help you during the postpartum period

You can find all of these tools at the back of this book. At the back you'll also find a "Terms You Should Know" section. This section defines the medical terms used in the book, terms that you may hear from your ob-gyn throughout your pregnancy.

In short, you hold in your hands a fully updated, factual guide that helps put you in control of your pregnancy and childbirth experience. ACOG hopes that *Your Pregnancy and Childbirth: Month to Month* becomes a trusted resource and a comforting presence throughout your pregnancy and postpartum period.

Finally, although the term "women" is used in this book, ACOG recognizes that ob-gyns treat people of all gender identities, including people who are cisgender, transgender, gender non-binary, or otherwise gender expansive and who may experience pregnancy. ACOG believes all people should have access to respectful, high-quality, and safe health care. The use of the term "women" in this book is intended to be used inclusively.

More to Explore Online

Looking for more on pregnancy, labor and delivery, and the postpartum period? Go to www.acog.org/MyPregnancy for the latest from the leading experts in women's health care. Online you'll find

- top patient questions answered by ACOG ob-gyns—and a tool to submit your own questions
- pregnancy stories from patients and ob-gyns
- an A–Z directory of health topics—covering pregnancy and beyond

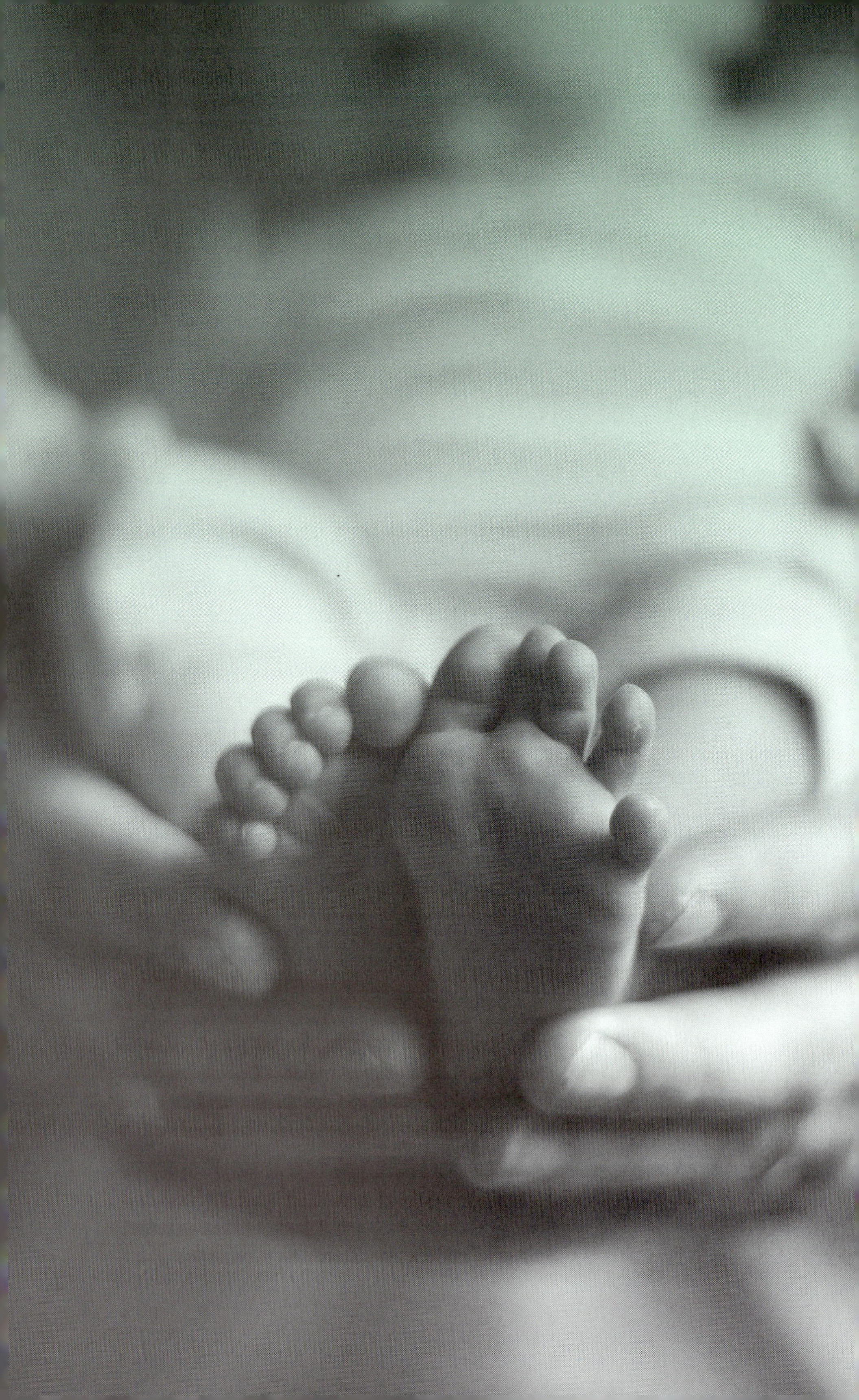

PART 1

Pregnancy
Month by Month

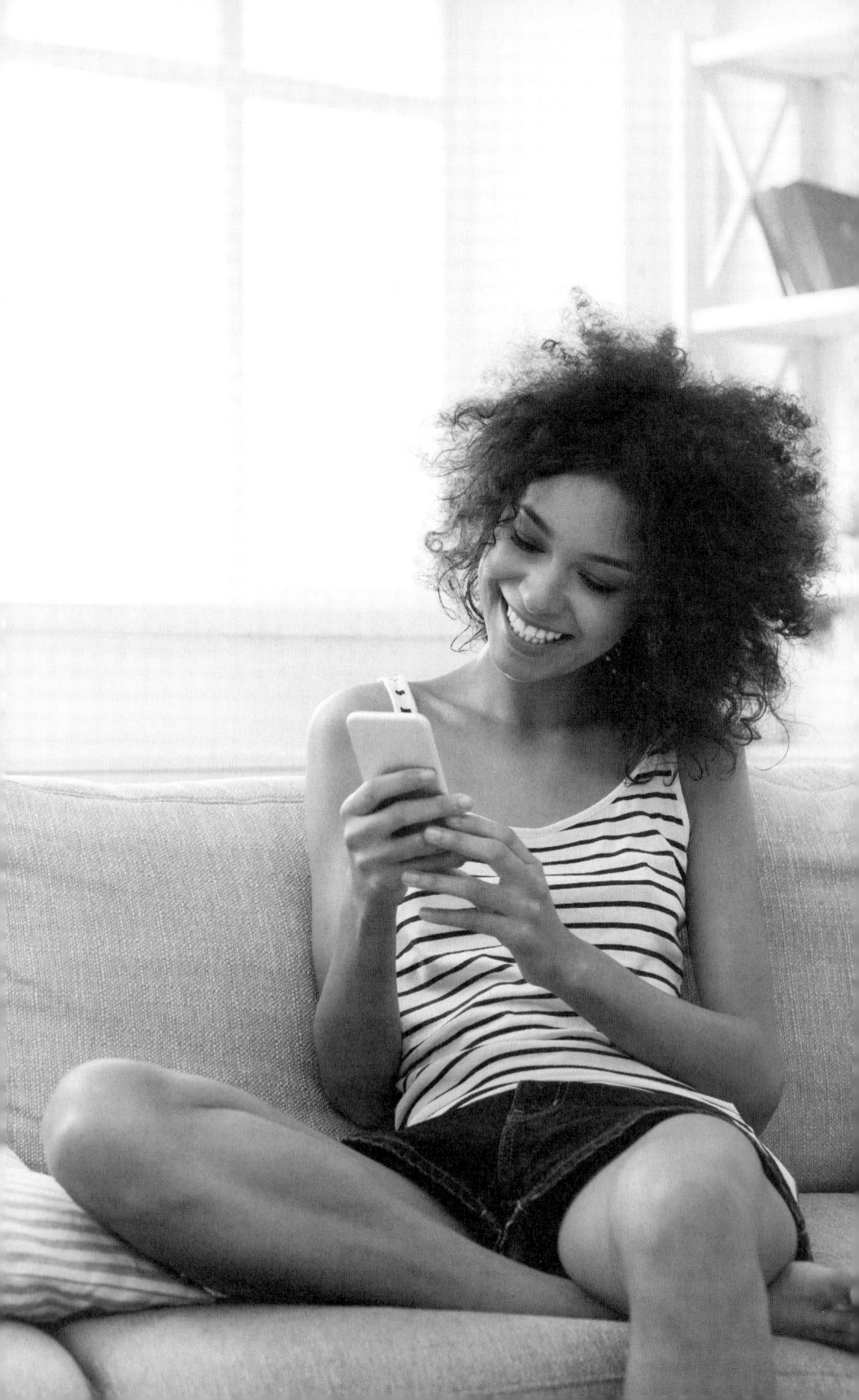

CHAPTER 1

Getting Ready for Pregnancy

Congratulations! You've decided to have a baby. Welcome to the first part of a journey that will change your life forever. Before you try to get pregnant, there are some important things you can do to give yourself the best chance of having a healthy pregnancy and a healthy baby. By planning ahead and making needed changes before you get pregnant, you are more likely to be prepared. That is why **prepregnancy care** is so important.

The Prepregnancy Visit

A prepregnancy care checkup is the first step in planning a healthy pregnancy. The goal of this checkup is to find things that could affect your pregnancy. Identifying these things is important because the first 8 weeks of pregnancy is the time when major organs have begun to form. You can see your primary care practitioner for your prepregnancy visit, or you can see the **obstetrician–gynecologist (ob-gyn)** you have chosen to care for you during your pregnancy (see Chapter 2, "Choosing Your Care Team").

During a prepregnancy care visit, you and your ob-gyn should talk about

- your diet and lifestyle (see the section "A Healthy Lifestyle" in this chapter)
- your medical and family history
- medications you take
- any past pregnancies

Together you'll review your **vaccinations** to be sure that you have had all the **vaccines** that are recommended for you. You'll go over the risks of **sexually** *transmitted infections (STIs)* and discuss how to protect yourself. You also may discuss screening for *genetic disorders* that may be in your or your partner's families.

Preexisting Health Conditions

Your ob-gyn should ask about any diseases or surgeries that you have had. He or she also should ask about any chronic conditions that you may have now. Medical conditions can cause problems during pregnancy. Some of these conditions include

- *depression*
- *diabetes mellitus*
- eating disorders
- *hypertension* (also called *high blood pressure*)
- *seizure disorders*

Some health conditions may increase the risk of problems for the baby, such as *birth defects*. Other conditions may increase the risk of health problems for you. Having one of these conditions does not mean that you cannot have a healthy pregnancy or baby. But good care before pregnancy may reduce pregnancy-related risks.

If you have a medical condition, you may need to make some changes to bring your condition under control before you try to get pregnant. For example, women with diabetes usually need to keep their *glucose* (blood sugar) levels in the normal range for some time before they get pregnant. If you are having trouble controlling your blood sugar, talk with your ob-gyn about diet, exercise, and medication, if needed.

Even if a health problem is well managed, the demands of pregnancy can cause it to get worse. To keep health problems in check, you may need to

- make lifestyle changes
- see your ob-gyn more often
- get other specialized care during pregnancy

Family Health History

Some health conditions are more common in certain families or ethnic groups. These conditions are called genetic disorders or inherited disorders. If a close relative has one of these medical conditions, you or your baby could be at greater risk of having it too. During your prepregnancy visit, your ob-gyn may ask you to complete a family history form. If you have a male partner, he also can complete the form. The form will ask for information such as

- your family medical history
- your race and ethnicity
- any problems you may have had in past pregnancies

Based on this information, your ob-gyn may suggest that you and your partner have **carrier screening** for certain genetic disorders (see the section "Prepregnancy Carrier Screening" in this chapter).

In some situations, your ob-gyn may recommend that you and your partner have genetic counseling. A **genetic counselor** is a health care professional who can help you understand your chances of having a baby with a genetic disorder. You also may see a doctor who is an expert in genetics. Genetic counseling involves taking a detailed family history. Sometimes physical exams and lab tests are done.

Medications and Supplements

The prepregnancy period is the time to review everything you take, including

- prescription medications
- over-the-counter medications
- vitamin supplements
- herbal supplements

Tell your ob-gyn about all the medications you take. Better yet, take the medications with you to your prepregnancy care checkup. Include all medications in their bottles, packs, or other packaging. You and your ob-gyn can discuss their safety when used during pregnancy.

You may need to stop using a certain medication or switch to another before you try to get pregnant. Some medications may increase the risk of birth defects, but the benefits of taking the medication during pregnancy may outweigh the risks to your baby. Do not stop taking a prescription medication until you have talked with your ob-gyn. See Chapter 24, "Reducing Risks of Birth Defects," for information on taking medication during pregnancy.

Past Pregnancies

During your prepregnancy care checkup, you and your ob-gyn should talk about any past pregnancies and any problems you may have had. Some past problems may increase the risk of having the same problem in a later pregnancy. These problems include

- *gestational diabetes*
- high blood pressure

- *preeclampsia*
- *preterm* birth

Getting proper care before and during pregnancy may lower the chances of these problems happening again.

Women who have had a **miscarriage** or **stillbirth** often fear that it will happen again. If this is a concern for you, discuss it with your ob-gyn. Most women who have lost a pregnancy go on to have healthy pregnancies and healthy babies.

Vaccinations

Certain infections during pregnancy can cause birth defects or pregnancy **complications**. Many infections can be prevented with vaccination. You should get all the shots recommended for your age group before you try to get pregnant. See information from the Centers for Disease Control and Prevention (CDC) in the "Resources" section at the end of this chapter.

Certain vaccines should not be given to pregnant women because they contain live, attenuated viruses. "Attenuated" means that the virus has been weakened so that it cannot cause disease in a healthy person. The vaccines that women should not get during pregnancy include

- **live, attenuated influenza (flu) vaccine** given as a nasal spray (but the flu shot is safe)
- **measles–mumps–rubella (MMR) vaccine**
- **varicella (chickenpox) vaccine**

If you need the MMR vaccine or the chickenpox vaccine, get these shots at least 1 month before getting pregnant. During this month, keep using birth control.

Most other vaccines contain killed versions of the viruses or **bacteria** that cause disease. These killed versions do not cause the disease itself when given as a vaccine. These shots are safe to get during pregnancy.

The CDC recommends that everyone 6 months and older get the flu shot each year. If you are pregnant or planning to get pregnant, it is especially important to get a flu shot as soon as the vaccine is available. The flu season is from October to May, and the flu vaccine is normally available shortly before it starts. A pregnant woman who gets the flu can get much sicker than a non-pregnant woman who gets the flu. The flu shot offers you the best protection. The shot also helps protect your baby from the flu until he or she can get a flu shot at 6 months.

Your ob-gyn also may mention the **tetanus toxoid, reduced diphtheria toxoid, and acellular pertussis (Tdap) vaccine**. This vaccine triggers your immune system to make **antibodies** against **pertussis** (whooping cough). This is important because whooping cough is dangerous for newborns. All pregnant women should get the Tdap shot, ideally between 27 and 36 weeks of each pregnancy. See Chapter 25, "Protecting Yourself From Infections," for information on infectious diseases and vaccinations.

Protection Against Sexually Transmitted Infections

Other infections that can be harmful during pregnancy are those passed through sexual contact. STIs can affect your ability to get pregnant. STIs also can harm your baby if you become infected while you are pregnant.

Before pregnancy, take steps to reduce your risk of getting an STI. Using a male or female condom every time you have **sexual intercourse** is important. But there are a few other recommendations:

- If you use sex toys, wash them before and after use and cover them with a condom during use.
- Use a **dental dam** during oral sex.
- Wash your hands before and after sex.

Urinating after sexual intercourse can reduce the chance of developing a **urinary tract infection (UTI)** but does not protect against STIs.

You are at higher risk of getting an STI if you have sex with more than one partner. You also are at higher risk if your partner has sex with someone else.

Some STIs do not have cures. These infections include

- *genital herpes*
- *human immunodeficiency virus (HIV)*
- *hepatitis B* and *hepatitis C*

Other STIs can be treated with medication. Because many STIs have no symptoms in the early stages, prepregnancy testing for the following is recommended:

- You should be tested for **chlamydia** if you are 25 or younger, or if you are over 25 with risk factors. Risk factors include having a new sex partner or multiple partners.

- You should be tested for **gonorrhea** if you are 25 or younger and you have certain risk factors. Risk factors include having gonorrhea or another STI in the past, having new or multiple sex partners and not using condoms every time, and living in an area where gonorrhea rates are high.

- All women should be tested for HIV. HIV cannot be cured, but if you know your HIV status, you can make important decisions about pregnancy. You also can learn about treatment options that may make it less likely you will pass the infection to your baby.

Screening tests for other STIs, including **syphilis** and **hepatitis B virus**, are recommended once you are pregnant. See Chapter 25, "Protecting Yourself From Infections."

Prepregnancy Carrier Screening

For some genetic disorders, carrier screening may be available. This **screening test** lets you and your male partner find out if you are **carriers** of certain disorders, even if you do not have any signs or symptoms. Carrier screening tests a sample of blood or saliva.

You and your partner can have carrier screening before pregnancy or during pregnancy. If you had carrier screening in a past pregnancy, testing does not have to be repeated. But if you have a new partner, your ob-gyn will want to know if your partner has any genetic conditions that run in the family. Additional screening may be recommended based on your partner's family history and your prior screening results.

In the past, carrier screening was recommended for people who are at higher risk of certain genetic disorders because of their family history, ethnicity, or race (see Table 1-1, "Recommended Carrier Screening Tests for People of Different Backgrounds"). Now all people should be offered carrier screening for **cystic fibrosis**, which is one of the most common genetic disorders, and for **spinal muscular atrophy (SMA)**.

If carrier screening is done before pregnancy, you have time to make decisions if you find out that you are a carrier of a genetic disorder:

- You may choose to get pregnant and ask if there is prenatal genetic testing for the condition you're concerned about.
- You may explore the option of **assisted reproductive technology (ART)**.
- You may choose not to have children.
- You may choose to adopt.

Once you are pregnant, there are **diagnostic tests** that can tell whether a baby has certain genetic disorders. It usually takes a long time to get the results of these tests. The pregnancy may be well along before the results are known. Because of this, your options are more limited. See Chapter 33, "Genetic Disorders, Screening, and Testing."

TABLE 1-1 **Recommended Carrier Screening Tests for People of Different Backgrounds***

Background and Ethnicity	Recommended Screening
All backgrounds	Cystic fibrosis Spinal muscular atrophy (SMA)
African descent	Alpha-*thalassemia* *Sickle cell disease*
Eastern or Central European Jewish descent	*Tay–Sachs disease*
French Canadian or Cajun descent	Tay–Sachs disease
Hispanic descent	Beta-thalassemia
Mediterranean descent (including Arab, Greek, southern Iranian, Italian, or Turkish)	Alpha-thalassemia Beta-thalassemia Sickle cell disease
Southeast Asian descent	Alpha-thalassemia Sickle cell disease
West Indian descent	Beta-thalassemia

*The tests that are available and who they should be offered to frequently change as a result of new research.

A Healthy Lifestyle

The months before you get pregnant are the best time to take steps to be healthier. These steps may include

- eating right
- getting regular exercise
- reaching and maintaining a healthy weight
- stopping unhealthy substances (tobacco, alcohol, marijuana, illegal drugs, and prescription drugs taken for a nonmedical reason)
- keeping your environment safe

Eating Right

A healthy diet is especially important before and during your pregnancy. The food you eat is the main source of **nutrients** and energy for you and your baby. As the baby grows and places new demands on your body, you will need more **calories** and nutrients. But simply doubling up on the amount that you eat—or "eating for two"—is not a healthy strategy. Experts stress the importance of

- eating nutrient-rich foods
- staying active
- gaining an appropriate amount of weight

At your prepregnancy visit, talk with your ob-gyn about any dietary concerns. He or she will need to know if you

- are a vegetarian, and if so, if you eat dairy products
- have any food allergies
- have trouble digesting milk and other dairy products
- have **celiac disease**
- routinely fast
- have ever had an eating disorder

If you want help planning a healthy diet, start with the U.S. Department of Agriculture's MyPlate food-planning guide (see the "Resources" section at the end of this chapter). The MyPlate website can help you learn how to make healthy food choices at every meal. MyPlate explains the five good groups:

1. Grains—Bread, pasta, oatmeal, cereal, and tortillas are all grains. Half of the grains you eat should be whole grains. Whole grains are those that have not been processed and include the whole grain kernel. They include oats, barley, quinoa, brown rice, and bulgur. Products made with these foods also count as whole grains. Look for the words "whole grain" on the product label.

2. Fruits—Fruits can be fresh, canned, frozen, or dried. Juice that is 100 percent fruit juice also counts. Make half of your plate fruits and vegetables.

3. Vegetables—Vegetables can be raw or cooked, frozen, canned, dried, or 100 percent vegetable juice. Use dark, leafy greens to make salads.

4. Protein foods—Protein foods include meat, poultry, seafood, beans and peas, eggs, processed soy products, nuts, and seeds. Include a variety of proteins and choose lean or low-fat meat and poultry.

5. Dairy—Milk and milk products, such as cheese, yogurt, and ice cream, make up the dairy group. Make sure any dairy foods you eat are pasteurized. Choose fat-free or low-fat (1 percent) varieties.

Oils and fats are another part of healthy eating. Oils in food come mainly from plant sources, such as olive oil, nut oils, and grapeseed oil. They also can be found in some fish, avocados, nuts, and olives. Most of the fats and oils in your diet should come from plant sources. Limit solid fats, which are found in animal fat, butter, shortening, cheese, fried potatoes, and many baked goods and desserts.

Getting Regular Exercise

Good health at any time in your life involves getting plenty of exercise, and that includes during pregnancy. Experts recommend that most pregnant women get at least 30 minutes of moderate exercise on most days of the week. Talk with your ob-gyn about how much exercise you can do safely during your pregnancy.

It is best to have an exercise routine in place before you get pregnant. If you are just starting out, good exercises to begin with include

- bicycling
- swimming
- walking

If you are not used to a lot of exercise, talk about safety with your ob-gyn and take it slow at first. Also, if you are overweight or obese, get your ob-gyn's approval before starting an exercise program. Many gyms and health clubs have fitness trainers who can help design a safe exercise program. There also may be trainers or classes at your local park district or YMCA. For more on exercise, see Chapter 23, "Exercise During Pregnancy."

Taking Folic Acid

Taking a prenatal vitamin with ***folic acid*** is important before and during pregnancy. Women should get 400 micrograms (mcg) for at least 1 month before pregnancy and during the first 12 weeks of pregnancy. If the vitamin label lists dietary folate equivalents (DFE) instead, it should have 667 mcg DFE.

Why is folic acid important? This vitamin reduces the risk of having a baby with birth defects of the brain and spine. These birth defects are called **neural tube defects (NTDs)**. Along with taking a prenatal vitamin (see the box "Focus on Folic Acid"), you also should eat foods rich in this vitamin every day, including

- fortified cereal
- enriched bread and pasta
- peanuts
- dark green leafy vegetables
- orange juice
- beans

Reaching and Maintaining a Healthy Weight

Being underweight or overweight can cause problems during pregnancy. For many people, it is hard to gain or lose weight. Talk with your ob-gyn about

> ## Focus on Folic Acid
>
> Folic acid, also known as folate or vitamin B$_9$, is a vitamin that helps prevent major birth defects of the baby's brain and spine called neural tube defects (NTDs). Current guidelines recommend that pregnant women get at least 600 mcg of folic acid per day, but it is hard to get enough from your diet alone. To reach this goal, take a prenatal vitamin with at least 400 mcg of folic acid every day and eat foods rich in this vitamin. The combination of folic acid in your vitamin and in your diet should help you reach the 600 mcg goal.
>
> Neural tube defects (NTDs), such as **spina bifida** and **anencephaly**, happen early in prenatal development when the coverings of the spinal cord do not close completely. You may have a higher risk of giving birth to a baby with an NTD if you
>
> - have already had a baby with an NTD
> - have certain health conditions, such as sickle cell disease
> - are taking certain medications, such as drugs for **epilepsy** (valproate)
>
> If any of these are true for you, your ob-gyn may recommend that you take 4 mg of folic acid each day—10 times the usual amount—as a separate vitamin supplement at least 3 months before pregnancy and for the first 3 months of pregnancy. You and your ob-gyn can discuss whether you need this amount of folic acid based on your health history.

whether your weight might be an issue for your pregnancy. Talking with a dietitian (an expert in healthy eating) also may be helpful.

If your ob-gyn suggests that you try to gain weight, start by taking in more calories each day than you burn through daily activity and exercise. Eat healthy high-calorie snacks every day. Some good choices include

- nuts
- granola bars
- meal replacement shakes
- fruit smoothies
- yogurt

If your ob-gyn suggests that you try to lose weight, keep in mind that losing even a small amount of weight can improve your overall health. This can pave the way for a healthier pregnancy. See Chapter 29, "Weight During Pregnancy: Obesity and Eating Disorders."

Stopping Use of Unhealthy Substances

Use of substances—tobacco, alcohol, marijuana, illegal drugs, and prescription drugs taken for a nonmedical reason—can cause serious problems for your pregnancy and your baby, including

- birth defects
- *low birth weight*
- preterm birth
- stillbirth

Substance use includes taking drugs such as heroin, cocaine, or methamphetamines. It also includes using oxycodone or other ***opioids*** in ways that were not prescribed for you.

When should you stop using these substances? It is best to quit smoking before you get pregnant. Avoid alcohol while trying to get pregnant and do not drink while pregnant. Stop using other harmful substances before you get pregnant as well.

Also, it's important to tell your ob-gyn how you use opioids, especially when you are or want to get pregnant. If you have an ***opioid use disorder***, treatment can start you on the road to recovery and a healthier pregnancy.

It's also important to know that states have different laws and policies. Some states consider opioid use during pregnancy a form of child abuse or neglect. Some states have created treatment programs specifically for pregnant women. Other states give pregnant women priority in general treatment programs. You can visit this site to learn about your state's laws and policies: www.guttmacher.org/state-policy/explore/substance-use-during-pregnancy.

The American College of Obstetricians and Gynecologists (ACOG) believes that pregnant women who have an opioid use disorder should receive medical care and counseling, not punishment. Seeking help is the first step in recovering from addiction and making a better life.

Your partner also should give up harmful substances. Living with someone who smokes means that you are likely to breathe in secondhand smoke. Secondhand smoke contains chemicals that are harmful to your health. These chemicals also can harm the health of your baby. Being around secondhand smoke while you are pregnant has been linked to a higher risk of

- low birth weight
- *sudden infant death syndrome (SIDS)*

Also, if you have a male partner, smoking and using illegal drugs can lower his fertility and damage *sperm*.

Keeping Your Environment Safe

Chemicals are all around us—in the air, water, soil, food we eat, and products we use. Before you get pregnant and during your pregnancy, you may have contact with chemicals at work, at home, or in your community.

A few chemicals are known to have harmful effects on a baby. These include lead, mercury, and certain pesticides. The effects of many other chemicals on pregnancy are not known. Some substances found in the home or the workplace may make it harder for you to get pregnant.

Tips for Partners

When a couple decides to have a baby, a lot of attention is given to the pregnant woman. The role of her partner, though, is just as important. Partners should be aware of a few things to make sure they are as healthy as possible for their new responsibilities:

- Get healthier. Join your partner in eating healthier and exercising every day. For example, if she needs to cut back on caffeine and unhealthy foods, you can too.

- Give up smoking and substance use. Secondhand smoke is dangerous for pregnant women and their babies.

- Be supportive. Trying to get pregnant can be an emotional rollercoaster. This can be especially true for a woman who is going through *in vitro fertilization (IVF)* or other treatment to help her get pregnant. Going to her appointments for infertility testing, prepregnancy care, and *prenatal care* will let your partner know she can lean on you.

- Get tested and treated for any sexually transmitted infections (STIs). Continue to protect yourself and your partner from STIs when she gets pregnant. While a woman is pregnant, she and the baby have no protection against these diseases. If she gets infected with an STI while pregnant, the results could be very serious for her and life threatening for the baby.

- Participate in genetic counseling and screening, if recommended. This will help your partner make decisions about the best approach to screening or diagnostic testing.

Take a look at your home and workplace. Tell your ob-gyn if you work

- on a farm
- in a factory
- in a dry-cleaning facility
- in a facility for printing or electronics
- any other location where you are exposed to chemicals

You also should discuss hobbies that might expose you to harmful agents, such as painting or pottery glazing. See Chapter 24, "Reducing Risks of Birth Defects."

Getting Pregnant

Knowing how pregnancy happens will help you find out when you are most fertile—that is, when you are most likely to get pregnant. To have a better chance of getting pregnant, sexual intercourse has to happen around the time of *ovulation*.

The Menstrual Cycle

The changes that happen during the ***menstrual cycle*** are caused by changing levels of ***hormones*** called ***estrogen*** and ***progesterone***. Each month, hormones signal your ***uterus*** to build up a blood-rich lining called the ***endometrium***. These hormones also send a signal to an ***egg***, causing it to mature in a ***follicle*** in one of your ***ovaries***.

When an egg is ready, it is released from the ovary and moves into a ***fallopian tube***, one of a pair of tubes that lead from the ovaries to the uterus. The release of the egg is called ovulation. Around the time an egg is released you also may notice

- breast tenderness
- an increase in vaginal discharge (the fluid that comes out of your ***vagina***)
- an increase in sexual desire

The average menstrual cycle lasts about 28 days, counting from the first day of one period (day 1) to the first day of the next. Cycles ranging from as few as 21 days to as many as 35 days are normal.

In an average 28-day menstrual cycle, ovulation happens around day 14. If pregnancy does not happen, your body absorbs the egg and hormone levels decrease. This decrease signals the lining of the uterus to shed. The shedding is your monthly period.

The Menstrual Cycle

Day 1

The first day of your menstrual period is considered day 1 of your menstrual cycle.

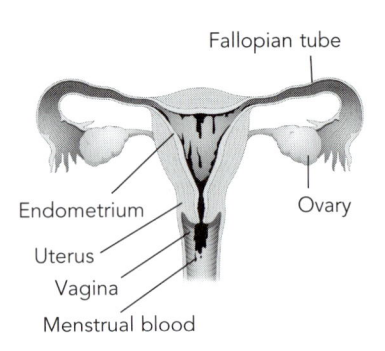

Fallopian tube
Endometrium
Ovary
Uterus
Vagina
Menstrual blood

Day 5

Estrogen levels start to increase. Estrogen causes the endometrium (the lining of the uterus) to grow and thicken.

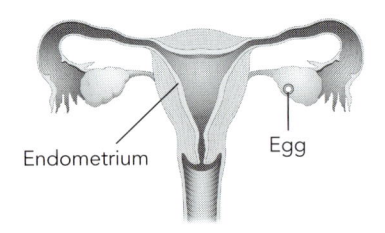

Endometrium
Egg

Day 14

An egg is released from the ovary and moves into one of the two fallopian tubes (ovulation). After ovulation, progesterone levels begin to increase, while estrogen levels decrease.

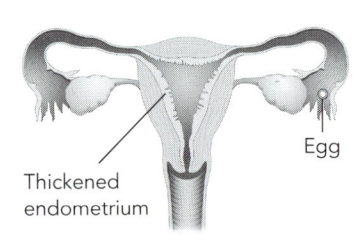

Thickened endometrium
Egg

Day 28

If the egg is not fertilized, progesterone and estrogen levels decrease, and the endometrium is shed during menstruation.

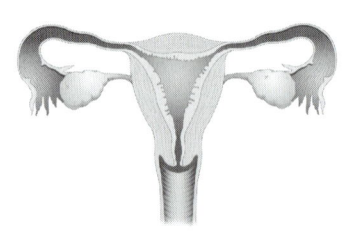

When Are You Most Fertile?

For pregnancy to happen, sperm must join with an egg while it is in the fallopian tube. When a man climaxes during sex and **ejaculates**, millions of sperm are deposited in a woman's vagina. After ejaculation, the sperm move through the **cervix** and into the uterus and fallopian tubes.

Sperm can live inside a woman's body for 3 days and sometimes up to 5 days. An egg's life span is much shorter—just 12 to 24 hours after ovulation. So pregnancy can happen if an egg is already in the fallopian tubes when you have sex. Or it can happen if you ovulate within a day or two after you have sex. This means that you are fertile anywhere from 3 to 5 days before ovulation until up to 1 day after ovulation.

There is no foolproof way to calculate your fertile days. But there are several methods that can help you predict when these days fall in your menstrual cycle. Smartphone apps also are available to help you keep track of your fertile times. Many of these apps use one or more of the methods discussed below.

Chart your cycle. One way to figure out your fertile days is to keep a menstrual calendar. This will help you learn how long your cycles tend to last. If your cycle is between 26 and 32 days long, days 8 through 19 are the days when you are most likely to get pregnant. For the best chance of getting pregnant, you should try to have sex between day 8 and day 19 either every day or every other day.

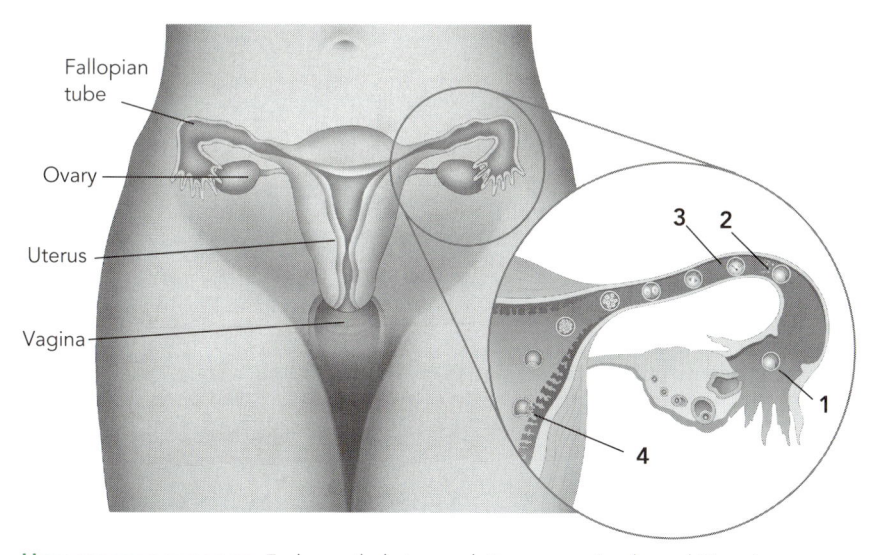

How pregnancy occurs. Each month during ovulation, an egg is released (*1*) and moves into one of the fallopian tubes. If a woman has sex around this time, and an egg and sperm meet in the fallopian tube (*2*), the two may join. If they join (*3*), the fertilized egg then moves through the fallopian tube into the uterus and attaches there to grow during pregnancy (*4*).

Keeping a Menstrual Calendar

When you are thinking about getting pregnant, you may want to keep track of your menstrual cycle. By charting your menstrual periods on a calendar for a few months, you can spot patterns in your cycle (how many days your menstrual periods last, for instance, and whether your cycle is typically 25 days or 30 days long). You also may be able to pinpoint the days that you are most fertile. To use the calendar, circle the days that you menstruate each month. If you can, chart your cycle for a few months and bring the calendar along with you to your prepregnancy care checkup. Smartphone apps also are available to help you chart your cycle.

Jan.	1	2	3	4	5	6	7	8	9	10	11	12	13	14	15	16	17	18	19	20	21	22	23	24	25	26	27	28	29	30	31
Feb.	1	2	3	4	5	6	7	8	9	10	11	12	13	14	15	16	17	18	19	20	21	22	23	24	25	26	27	28	29		
March	1	2	3	4	5	6	7	8	9	10	11	12	13	14	15	16	17	18	19	20	21	22	23	24	25	26	27	28	29	30	31
April	1	2	3	4	5	6	7	8	9	10	11	12	13	14	15	16	17	18	19	20	21	22	23	24	25	26	27	28	29	30	
May	1	2	3	4	5	6	7	8	9	10	11	12	13	14	15	16	17	18	19	20	21	22	23	24	25	26	27	28	29	30	31
June	1	2	3	4	5	6	7	8	9	10	11	12	13	14	15	16	17	18	19	20	21	22	23	24	25	26	27	28	29	30	
July	1	2	3	4	5	6	7	8	9	10	11	12	13	14	15	16	17	18	19	20	21	22	23	24	25	26	27	28	29	30	31
Aug.	1	2	3	4	5	6	7	8	9	10	11	12	13	14	15	16	17	18	19	20	21	22	23	24	25	26	27	28	29	30	31
Sept.	1	2	3	4	5	6	7	8	9	10	11	12	13	14	15	16	17	18	19	20	21	22	23	24	25	26	27	28	29	30	
Oct.	1	2	3	4	5	6	7	8	9	10	11	12	13	14	15	16	17	18	19	20	21	22	23	24	25	26	27	28	29	30	31
Nov.	1	2	3	4	5	6	7	8	9	10	11	12	13	14	15	16	17	18	19	20	21	22	23	24	25	26	27	28	29	30	
Dec.	1	2	3	4	5	6	7	8	9	10	11	12	13	14	15	16	17	18	19	20	21	22	23	24	25	26	27	28	29	30	31

Use an ovulation predictor kit. These are sold over-the-counter at pharmacies and test the level of *luteinizing hormone (LH)* in your urine. When your LH levels rise, it means that one of your ovaries is about to release an egg.

Monitor your cervical mucus. Your cervix makes mucus, which changes at different points in your cycle. Just before ovulation, the amount of mucus made by the cervix increases, and the mucus gets thin and slippery. The last day of this thin and slippery mucus is called the "peak day." Ovulation happens within 24 to 48 hours of the peak day. Just after ovulation, the amount of mucus decreases, and it gets thicker and less noticeable.

To use this method, check the mucus at the opening of your vagina each time you urinate, starting on the first day after your period bleeding stops. For the best chance of getting pregnant, you should try to have sex every day or every other day when cervical mucus is present.

Track your temperature. Most women's *basal body temperature (BBT)* increases slightly—about half a degree—after they ovulate. To use this method, take your temperature at the same time every morning before you get out of bed. You'll need a thermometer that measures by tenths of degrees. Chart the temperature on a graph that also shows the days you have your period. Your temperature will go up 24 to 48 hours after you ovulate.

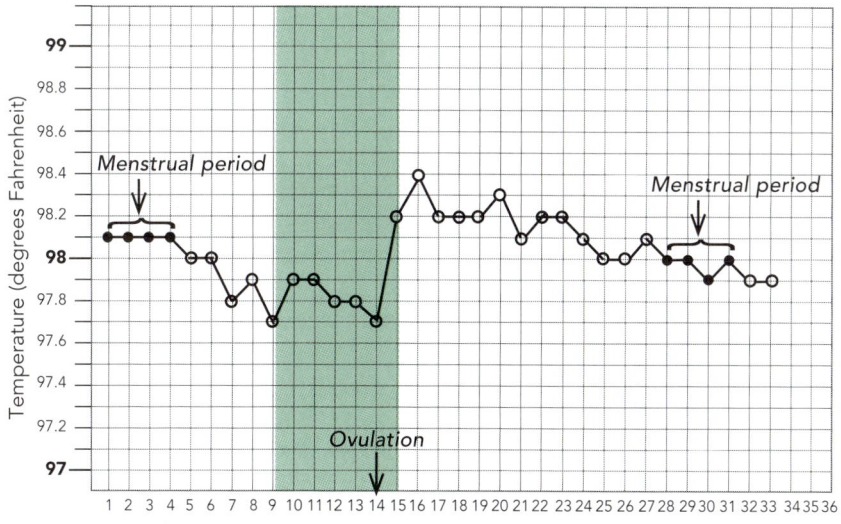

Sample basal body temperature chart. Keeping a basal body temperature chart for several months may help you predict when you will ovulate. Body temperature rises 24 to 48 hours after ovulation and stays high for at least 3 days.

By itself, tracking your temperature is not a good way to time when to have sex. The temperature change shows only when ovulation has happened, not when it is going to happen. Combining methods may work best. For example, a cervical mucus method can be used to find out when your fertile time begins, and the temperature method can be used to find out when your fertile time ends.

Stopping Birth Control

You can start trying to get pregnant right after stopping hormonal birth control. With most hormonal methods, such as birth control pills, the patch, and the hormonal **intrauterine device (IUD)**, ovulation can happen within 2 weeks of stopping. This also is true for the copper IUD. If you use the birth control injection, it may take up to 10 months or longer for normal ovulation to come back.

If you get pregnant while using a hormonal birth control method, do not worry. It does not increase the risk of birth defects. But once you know that you are pregnant, you should stop using your method right away.

Rarely, pregnancy may happen with an IUD in place. If it does, the IUD should be removed if it is possible to do so without surgery. Talk with your ob-gyn if you have an IUD and you think you might be pregnant.

RESOURCES

Before Pregnancy
www.cdc.gov/preconception
Information from the Centers for Disease Control and Prevention (CDC). Offers tips for women who are planning a pregnancy. Includes information for men.

MyPlate
www.ChooseMyPlate.gov
Website from the U.S. Department of Agriculture. The customized MyPlate Plan lets you enter your information for tips on what and how much to eat.

My Family Health Portrait Tool
https://phgkb.cdc.gov/FHH/html/index.html
Website from the CDC that helps you create a personalized family health history. Creates a drawing of your family tree and a health history chart based on the information you enter.

Pregnancy and Vaccination
www.cdc.gov/vaccines/pregnancy/pregnant-women
Information from the CDC on vaccination before, during, and after pregnancy. Includes a quiz to help you figure out which vaccines you need.

Smokefree Women: Pregnancy and Motherhood
https://women.smokefree.gov/pregnancy-motherhood
Website from the National Cancer Institute. Offers tools and tips for quitting smoking. Includes a text message program to help women cut down or quit smoking during pregnancy.

Your Pregnancy and Childbirth
www.acog.org/MyPregnancy
Website from ACOG with information on pregnancy, labor, delivery, and postpartum care. Includes the latest information from the experts in women's health care, questions answered by ACOG ob-gyns, pregnancy stories from real women, and an A–Z directory of health topics covering pregnancy and beyond.

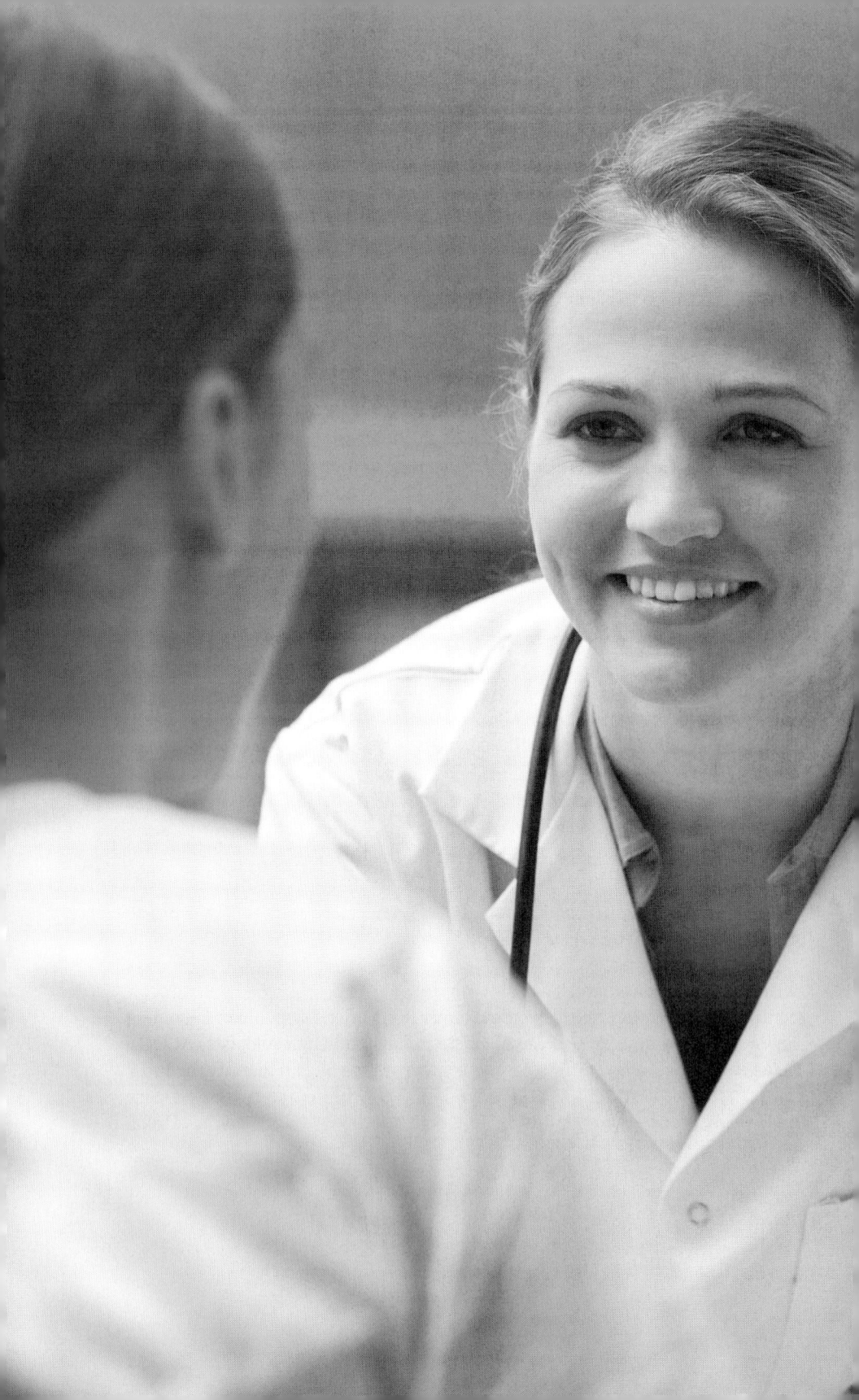

CHAPTER 2

Choosing Your Care Team

Choosing who will care for you during pregnancy is one of the most important decisions you'll make. You should choose someone you are comfortable with. It's also important to understand the types of practitioners, how they are trained, and how they can work together.

Types of Pregnancy Doctors

There are different types of doctors who are licensed to provide prenatal, pregnancy, and *postpartum* care.

Obstetrician–Gynecologists

Obstetrician–gynecologists (ob-gyns) are doctors who specialize in the health care of women. After medical school, ob-gyns take 4 years of specialized training in *obstetrics* and *gynecology*. To be board-certified, ob-gyns must pass written and spoken exams. They also must maintain their certification through continuing education and periodic exams. A certified ob-gyn can become a Fellow of the American College of Obstetricians and Gynecologists (ACOG). Fellows of ACOG use "FACOG" after their names so you can identify them.

ACOG recommends that an ob-gyn be on every pregnant woman's care team. Ob-gyns practice "evidence-based medicine." This means they rely on up-to-date and scientifically proven information. You and your ob-gyn can talk about the most current information, discuss your expectations, and agree on all aspects of your care during pregnancy.

Ob-gyns are trained to manage all pregnancies, including pregnancies that develop *complications*. Ob-gyns can coordinate care with other practitioners on your care team. Also, after your pregnancy and postpartum period, your ob-gyn can provide ongoing care to help you stay healthy throughout your life. Having one doctor who knows your health history can help you maintain control of your future care.

Maternal–Fetal Medicine Specialists

Maternal-fetal medicine (MFM) specialists are ob-gyns who specialize in high-risk pregnancies. MFMs have 4 years of training in obstetrics and gynecology. They then go on to 3 years of training in high-risk pregnancies. MFMs must pass written and spoken exams to be certified.

MFMs can play different roles during pregnancy. A woman with a high-risk pregnancy may see her ob-gyn and have a one-time consultation with an MFM. Or she may be managed by her ob-gyn and an MFM at the same time. Another option would be having care transferred to an MFM for the rest of a high-risk pregnancy. And in some cases, an MFM may do a fetal ultrasound instead of the primary ob-gyn.

Family Medicine Doctors

Doctors in family medicine (also known as family practice doctors) offer general care for most conditions, including pregnancy. After medical school, these doctors complete 3 years of training in family medicine, which includes time spent on obstetrics. They are certified by passing a written exam.

Family medicine doctors can care for women with low-risk pregnancies and deliveries. They also may care for the baby after birth. If a woman develops complications during pregnancy, her care may be transferred to an ob-gyn.

Other Practitioners

There are other practitioners who can provide prenatal, pregnancy, and postpartum care. These practitioners can manage low-risk pregnancies and can be part of your care team, along with your ob-gyn.

Certified Nurse–Midwives and Certified Midwives

Certified nurse–midwives (CNMs) and certified midwives (CMs) are specially trained practitioners. They offer care for women with low-risk pregnancies and their babies from early pregnancy through labor, delivery, and the weeks after birth. CNMs and CMs usually work with ob-gyns as part of a care team.

CNMs are registered nurses who have completed an accredited nursing program and have a graduate degree in midwifery. To be certified, they must pass a national written exam from the American Midwifery Certification Board (AMCB) and must maintain an active nursing license.

CMs have graduated from a midwifery education program accredited by the American College of Nurse–Midwives Division of Accreditation. They have completed the same requirements, have passed the same AMCB national certification exam, and follow the same professional standards as CNMs.

Certified Professional Midwives

Certified professional midwives (CPMs) are medical practitioners who are recognized in some U.S. states but not in others. CPMs also may be called "licensed direct-entry midwives," "registered midwives," or "licensed midwives."

There is no standard education program for CPMs. CPMs can learn by following a training program, through an apprenticeship, or through self-study. They receive certification through the North American Registry of Midwives (NARM).

Types of Practices

Another factor to think about is whether your ob-gyn is in a solo practice, group practice, or collaborative practice:

- In a solo practice, an ob-gyn works alone. He or she may have help from other ob-gyns to cover deliveries.

- In a group practice, two or more ob-gyns share duties.

> ### How to Find Pregnancy Care
>
> There are different ways to find ob-gyns and other practitioners who specialize in pregnancy and postpartum care:
>
> - Ask your primary care doctor or other health care practitioner for recommendations.
> - Ask friends and family members about their experiences with their pregnancy care teams.
> - Look for the "find a doctor" service at the website of your health insurance plan.
> - Look for the "Find an Ob-Gyn" tool at the ACOG website. See the "Resources" section at the end of this chapter.
>
> You can use the internet to learn about the education, qualifications, and certifications of the ob-gyns and practitioners you are interested in. You also can call their offices with questions.

- A collaborative practice brings together a team of professionals. These can include ob-gyns, nurses, CNMs or CMs, **laborists**, nurse practitioners, physician assistants, social workers, and childbirth educators. The contributions of each member are key to patient care.

There also is group prenatal care. Instead of individual medical appointments, a group of women with similar due dates meets regularly with an ob-gyn for health assessments, education, and support. Physical exams with a practitioner are done in a private room. If this model of prenatal care appeals to you, ask your ob-gyn for more information.

Questions to Ask

Once you find an ob-gyn who seems promising, ask questions that are important to you. Write down a list of your concerns to take to your first prenatal care visit. Use this list as a guide for some questions you may want to ask:

- Do you accept my health insurance?
- Are you in practice alone, or is there a group?
- If it is a group, how often will I see the same person when I come for my prenatal care visits?
- If you are in solo practice, who covers when you are not available?
- How can I get in touch with you during business hours?
- Do you have an after-hours phone number that I can call in case of an emergency or if I have concerns?
- Who takes the after-hours calls?
- Which hospital will I go to when I give birth?
- Who will deliver my baby?
- What are your views on anesthesia during labor, **episiotomy**, alternative birthing positions, **cesarean birth**, and assisted vaginal delivery?
- Who can be with me during delivery?

See Chapter 12, "Preparing for Birth," for more discussion of some of these questions.

Prenatal Care Visits

You'll have regular prenatal care appointments throughout your pregnancy. What happens during a visit, and how often you have appointments, will depend on factors such as

Making the Most of Your Prenatal Care Visits

Can I bring another person with me to the appointment?
Yes, you can bring a partner, friend, or family member with you to your appointment. This person can act as your advocate—someone who knows you and has your best interests in mind. This person may help you remember something during or after the visit. Make sure that you are comfortable sharing private information with this person. If you need to bring young children with you, also bring someone to take care of them.

What if I need an interpreter?
You may need an interpreter if your ob-gyn does not speak your preferred language. Before your visit, ask the office staff whether they can find an interpreter who is familiar with medical terms. Or ask if the office can provide medical translation via phone. Office visits with translation take longer, and the office will need to be aware for scheduling. Be sure to give them enough notice. Also, if you need a sign-language interpreter, be sure to make this request in advance.

Friends or family members may not make the best interpreters. They may not understand medical terms. Also, you may discuss concerns with your ob-gyn that you want to keep private.

What if I have vision or hearing problems?
If you use eyeglasses, take them with you to the office. If you use a hearing aid, wear it and make sure that it works before the office visit. Let your ob-gyn know if you have trouble seeing or hearing. Ask if you need someone to speak slowly.

How should I talk with my ob-gyn?
If you have questions, ask them. You have a right to ask questions of everyone who is involved in your health care. Feel free to ask anything about the health care process. If your ob-gyn asks you questions, answer them as best you can.

It is important to make sure you understand everything your ob-gyn says. Ask for simple, clear explanations. Ask him or her to draw a picture if you think that might help. Take notes. If you have someone with you, ask that person to take notes so you can listen closely to what is being said. Remember, you and your ob-gyn have the same goal: a healthy pregnancy for you and your baby.

- how far along you are in your pregnancy
- your health
- your baby's health

You will need to have a physical exam during one or more prenatal care visits, so it's important that you feel comfortable with your ob-gyn. Suggestions for making your visits more comfortable are discussed in this section.

What Happens During a Visit?

At each visit, your ob-gyn will monitor your health and your baby's health. Your first or second prenatal care visit will probably be one of your longest visits. Your ob-gyn will ask a lot of questions about your health and do several tests.

It's important to answer all questions honestly and with as much detail as you can. A medical history form is provided in the back of this book. You can use this form to help you prepare. Fill out the form before your visit and bring it with you, or just read through it to see some of the questions that will be asked.

Prenatal care visits are also a good time for you to ask questions and learn. If you have questions between visits, write them down for your next visit. It may be helpful to bring a support person with you for your prenatal care visits (see the box "Making the Most of Your Prenatal Care Visits" on the previous page). This person can take notes for you and remind you of questions you may have.

How Often Should You See Your Ob-Gyn?

How often you will see your ob-gyn for prenatal care depends on your health history, pregnancy history, and other factors:

- If this is your first pregnancy and you do not have any complications, you likely will see your ob-gyn every 4 weeks for the first 28 weeks of pregnancy, every 2 weeks until 36 weeks, and then weekly.
- If you're healthy and you have had a successful pregnancy before, you may be able to have fewer visits as long as you can see your ob-gyn on an as-needed basis.
- If you have health issues or pregnancy complications, you may need to see your ob-gyn more often, and you may need to have extra tests.

The month-by-month chapters in this book discuss what you can expect each month. Also, in some cases it may be possible to use telehealth for prenatal care visits. See the box "Telehealth and Your Ob-Gyn Visits."

Making Your Physical Exam More Comfortable

To check your health and the health of the baby, your ob-gyn will need to do a physical exam. He or she will need to touch different parts of your body, including your

- arm, to measure blood pressure
- chest or back, to listen to your heart and lungs with a stethoscope
- abdomen and **genitals**, to do a **pelvic exam**

Telehealth and Your Ob-Gyn Visits

In recent years, telehealth has become more available as a form of health care. During the coronavirus (COVID-19) health crisis, telehealth has been a safe way for people to get health care without going to an office. But telehealth also is a good choice for people who need to travel long distances to see a doctor. In some cases, telehealth can be used to reduce the number of in-person visits needed during pregnancy. But keep in mind that if your ob-gyn thinks it would be better for you to be seen in person, you may be asked to schedule an office visit.

To visit with your ob-gyn using telehealth, you need a phone, computer, or tablet. If your visit is just by phone, you and your doctor will speak on the phone like any typical phone call. If your visit is through a video connection, your ob-gyn's office will give you instructions for how to download and use a video app on your smartphone, computer, or tablet. With a video connection you and your ob-gyn will see each other on screen.

When You Schedule the Telehealth Visit
- Ask your ob-gyn's office how the visit will work. Will your ob-gyn call your phone? Or will the office send you a link to a website or ask you to download an app for video chat? Let the office know if you would prefer to do your telehealth visit by phone only.
- Talk with your ob-gyn's office about how they will keep the visit private and secure.
- Ask what you will need to have with you during the visit, and if you will need to do anything like take your temperature or blood pressure at home.
- Ask about the fee for the telehealth visit. If you have insurance, ask your insurance carrier how much they will cover.

Before the Telehealth Visit
- If possible, find a quiet, safe, and private place for your visit. If you have headphones, you can use them to lessen noise and help with privacy. Try to choose a spot that has good cell phone service or internet connection.
- If needed, try to make plans for child care during your visit.
- Try out any technology you need for the visit ahead of time. If you are using an app or website, test it out and make sure you can log in.
- Prepare like you would for an in-person visit. Write down your symptoms, health history, medications, and questions for your ob-gyn.

After the Telehealth Visit
- Follow up with your ob-gyn's office if you think of any more questions about your care. If you and your ob-gyn discussed any tests or follow-up visits, ask how and when these will be scheduled.
- Let your ob-gyn's office know if you have any feedback about how the visit went.

During a pelvic exam, your ob-gyn checks your internal organs by inserting one or two fingers into the *vagina* while pressing on your belly with the other hand. If you are nervous or uncomfortable about any of this, let your ob-gyn know. Together you can discuss ways to make you feel more comfortable.

Your ob-gyn should have a chaperone in the exam room. This person usually is a nurse or medical assistant. You can decline to have the chaperone in the room. You also can have your partner or another family member with you during the exam. Make your wishes known.

Special Concerns for Survivors of Sexual Abuse

About 1 in 5 women were sexually abused in childhood or their teen years. Because these experiences can affect health, many ob-gyns ask their patients if they have had unwanted sexual experiences.

Pregnancy and childbirth may be difficult for *sexual abuse* survivors. You may find it helpful to work with a counselor or therapist with experience in abuse or trauma. Ask your ob-gyn if he or she can give you a referral. You also can call the National Sexual Assault Telephone Hotline at 1-800-656-HOPE (4673) to find services in your area.

Pelvic exams can be painful or triggering for abuse survivors. If this is true for you, let your ob-gyn know. These things may help make the pelvic exam easier:

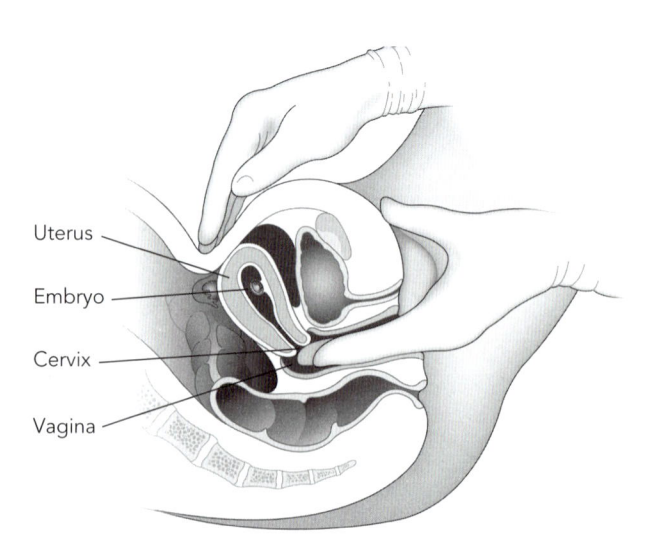

Pelvic exam. During a pelvic exam, your ob-gyn checks your internal organs by inserting one or two fingers into the vagina while pressing on your belly with the other hand.

- Your ob-gyn should explain what he or she will be doing ahead of time and talk you through the steps as they happen.

- Your ob-gyn should always ask permission before touching you.

- Some things may help you feel more in control, like controlling the pace of the exam, being able to see more (such as with a mirror), or putting your hand over your ob-gyn's hand to guide the exam.

- You may want to have a partner, friend, or family member in the room during the exam to help you feel more comfortable.

If you think one or more of these might help, tell your ob-gyn.

RESOURCES

Choosing a Family Doctor
https://familydoctor.org/choosing-a-family-doctor/
Website from the American Academy of Family Physicians. This page discusses the role of the family doctor and gives advice on finding the right doctor for you and your family.

Find a Midwifery Practice Near You
www.midwife.org/find-a-midwife
This directory from the American College of Nurse–Midwives (ACNM) helps you find practices near you with at least one certified nurse–midwife or certified midwife who is a member of the ACNM.

Find an MFM Specialist
www.smfm.org/members/search
This directory from the Society for Maternal-Fetal Medicine can help you find an MFM specialist near you.

Find an Ob-Gyn
www.acog.org/FindAnObGyn
This directory from the American College of Obstetricians and Gynecologists (ACOG) can help you find an ob-gyn near you.

National Sexual Assault Telephone Hotline
1-800-656-HOPE (4673)
https://hotline.rainn.org/online/
Hotline that connects survivors of sexual assault with help and resources from trained service providers in their area.

Your Pregnancy and Childbirth
www.acog.org/MyPregnancy
Website from ACOG with information on pregnancy, labor, delivery, and postpartum care. Includes the latest information from the experts in women's health care, questions answered by ACOG ob-gyns, pregnancy stories from real women, and an A–Z directory of health topics covering pregnancy and beyond.

The following illustrations show fetal development and the changes that occur in a woman's body throughout pregnancy. Seeing them all together gives you an idea of how the body adjusts as a baby grows. These illustrations also are found in each of the month-to-month chapters.

PREGNANCY MONTH BY MONTH • 33

Mother and baby: Weeks 1 to 8

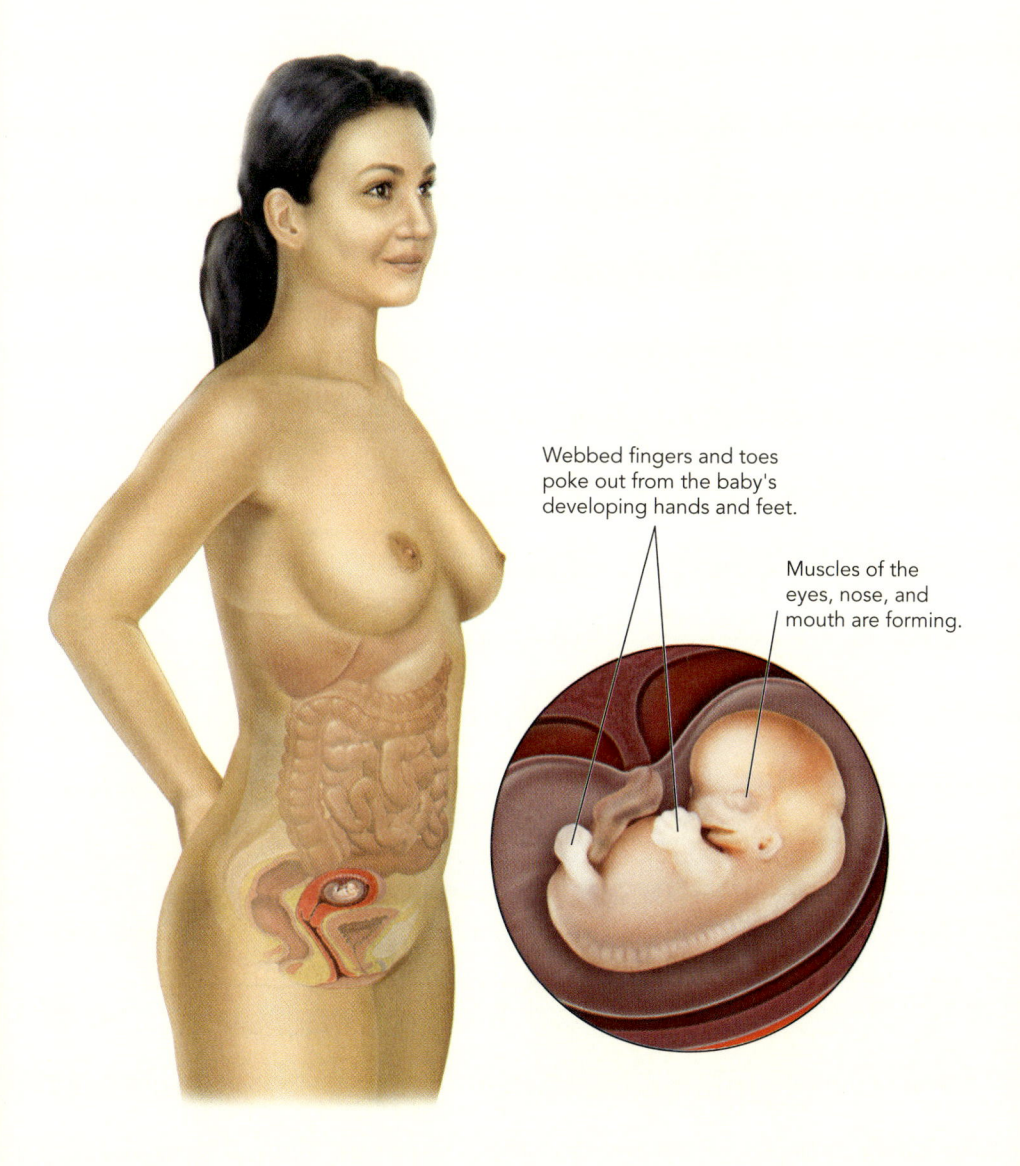

Webbed fingers and toes poke out from the baby's developing hands and feet.

Muscles of the eyes, nose, and mouth are forming.

The first 8 weeks of pregnancy are a time of rapid growth for your baby. Most of the organs have begun to form during these weeks. By the end of week 8, the baby—called an embryo at this stage—is about half an inch long.

Mother and baby: Weeks 9 to 12

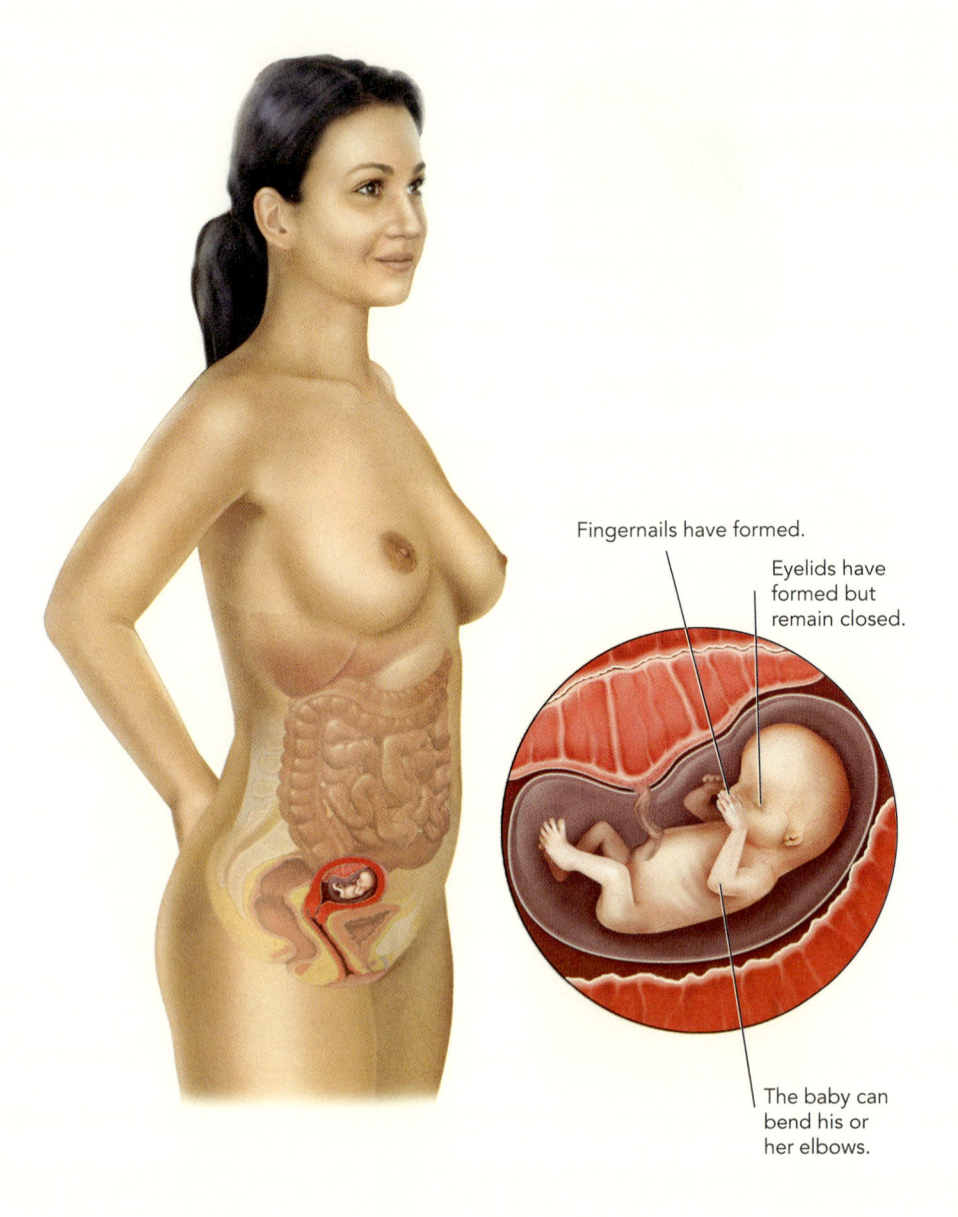

Fingernails have formed.

Eyelids have formed but remain closed.

The baby can bend his or her elbows.

By the end of week 12, the baby—now called a fetus—is about 2 inches long and weighs about half an ounce.

PREGNANCY MONTH BY MONTH • 35

Mother and baby: Weeks 13 to 16

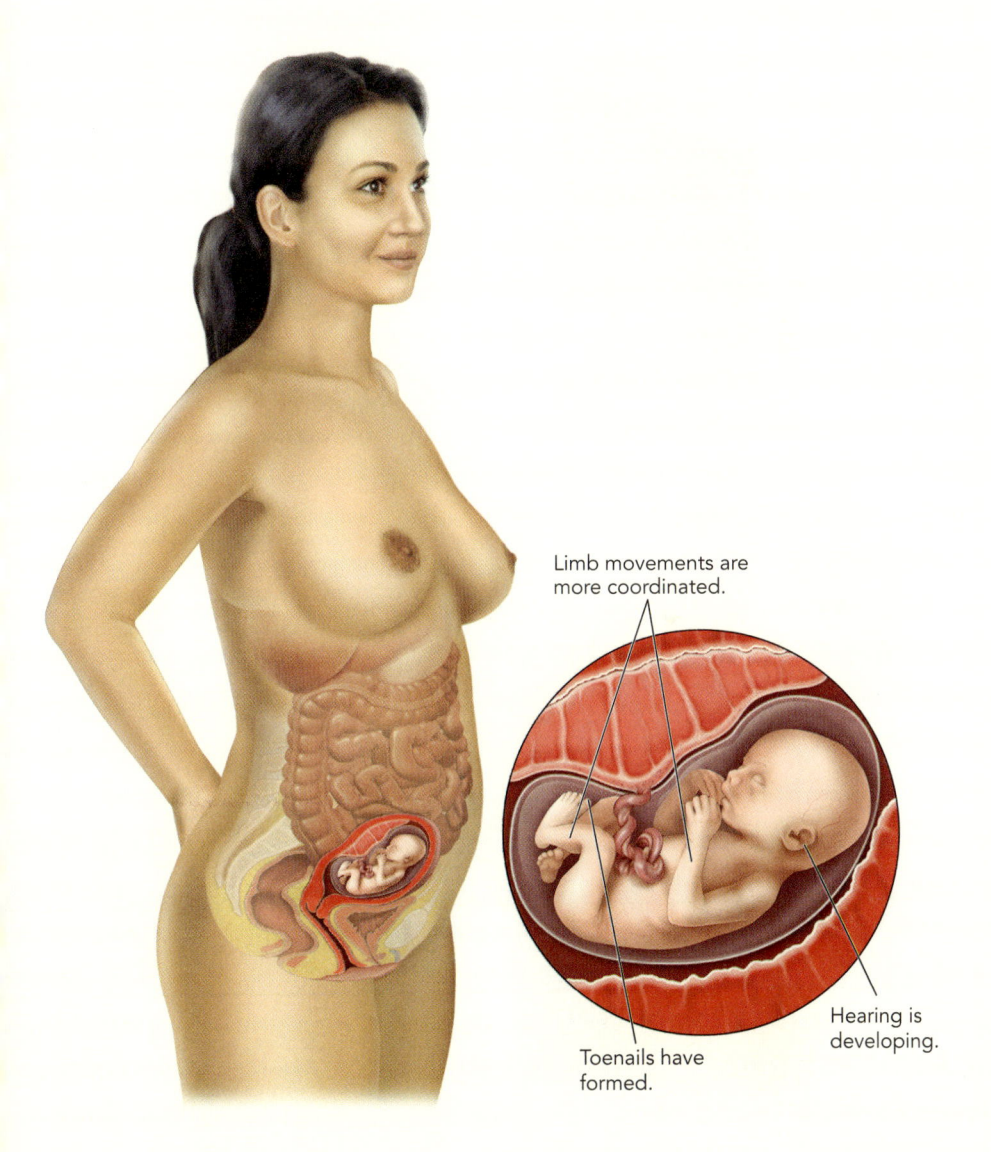

Limb movements are more coordinated.

Toenails have formed.

Hearing is developing.

By the end of week 16, the baby is more than 4 inches long and weighs more than 3 ounces.

36 • PREGNANCY MONTH BY MONTH

Mother and baby: Weeks 17 to 20

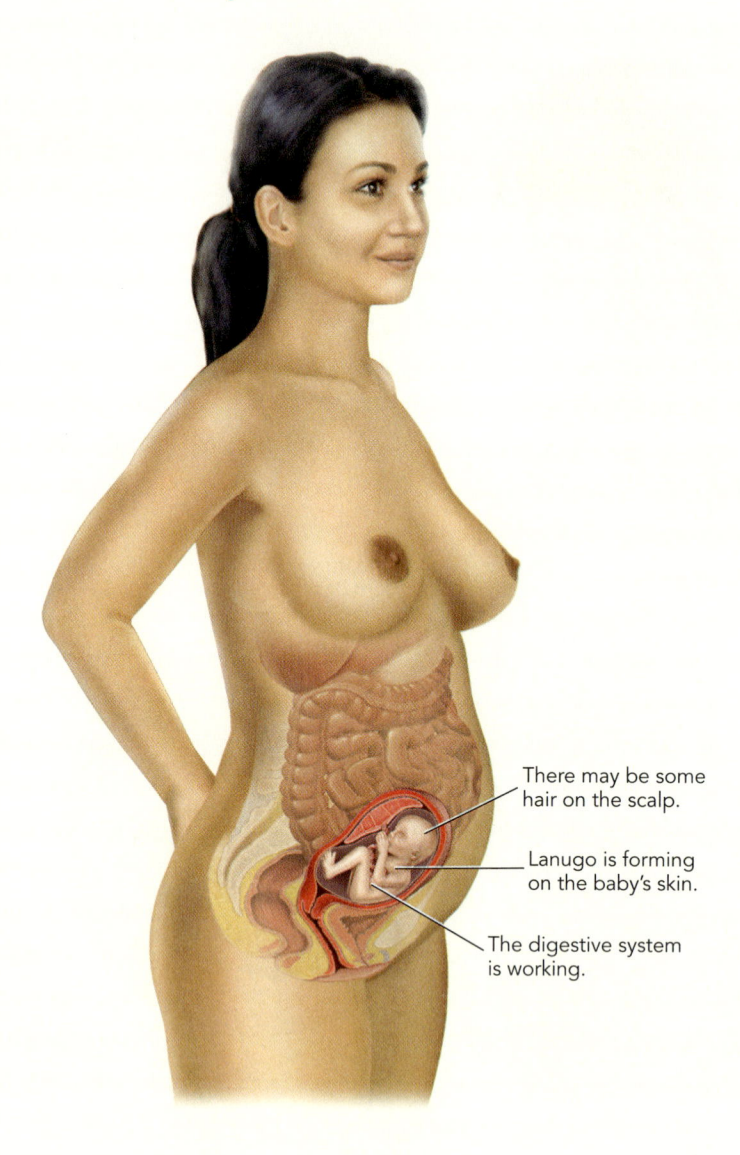

There may be some hair on the scalp.

Lanugo is forming on the baby's skin.

The digestive system is working.

By the end of week 20, the baby is more than 6 inches long and weighs less than 11 ounces.

PREGNANCY MONTH BY MONTH • 37

Mother and baby: Weeks 21 to 24

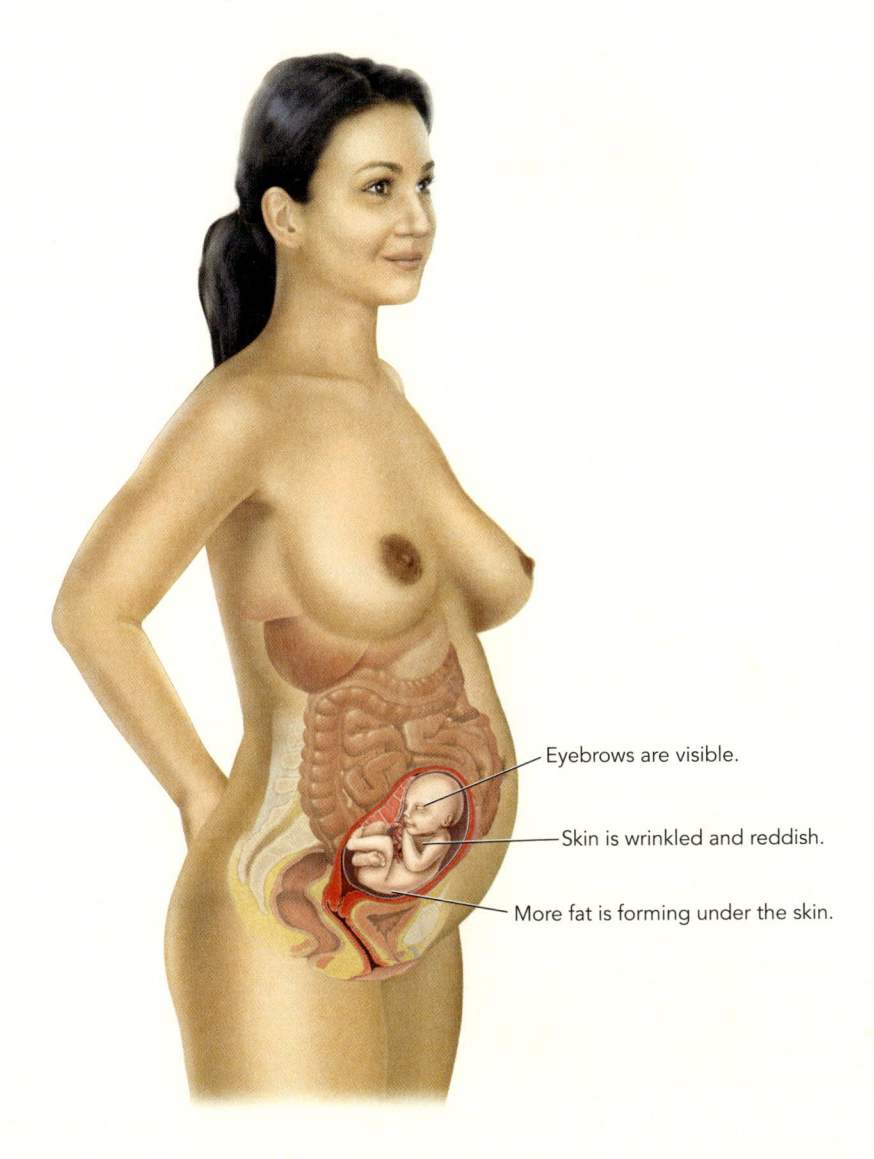

Eyebrows are visible.

Skin is wrinkled and reddish.

More fat is forming under the skin.

By the end of week 24, the baby is about 12 inches long and weighs about 1½ pounds.

Mother and baby: Weeks 25 to 28

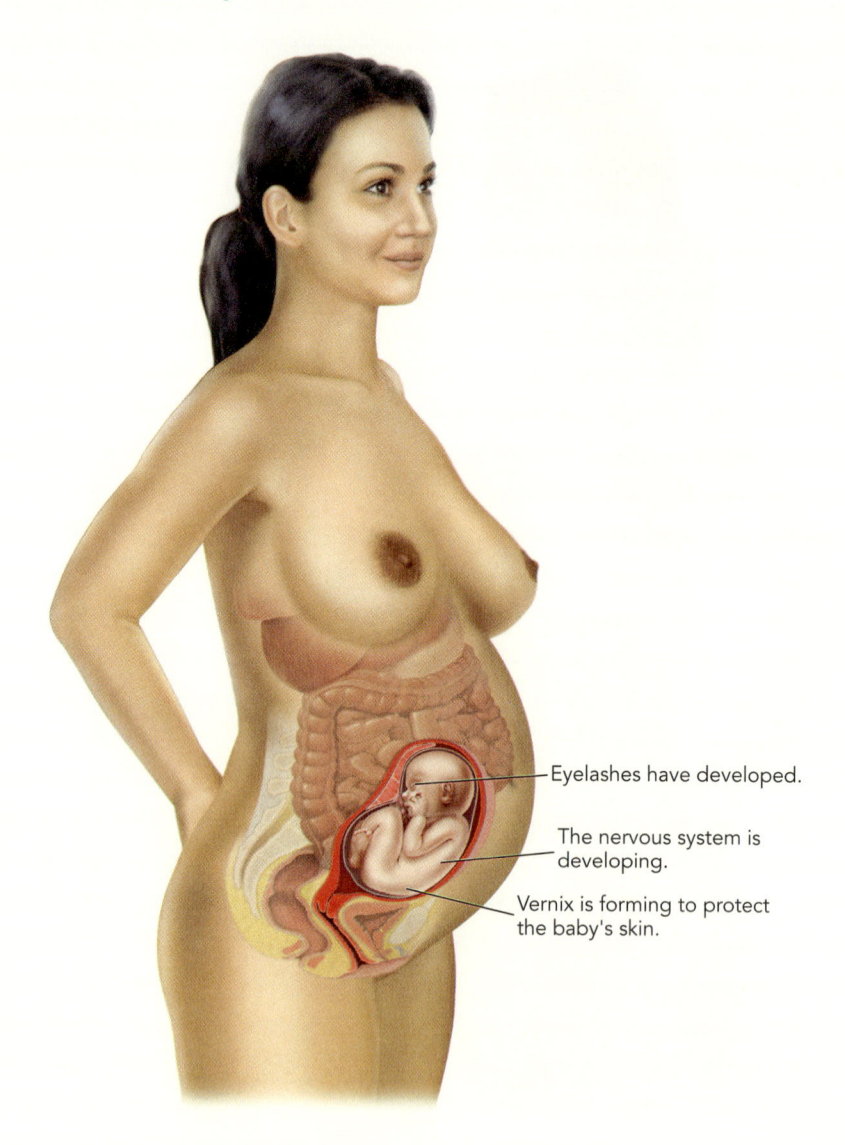

- Eyelashes have developed.
- The nervous system is developing.
- Vernix is forming to protect the baby's skin.

By the end of week 28, the baby is nearly 15 inches long and weighs about 2½ pounds.

PREGNANCY MONTH BY MONTH • 39

Mother and baby: Weeks 29 to 32

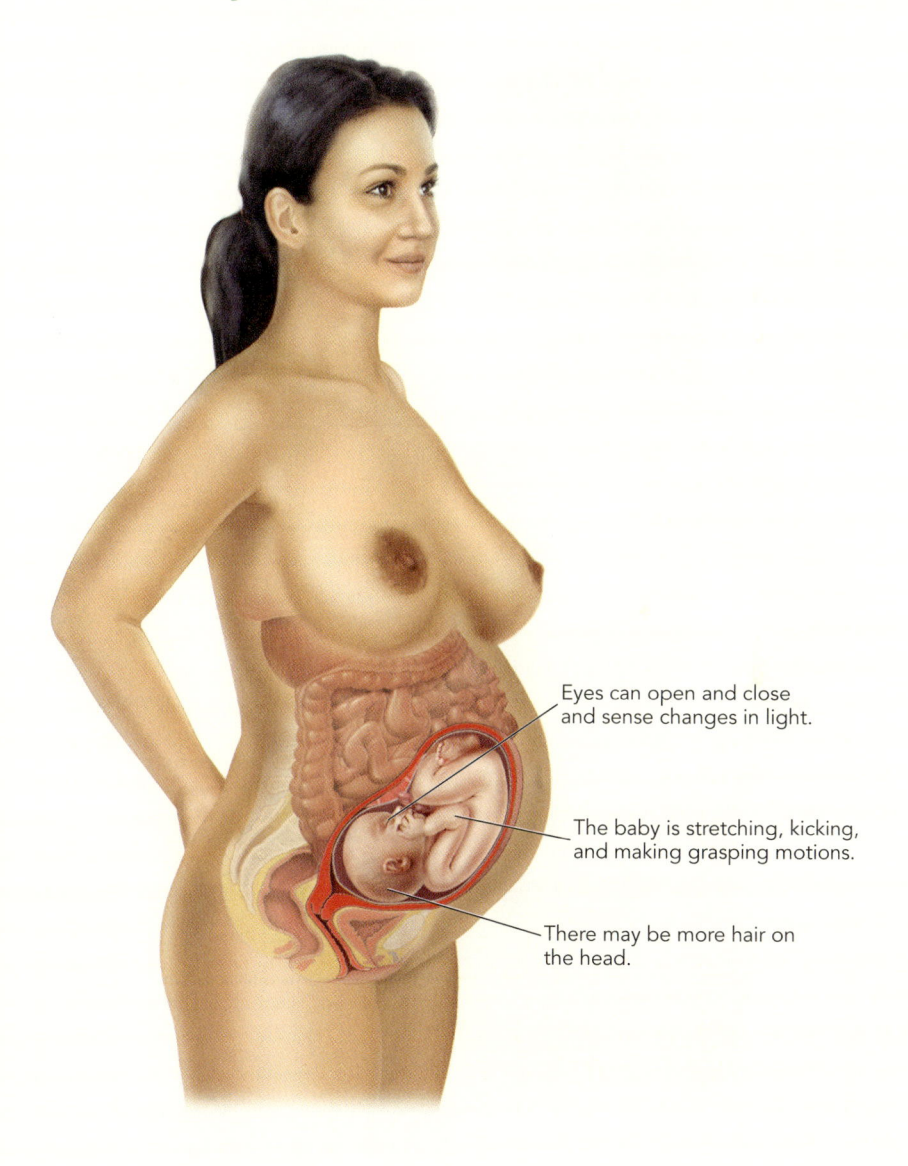

Eyes can open and close and sense changes in light.

The baby is stretching, kicking, and making grasping motions.

There may be more hair on the head.

By the end of week 32, the baby is almost 17 inches long and weighs nearly 4 pounds.

Mother and baby: Weeks 33 to 36

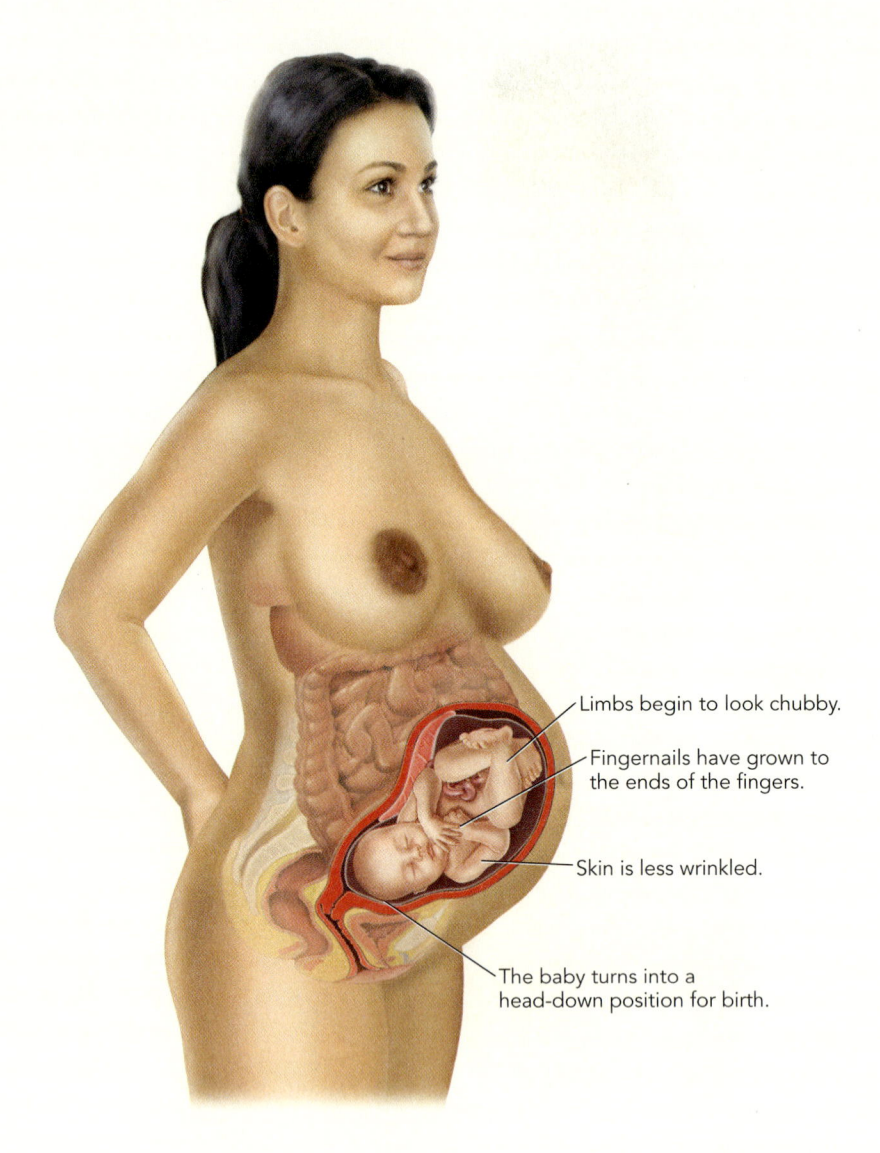

- Limbs begin to look chubby.
- Fingernails have grown to the ends of the fingers.
- Skin is less wrinkled.
- The baby turns into a head-down position for birth.

By the end of week 36, the baby is about 18 inches long and weighs a little more than 6 pounds.

PREGNANCY MONTH BY MONTH • 41

Mother and baby: Weeks 37 to 40

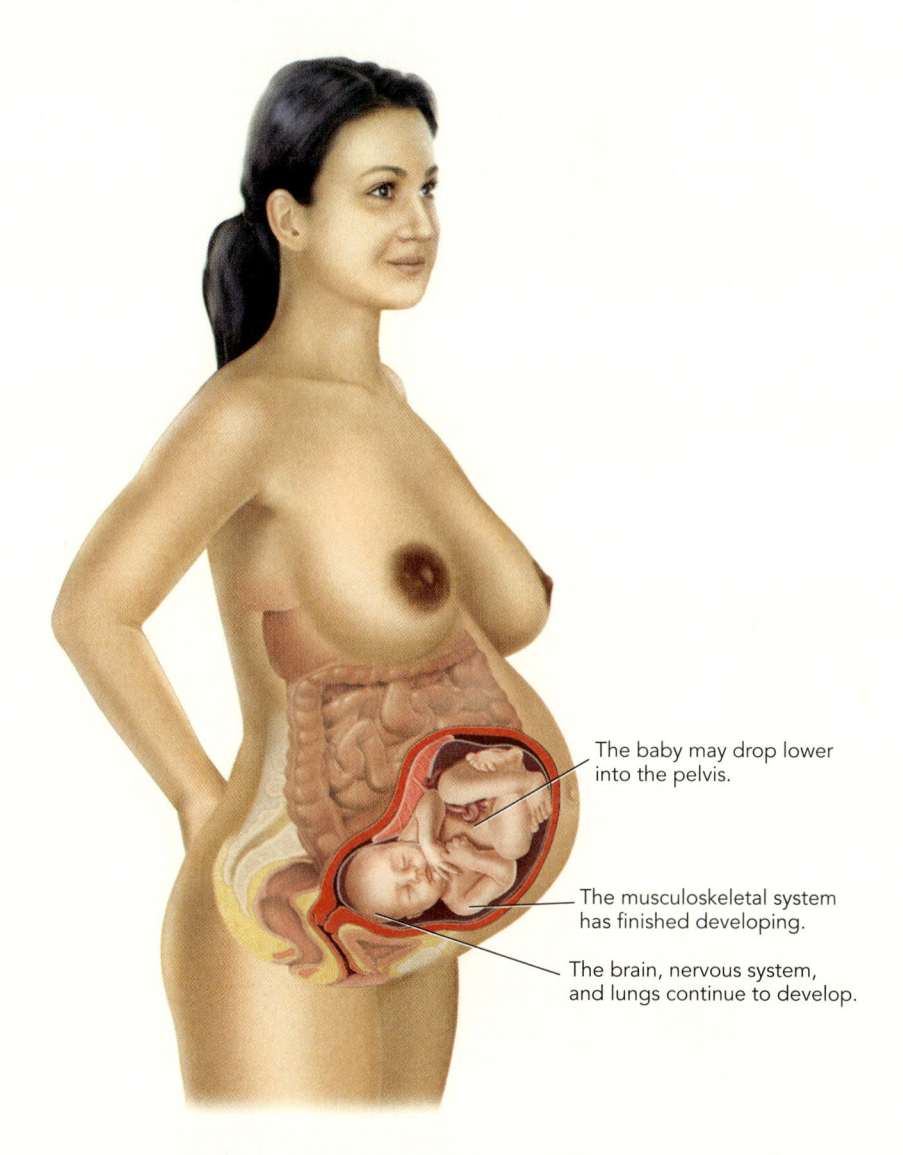

The baby may drop lower into the pelvis.

The musculoskeletal system has finished developing.

The brain, nervous system, and lungs continue to develop.

By the end of week 40, the baby is 20 inches long and may weigh 7½ to 8 pounds. The baby is now ready to be born.

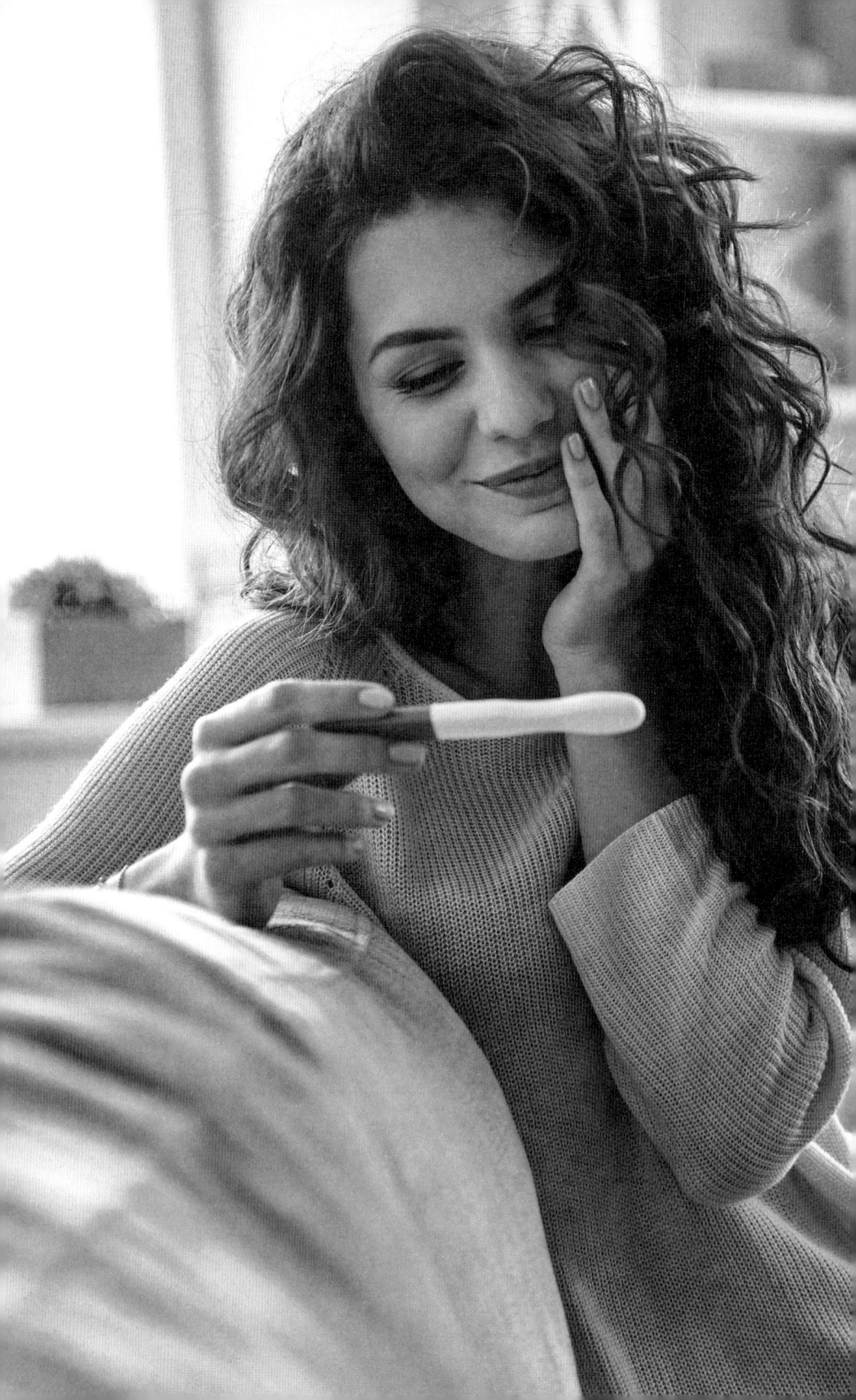

CHAPTER 3

Months 1 and 2
(Weeks 1 to 8)

YOUR BABY

➤ WEEK 1

The countdown of your pregnancy begins this week, but not because you're pregnant. This is the week of your **last menstrual period (LMP)** before getting pregnant. Because most women know the date of their LMP, **obstetrician–gynecologists (ob-gyns)** generally calculate the **estimated due date (EDD)** as 40 weeks from the first day of the LMP.

➤ WEEK 2

During this week, **eggs** are maturing in the **ovaries,** and the lining of the **uterus** is thickening. At the end of this week, **ovulation** takes place. This is the release of a mature egg from an ovary. After its release, the egg begins to travel down a **fallopian tube.**

➤ WEEK 3

This is the week of **fertilization**, the union of an egg and a sperm. When the egg and sperm come together, they form a single **cell** called a **zygote**. Fertilization takes place in one of the woman's fallopian tubes. After fertilization, the zygote divides, forming two cells. These cells then divide, forming four cells, and then eight cells, and so on. At the same time, the mass of dividing cells continues to move down the fallopian tube toward the uterus.

➤ WEEK 4

About 8 to 9 days after fertilization, the rapidly dividing group of cells, now called a **blastocyst,** enters the uterus. The blastocyst has started to make an important pregnancy **hormone** called **human chorionic gonadotropin (hCG)**. The **endometrium**, or uterine lining, has prepared itself for pregnancy. The blastocyst burrows deep into the uterine lining. This is called **implantation.**

> This week, the blastocyst is about the size of a single poppy seed.

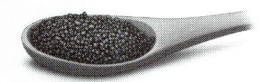

▶ WEEK 5
This week begins the **embryo** stage of development. The brain and spine have begun to form. Cardiac muscle also starts to develop.

> This week, the embryo is about the size of a single sesame seed.

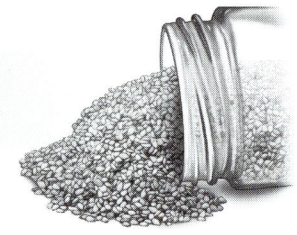

▶ WEEK 6
Parts of the face are taking shape now, including the eyes and nostrils. Cardiac activity can sometimes be seen during an **ultrasound exam** this week. The neural tube, from which the brain, spinal cord, and backbone will form, is completing its development.

> This week, the embryo is about the size of a single pea.

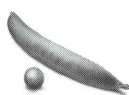

▶ WEEK 7
This week the mouth and face continue to develop. Arm and leg buds appear. The lungs start to develop the tubes that will carry air in and out after birth. The long tube that will become the digestive tract has taken shape.

> This week, the embryo is about the size of a single blueberry.

▶ WEEK 8
Webbed fingers and toes are now poking out from the developing hands and feet. The inner ear begins to develop. Muscles of eyes, nose, and mouth are developing.

> This week, the embryo is about the size of a single raspberry.

MONTHS 1 AND 2 • **45**

Webbed fingers and toes poke out from the baby's developing hands and feet.

Muscles of the eyes, nose, and mouth are forming.

Mother and baby: Weeks 1 to 8
By the end of week 8, the baby—called an embryo at this stage—is about half an inch long.

Months 1 and 2

YOUR PREGNANCY

Your Changing Body

Many signs and symptoms of pregnancy are thought to be caused by changing hormone levels. These early signs and symptoms can be subtle. Some women are not even aware of them, while others notice them right away.

Signs and Symptoms of Pregnancy

Most likely you will not have symptoms until about the time you've missed your period or even about 1 or 2 weeks later. Some women notice symptoms earlier than others. Here are the six most common signs and symptoms of pregnancy:

1. Tender, swollen breasts—One of the early signs of pregnancy is sore breasts. This soreness is caused by increasing levels of hormones. The soreness may feel like a more intense version of how your breasts feel before your period. The pain and discomfort should lessen after the first few weeks as your body adjusts to the hormonal changes.

2. Frequent urination—Soon after you get pregnant, you may find yourself rushing to the bathroom more often. During pregnancy, the amount of blood in your body increases, which leads to extra fluid being processed by your **kidneys** and ending up in your **bladder**. This symptom usually continues as your pregnancy gets farther along and your baby puts more pressure on your bladder.

3. Nausea or vomiting—Most women do not experience a queasy stomach and vomiting until about 1 month after getting pregnant. But some women start to feel nausea a bit earlier. Other women never experience nausea or vomiting.

4. Fatigue—Feeling tired is a common symptom of early pregnancy. No one knows for sure what causes early-pregnancy fatigue. Rapidly rising levels of the hormone *progesterone* may contribute to sleepiness. You should start to feel more energetic once you enter your second *trimester*. Fatigue usually returns late in pregnancy.

5. Moodiness—You may notice that your emotions are up one moment and down the next. Having mood swings during this time is normal.

6. Bloating—Hormonal changes in early pregnancy may leave you feeling bloated, similar to the feeling some women have just before their periods start. The bloating may cause your clothes to fit tighter around the waist, even early on when your uterus is still quite small.

Pregnancy Tests

If you've missed your period and have some of the symptoms of pregnancy, you may want to take a pregnancy test. There are several brands of home pregnancy tests you can buy. All of them are easy to use and can be done at home. Results are ready in a few minutes.

With home pregnancy tests, you urinate on a stick that detects the hormone hCG in your urine. About 6 to 7 days after fertilization, the blastocyst (fertilized egg) starts to make hCG as it moves down the fallopian tube toward the uterus. After the blastocyst implants in the uterus, production of hCG increases rapidly.

Home pregnancy tests measure hCG as milli-international units per milliliter (mIU/mL). Depending on the brand, home pregnancy tests can detect 20 mIU/mL, 50 mIU/mL, or 100 mIU/mL of hCG in the urine. It's important to read the label on the test, because not all tests can detect the same level of hCG. In general, the lower the level of hCG that the test can detect, the better the test is at accurately detecting pregnancy.

Many home pregnancy tests claim to be around 99 percent accurate in detecting pregnancy on the first day after your missed period. But in research studies of these tests, it was found that most brands of tests do not consistently detect pregnancy that early. A ***false-negative*** result is a result that says you are not pregnant when you actually are pregnant. Most false-negative results are caused by taking the test too early, when there is not enough hCG in the urine. If you get a negative result and you have some pregnancy symptoms, you may want to take the test again when your period is at least 1 week late.

Also, make sure that you follow the directions for taking the test exactly. Doing so may lead to more accurate results. For example, most tests say to take the test with the first urine of the day, when hCG levels are highest.

Home pregnancy tests also can give a ***false-positive*** result. This means that the test says you are pregnant even though you are not pregnant. The most common reasons for a false-positive home pregnancy test result are not following the test's directions or reading the results incorrectly.

If you have a positive home pregnancy test result or if your result is negative and you really want to be sure, you can see your ob-gyn to have a blood test and a physical exam. The blood test for pregnancy is more sensitive than most urine tests for two reasons:

1. It can detect low hCG levels of 5 to 10 mIU/mL.
2. More hCG is present in the blood than in the urine.

These two factors allow the blood test to detect pregnancy 6 to 10 days after ovulation. For many women, this is before a period is missed.

By the end of week 2, you probably don't know that you are pregnant. You may notice a little spotting. This spotting, known as ***implantation bleeding***, can occur when the fertilized egg attaches to the lining of the uterus. The spotting is very light, and not all women have it. Some women mistake it for menstrual bleeding. Implantation bleeding is normal and usually doesn't signal a problem.

Hormones

Hormones are the chemical messengers that guide the body's functions. The following hormones play a leading role in reproduction, pregnancy, and birth:

- ***Estrogen*** and progesterone—These hormones are produced by the ovaries. They trigger the lining of the uterus to thicken during each ***menstrual cycle*** and to be shed if pregnancy doesn't occur. After an egg is fertilized, higher estrogen and progesterone levels stop the ovaries from releasing any eggs until the end of the pregnancy.

- ***Follicle-stimulating hormone (FSH)*** and ***luteinizing hormone (LH)***—These hormones are made by the ***pituitary gland***, a small organ at the base of the brain. FSH causes an egg to mature in one of the ***ovaries***. LH triggers the egg's release.

- ***Gonadotropin-releasing hormone (GnRH)***—This hormone is made in a part of the brain called the hypothalamus. It signals the pituitary gland to produce FSH and LH.

- Human chorionic gonadotropin (hCG)—This hormone causes the body to increase estrogen and progesterone. This is the hormone that is detected by pregnancy tests.

Your Estimated Due Date

Because most women know when their last menstrual period (LMP) occurred, and because babies typically are born 40 weeks later, ob-gyns usually count pregnancy from the first day of your LMP. The day your baby is due is called the estimated due date (EDD).

Your EDD can be calculated by counting 280 days from the first day of your LMP (see the box "Estimating Your Due Date"). In some cases, there are better ways of estimating your due date than using your LMP. Your ob-gyn may use an ultrasound exam in your first trimester to calculate your EDD if

- you are not sure of the first day of your LMP
- your periods are not regular

- you were using hormonal **birth control** when you got pregnant
- your menstrual cycles are very short or very long

It's important to know that the EDD gives only a rough idea of when your baby will be born, as only about 1 in 20 women give birth on their EDD. Most women go into labor within about 2 weeks of their due date—either before or after.

Your ob-gyn will use your EDD to calculate the baby's **gestational age.** Gestational age is measured in weeks, months, and trimesters. Ob-gyns also divide the weeks of pregnancy into days. For example, "24 and 3/7 weeks" means "24 completed weeks plus 3 days of pregnancy."

Remember that women typically ovulate about 2 weeks after the beginning of their LMP. So, from the first day of your LMP through about day 14, the body is preparing for pregnancy, but you aren't pregnant yet. This means that pregnancy can last up to 10 months because of these extra weeks. Here's how the trimesters are defined:

- First trimester (first day of LMP to 13 weeks and 6 days): The time when fertilization and major organ development occurs.

- Second trimester (14 weeks and 0 days to 27 weeks and 6 days): The time of rapid growth and development. There is some chance of survival if the baby is born in the later weeks of the second trimester.

- Third trimester (28 weeks and 0 days to 40 weeks and 6 days): The time when the baby's weight increases and the organs mature so they will be ready to function after birth.

Estimating Your Due Date

1. Take the date that your last normal menstrual period started.
2. Add 7 days.
3. Count back 3 months.

Example: The first day of your last menstrual period was January 1. Add 7 days to get January 8. Then count back 3 months. Your estimated due date is October 8.

Discomforts and How to Manage Them

The signs and symptoms of early pregnancy are mere annoyances for some women. For others, symptoms can be severe. It's not possible to predict which women will have more severe symptoms. Also, a woman may have different symptoms during each of her pregnancies. Whether they are mild or severe, there are ways to manage these discomforts safely and effectively.

Morning Sickness

Morning sickness is not just a feeling that happens before noon. The nausea and vomiting that define morning sickness can strike at any time of day—morning, afternoon, or night—and may last all day long. As many as 8 in 10 pregnant women have morning sickness during their first trimester. The nausea usually starts between 4 and 9 weeks of pregnancy.

Most women who experience nausea and vomiting usually feel complete relief by about 16 weeks of pregnancy. But for some women, nausea and vomiting continue for several weeks or months. And for a few women, morning sickness lasts throughout the entire pregnancy.

If you have morning sickness, there are a few things that you can try to help make it more bearable and to make sure you are getting enough nutrients and fluids:

- Take a prenatal vitamin—Taking a prenatal vitamin before and during pregnancy may reduce the risk of severe morning sickness.

- Keep snacks by the bed—Try eating crackers in the morning before you get out of bed. This avoids moving around on an empty stomach.

- Drink fluids—Your body needs more water in the early months, so aim to drink fluids often during the day. Not drinking can lead to **dehydration,** which can make nausea worse. If you are having trouble drinking water because of a bad taste in your mouth, try chewing gum or eating hard candies.

- Avoid smells that bother you—Foods or odors that may never have bothered you before may now trigger nausea. Do your best to stay away from them. Use a fan when cooking. Have someone else empty the trash.

- Eat small and often—Make sure your stomach is never empty. Eat five or six small meals each day.

- Try bland foods—The "BRATT" diet (bananas, rice, applesauce, toast, and tea) is low in fat and easy to digest. If these foods don't appeal to you, try others that do. The goal is to find foods that you can eat and that stay down. If you can, try to add a protein food at each meal. Good nonmeat sources of protein are dairy foods (milk, ice cream, yogurt), nuts and seeds (including nut butters), and protein powders and shakes.

- Try ginger—Ginger ale made with real ginger, ginger tea made from fresh grated ginger, ginger capsules, and ginger candies may help settle a queasy stomach.

If you try these remedies and they don't work, your ob-gyn may recommend medication. A combination of vitamin B_6 with or without another medication called doxylamine usually is recommended first. If this does not work, other medications may be tried.

About 1 in 50 women who have morning sickness have a severe form called **hyperemesis gravidarum**. No one knows what causes this condition, and it can be serious if it is not treated right away. Call your ob-gyn if you have any of the following signs or symptoms:

- You have not been able to keep any food or fluids down for 24 hours or more.
- Your lips, mouth, and skin are very dry.
- You are urinating less often (less than three times a day), you are not producing much urine, or your urine is dark and has an odor.
- You are not gaining weight or have lost 5 or more pounds over a 1- to 2-week period.

Your ob-gyn most likely will examine you to rule out other causes of your symptoms. If hyperemesis gravidarum is diagnosed, you may be given medication to help control your nausea and vomiting. If you have a severe case of hyperemesis gravidarum, you may need to get fluids through an ***intravenous (IV) line***.

Fatigue

During your first trimester, you may feel totally wiped out. You may find it hard just to get out of bed in the morning. This is normal. Being pregnant puts a strain on your entire body, which can make you feel very tired. Your hormone levels have increased. Your ***metabolism*** is running high and burning energy, even while you sleep. Women who are pregnant for the second time or more may experience even more fatigue than during their first pregnancy because of the need to take care of the other children as well as other demands on their time.

To help with fatigue, listen to your body. Slow down and get the rest you need. Try going to bed earlier than usual or take a 15-minute nap during the day. Don't forget that during these first couple of months, getting enough rest is important. So, if need be, let some things go undone until you have the energy to do them, or get help from your partner, friends, or family members. A healthy diet and exercise also may help boost your energy.

Fatigue usually begins to go away after the first trimester. By your fourth month of pregnancy, most of your energy will come back. But many women begin to feel tired again in the last months of pregnancy.

Nutrition

For some women, pregnancy is a planned event. They've been exercising, eating healthy foods, and taking vitamins for months beforehand. For others, pregnancy is a surprise. One of the most important things you need to do in early pregnancy (and, ideally, before pregnancy) is make sure that you are getting enough **folic acid**, a vitamin that helps reduce the risk of certain **birth defects**.

Prenatal Vitamins

If you weren't already taking a prenatal vitamin, start taking one when you find out you are pregnant. This vitamin supplement is available without a prescription. Prenatal vitamins contain the recommended daily allowances for the vitamins and minerals you will need during your pregnancy, such as

- vitamins A, C, and D
- folic acid
- iron

Taking prenatal vitamins can ensure that you're getting the important nutrients you need. This is especially important if you're battling nausea and finding it hard to eat. Also, take your prenatal vitamin only as directed on the bottle. Some prenatal vitamins are meant to be taken two or three times a day to get the full doses of vitamins and minerals. Do not take more than recommended per day.

At your first **prenatal care** visit, tell your ob-gyn if you have been taking prenatal vitamins and any other vitamins. You may want to bring the bottles with you. It's important to talk with your ob-gyn about all of the vitamins and supplements you take because excess amounts of some vitamins can be harmful. Some ingredients, such as vitamin A, are safe at low doses but can cause birth defects at higher doses.

Focus on Folic Acid

Folic acid, also known as folate or vitamin B_9, is a vitamin that helps prevent major birth defects of the baby's brain and spine called **neural tube defects (NTDs).** Current guidelines recommend that pregnant women get at least 600 mcg of folic acid per day, but it is hard to get enough from your diet alone. To reach this goal, take a prenatal vitamin with at least 400 mcg of folic acid every day and eat foods rich in this vitamin. The combination of folic acid in your vitamin and in your diet should help you reach the 600 mcg goal.

Neural tube defects, such as **spina bifida** and **anencephaly**, happen early in prenatal development when the coverings of the spinal cord do not close completely. You may have a higher risk of giving birth to a baby with a neural tube defect if you

- have already had a baby with a neural tube defect
- have certain health conditions, such as **sickle cell disease**
- are taking certain medications, such as anti-epilepsy drugs (especially valproate)

If any of these are true for you, your ob-gyn may recommend that you take 4 mg of folic acid each day—10 times the usual amount—as a separate supplement at least 3 months before pregnancy and for the first 3 months of pregnancy. You and your ob-gyn can discuss whether you need this amount of folic acid based on your health history.

Weight Gain

How much weight you should gain during pregnancy depends on your weight before you got pregnant. Your **body mass index (BMI)** is an indication of whether you are at a healthy weight for your height. If your BMI before pregnancy falls between 18.5 and 24.9, you are at a normal, healthy weight. A BMI below 18.5 is considered underweight, and a BMI of 25 or greater is considered overweight.

Use the "Body Mass Index Chart" at the back of this book to look up your prepregnancy BMI. In this chapter, Table 3-1, "Weight Gain During Pregnancy," shows recommended weight gain based on prepregnancy BMI.

Too much or too little weight gain can be a problem. Your ob-gyn should check your weight gain at each of your prenatal care visits and will let you

TABLE 3-1 Weight Gain During Pregnancy

Body Mass Index (BMI) Before Pregnancy	Recommended Total Weight Gain With a Single Baby (in Pounds)	Recommended Rate of Weight Gain per Week in the Second and Third Trimesters* (in Pounds)
Less than 18.5 (underweight)	28 to 40	1.0 to 1.3
18.5 to 24.9 (normal weight)	25 to 35	0.8 to 1.0
25.0 to 29.9 (overweight)	15 to 25	0.5 to 0.7
30.0 and above (obese)	11 to 20	0.4 to 0.6

*Assumes a first-trimester weight gain between 1.1 pounds and 4.4 pounds

Source: Institute of Medicine and National Research Council. 2009. *Weight Gain During Pregnancy: Reexamining the Guidelines.* Washington, DC: The National Academies Press.

know whether you are on a healthy track. Do not worry about how much weight other pregnant women gain.

Keep in mind that you will gain weight differently throughout the different months of your pregnancy. During the first 3 months, you may see little gain. In fact, some women lose a few pounds because of morning sickness. You will gain most of your weight during the second and third trimesters, when your baby is growing at a faster rate. But your rate of weight gain should stay within a certain range. Also, if you are pregnant for the second time, you may gain weight differently.

If you have an eating disorder, even if it is under control, it is important to tell your ob-gyn. Together, you and your ob-gyn can monitor your feelings and be alert to any signs that the disorder has returned. It may be helpful to continue with counseling or start counseling when you get pregnant.

Also, you may want to ask your ob-gyn to refer you to a nutritionist who can help you plan for healthy eating during your pregnancy. Remember that gaining the right amount of weight is crucial to having a healthy baby. If you need more support, ask for it. See Chapter 29, "Weight During Pregnancy: Obesity and Eating Disorders."

Exercise

Being active and exercising—even just walking—at least 30 minutes on most days of the week can benefit your pregnancy. Exercise can

> ### Where Does the Weight Come From?
>
> The average newborn weighs about 7½ pounds, yet most women are advised to gain 25 to 35 pounds when they are pregnant. Where do the other pounds come from? Here's a breakdown of the weight gain for an average-weight woman who gains 30 lbs. during pregnancy:
>
> - Baby—7½ lbs.
> - Amniotic fluid—2 lbs.
> - Placenta—1½ lbs.
> - Uterus—2 lbs.
> - Breasts—2 lbs.
> - Body fluids—4 lbs.
> - Blood—4 lbs.
> - Maternal stores of fat, protein, and other nutrients—7 lbs.

- reduce backache, constipation, bloating, and swelling
- boost your mood
- promote muscle tone, strength, and endurance
- help you sleep better

Before you start an exercise program, talk with your ob-gyn to make sure you do not have any health conditions that may limit your activity. If you have heart disease, are at risk of **preterm** labor, or have vaginal bleeding, your ob-gyn may advise you not to exercise. See Chapter 23, "Exercise During Pregnancy," to learn about staying active during your pregnancy.

Healthy Decisions

In the first 2 months of pregnancy, you may have a lot of questions to ask and decisions to make. The decisions facing you now may include making important lifestyle changes and deciding when to tell others your news. If you haven't already done so, you'll also want to choose a practitioner who will care for you during your pregnancy (see Chapter 2, "Choosing Your Care Team").

Things to Avoid During Pregnancy

It's normal to be anxious about what you can and cannot do while you are pregnant. The list of "don'ts" may seem long, but most are easy to remember.

Using Tobacco. Cigarette smoke contains thousands of harmful chemicals, including lead, tar, nicotine, and carbon dioxide. When you smoke, these *toxins* increase the risk of pregnancy *complications*, including

- vaginal bleeding
- preterm birth
- *low birth weight*
- *stillbirth*
- *sudden infant death syndrome (SIDS)*

It is best to stop smoking before pregnancy or as soon as you find out you are pregnant.

If you are pregnant and you smoke, tell your ob-gyn. He or she can help you find support and quitting programs in your area. You also can call the national "quit line" at 1-800-QUIT-NOW. To find out more about quitting programs in your area, to get information about quitting, or to find support, see the "Resources" section at the end of this chapter.

Also, electronic cigarettes (known as "e-cigarettes") contain many harmful substances, including nicotine. Using them is called "vaping." E-cigarettes are not safe substitutes for cigarettes and should not be used during pregnancy.

Being Around Secondhand Smoke. Smoke from cigarettes smoked by other people can be harmful as well. Breathing secondhand smoke during pregnancy increases the risk of having a smaller baby. Babies who are exposed to secondhand smoke have an increased risk of SIDS. They also are more likely to have respiratory illnesses than those not exposed to secondhand smoke. If you live or work around smokers, take steps to avoid secondhand smoke. You may want to ask family members who smoke to smoke outside or quit altogether.

Drinking Alcohol. It's best to stop drinking before you get pregnant. If you did have some alcohol before you knew you were pregnant, it most likely will not cause serious harm to your baby. The important thing is to avoid alcohol once you know you're pregnant.

When a pregnant woman drinks alcohol, it quickly reaches the baby. Alcohol is much more harmful to a baby than it is to an adult. In an adult, the liver breaks down the alcohol. A baby's liver is not fully developed and is not able to break down alcohol.

Fetal alcohol spectrum disorder (FASD) is a term that describes different effects that can occur in a baby when a woman drinks during pregnancy. These effects may include physical, mental, behavioral, and learning disabilities that can last a lifetime. Even moderate alcohol use during pregnancy (defined as one alcoholic drink per day) can cause lifelong learning and behavioral problems in a child.

It is not known how much alcohol it takes to harm the baby. The best course is not to drink at all during pregnancy. Also, there are no types of drinks that are safe. One beer, one shot of liquor, one mixed drink, or one glass of wine all contain about the same amount of alcohol.

Talk with your ob-gyn about your drinking habits. If you are dependent on alcohol, you may need specialized counseling and medical care. Your ob-gyn can help you connect with these resources.

Do You Have a Drinking Problem?

Do you use alcohol or abuse it? Sometimes it's hard to tell. If you're not sure, ask yourself these questions:

1. On average, how many standard-sized drinks containing alcohol do you have in a week? If your answer is more than 7 drinks per week, that is at-risk alcohol use.

2. When you drink, what is the maximum number of standard-sized drinks you have at one time? If your answer is 3 drinks or more, that is at-risk alcohol use.

If you do drink alcohol, answer the following questions:

T How many drinks does it take to make you feel high? (TOLERANCE)

A Have people ANNOYED you by criticizing your drinking?

C Have you felt you ought to CUT DOWN on your drinking?

E Have you ever had a drink first thing in the morning to steady your nerves or get rid of a hangover? (EYE OPENER)

Scoring:
- 2 points if your answer to the first question is more than 2 drinks.
- 1 point for every "yes" response to the other questions.

If your total score is 2 or more, you may have an alcohol problem.

Modified from Sokol RJ, Martier SS, Ager JW. The T-ACE questions: practical prenatal detection of risk drinking. Am J Obstet Gynecol 1989;160:865.

Using Marijuana. Recreational marijuana use is legal in some states, and even more states have legalized medical marijuana. But both are illegal under federal law, and neither should be used during pregnancy.

When marijuana is smoked or eaten, the chemicals reach the baby by crossing the placenta. Research is limited on the harms of marijuana use during pregnancy. But there are possible risks of marijuana use to your baby, including problems with brain development and increased risk of stillbirth and preterm birth.

If you use medical marijuana, talk with your ob-gyn. He or she should recommend other treatments you can try that are safe to use during pregnancy.

Using Opioids. *Opioids* are a type of medication that relieves pain. They also release chemicals in the brain that have a calming effect. Doctors may prescribe opioids for people who have had surgery, dental work, or an injury.

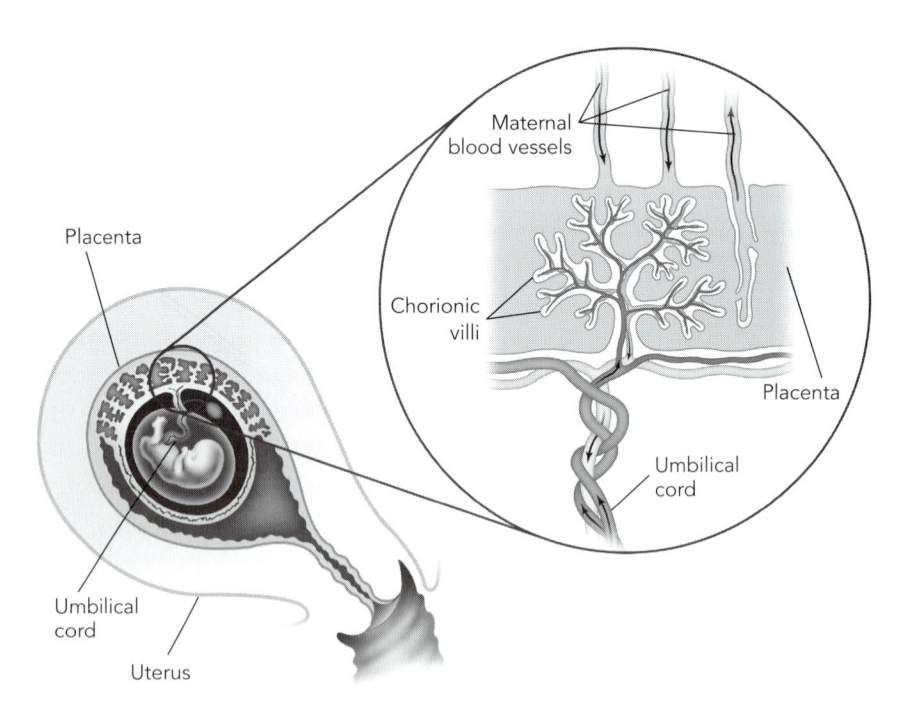

The placenta. The placenta connects the baby to the wall of the uterus. Finger-like projections, called chorionic villi, contain blood vessels that allow the exchange of nutrients, oxygen, and waste products between the pregnant woman's blood supply and the baby. The umbilical cord bridges the connection between the placenta and the baby. The cord is attached to the baby in the center of the belly.

Most people who use a prescription opioid have no trouble stopping their use, but some people develop an *opioid use disorder*. Pregnant women with opioid use disorder have an increased risk of serious complications, including

- *placental abruption*
- growth problems for the baby
- preterm birth
- stillbirth

When you are pregnant and have an opioid use disorder, you should not stop using the drug without medical help. Quitting without a doctor's help, especially when done suddenly, often leads to relapse (return to drug use). This can be dangerous for you and your baby.

The best treatment for opioid use disorder during pregnancy includes opioid replacement medication, behavioral therapy, and counseling. The medications that are given are called methadone and buprenorphine. They reduce cravings but do not cause the good feelings that other opioids cause. Behavioral therapy and counseling may help people avoid and cope with situations that might lead to relapse.

Using Other Substances. Substance use is the use of illegal drugs such as heroin, cocaine, and methamphetamines, or prescription drugs used for a nonmedical reason. Use of these substances during pregnancy increases the risk of several problems, including

- birth defects
- *miscarriage*
- preterm birth
- growth problems for the baby
- stillbirth

The bottom line is that you should make all substance use off-limits while you are pregnant. If you are addicted to any drugs, tell your ob-gyn that you need help.

Some states have substance use treatment programs tailored for pregnant women. These programs offer prenatal care, counseling and family therapy, nutritional education, and other services. Your ob-gyn can help you enroll in one of these programs. To find a program in your area, contact the Substance Abuse and Mental Health Services Administration's website (see the "Resources" section at the end of this chapter).

What Should I Do About Medications?

Most medications do not cause harm during pregnancy. But it is a good idea to tell your ob-gyn about all of the medications that you are taking. This includes prescription medications, over-the-counter drugs, and herbal remedies.

Do not stop taking a medication prescribed for you until you have talked with your ob-gyn. The risks of taking some medicines during pregnancy may be outweighed by the effects of not taking them. If a medication you are taking poses a risk, your ob-gyn may recommend switching to a safer drug while you are pregnant.

You also should check with your ob-gyn before taking over-the-counter pain relievers, **laxatives**, cold or allergy remedies, and skin treatments. But you don't have to go through the discomfort of headaches or colds without relief. Your ob-gyn can give you advice about medicines that are safe for pregnant women to use. See Chapter 24, "Reducing Risks of Birth Defects."

Other Considerations

Pregnant women often work right up until delivery and return to their jobs within weeks or months of a baby's birth. But some jobs may not be safe for a pregnant woman. Also, fatigue, nausea, and other discomforts can make working during early pregnancy a challenge.

A Safe Workplace

Most women can continue working throughout their pregnancies. But small changes may be needed depending on the work that you do. Jobs that require heavy lifting, climbing, carrying, or standing may not be safe during pregnancy. That's because the dizziness, nausea, and fatigue common in early pregnancy can increase the chance of injury. Later on, the change in body shape can throw off balance and lead to falls.

Being exposed to harmful substances on the job is rare. But it makes sense to think about the things you have contact with during your workday. Some substances found in the workplace pose a risk during pregnancy. These substances include

- lead
- mercury
- arsenic
- pesticides

- some solvents
- ionizing **radiation**
- certain drugs used for cancer treatment (**chemotherapy**)

You also may come into contact with harmful substances through a hobby. See Chapter 24, "Reducing Risks of Birth Defects," to learn more about things that may be a risk to pregnancy.

If you think your job may bring you into contact with something harmful, find out for sure by asking your personnel office, employee clinic, or union. Let your ob-gyn know right away if you think you and your baby are at risk. Workplace hazards and safety tips can be found at the websites of the Occupational Safety and Health Administration (OSHA) and the National Institute for Occupational Safety and Health (NIOSH). See the "Resources" section at the end of this chapter and in Chapter 26, "Work and Travel During Pregnancy."

Tips for Working During Early Pregnancy

Working when you have nausea and fatigue can be difficult. To cope, try the following:

- Take advantage of flex time—If your workplace has flex time, use this benefit to your advantage. What is the time of day when you feel the most energized? Consider coming in later if the early morning is bad for you. If afternoons are a problem, arrive earlier so that you can leave earlier.

- Bring snacks with you—Healthy snacks throughout the day may help keep nausea at bay and give you energy. Crackers, raw vegetables, or fruit and cheese are good choices.

- Nap, if you can—If you have an office, you can shut the door and rest during your lunch hour.

- Stay hydrated—Being dehydrated can make you feel worse. Make sure you are drinking enough fluids throughout the day.

Prenatal Care Visits

As soon as you know you're pregnant, call your ob-gyn to schedule an appointment so you can start prenatal care right away. You'll have regular appointments throughout your pregnancy. At each visit, your ob-gyn should monitor your health and the health of your baby. See Chapter 2, "Choosing Your Care Team," if you don't have an ob-gyn yet.

Your first or second prenatal care visit will probably be one of your longest visits. Your ob-gyn will need to ask a lot of questions about your health and do several tests. It's important to answer all questions honestly and with as much detail as you can.

A medical history form is provided in the back of this book. You can use this form to help you prepare. Fill out the form before your visit and bring the book with you, or just read it through to see some of the questions that will be asked. It also may be helpful to bring your partner or a support person with you on your prenatal care visits.

During these early visits, your ob-gyn may

- ask about your health history, including past pregnancies, surgeries, or medical problems
- ask about any prescription and over-the-counter medications you're taking (bring them with you, if possible)
- ask about the health history of your family and the family of the baby's father
- do a complete physical exam with blood and urine tests
- do a *pelvic exam*
- measure your blood pressure, height, and weight
- calculate the baby's estimated due date

Some ob-gyns do an ultrasound exam to confirm pregnancy. This may be a *transvaginal ultrasound* exam, in which a special *transducer* is placed in the *vagina*. If you are less than 5 weeks pregnant, the embryo may not be visible. Even if you are more than 5 weeks pregnant, don't expect to see much more than a small, circular shape that represents the *amniotic sac.* You will not be able to see arms or legs or any other distinct features until later in pregnancy.

A first-trimester ultrasound exam is used to estimate gestational age and due date. The gestational age can be estimated using a measurement called "crown–rump length." This is the length of the embryo or *fetus* measured from the top of the head ("crown") to the bottom of the area that will become the buttocks ("rump"). If you are less than 7 weeks pregnant, it is not possible to see the embryo's crown or rump, so the greatest length of the embryo is measured. A formula then is used to estimate the gestational age based on this measurement. Cardiac activity also can be detected at about 6 weeks of pregnancy during an ultrasound exam.

Special Concerns

Although it's normal for pregnant women to worry about complications, most women have healthy pregnancies and give birth to healthy babies. But it's best to be alert to signs and symptoms that may signal a problem. Often, the earlier you see your ob-gyn, the more likely that the complication can be managed successfully.

Miscarriage

The loss of a pregnancy before 20 completed weeks is called ***miscarriage***. About 1 in 5 or 6 pregnancies ends this way. Some miscarriages take place before a woman misses her period or even knows that she is pregnant.

The most common sign of a miscarriage is bleeding. Call your ob-gyn if you have

- spotting or bleeding without pain
- heavy or persistent bleeding with abdominal pain or cramping
- a gush of fluid from your vagina but no pain or bleeding
- passed fetal tissue

Most miscarriages are caused by a problem with the ***chromosomes*** of the fertilized egg. These problems occur by chance and are not likely to happen again in a later pregnancy. In most cases, there is nothing wrong with the woman's or man's health. Most women who have a miscarriage go on to have healthy pregnancies. See Chapter 40, "Early Pregnancy Loss: Miscarriage, Ectopic Pregnancy, and Gestational Trophoblastic Disease."

Ectopic Pregnancy

An ***ectopic pregnancy*** occurs when a fertilized egg grows outside of the uterus. Almost all ectopic pregnancies—more than 90 percent—occur in a fallopian tube. As the pregnancy grows, it can cause the tube to burst (rupture). A rupture can cause major internal bleeding. This can be a life-threatening emergency that needs immediate surgery.

At first, an ectopic pregnancy may feel like a typical pregnancy with some of the same signs, such as a missed period, tender breasts, or an upset stomach. Other signs may include

- abnormal vaginal bleeding
- low back pain
- mild pain in the abdomen or pelvis
- mild cramping on one side of the pelvis

At this stage, it may be hard to know if you are experiencing a typical pregnancy or an ectopic pregnancy. Call your ob-gyn if you have abnormal bleeding and pelvic pain.

As an ectopic pregnancy grows, more serious symptoms may develop, especially if a fallopian tube ruptures. Symptoms may include

- sudden, severe pain in the abdomen or pelvis
- shoulder pain
- weakness, dizziness, or fainting

If you have sudden pain that is severe, shoulder pain, or weakness, go to an emergency room. See Chapter 40, "Early Pregnancy Loss: Miscarriage, Ectopic Pregnancy, and Gestational Trophoblastic Disease."

When to Share the News

When to tell family and friends that you're pregnant is your choice. Many women choose to wait until after the first 12 weeks have passed. Others decide to tell as soon as they get the positive pregnancy test result. Deciding when to deliver the news is a personal decision, but you may want to keep a few things in mind:

- The risk of miscarriage is highest in the first 3 months of pregnancy. You may want to wait until your second trimester to tell friends, coworkers, and extended family members that you're pregnant.

- Discrimination against pregnant women is illegal. But you may want to wait to spread the news on your job until you've worked out the details of your maternity leave with your supervisor.

- Women who have had problems with past pregnancies, especially early problems, may prefer to tell others early, as the support of friends and family can be very helpful if there is another problem. On the other hand, some women feel more secure waiting until the second trimester to tell others. There is no right or wrong answer, so consider what is best for you.

RESOURCES

Find an Ob-Gyn
www.acog.org/FindAnObGyn
This directory from the American College of Obstetricians and Gynecologists (ACOG) can help you find an ob-gyn near you.

SAMHSA's Treatment Services Locator
https://findtreatment.samhsa.gov
1-800-662-HELP (4357)
Website from the Substance Abuse and Mental Health Services Administration. Find substance use treatment programs in your area and links to self-help and support groups.

Smokefree Women: Pregnancy and Motherhood
https://women.smokefree.gov/pregnancy-motherhood
Website from the National Cancer Institute. Offers tools and tips for quitting smoking. Includes a text message program to help women cut down or quit smoking during pregnancy.

Workplace Safety and Health
National Institute for Occupational Safety and Health: www.cdc.gov/niosh
Occupational Safety and Health Administration: www.osha.gov/workers
These government websites provide information about workers' rights, workplace safety, and occupational health. Includes information about hazardous chemicals in the workplace.

Your Pregnancy and Childbirth
www.acog.org/MyPregnancy
Website from ACOG with information on pregnancy, labor, delivery, and postpartum care. Includes the latest information from the experts in women's health care, questions answered by ACOG ob-gyns, pregnancy stories from real women, and an A–Z directory of health topics covering pregnancy and beyond.

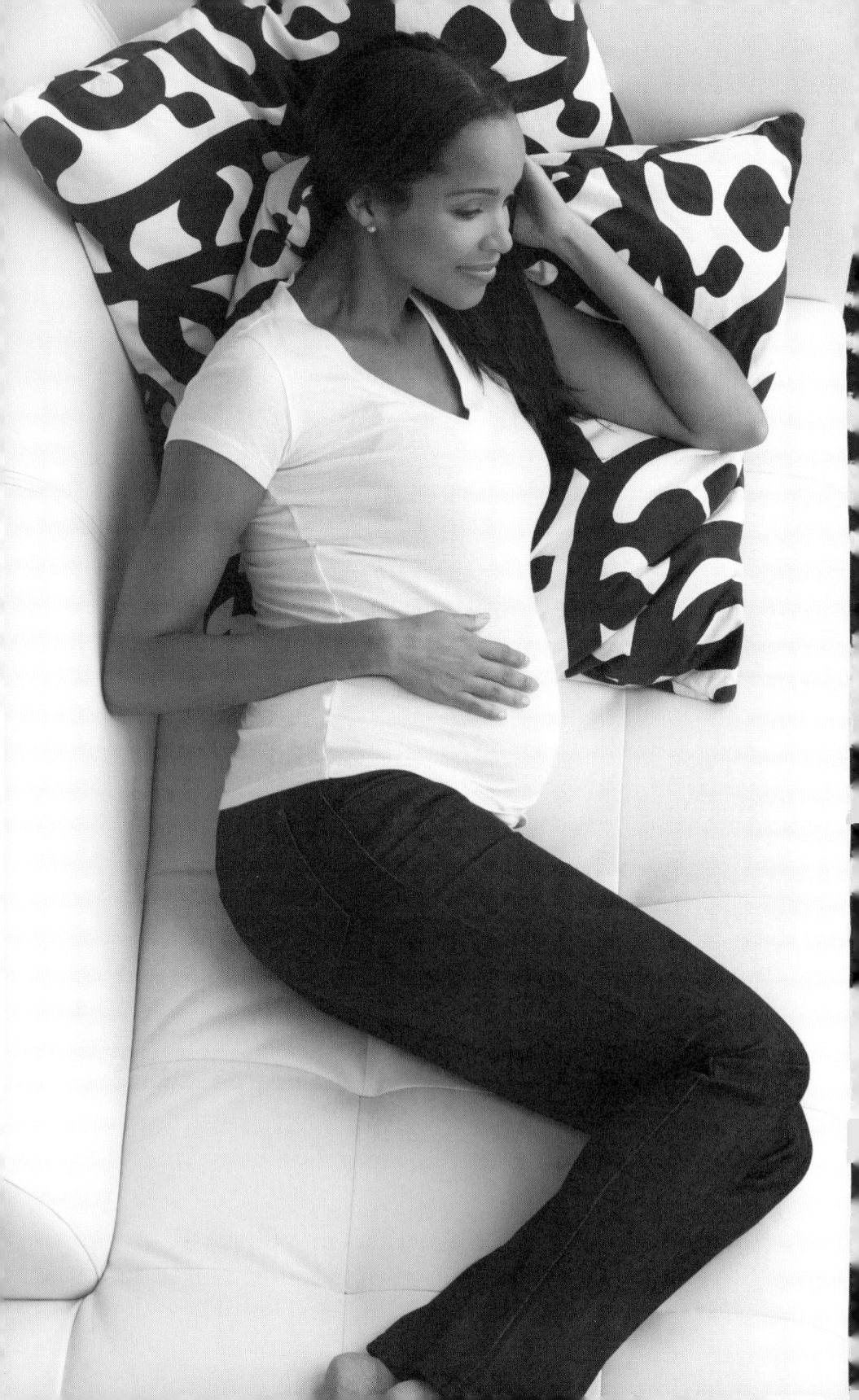

CHAPTER 4

Month 3
(Weeks 9 to 12)

YOUR BABY

▶ WEEK 9
This week continues the development of the ***embryo***, though you may already be calling it a baby. Cartilage for the limbs, hands, and feet is forming but won't harden into bones for a few weeks. Eyelids form but remain closed.

> This week, your baby is about the size of a single grape.

▶ WEEK 10
At 10 weeks—8 weeks since ***fertilization***—the embryo is about 1 inch long. The head has developed a more rounded shape. Bone cells start to replace cartilage, and the baby can bend his or her elbows.

> This week, your baby is about the size of a kumquat.

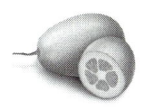

▶ WEEK 11
This week, the ninth week after fertilization, the baby is officially called a ***fetus***. At a little more than 1½ inches long, the baby is making breathing-like

movements and swallowing **amniotic fluid**. By the end of this week, the baby's external **genitals** will start developing. The liver is forming blood cells.

> This week, your baby is about the size of a fig.

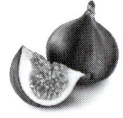

▶ WEEK 12

As you near the end of your third month, the baby's kidneys are making urine. The pancreas is making insulin. The baby moves on his or her own now, but it is still too early to feel these movements. Fingernails have formed. The baby is now about 2 inches long.

> This week, your baby is about the size of a small lime.

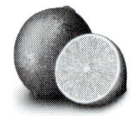

YOUR PREGNANCY

Your Changing Body

You still may not look pregnant to others, but you may be able to tell your waist is getting a little thicker. When you are not pregnant, the **uterus** is about the size of a small pear. By around week 12, the uterus is as big as a grapefruit.

Discomforts and How to Manage Them

As you begin your third month of pregnancy, you may notice that your morning sickness is not as bad. At the same time, you may notice changes in your breasts, skin, and digestion. Also, your mood may be up one minute and down the next. These changes are normal early in pregnancy.

Nausea

Most women start to feel relief from nausea this month. If there are remedies that help you, keep them handy. Remember to drink as much fluid as you can during the day. If you still have severe nausea and vomiting, talk with your **obstetrician–gynecologist (ob-gyn)**. See Chapter 3, "Months 1 and 2 (Weeks 1 to 8)," for more on nausea and vomiting.

Fatigue and Sleep Problems

You may still be tired during the day from all the changes happening in your body. But as time goes on, it may be more difficult to get a good night's sleep.

MONTH 3 • **69**

Fingernails have formed.

Eyelids have formed but remain closed.

The baby can bend his or her elbows.

Mother and baby: Weeks 9 to 12
By the end of week 12, the baby—now called a fetus—is about 2 inches long and weighs about half an ounce.

As your belly grows larger, it will be harder to find a comfortable position. To help you get the rest you need, you may find the following suggestions helpful:

- Try sleeping on your side with a pillow under your belly and another pillow between your legs. A full-body pillow is another option.

- Take a warm (not hot) shower or bath at bedtime to help you relax.

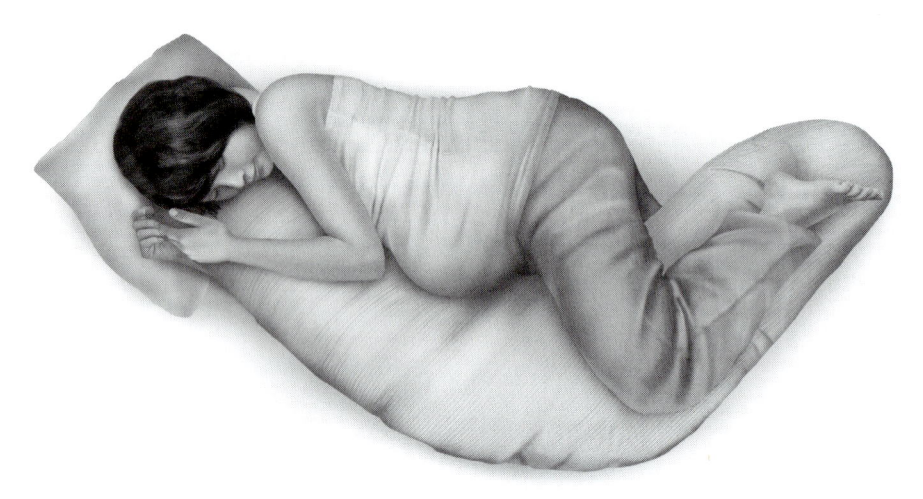

Comfortable sleeping. A full-body pillow can help support your neck, back, hips, and belly during sleep.

- Exercise daily. Aerobic exercise during the day, such as walking and swimming, helps with sleep at night. Yoga and meditation also are good. These can be done right before bed to help clear your mind and relax.
- Make your bedroom relaxing. The bed should be comfortable, and the room should not be too hot, cold, or bright.

Acne

Acne is common during pregnancy. If you are prone to acne, you may notice that it is getting worse. If you've never had it, you may find yourself dealing with acne breakouts during these months. If you get acne during pregnancy, you can take the following steps to care for your skin:

- Wash your face twice a day with a mild cleanser and lukewarm water.
- If you have oily hair, shampoo every day and try to keep your hair off your face.
- Avoid picking or squeezing acne sores to lessen possible scarring.
- Choose oil-free cosmetics and sunscreens.

Many medications can be used to treat acne. Some are available as the active ingredients in over-the-counter products. Others are available only by prescription. Ask your ob-gyn before trying any over-the-counter product. Also, tell any health care practitioner who is treating you for acne that you are pregnant.

Most over-the-counter acne products are applied directly on the skin (topical). The amount of medication absorbed through the skin is very low. For this reason, these products are considered safe to use during pregnancy. Over-the-counter products with the following ingredients can be used during pregnancy:

- Topical benzoyl peroxide
- Azelaic acid
- Topical salicylic acid
- Glycolic acid

If you want to use an over-the-counter product that has an ingredient not on this list, talk with your ob-gyn before buying it.

Some acne medications can seriously harm your baby. The following medications should not be used while you are pregnant:

- Hormonal therapy
- **Isotretinoin**
- Oral tetracyclines
- Topical retinoids

Some topical retinoids are available by prescription (tretinoin). But some also can be found in some over-the-counter products. Read labels carefully. If you are concerned about which products to use to treat your acne, talk with your dermatologist or ob-gyn. Together you can decide which option is best for you. See Chapter 24, "Reducing Risks of Birth Defects."

Skin Color Changes

During pregnancy, higher **estrogen** levels cause your body to make more **melanin**—the pigment that gives color to skin. This increase in melanin is the reason your nipples become darker, for example. It also causes the skin condition known as **melasma** during pregnancy. Melasma causes brown patches on the face around the cheeks, nose, and forehead.

Spending time in the sun can make melasma worse. Protect yourself from the sun by wearing sun block and a hat. Also, limit your exposure to direct sunlight. The good news is that melasma usually fades on its own after you give birth. Some women, though, may have dark patches that last for years.

Some women also notice a faint, dark line that runs from their belly button to their pubic hair. This is called the **linea nigra**. This line is always there, but before you get pregnant it is the same color as the skin around it.

Breast Changes

Early in pregnancy, your breasts begin changing to get ready for feeding the baby. By now, your breasts may even have grown a whole bra-cup size. They may be very sore. Many changes are taking place:

- Fat builds up in the breasts, making your normal bra too tight.
- Milk glands expand as your body prepares for making milk.
- The nipples and **areolas** (the pink or brownish skin around your nipples) get darker.
- Your nipples may begin to stick out more, and the areolas will grow larger.

Your breasts may keep growing in size and weight during these first 3 months. If they are making you uncomfortable, switch to a good maternity bra. These bras have wide straps, more coverage in the cups, and extra rows of hooks so you can adjust the band size. Consider a special sleep bra for nighttime support. When you exercise, wear an athletic bra with good support.

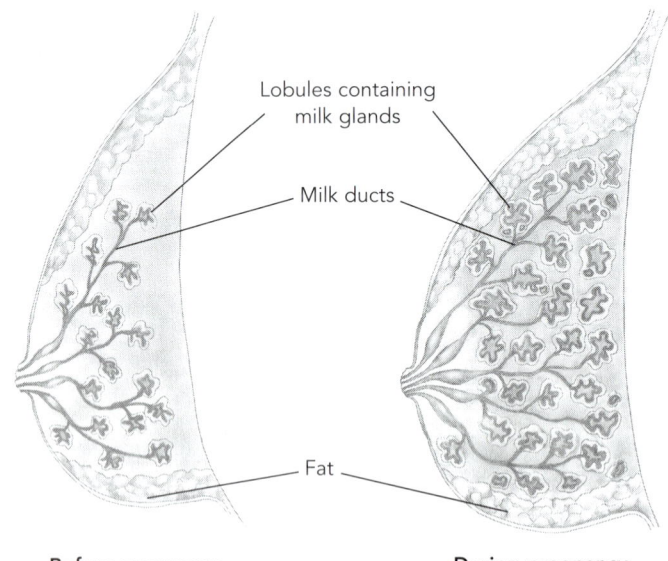

Before pregnancy | During pregnancy

Breast changes during pregnancy. During pregnancy, the fat layer of your breasts thickens, and the milk glands expand. Because of these changes, your breasts enlarge.

Constipation

Rising levels of **hormones** cause your digestive system to slow. This may lead to constipation. The iron in prenatal vitamin supplements also can cause constipation. To help ease this problem, exercise regularly and increase your intake of fiber. Fiber is found in fruits, vegetables, and whole grains. Staying hydrated helps with constipation too. You should drink 8 to 12 cups (64 to 96 ounces) of water a day during pregnancy.

Unfortunately, a side effect of increased fiber consumption is gas formation. To combat this problem, try eating your meals more slowly. Avoid anything that causes you to swallow air, such as gum chewing and carbonated drinks. Your body eventually will adjust to the dietary changes. Talk with your ob-gyn if these approaches don't ease constipation.

Emotional Changes

Your body is going through big changes now, and so are your emotions. You may feel down or moody. The emotions you are feeling—happy or sad—are normal. Ask loved ones to support you and be patient. If your emotions are affecting your work or personal relationships and you're concerned about these issues, talk with your ob-gyn.

Nutrition

You should continue eating nutritious meals this month. As you plan your meals, make sure that you are getting enough iron—a key mineral that most women need more of during pregnancy. Iron is used by your body to make the extra blood that you and your baby need during pregnancy. Pregnant women need 27 mg of iron a day, an amount that is found in most prenatal vitamins. See the box "Focus on Iron" on the next page.

Weight Gain

You may notice that your clothes are starting to fit more snugly around the waist. By the end of week 12, most women have gained between 1½ and 4½ pounds, although some women will have lost weight due to morning sickness. Don't worry if you have lost a pound or two. You will gain it back in the coming months.

Your ob-gyn should track your weight each month. The amount of weight you should gain depends on your health and your **body mass index (BMI)** before pregnancy. Use the "Body Mass Index Chart" at the back of this book to look up your prepregnancy BMI. Also see Chapter 22, "Nutrition During Pregnancy," for more on healthy weight gain during pregnancy.

Focus on Iron

Iron is used by your body to make the extra blood that you and your baby need during pregnancy. Women who are not pregnant need 18 milligrams (mg) of iron per day. Pregnant women need more, 27 mg per day. This increased amount is found in most prenatal vitamins. Vitamin supplements with higher iron levels may cause digestion problems, such as constipation.

You also can eat foods rich in a certain type of iron called heme iron. Heme iron is absorbed more easily by the body. It is found in animal foods, such as red meat, poultry, and fish. Non-heme iron is found in vegetables and legumes, such as soybeans, spinach, and lentils. Although it is not as easily absorbed as heme iron, non-heme iron is a good way to get extra iron if you are a vegetarian. Iron also can be absorbed more easily if iron-rich foods are eaten with vitamin C-rich foods, such as citrus fruits and tomatoes.

Your blood should be tested during pregnancy to check for anemia. If you have anemia, your ob-gyn may recommend extra iron supplements. The body can absorb supplemental iron only when it's part of a chemical compound. Look at the label to see how much elemental iron is in a supplement. There may be two numbers on the label: the weight of the compound, and the weight of the iron alone.

For example, you may see these compounds and how much elemental iron they contain:

- Ferrous fumarate 200 mg contains 66 mg of elemental iron.
- Ferrous gluconate 325 mg contains 38 mg of elemental iron.
- Ferrous sulfate 325 mg contains 65 mg of elemental iron.

Knowing how much and what formulation of iron to take for anemia can be confusing. Check with your ob-gyn to see what he or she recommends.

Sugar and Sugar Substitutes

It's important to limit the amount of simple sugars you eat. Simple sugars are found in foods such as table sugar, honey, syrup, fruit juices, soft drinks, and many processed foods. Although they may give you a quick energy boost, these foods have more calories than other nutrients. The energy they provide is used up quickly. They also can cause extra weight gain.

Artificial sweeteners, which are 200 to 600 times sweeter than sugar, are safe to use while you're pregnant as long as you use them in moderation. These sweeteners include

- saccharin (Sweet'n Low)
- aspartame (Equal and NutraSweet)
- sucralose (Splenda)
- acesulfame-K (Sunett)
- stevia (Truvia and SweetLeaf)

Prenatal Care Visits

Prenatal care involves lab tests, physical exams, and **ultrasound exams.** These tests are done to assess the health and well-being of you and your baby. Some of the tests that are done during pregnancy may be mandated by state law. Most commonly, state-regulated tests are those that screen for certain **sexually transmitted infections (STIs)**. Prenatal visits also give you time to learn about your pregnancy and ask questions.

How often you will see your ob-gyn for prenatal care depends on your health history, past pregnancies, and other factors. If this is your first pregnancy and you do not have any **complications**, you will see your ob-gyn

- every 4 weeks for the first 28 weeks
- every 2 weeks until 36 weeks
- weekly after 36 weeks

If you've had a successful pregnancy before and you're healthy, you may be able to have scheduled visits less often. On the other hand, if you have a high-risk pregnancy, you may need to see your ob-gyn more often as you get closer to delivery.

It's important that you feel comfortable with your ob-gyn. During a physical exam, he or she will need to examine various parts of your body, including your breasts and **genitals**. If you are uncomfortable about anything, let your ob-gyn know.

Your ob-gyn should have a chaperone in the exam room. This person usually is a nurse. You also can have a partner, friend, or family member with you during the exam. See Chapter 2, "Choosing Your Care Team," for more discussion about feeling comfortable during exams.

Ultrasound Exam

An ultrasound exam makes an image of your baby from sound waves. These sound waves are produced by a device called a **transducer**. The transducer is either moved across your belly, which is called a **transabdominal ultrasound exam**, or placed in your **vagina**, which is called a **transvaginal ultrasound exam**. The method chosen depends on the reason for the exam and the **gestational age** of the fetus.

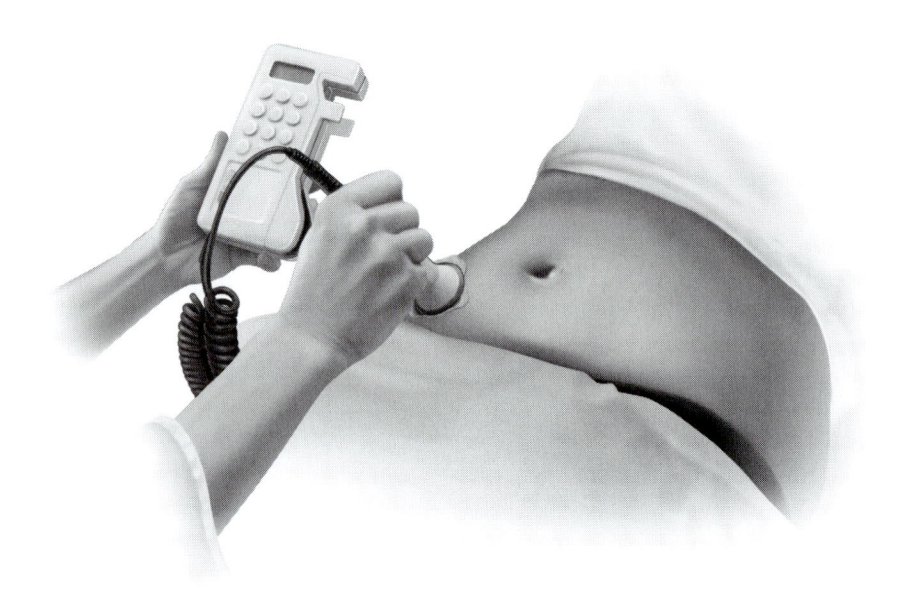

Listening to cardiac activity. Early in pregnancy, it may be possible to hear the baby's cardiac activity. Your ob-gyn may use a handheld Doppler device pressed against your belly to hear cardiac sounds.

Some women have an ultrasound exam early in pregnancy. This exam often is done to confirm the pregnancy and to help estimate the gestational age. A first-*trimester* ultrasound exam also may be done to

- hear cardiac sounds
- determine if there is more than one baby
- screen for genetic problems, such as **Down syndrome (trisomy 21)** (in combination with a blood test)
- examine your uterus and *ovaries*

It's important to know that an ultrasound exam uses only sound waves. There are no X-rays and no *radiation* used with this test.

Lab Tests

The following tests are performed early in pregnancy and may not all be done at the same prenatal care visit:

- ***Complete blood count (CBC)***—The CBC measures and describes different *cell* types in the blood. The number of red blood cells can show whether

MONTH 3 • 77

Transducer

Uterus

Vagina

Transabdominal
ultrasound exam

Uterus

Vagina

Transducer

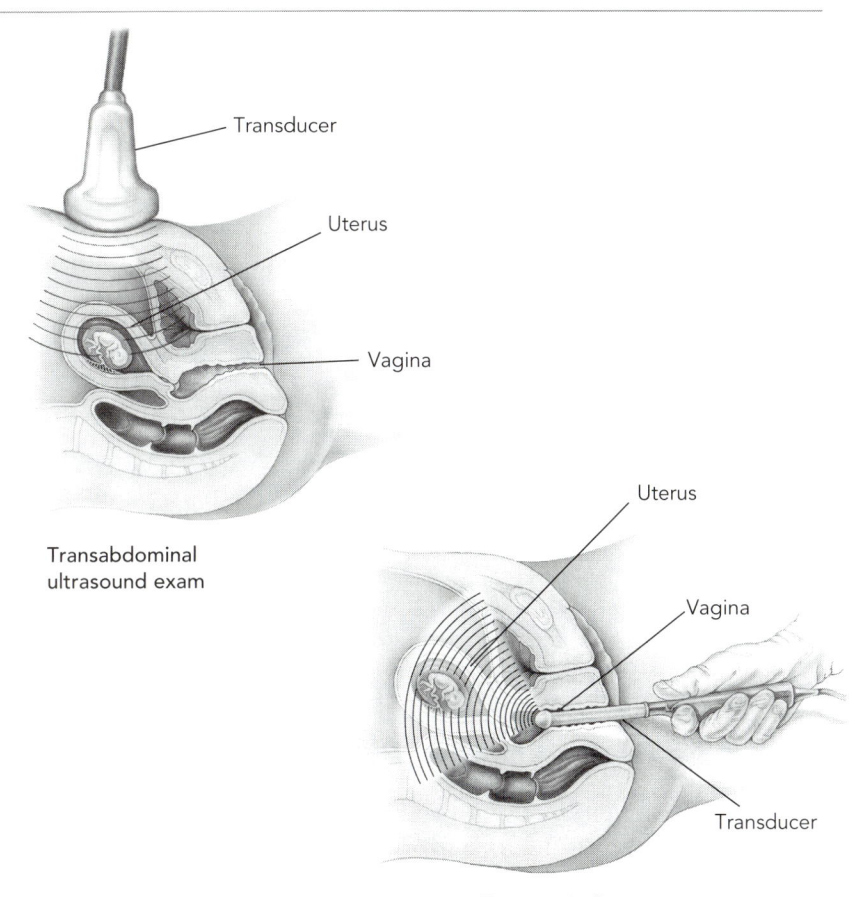

Transvaginal
ultrasound exam

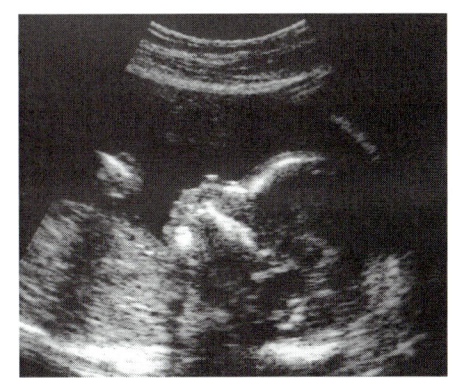

Ultrasound image of a baby between 11 and
13 weeks of gestation

Ultrasound exam. During an ultrasound exam, sound waves are produced by a transducer. These sound waves are reflected off the baby. The reflected sound waves are changed into pictures that you and your ob-gyn can view on a screen.

Month 3

you have **anemia**. The number of white blood cells shows how many disease-fighting cells are in your blood. The number of **platelets** can show if you have a problem with blood clotting.

- Blood type—During the first trimester of pregnancy, you should have a blood test to find out your blood type and whether you are Rh positive or Rh negative. Just as there are different major blood groups, such as type A, B, and O, there also is an **Rh factor**. The Rh factor is a protein that is found on the surface of red blood cells. Most people have the Rh factor—they are Rh positive. Others do not have the Rh factor—they are Rh negative.

If the baby is Rh positive and the woman is Rh negative, the woman's body can make **antibodies** against the Rh factor. These antibodies can damage the baby's red blood cells. Problems usually do not occur in a first affected pregnancy, when only a small number of antibodies are made. But problems can occur in a later pregnancy. These problems can be prevented by giving **Rh immunoglobulin (RhIg)** to the woman during pregnancy or after delivery if the baby's blood type is determined to be Rh positive. See Chapter 36, "Blood Type Incompatibility."

- Urinalysis—Your urine should be tested for **glucose** (blood sugar) and protein at every visit. High blood sugar may be a sign of **diabetes mellitus**. High protein may be a sign of **preeclampsia**. Your urine also may be tested to see if you have a **urinary tract infection (UTI),** especially if you have symptoms.

- Urine culture—This test looks for **bacteria** in your urine, which can be a sign of a UTI. Sometimes these infections do not cause symptoms. Your urine should be tested early in pregnancy and again later in pregnancy. If your test result shows that you have bacteria in your urine, you will be treated with **antibiotics**. There are antibiotics that can be used safely during pregnancy. After you finish treatment, you may have a repeat test to confirm the infection is gone.

- Rubella—Your blood should be tested to see if you have had a past infection with or have been vaccinated against rubella (sometimes called German measles). Rubella spreads easily and can cause birth defects if a woman is infected during pregnancy.

If you had this infection before or you have been vaccinated, you are not likely to get it again—you are **immune** to the disease. If your blood test shows you are not immune, you should avoid anyone who has rubella while you are pregnant. If you get rubella or are exposed to rubella while you are pregnant, contact your ob-gyn right away.

The vaccine for rubella is part of the **measles–mumps–rubella (MMR) vaccine.** This vaccine contains live viruses and is not recommended for pregnant women. If you have not had the MMR vaccine, you should get it right after you give birth. The vaccine is safe to get if you are breastfeeding.

- *Hepatitis*—**Hepatitis B** and **hepatitis C** are viruses that infect the liver. Pregnant women who are infected with either virus can pass it to their babies. All pregnant women are tested for hepatitis B infection. The Centers for Disease Control and Prevention (CDC) also recommends testing for hepatitis C. If you are infected with either virus, you may need special care during pregnancy. Your baby also may need specialized care after birth. You can breastfeed if you have either infection.

  A vaccine that protects against hepatitis B is available. The vaccine is given in a series of three shots, with the first dose given to the baby within a few hours of birth. This vaccine is not given to pregnant women.

- STIs—All women are tested for **syphilis** and **chlamydia** early in pregnancy. Tests for these STIs may be repeated later in pregnancy if you have certain risk factors. If you have risk factors for **gonorrhea** (you are 25 or younger, have multiple sex partners, or live in an area where gonorrhea is common), you also should be tested for this STI. If you have an STI, get treated right away. STIs can cause serious birth defects and pregnancy problems.

- *Human immunodeficiency virus (HIV)*—This virus attacks cells of the body's immune system and causes *acquired immunodeficiency syndrome (AIDS)*. If you are infected with HIV, there is a chance you could pass it to your baby. While you are pregnant, you can be given medication that can greatly reduce this risk. You also may get specialized care to help you stay as healthy as possible. Your baby may receive specialized care after birth.

- *Tuberculosis (TB)*—Women at high risk of TB should be tested for this infection. Women at high risk are those who are infected with HIV or live in close contact with someone who has TB.

Screening for Birth Defects

First-trimester **screening tests** for chromosomal defects and other birth defects may be done this month. So may certain **diagnostic tests**. You and your ob-gyn should talk about the testing options. It is your choice whether you want to have testing.

Discussions With Your Ob-Gyn

If you had a ***cesarean birth*** with another pregnancy, think about how you will deliver your baby this time. Discuss your options with your ob-gyn. Another important decision to consider is ***genetic screening*** for birth defects.

Vaginal Birth After Cesarean Delivery

If you have had a baby by cesarean in the past, it is important to talk about your delivery plans with your ob-gyn early in your prenatal care. Some women who have had a past cesarean birth can try to have a ***vaginal birth after cesarean (VBAC) delivery***. A successful VBAC offers several benefits, including

- no abdominal surgery
- shorter recovery period
- lower risk of infection
- less blood loss

Many women would like to have the experience of vaginal birth, and when successful, VBAC allows this to happen. For women planning to have more children, VBAC may help them avoid certain complications linked to multiple cesarean births, including

- bowel or ***bladder*** injury
- ***hysterectomy***
- problems with the ***placenta*** in future pregnancies

If you know that you want more children, this may figure into your decision.

There are risks involved with a VBAC. It may not be the right choice for every woman. Some risks of a VBAC are infection, blood loss, and other complications. One rare but serious risk with VBAC is that the cesarean scar on the ***uterus*** may rupture (break open). Although a rupture of the uterus is rare, it is very serious and may harm both you and your baby. If you are at high risk of rupture of the uterus, VBAC should not be tried.

The decision of whether to try a vaginal delivery or to have a repeat cesarean birth can be complex. Let your ob-gyn know if you're interested in trying to have a VBAC with this pregnancy. Together, you can consider the risks and benefits that apply to your situation. You also should discuss the resources available at the hospital where you will give birth. Some hospitals may not offer VBAC because they don't have the resources to provide proper care if there is an emergency during a VBAC. See Chapter 17, "Cesarean Delivery and Vaginal Birth After Cesarean Delivery," for detailed information about VBAC.

Prenatal Genetic Screening and Diagnosis

There are now many ways to screen for certain birth defects and **genetic disorders** during pregnancy, and to provide diagnostic testing for those who desire it. Your ob-gyn can explain the options and help you decide which tests are best for you. See Table 4–1, "Prenatal Screening and Diagnostic Tests," for a comparison of tests.

Deciding if you want to be tested—and if so, what types of tests to have—depends on a lot of factors. Here are some important things to consider:

- Getting results in the first trimester from a diagnostic procedure is appealing to many parents-to-be because it gives more time to make decisions.

TABLE 4–1 Prenatal Screening and Diagnostic Tests

Prenatal Screening Tests	Prenatal Diagnostic Tests
Offered to all pregnant women	Available for all pregnant women, even for those who do not have risk factors
Can tell you whether you are at increased risk of having a child with a certain birth defect, but cannot tell you for sure whether your baby has the disorder or not	Can tell you whether the baby has a certain birth defect. Results are either "positive" (a defect is present) or "negative" (no defect is present).
Available for certain chromosomal defects such as Down syndrome (trisomy 21) and for **neural tube defects (NTDs)** such as **spina bifida**	Available for chromosomal defects as well as many specific inherited disorders, such as **cystic fibrosis, sickle cell disease,** Tay–Sachs disease, and **thalassemias**
Done using a specialized ultrasound exam called a **nuchal translucency screening** and a sample of your blood	Done using **chorionic villus sampling (CVS),** which takes a sample of tissue from the **placenta,** or using **amniocentesis,** which takes a sample of amniotic fluid
Can be done in the first or second trimester	*CVS:* done in the first trimester (between 10 and 13 weeks) *Amniocentesis:* done in the second trimester (between 15 and 20 weeks)
No risks for the fetus	*CVS:* risk of miscarriage is 1 in 455 procedures *Amniocentesis:* risk of miscarriage is 1 in 900 procedures

- First-trimester screening tests can detect about 85 percent of cases of Down syndrome. Second-trimester screening tests can detect about 80 percent of cases of Down syndrome. Combining results of first-trimester and second-trimester screening tests provides a Down syndrome detection rate of 94 to 96 percent. Diagnostic testing has a detection rate of more than 99 percent for many disorders.

- Some parents want to know if their child will have a birth defect so that they can be prepared. Knowing also gives you the opportunity to learn about the disorder and to organize the care that the child will need.

- Some parents may decide to end the pregnancy in certain situations. Ending a pregnancy carries less risk of complications if it is done before 13 weeks of pregnancy. This timing may affect which tests a woman chooses to have.

Your personal beliefs and values are important factors in any decision. The choice that's right for one woman may not be right for another.

A *genetic counselor* or physician with special training in genetics can help you understand whether you are at risk of having a child with certain genetic disorders. In genetic counseling, the counselor asks you and the baby's father for a detailed family history. If a family member has a problem, the counselor may ask to see that person's medical records. You also may be referred for additional physical exams or tests.

Using all the information gathered, the counselor will assess the baby's risk of having a disorder. The counselor then will discuss the options for prenatal testing. It is your choice whether you want to have testing. See Chapter 33, "Genetic Disorders, Screening, and Testing," for a detailed discussion of screening and testing.

RESOURCES

Making Sense of Your Genes: A Guide to Genetic Counseling
www.geneticalliance.org/publications/guidetogeneticcounseling
Guide from the Genetic Alliance. Discusses genetic counseling and how it is used in different situations, including during pregnancy.

Skin and Hair Changes During Pregnancy
www.nlm.nih.gov/medlineplus/ency/patientinstructions/000611.htm
Webpage from the U.S. National Library of Medicine. Describes the normal changes that can happen to skin and hair during pregnancy. Provides guidance about when to call your ob-gyn.

Your Pregnancy and Childbirth
www.acog.org/MyPregnancy
Website from the American College of Obstetricians and Gynecologists (ACOG) with information on pregnancy, labor, delivery, and postpartum care. Includes the latest information from the experts in women's health care, questions answered by ACOG ob-gyns, pregnancy stories from real women, and an A–Z directory of health topics covering pregnancy and beyond.

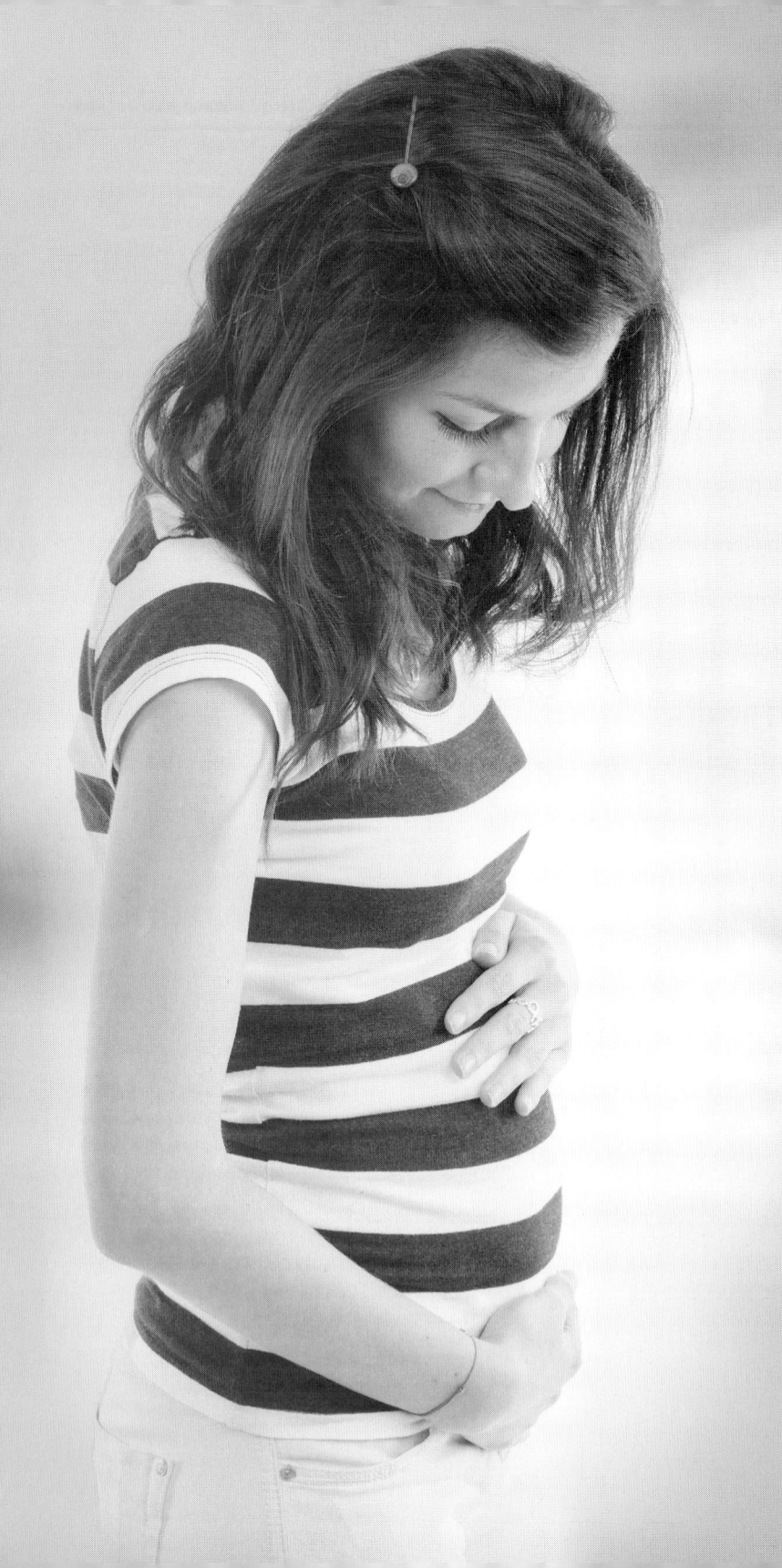

CHAPTER 5

Month 4
(Weeks 13 to 16)

YOUR BABY

▸ WEEK 13
All major organs have formed and will continue to develop. Bones are hardening, especially the long bones. The skin is thin and see-through but will start to thicken soon.

> This week, your baby is about as long as a peapod.

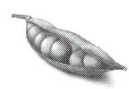

▸ WEEK 14
This week is the beginning of the second **trimester** of pregnancy. At this point, your baby is about 3 inches long. The **genitals** may be seen on an **ultrasound exam**, if the baby is in the right position. But it is too early to tell for sure if it is a girl or a boy. Toenails are forming. The neck is defined, and the lower limbs are developed.

> This week, your baby is about the size of a lemon.

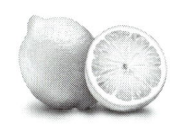

▸ WEEK 15
The baby is beginning to grow at a quicker pace and now is about 4 inches long. You may be able to feel movement this week, often just a sensation like little bubbles in your pelvis. This is called **quickening**. But don't worry if you

don't feel anything. Some women may not feel their babies moving for up to another 10 weeks.

> This week, your baby is about the size of a small apple.

▶ WEEK 16

The baby's hearing is starting to develop this week. The lungs begin to form the tissue that will allow them to exchange **oxygen** and carbon dioxide when the baby is breathing after birth. The baby's limb movements are becoming more coordinated. The baby is now more than 4 inches long.

> This week, your baby is about the size of an avocado.

YOUR PREGNANCY

Your Changing Body

Most women feel their best during these next couple of months, which is why the second trimester is often called the "honeymoon period" of pregnancy. Your morning sickness has probably lessened. Your energy level may be back to normal, and your pregnancy may be starting to show.

The second trimester also marks the time when many women worry a little less because the risk of **miscarriage** is lower. And beginning this month, your **uterus** is large enough that it is no longer completely within the pelvis.

Discomforts and How to Manage Them

This month's discomforts may include spider veins and changes in your gums, teeth, and mouth—even strange dreams. You also may have aches and pains in your abdomen. It helps to know what pain is normal and what isn't, and when you should call your **obstetrician–gynecologist (ob-gyn)**.

Lower Abdominal Pain

As the uterus grows, the round **ligaments** (bands of tissue that support the uterus on both sides) are pulled and stretched. You may feel this stretching as either a dull ache or a sharp pain on one side of your belly. The pain may be most noticeable when you cough or sneeze. Not moving for a short time or changing position may help relieve the pain.

MONTH 4 • 87

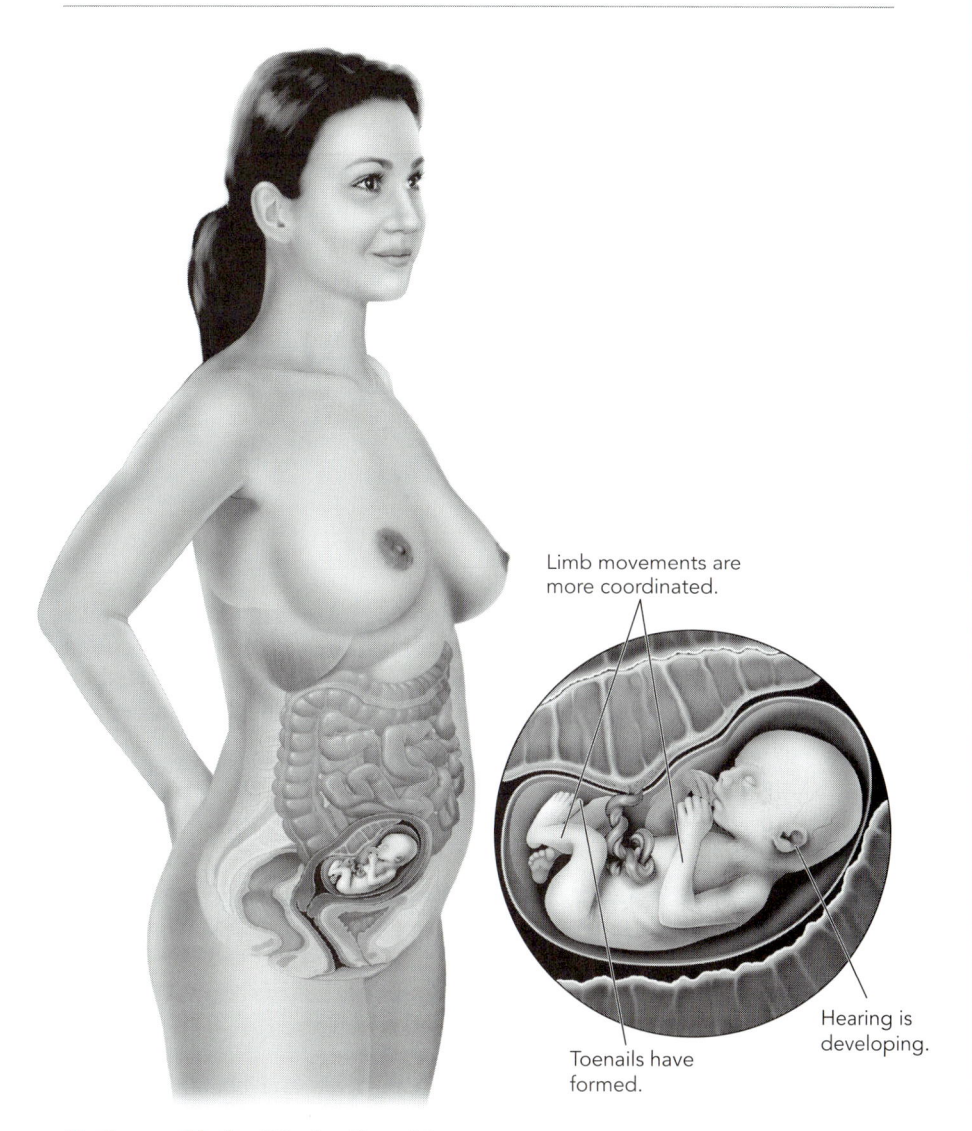

Limb movements are more coordinated.

Hearing is developing.

Toenails have formed.

Mother and baby: Weeks 13 to 16
By the end of week 16, the baby is more than 4 inches long and weighs more than 3 ounces.

If abdominal pain doesn't go away or gets worse, call your ob-gyn. It could be a sign of a problem.

Mouth and Dental Changes

Another surprising thing that you may not have expected during pregnancy are changes in your mouth, teeth, and gums. Pregnancy can cause a variety of changes, including

- swelling or bleeding gums (***gingivitis***)
- sores in your mouth (***granuloma gravidarum***)
- looser teeth caused by hormone changes
- tooth erosion, especially if you have been vomiting often

It's important to continue your usual dental routine during pregnancy. This includes

- brushing with a soft-bristled brush and fluoride toothpaste
- flossing between your teeth every day
- eating healthy foods without too many sugary foods and drinks

See your dentist for routine checkups every 6 months.

If you have mouth irritation, rinsing with saltwater and switching to a softer toothbrush may help. A saltwater rinse can be 1 teaspoon of salt in 1 cup of warm water. If you vomit, don't brush your teeth right away. Instead, rinse your mouth with 1 teaspoon of baking soda dissolved in 1 cup of water. This neutralizes the acid and helps protect your teeth.

Good dental health is good for you. It also may reduce your baby's risk of cavities in the future. If needed, procedures like filling cavities, tooth extractions, and root canals should all be done as soon as possible.

Dental care is safe throughout pregnancy. This includes mouth X-rays and ***local anesthesia***. If you will need ***general anesthesia*** for a dental procedure, your dentist should consult with your ob-gyn.

Some dentists require a letter from your ob-gyn that says it is safe for you to have dental care. The letter also may say what procedures and medications to avoid. Check with the dentist's office ahead of time and ask your ob-gyn for a letter if needed. If you do not have a dentist, ask your ob-gyn if he or she can refer you to one.

Excessive Salivation

Some women notice that they have extra saliva during pregnancy, especially when they're nauseated. This is more common among women who have severe morning sickness.

The exact cause of excessive salivation is not known. Hormonal changes may be a cause. Also, nausea might make some women try to swallow less, causing saliva to build up in the mouth. If this is a problem for you, talk with your ob-gyn.

Pregnancy-Related Stress

It is normal to worry about your pregnancy and whether you are doing all the right things for the baby. The changes happening in your life can be stressful. So can thoughts about how your life will change after the baby arrives. But it's important to make sure this type of normal stress doesn't lead to making you anxious or upset every day.

If you think your stress is becoming too much to handle, talk with your family, friends, and especially your ob-gyn. You will need help to ease your feelings. Know that you can't do everything and may need to ask for help sometimes—from your partner, family, and friends. Here are a few more tips that can help reduce your stress:

- Let the household chores go undone sometimes. Use that time to do something relaxing.
- Take advantage of sick days or vacation whenever possible. Spending a day, or even an afternoon, resting at home will help you get through a tough work week.
- Get regular exercise. Yoga especially helps to reduce stress.
- Go to bed early. Your body is working overtime to nourish your baby. You need all the sleep you can get.

Depression is common in pregnant women. It's important to get help if you need it. Talk with your ob-gyn if it seems like more than just stress or if you have any warning signs of depression. See the Depression Screening Test in Chapter 8, "Month 7 (Weeks 25 to 28)".

Spider Veins

You may have tiny red veins that show up under the skin of your face or legs. Spider veins are a normal part of the changes in your circulation. These veins usually fade after you give birth.

As your pregnancy goes on, you may develop **varicose veins**. These are swollen veins in the lower legs. For some women, varicose veins shrink or go away after giving birth. In the meantime, prop up your legs when you can. If you must sit or stand for long periods, move around often. This will help reduce swelling.

Strange Dreams

It's normal to have unusual dreams that may be vivid and scary. Experts believe these types of dreams may provide a way for your subconscious to cope with any fears and doubts you have about pregnancy and becoming a mother.

Urinary Problems

It's normal to urinate often while you're pregnant. But some urinary problems may be a sign of a **urinary tract infection (UTI)**. Be alert to the signs and symptoms of a UTI, which include

- pain when you urinate
- urge to urinate right away
- urine that is cloudy or has blood in it
- urine that has a strong smell
- fever
- back pain

Call your ob-gyn if you have any of these symptoms. If you have a UTI, your ob-gyn may prescribe an **antibiotic** that is safe for you to take during pregnancy.

Vaginal Discharge

Vaginal discharge (the fluid that comes out of your **vagina**) often increases during pregnancy. This is caused by normal changes in the vagina and **cervix**. A sticky, clear, or white discharge is normal, and it's usually nothing to worry about. But some changes could mean you have an infection, such as **bacterial vaginosis (BV)** or a **yeast infection**. Call your ob-gyn if you have symptoms, including

- discharge that has changed from its normal color
- discharge that has a bad smell
- pain, soreness, or itching in the vaginal area

If an infection is diagnosed, your ob-gyn may prescribe medication for treatment. Even if you have had a yeast infection before, talk with your ob-gyn before using an over-the-counter medication.

Nutrition

This month may bring food cravings that you didn't expect, which can be a challenge when you are trying to eat healthy foods.

Month 4: When to Call Your Ob-Gyn

- You have abdominal pain that doesn't go away or gets worse.
- You have discharge from your vagina that has changed from its normal color or has a bad smell.
- You have pain, soreness, or itching in the vaginal area.
- You have symptoms of a urinary tract infection (UTI).
- You are craving or eating things that are not food, like chalk or clay.
- You feel very stressed, anxious, or depressed. See the Depression Screening Test in Chapter 8, "Month 7 (Weeks 25 to 28)".

Weight Gain

Eating a healthy diet and gaining a healthy amount of weight during pregnancy are important for you and your baby. During your second trimester, your appetite increases. Stick to a healthy diet to be sure you and your baby are getting all of the **nutrients** you need. It's a balancing act that may be challenging.

See Chapter 22, "Nutrition During Pregnancy," for information about how to keep eating a healthy diet throughout your pregnancy. Also see Table 3-1, "Weight Gain During Pregnancy," in Chapter 3, "Months 1 and 2 (Weeks 1 to 8)," for the recommended weight gain based on **body mass index (BMI)** before pregnancy. Your ob-gyn will let you know if your weight gain is on track.

Food Cravings

Pregnant women often have food cravings. Giving in to these cravings is OK sometimes. But cravings can cause problems if you eat only a few types of food for long periods. It also can be a problem if you indulge your cravings for one type of food and neglect the rest of your diet. Eating lots of sugary foods, for instance, can lead to too much weight gain and tooth problems.

Some women may feel a strong urge to eat nonfood items, such as clay, chalk, or laundry starch. This condition is called **pica** (pronounced "pike-uh"). If you feel these urges, don't indulge in them. Eating nonfood items can be harmful and can keep you from getting the nutrients you need. Pica can also be a sign that you lack one or more nutrients, such as iron or **zinc**. You may need to be tested for **anemia** or other health problems. Call your ob-gyn if you think you have pica.

Prenatal Care Visits

Your **prenatal care** visit in your fourth month will be much shorter than your first visit. Still, you will have some tests and procedures to check your health and your baby's health. Your ob-gyn should do a routine check of your weight and blood pressure. He or she also may do a urine test to check for protein and possibly for **glucose** (blood sugar).

You may have additional **screening tests** for **birth defects** or **chromosome abnormalities**. For example, the "quad" or "quadruple" blood test and a **cell-free DNA** screening test can be used to screen for **Down syndrome (trisomy 21)** and **Edwards Syndrome (trisomy 18)**. The quad screen measures the levels of four different substances in your blood. This test is normally done between 15 and 22 weeks of pregnancy. One of the four substances that is measured in the quad screen can also be used to screen for **neural tube defects (NTDs)** and some other birth defects.

Another blood test also screens for NTDs. It measures the levels of a substance called **alpha-fetoprotein (AFP)** in your blood. This test is normally done between 15 and 18 weeks, sometimes in combination with other tests. And if you have chosen to have diagnostic testing with **amniocentesis**, this usually can be done after 15 weeks. See Chapter 33, "Genetic Disorders, Screening, and Testing."

Also, if you have not talked about possible health risks in your workplace, you may want to bring this up with your ob-gyn now. Exposure to lead and other chemicals may be a concern for some pregnant women, such as those who work in certain industries or who live with someone who does. A screening test for lead is recommended for women with at least one risk factor for lead exposure. See Chapter 24, "Reducing Risks of Birth Defects," to learn more about things that may be a risk to pregnancy.

Discussions With Your Ob-Gyn

Although it's still early in your pregnancy, you may want to start thinking about where you want to have your baby when the time comes.

Birth Places

The safest places to give birth are thought to be:

- A hospital that offers various levels of care
- A birth center within the hospital complex that meets the standards outlined by the American Academy of Pediatrics and the American College of Obstetricians and Gynecologists (ACOG)

- An accredited freestanding birth center that meets the standards of the Accreditation Association for Ambulatory Health Care, the Joint Commission, or the American Association of Birth Centers

Some things to keep in mind:

- Women with low-risk, uncomplicated pregnancies may be able to give birth at a freestanding birth center staffed by qualified ob-gyns.
- Women with complicated pregnancies (carrying more than one baby, for example) or health problems (like **preeclampsia**) need more advanced care, either in a hospital or in a birth center attached to a hospital.

Your ob-gyn will let you know about the choices available in your area. You also may discuss where he or she does deliveries and what your health insurance will cover. You can tour the hospitals in your area to see which settings appeal to you. See Chapter 12, "Preparing for Birth."

Home Birth

What about giving birth at home? **Complications** during labor and delivery can happen to anyone, even women with healthy pregnancies. If problems happen, a hospital setting offers the expert staff and equipment to give you and the baby the best care in a hurry. For this reason, ACOG says that the safest place for you and your baby during labor, delivery, and the days after is a hospital, hospital-based birth center, or accredited freestanding birth center.

RESOURCES

Depression During Pregnancy
www.marchofdimes.org/complications/depression-during-pregnancy.aspx
March of Dimes website that explains symptoms of depression during pregnancy and how you can get help.

Oral Health Topics: Pregnancy
www.ada.org/en/member-center/oral-health-topics/pregnancy
Discussion of dental care during pregnancy from the American Dental Association.

Your Pregnancy and Childbirth
www.acog.org/MyPregnancy
Website from the American College of Obstetricians and Gynecologists (ACOG) with information on pregnancy, labor, delivery, and postpartum care. Includes the latest information from the experts in women's health care, questions answered by ACOG ob-gyns, pregnancy stories from real women, and an A–Z directory of health topics covering pregnancy and beyond.

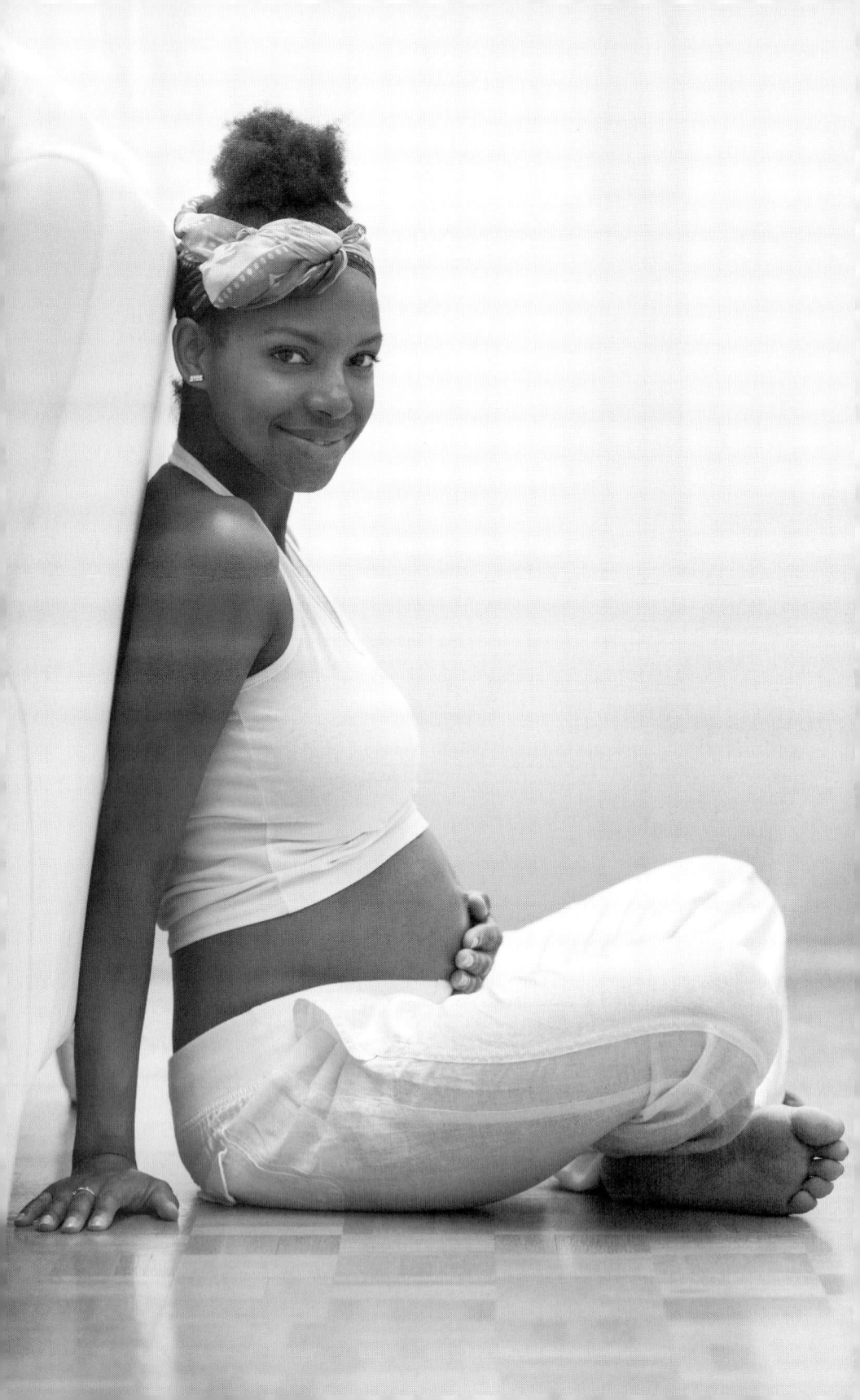

CHAPTER 6

Month 5
(Weeks 17 to 20)

YOUR BABY

▶ WEEK 17
The baby is getting more active now in the **amniotic sac**, rolling around and doing flips. Cardiac activity may be seen via an **ultrasound exam**. The baby is about 5 inches long now.

> This week, your baby is about the size of a pear.

▶ WEEK 18
This week the baby can hear sounds. The part of the brain that controls motor movements is fully formed. The digestive system is working now.

> This week, your baby is about the size of a bell pepper.

▶ WEEK 19
During this month, the ears, nose, and lips are recognizable on an ultrasound exam. In girls, the **uterus** and **vagina** are starting to form.

> This week, your baby is about the size of a mango.

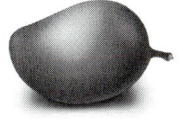

► WEEK 20

Soft, downy hair called **lanugo** is starting to form and will cover your baby's body. There also may be some hair on the scalp. The baby is now more than 6 inches long.

> This week, your baby is about as long as a small banana.

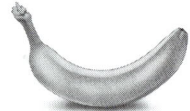

YOUR PREGNANCY

Your Changing Body

Some women feel the baby move for the first time during this month. This is known as **quickening**. Some women, especially those who have had a baby before, feel quickening as early as 16 weeks of pregnancy. If this is your first baby, you may not be aware of your baby's movements for a few more weeks. The location of the **placenta** and baby's position can affect when you first feel movements.

Another thing you may be noticing now is that your feet are getting bigger. They may continue to increase in size until late in pregnancy. The growth in your feet is partly caused by your weight gain and swelling from the extra fluid your body retains while you're pregnant.

The swelling also could be caused by a **hormone** called relaxin, which loosens the joints around your pelvis. This loosening helps make more room for the baby to travel down the birth canal during delivery. Relaxin also loosens the ligaments in your feet, causing the foot bones to spread. To help with the swelling, you can soak your feet in cool water and prop them on a pillow when you can. You may have to buy new shoes in a bigger size.

Your Baby's Movement

For many women, feeling their babies move is reassuring, and not feeling their babies move for a while is worrying. Remember that while some women feel movement this month, many will not feel movement until after 20 weeks of pregnancy. If you have felt movement this month, your baby's movements should be similar from day to day. Once you reliably feel a baby's movements every day, he or she should not "take a day off."

Remember that worrying too much about how often your baby moves is not good for you or the baby. Feeling less movement from your baby does not necessarily mean that something is wrong. There is no guideline about how much movement is normal. But if you have felt movement at this stage and

MONTH 5 • 97

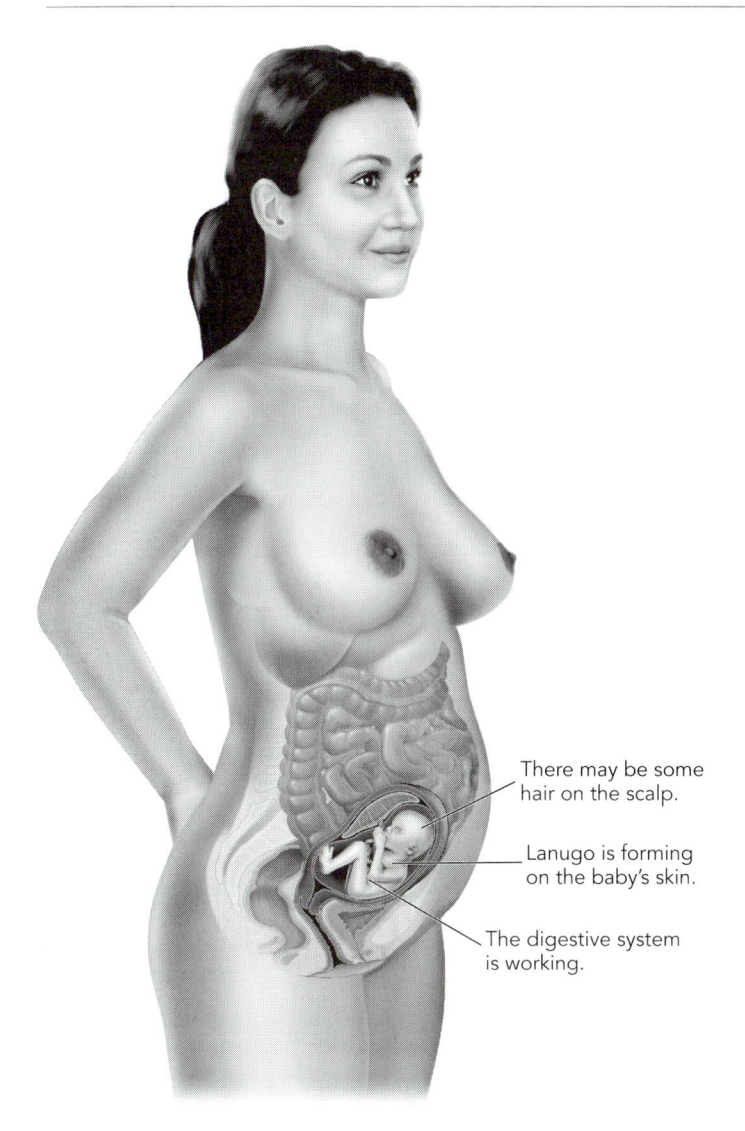

Mother and baby: Weeks 17 to 20
By the end of week 20, the baby is more than 6 inches long and weighs less than 11 ounces.

Labels on illustration:
- There may be some hair on the scalp.
- Lanugo is forming on the baby's skin.
- The digestive system is working.

you think that your baby is less active now than before, tell your ***obstetrician–gynecologist (ob-gyn)***.

Discomforts and How to Manage Them

If you were not expecting it, nasal congestion may seem like a strange pregnancy symptom. But there is an explanation for that stuffy feeling. You also may feel dizzy or forgetful at times. You may have trouble finding a comfortable sleeping position. And another uncomfortable symptom—one that may stay with you through the rest of your pregnancy—is low back pain.

Congestion and Nosebleeds

During pregnancy, some of your hormone levels increase, and your body makes extra blood. Both of these changes cause the mucous membranes inside your nose to swell up, dry out, and bleed easily. This may cause a stuffy or runny nose. You also may get nosebleeds from time to time. Here are some remedies:

- Try saline drops or a saline rinse to relieve congestion. (Do not use other types of nose drops, nasal sprays, or decongestants until you talk with your ob-gyn.)
- Drink plenty of liquids.
- Use a humidifier to moisten the air in your home.
- Dab petroleum jelly around the edges of your nostrils to keep the skin moist.

Dizziness

Early in your second *trimester*, it's normal to feel dizzy or lightheaded at times. Your blood circulation is changing. There can be less blood flow to your head and upper body, especially when you first sit or stand or if you stand for a long time. To prevent dizziness, move slowly when you stand up or change positions. Drinking a lot of fluids may help. Also, avoid standing for a long time or getting too hot. If you feel dizzy, lie down on your side.

Month 5: When to Call Your Ob-Gyn

- You think your baby is moving less than normal (if you have felt movement at this stage of your pregnancy). Keep in mind that many women will not feel movement until next month.
- You are concerned about your exposure to lead or other chemicals at home or at work.
- You are planning to travel, especially to an area where *Zika* virus is active.
- You or your partner has traveled to an area where there is Zika virus.

Memory Changes

If you're finding it harder to remember things these days, you're not alone. Many women have memory changes during pregnancy. Some women refer to this as "pregnancy brain." You may be forgetful or absentminded. You also may have trouble concentrating or reading.

Researchers are still learning why pregnancy causes memory changes. In the meantime, don't be worried. It may help to keep lists of things to do at work or home.

Sleeping Positions

You may be finding it hard to get comfortable for sleep. Your belly has grown, which means sleeping face down is uncomfortable. Sleeping on your back may not be good for you either because it puts the weight of your uterus on your spine and back muscles. In the second and third trimesters, lying on your back may compress a major blood vessel that takes blood to your uterus, making you feel dizzy and possibly reducing blood flow to your baby.

Sleeping on your side during your second and third trimesters may be best. Keep one or both knees bent. It may also help to place a pillow between your knees and another under your belly. You also can try a full-length body pillow. Trust your body. Some pregnant women find that their bodies automatically find the best positions for sleep.

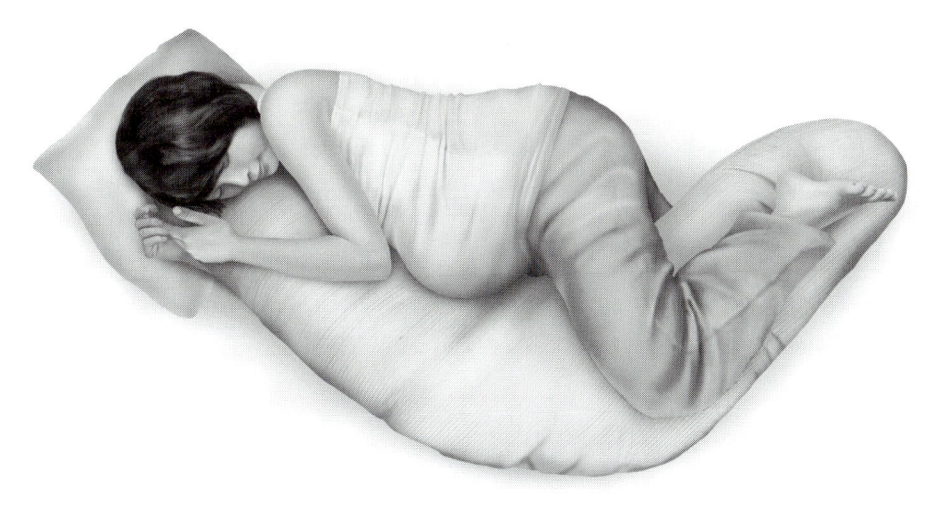

Comfortable sleeping. A full-body pillow can help support your neck, back, hips, and belly during sleep.

Lower Back Pain

Backache is one of the most common pregnancy problems, especially in the later months. You can blame your growing uterus and hormonal changes for your aching back. Your expanding uterus shifts your center of gravity and stretches out and weakens your abdominal muscles. This changes your posture and puts a strain on your back. The extra weight you're carrying means more work for your muscles and increased stress on your joints, which is why your back may feel worse at the end of the day. Here are some tips to help lessen back pain:

- Wear low-heeled (but not flat) shoes with good arch support, such as walking shoes or athletic shoes. Avoid high heels—they tilt your body forward and strain your lower back muscles.
- Do exercises to stretch and strengthen your back muscles. Many of the exercises in this book are designed to do just that (see Chapter 23, "Exercise During Pregnancy").
- If you must lift something, squat down, bend your knees, and keep your back straight. Do not bend at the waist to pick up things.
- Get off your feet. If you need to stand for a long time, rest one foot on a stool or a box to take the strain off your back.
- Sit in chairs with good back support or tuck a small pillow behind your lower back.
- Use an abdominal support garment (for sale in maternity stores and catalogs). It looks like a girdle and helps take the weight of your belly off your back muscles. Also, some maternity pants come with a wide elastic band that fits under the curve of your belly to help support its weight.
- Apply a heating pad or warm-water bottle. Heating pads should be set at the lowest possible temperature setting. Wrap your heating pad or warm-water bottle in a towel to help prevent burns. Cold compresses also can help ease pain.

Nutrition

As your appetite increases in the second trimester, you may be wondering which snack foods pack the most nutritional punch.

Healthy Snacking

Snacking is a good way to get the extra calories you need during pregnancy, as long as you choose some snacks that are low in fat and good for you, including

- whole-grain crackers, pretzels, and crisp breads
- fruits and vegetables
- nuts and seeds
- low-fat cheese and yogurt
- fruit smoothies (for example, whip together frozen yogurt, a banana, a splash of fruit juice, and a handful of berries in a blender)

Remember to count any snacks in your total calorie count for the day. See Chapter 22, "Nutrition During Pregnancy."

Weight Gain

Steady weight gain is more important in the second and third trimesters, especially if you start out at a healthy weight or you're underweight. In general, you should gain about one third of your total pregnancy weight by your 20th week of pregnancy.

If you are gaining weight too quickly, you may have to adjust how much food you're eating and get more exercise. See Table 3-1, "Weight Gain During Pregnancy," in Chapter 3, "Months 1 and 2 (Weeks 1 to 8)," for the recommended weight gain based on **body mass index (BMI)** before pregnancy. You and your ob-gyn should talk about whether your weight gain is on track.

Prenatal Care Visits

The timing of your **prenatal care** visits during your second trimester depends on your health and any special needs you may have during your pregnancy. Healthy women with no known risk factors may need fewer visits than women with health conditions or pregnancy problems.

If your pregnancy is healthy, you likely will have a checkup every 4 weeks from your first prenatal visit until 28 weeks. During your second-trimester visits, you may have the following:

- Ultrasound exam—A standard ultrasound exam usually is done between 18 and 22 weeks of pregnancy. The exam looks at your baby's basic anatomy. Your ob-gyn may be able to tell the sex if the baby is in a good position for the *genitals* to be seen. The amount of **amniotic fluid** and the baby's cardiac activity are checked. Although ultrasound doesn't find all problems, it is important to remember that a normal ultrasound is reassuring.

- *Fundal height* measurement—As your baby grows, the top of the uterus (the fundus) grows up and out of the pelvic area. At about 12 weeks of pregnancy, it can be felt just above the pubic bone. At 20 weeks, the fundus reaches the navel. Starting at this prenatal care visit, your ob-gyn should measure the fundal height. This measurement allows your ob-gyn to check your baby's size and growth rate. The fundal height in centimeters should roughly equal the weeks of pregnancy. For example, at 20 weeks, the fundal height should be about 18 to 22 centimeters. In women who are obese, it may be hard to accurately measure fundal height, so ultrasound exams may be done instead.

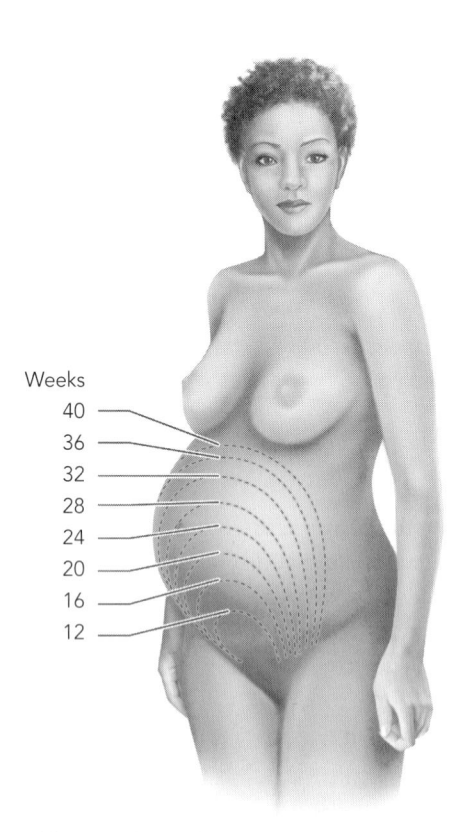

Changes in uterine size. The size of the uterus can help show how long you have been pregnant.

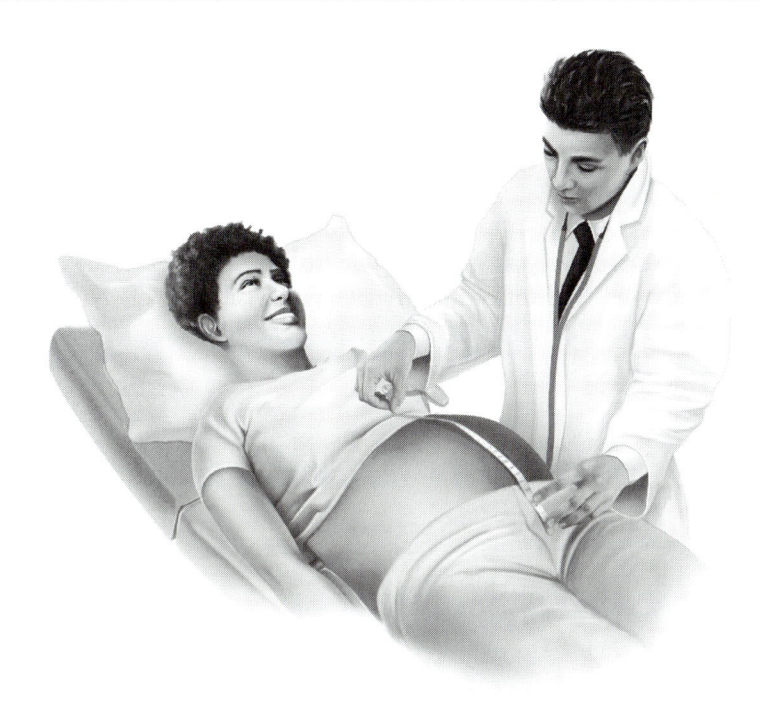

Measuring fundal height. Starting at around the fifth month of pregnancy, your ob-gyn should measure the height of your uterus to check your baby's growth. The fundal height will be measured during each prenatal care visit.

- *Amniocentesis*—If you decided to have amniocentesis but didn't have the test last month, you can still have it this month (see Chapter 33, "Genetic Disorders, Screening, and Testing").

Discussions With Your Ob-Gyn

Do you want to know the baby's sex? You may be able to find out during this month's ultrasound exam. Now is also a good time to start thinking about choosing your baby's doctor.

Learning the Baby's Sex

If you want to know the sex of your baby, this month's ultrasound exam may tell you. Sometimes it's not possible to determine the sex because the baby is not facing the right way during the exam. If the baby's genitals cannot be seen, an ultrasound exam later in pregnancy may be able to reveal the baby's sex.

Choosing Your Baby's Doctor

Now is a good time to decide who will care for your baby after birth. Most parents choose a **pediatrician,** a doctor who specializes in the health care of children from birth until young adulthood. Other parents use a family practice doctor who treats the entire family.

Not sure how to find a doctor for your baby? Talk with friends and family members who are parents. Ask your ob-gyn for a referral. You also can search your health insurance plan's network of practitioners. Make sure the doctor you want

- is accepting new patients
- has an office near your home
- accepts your health insurance
- is on staff at the hospital or birth center where you plan to deliver

Some pediatricians will meet with parents-to-be for brief interviews to answer questions. During the interview, ask yourself whether you feel comfortable with the doctor. Do you like his or her manner and communication style? Here are some other questions you might ask:

- When will the doctor see your baby for the first time? Will he or she come to the hospital to see your newborn?
- How often will your baby be seen for checkups?
- Is the doctor available by phone or email for questions? If not, is there a nurse who can answer your questions without an office visit?
- Does the doctor take calls after hours (nighttime or weekends), or do you need to visit an urgent care center or emergency room?
- Are there extra fees for sick visits, routine exams, and vaccinations?

See the "Resources" section at the end of this chapter for information about pediatricians and how to choose one.

Special Concerns

Exposure to lead and other chemicals may be a concern for some pregnant women, such as those who work in certain industries or who live with someone who does. A screening test for lead is recommended for women with at least one risk factor for lead exposure.

Prenatal Lead Exposure

Lead is a heavy metal that is used in certain industries (battery manufacturing, construction, and printing). Until the late 1970s, lead also was used in paint.

Today, the United States strictly regulates the use of lead in industry. Standards are in place to help reduce workers' exposure. But older houses may still contain lead in paint, pipes, and fixtures. Areas of some cities still have lead water mains. Some things made in other countries also may have lead in them, including pottery and jewelry. Certain folk remedies and medicines used in other cultures also may contain high levels of lead.

Lead can be inhaled in dust, absorbed through the skin, or swallowed. It easily crosses the *placenta* in pregnant women. The risks of lead exposure during pregnancy include

- *miscarriage*
- *low birth weight*
- *preterm* birth

Studies show that children exposed to high levels of lead before birth have an increased risk of learning and behavioral problems.

A blood test that measures the level of lead in your body is available. This test can be used to see how much lead you have been exposed to. Pregnant women who have at least one risk factor for lead exposure should have this blood test. If any of the following apply to you, tell your ob-gyn:

- You are renovating an older home without lead hazard controls in place. It's very easy to accidentally absorb lead from paint chips or paint dust.

- Your home has lead pipes or water sources that are lined with lead (this is more likely in houses built before 1986).

- Your neighborhood has lead water mains.

- You have recently relocated from a country or area where lead is common, such as countries where leaded gasoline is still being used (or was recently phased out) or where pollution is not well controlled.

- You live near a source of lead (even if it is closed), such as a lead mine, smelter, or battery recycling plant.

- You work in an industry that uses lead (lead production, battery manufacturing, paint manufacturing, ship building, ammunition production, or plastic manufacturing).

- You have a hobby that may expose you to lead (stained glass production or pottery making with certain leaded glazes and paint).
- You live with someone who works with lead or who has a hobby with potential lead exposure.
- You cook, store, or serve food in lead-glazed ceramic pottery made in a traditional process.
- You use imported spices, foods, ceremonial powders, herbal remedies, or cosmetics (kohl or surma). Items at highest risk of containing lead come from East India, India, the Middle East, West Asia, and some areas of Latin America.
- You have *pica* (a condition in which a pregnant woman eats things that are not food, such as soil).
- You have a history of lead exposure or elevated lead level, or you live with someone with an elevated lead level.

If your lead level is elevated, steps may need to be taken to identify the source of lead exposure and to avoid future exposure. Depending on how much lead is found in your body, you may need ongoing follow-up testing of your lead levels for the rest of your pregnancy. You also may need treatment to prevent problems for you and your baby. See Chapter 24, "Reducing Risks of Birth Defects."

RESOURCES

Choosing a Family Doctor
https://familydoctor.org/choosing-a-family-doctor/
Webpage from the American Academy of Family Physicians that discusses the role of the family doctor. Gives advice on finding the right doctor for you and your family.

Find a Pediatrician or Pediatric Specialist
www.healthychildren.org/English/tips-tools/find-pediatrician/Pages/Pediatrician-Referral-Service.aspx
Online tool from the American Academy of Pediatrics. Helps you find a doctor for your baby or older children.

Lead
www.epa.gov/lead
Information from the U.S. Environmental Protection Agency about lead and how to protect yourself and your family.

Your Pregnancy and Childbirth
www.acog.org/MyPregnancy
Website from the American College of Obstetricians and Gynecologists (ACOG) with information on pregnancy, labor, delivery, and postpartum care. Includes the latest information from the experts in women's health care, questions answered by ACOG ob-gyns, pregnancy stories from real women, and an A–Z directory of health topics covering pregnancy and beyond.

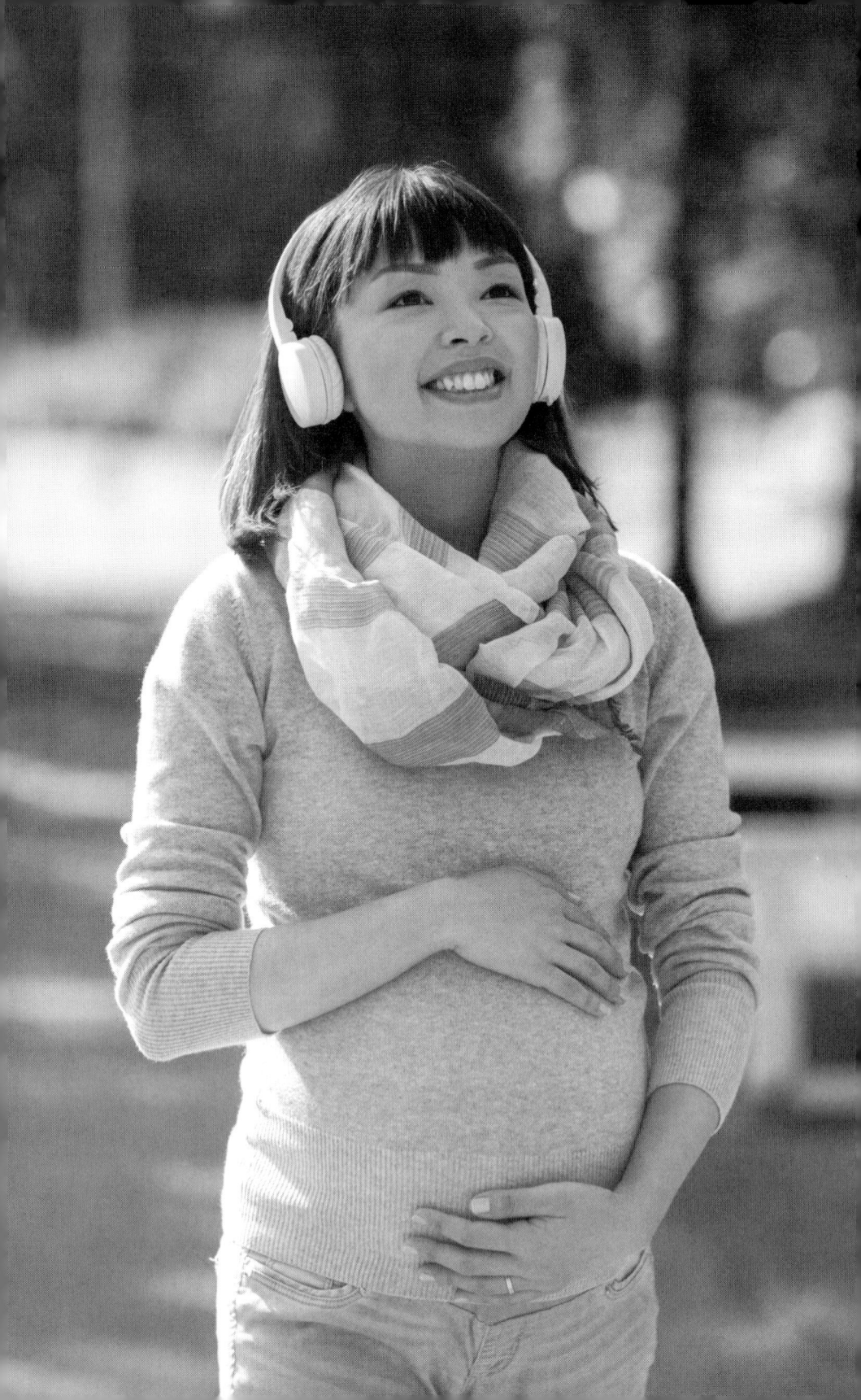

CHAPTER 7

Month 6
(Weeks 21 to 24)

YOUR BABY

▶ WEEK 21
The baby's kicks and turns are stronger now. If you have already felt the baby move, the movements are more noticeable now. The sucking reflex is developing. If the hand floats to the mouth, the baby may suck his or her thumb. You may notice jerking movements—it's likely the baby having hiccups.

> This week, your baby is about as long as a carrot.

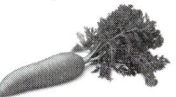

▶ WEEK 22
The baby now weighs about 1 pound and is 11 inches long. Eyebrows are visible. More fat is forming under the skin to keep the baby warm.

> This week, your baby is about the size of a small spaghetti squash.

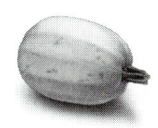

▶ WEEK 23
Most of the baby's sleep time is now spent in rapid eye movement (REM) sleep. During this stage of sleep, the eyes move and the brain is very active. Ridges are forming in the hands and feet that later will be fingerprints and footprints.

> This week, your baby is about the size of a large grapefruit.

➤ WEEK 24

The baby's skin is wrinkled and reddish, thanks to blood vessels under the skin. The lungs continue to develop. The baby now weighs about 1½ pounds.

This week, your baby is about as long as an ear of corn.

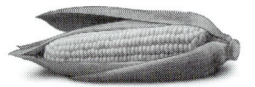

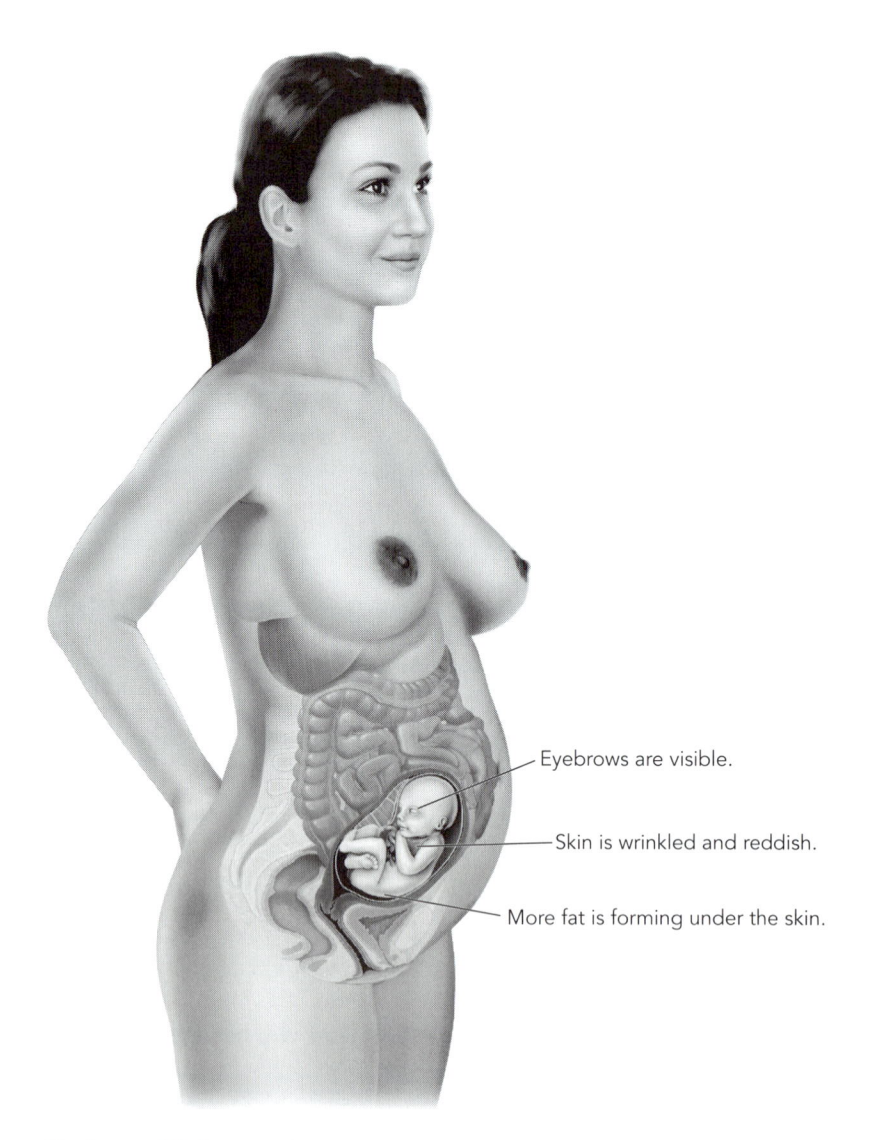

Eyebrows are visible.

Skin is wrinkled and reddish.

More fat is forming under the skin.

Mother and baby: Weeks 21 to 24
By the end of week 24, the baby is about 12 inches long and weighs about 1½ pounds.

YOUR PREGNANCY

Your Changing Body

At week 21, you have started the second half of your pregnancy. If you have felt movement before now, you may feel the baby moving even more now. But don't worry if you don't feel anything. Some women may not feel their babies moving for another few weeks.

Body Image

Some women love the way they look during pregnancy. Other women don't. Mixed feelings about your pregnant body are normal. Some days, you may love your growing body. Other days, though, you may wonder if your body will ever be the same.

Eating a healthy diet and exercising will help you feel better about how you look. If you're in good shape and don't gain more than the suggested weight during pregnancy, you'll have an easier time losing weight after delivery.

Sexual Activity

If you're having a healthy pregnancy, most sexual activity is safe, including **penetration** with fingers or sex toys. If you have a male partner, **sexual intercourse** is safe, too. You won't hurt the baby. The **amniotic sac** and the strong muscles of the **uterus** keep the baby protected.

It's up to you whether you feel up to having sex. Some women do, and some don't. During the first **trimester**, you may have felt too nauseated and tired to have sex. But you may find that your sex drive comes back during the second trimester after morning sickness goes away and you have your energy again. It's also normal for desire to wane again during the third trimester. Whatever your mood, talk with your partner.

It is normal to have cramps or spotting after sex with penetration. Also, **orgasm** can cause cramps. If you have severe, persistent cramping, or if your bleeding is heavy (like normal menstrual bleeding), call your **obstetrician–gynecologist (ob-gyn).**

As your belly grows, you'll have to find a position that is most comfortable for you. Let your partner know if anything feels uncomfortable, even if it's something you're used to doing all the time. You may want to try these positions:

- Side-by-side—You and your partner can face each other.
- You on top—This position takes the pressure off your belly.
- Partner behind—Support yourself on your knees and elbows.

If you have pregnancy **complications** or you have a history of **preterm** labor, you may need to limit sexual activity. You also may need to monitor yourself for contractions after sex. In some (rare) cases, you may be told to avoid orgasm. Ask your ob-gyn what sexual activity is safe for you.

Weight Gain

You may have gained between 10 and 15 pounds by this month. If your ob-gyn thinks you are gaining weight too quickly, you may have to adjust how much food you're eating and get more exercise. See Table 3-1, "Weight Gain During Pregnancy," in Chapter 3, "Months 1 and 2 (Weeks 1 to 8)," for the recommended weight gain based on **body mass index (BMI)** before pregnancy. You and your ob-gyn will discuss whether your weight gain is on track.

Discomforts and How to Manage Them

You may already have experienced acid reflux—otherwise known as heartburn—earlier in your pregnancy. But now, as your uterus grows larger and pushes up against your stomach, you may have heartburn more often. Other discomforts include hot flashes (caused by pregnancy **hormones**) and aches and pains (caused by the increased weight of your uterus). Most of these discomforts are normal. But some may be signs of something more serious. Tell your ob-gyn if you have shortness of breath or a severe headache.

Heartburn

Heartburn is pain or a burning feeling in the throat and chest and is common among pregnant women. Pregnancy hormones, which relax the valve between your stomach and esophagus (the tube leading from the mouth to the stomach), are a main cause of heartburn. When the valve between your esophagus and stomach doesn't close, stomach acids leak into the esophagus. As your uterus grows, it adds to the problem by pressing up against your stomach.

If you are bothered by heartburn, try these remedies:

- Eat six small meals per day instead of three big ones.
- Eat slowly and chew your food well.
- Do not drink a lot of liquid with your meals. Drink liquid between meals instead.

- Do not eat or drink within a few hours of bedtime. Do not lie down right after meals.
- Try raising the head of your bed. Place a few extra pillows under your shoulders or put a couple of books or wood blocks under the legs at the head of the bed.
- Avoid foods that are known to make acid reflux worse. These include citrus fruits, chocolate, and spicy or fried foods.

Several antacids are available over-the-counter. These typically contain aluminum, calcium, and magnesium. These products are considered safe to use during pregnancy, but do not overdo it. If you have tried these remedies and your acid reflux continues or gets worse, see your ob-gyn.

Hot Flashes

If you're feeling hot and sweaty when everyone else says they feel fine, blame your pregnancy hormones and your increased **metabolism**. You are burning more **calories** and generating more heat. Try to stay cool just as you would on the hottest summer days:

- Wear loose clothing.
- Drink plenty of water.
- Stay close to a fan or air conditioner for a blast of cool air.

Month 6: When to Call Your Ob-Gyn

- You have heartburn that won't go away.
- You have a racing heartbeat that doesn't go away at rest.
- You have severe, persistent cramping or heavy bleeding.
- You have signs of **preeclampsia**, such as swelling of the face or hands, headache that will not go away, and trouble breathing (see the "Preeclampsia" section in this chapter).
- You have signs of preterm labor, including a change in vaginal discharge, constant low backache, and frequent contractions (see the "Signs of Preterm Labor" section in this chapter).

Aches and Pains

It is normal for the extra weight of your growing belly to cause aches and pains as you move around during the day or when you're trying to rest. You may not be able to take the medications you normally would for pain, but you can take acetaminophen. To be sure that you don't take too much acetaminophen, check with your ob-gyn. Together you can review whether you are taking any other medications that contain acetaminophen.

Avoid taking aspirin or **nonsteroidal anti-inflammatory drugs (NSAIDs)**, such as ibuprofen, during pregnancy. Some studies have suggested that they may increase the risk of certain **birth defects** when they are taken in the third trimester.

There may be other ways to relieve the pain. If your muscles are sore and aching, try a warm bath or massage. A heating pad or a heat wrap may help. For mild headaches, try lying down with a cool pack on your head. If you have a severe headache or if a headache doesn't go away, call your ob-gyn right away.

Fast or Racing Heartbeat

You may notice throughout your pregnancy that your heart is beating faster. This is normal. It happens because your heart is pumping more blood faster than normal. As your pregnancy goes on, your heart pumps up to 30 to 50 percent more blood than when you aren't pregnant. These increases in heart rate and blood volume help deliver **oxygen** and **nutrients** to the baby through the **placenta**.

Another reason for the faster heartbeat may be sensitivity to caffeine. Pregnant women may be more sensitive to the effects of caffeine. If you notice that your heart rate stays fast or if you also have shortness of breath, call your ob-gyn right away.

Exercise

It's important to stay active this month. See Chapter 23, "Exercise During Pregnancy," for exercise tips. Also, from now on be aware of how your growing belly affects your balance.

Loss of Balance

As you continue to exercise in your second and third trimesters, be aware that your growing belly changes how your weight is balanced when you move around. The weight you gain in the front of your body shifts your center of gravity. This puts stress on your joints and muscles—mostly those in the lower back and pelvis. It also can make you less stable and more likely to fall. If you do fall, call your ob-gyn or go to the hospital if you have bleeding or contractions.

Prenatal Care Visits

Your prenatal visit this month will focus on checking your baby's growth and making sure you are not having any complications. Your weight and blood pressure will be checked, and the ***fundal height***—the distance from your pubic bone to the top of your uterus—also will be measured. It should now be around 21 to 24 centimeters.

Be sure to tell your ob-gyn if you are experiencing any symptoms that are causing discomfort. Ask questions and share your concerns.

Discussions With Your Ob-Gyn

With about 3 months to go, now is a good time to think about labor, delivery, and your baby's care after birth. You have quite a few decisions to make, including how you will feed your baby.

Labor and Delivery: Things to Start Thinking About

It is best to think about your childbirth options and resolve as much as you can well before you give birth. You also should make choices about your baby's birth and care after delivery. Some options you may want to think about ahead of time include the following:

- What kind of childbirth preparation classes do you want?
- Do you want pain relief during labor, or will you try natural childbirth?
- If you have a boy, do you want him circumcised?
- Will you breastfeed your baby? Are there lactation classes in your area?

Another thing to think about is who you want at your side during labor and delivery. A childbirth partner can be anyone you want—a spouse, partner, relative, or close friend. If possible, your childbirth partner should come with you to ***prenatal care*** visits and tests. Your partner also needs to attend childbirth classes with you because this person has almost as much to learn as you do. When you're in labor, your childbirth partner will coach you through contractions and help you carry out what you learned in class. See Chapter 12, "Preparing for Birth," for information about childbirth classes, *circumcision,* breastfeeding, and more.

Special Concerns

Preterm birth can happen if labor starts before 37 weeks of pregnancy. It's important to recognize the signs and symptoms of preterm labor. If preterm labor is diagnosed early, your ob-gyn may try to postpone birth to give your baby extra time to grow. Even a few more days in the uterus may mean a healthier baby.

Preeclampsia is another concern that you should be aware of. It is most common in the third trimester, but it can happen any time after 20 weeks of pregnancy. It also can develop during the *postpartum* period.

Early Preterm Birth

A baby is preterm (premature) when he or she is born before 37 weeks of pregnancy. When babies are born before 34 weeks, they are called early preterm. Early preterm babies are at risk of many short-term and long-term problems, including

- breathing problems
- bleeding in the brain
- *cerebral palsy* and other *neurological* problems
- vision problems
- learning disabilities

Babies born before 23 weeks of pregnancy are not likely to survive. By week 26, the chances of survival are higher, but serious lifelong health problems are likely. Survival at 26 weeks depends on several factors, including

- the type of hospital the baby is born in
- the baby's sex and weight
- whether medications have been given before birth to help with the baby's development
- whether there is more than one baby

Signs of Preterm Labor

Call your ob-gyn right away if you notice signs of preterm labor, including

- change in vaginal discharge (watery, mucus-like, or bloody)
- increase in amount of vaginal discharge
- pelvic or lower abdominal pressure
- constant, low, dull backache
- mild abdominal cramps, with or without diarrhea
- regular or frequent contractions or uterine tightening, often painless (four times every 20 minutes or eight times an hour for more than 1 hour)
- ruptured membranes (your water breaks—either a gush or a trickle)

There may be treatment if you are at risk of preterm labor or have symptoms of preterm labor. See Chapter 35, "When Labor Starts Too Soon: Preterm Labor, Prelabor Rupture of Membranes, and Preterm Birth," for details about how preterm labor is diagnosed and treated.

Preeclampsia

Preeclampsia is a medical condition that can happen after 20 weeks of pregnancy or after childbirth. This condition can affect all organs of a woman's body, including the **kidneys**, liver, brain, and eyes. It also affects the placenta. Preeclampsia is a serious condition that requires diagnosis and treatment right away.

Preeclampsia is diagnosed when your blood pressure is higher than a certain level and you have signs of organ injury, such as

- an abnormal amount of protein in your urine
- low number of **platelets**
- abnormal kidney or liver function
- pain over the upper abdomen
- fluid in the lungs
- severe headache or changes in vision

Preeclampsia may cause

- swelling of the face or hands
- headache that will not go away
- seeing spots or changes in eyesight
- pain in the upper abdomen (near your ribs) or shoulder
- nausea and vomiting (in the second half of pregnancy)
- sudden weight gain
- difficulty breathing

If you notice any of these symptoms, call your ob-gyn right away. See Chapter 30, "Hypertension and Preeclampsia."

Involving Your Other Children in Your Pregnancy

If you already have children, they may have many different feelings about your pregnancy and a new baby. Some children may have questions about where babies come from. Others may not want to talk about the baby at all. Some children are eager to be a big brother or sister. Others resent losing center stage to the new baby. A busy teenager with his or her own hobbies and friends may show little interest in your pregnancy and the baby.

When is the best time to share the news about your pregnancy? It really depends on your child. You may want to tell your school-aged children before you tell people outside your family. This way, they will hear the news from you, and not others.

With young children, it may be a good idea to wait until they ask about your changing body. The idea of a baby growing inside of you may be too hard for small children to understand before they can see your bigger belly.

RESOURCES

Preeclampsia Foundation
www.preeclampsia.org
Provides in-depth information about signs and symptoms, diagnosis, and treatment of preeclampsia. Offers a community for women who have had this condition.

Preparing Your Child for a New Sibling
http://kidshealth.org/parent/emotions/feelings/sibling_prep.html
Tips and advice from KidsHealth for getting your kids ready for a new baby.

Reproductive Health: Preterm Birth
www.cdc.gov/reproductivehealth/maternalinfanthealth/pretermbirth.htm
Website from the Centers for Disease Control and Prevention that answers frequently asked questions about preterm birth.

Your Pregnancy and Childbirth
www.acog.org/MyPregnancy
Website from the American College of Obstetricians and Gynecologists (ACOG) with information on pregnancy, labor, delivery, and postpartum care. Includes the latest information from the experts in women's health care, questions answered by ACOG ob-gyns, pregnancy stories from real women, and an A–Z directory of health topics covering pregnancy and beyond.

Month 6

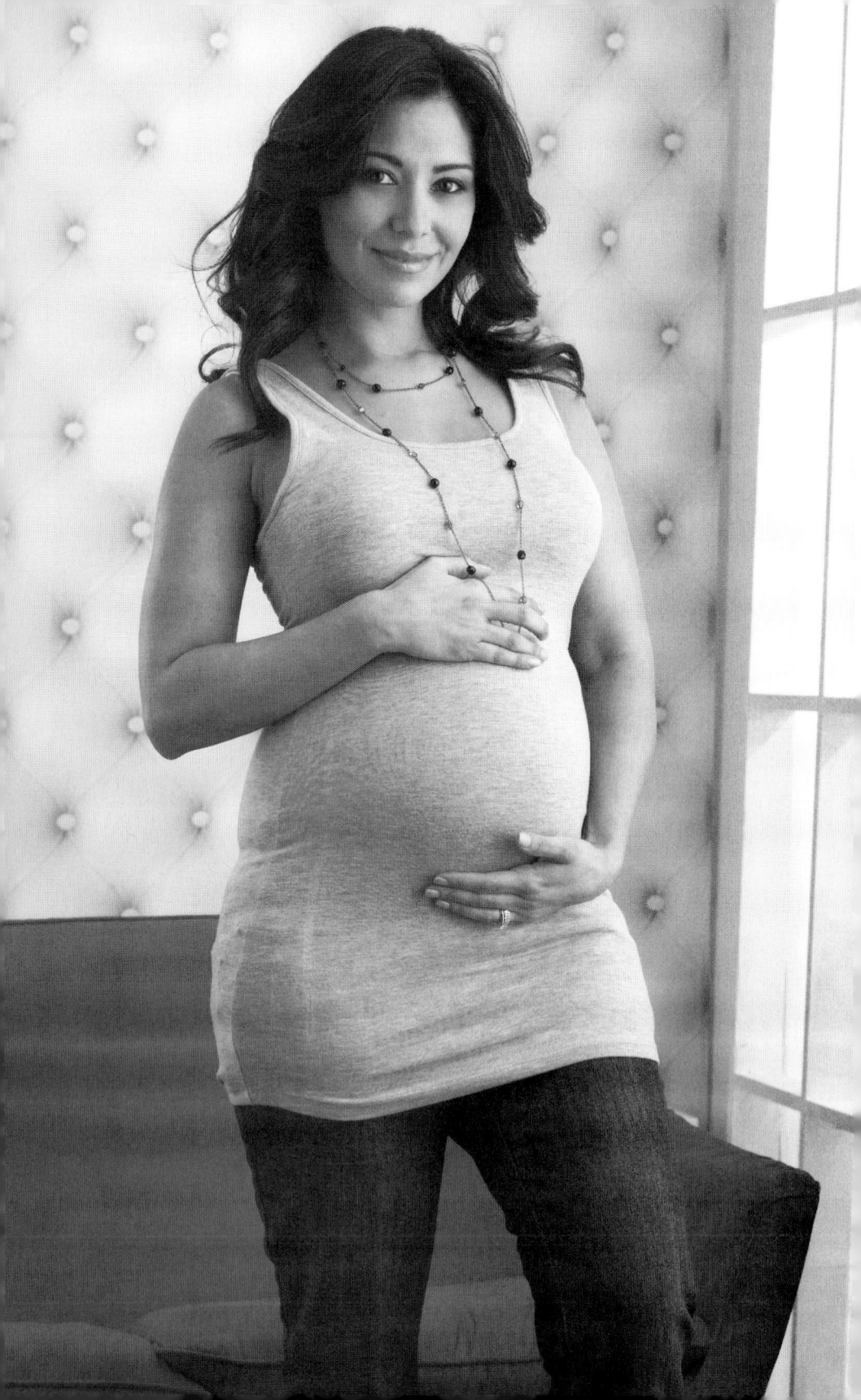

CHAPTER 8

Month 7
(Weeks 25 to 28)

YOUR BABY

▶ WEEK 25
Your baby can respond with movement to familiar sounds, such as the sound of your voice. The lungs are now fully formed but not yet ready to function outside the **uterus**.

> This week, your baby is about the size of a rutabaga, a larger cousin of the turnip.

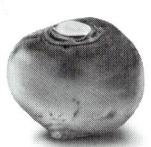

▶ WEEK 26
Loud sounds may make your baby respond with a startled movement and pull in his or her arms and legs. Eyelids can open and close. The lungs begin making **surfactant**, a substance needed for breathing after birth. The baby is closing in on 2 pounds and is about 14 inches long.

> This week, your baby is about as long as a scallion, also known as green onion.

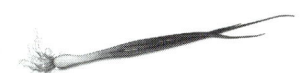

➤ WEEK 27

Your baby is growing rapidly now. The nervous system is developing. More fat is being added too, which will make the baby's skin look smoother.

> This week, your baby is about the size of a cauliflower.

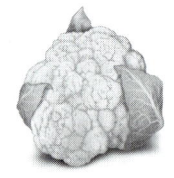

➤ WEEK 28

This week is the beginning of the third **trimester** of pregnancy. A greasy material called **vernix** has started to develop. Vernix acts as a waterproof barrier that protects the baby's skin. The skin will be completely covered with vernix by the time the baby is born. Eyelashes have developed. The baby is now nearly 15 inches long.

> This week, your baby is about the size of a standard eggplant.

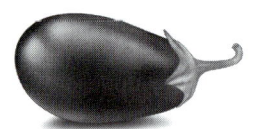

YOUR PREGNANCY

Your Changing Body

At 28 weeks of pregnancy, you will start the third—and last—trimester. The end is finally in sight. Now's the time to start making plans for the baby's birth and think more about what your life will be like after the baby is born.

Body Image and Weight Gain

Sometimes people, including family members, comment on a pregnant woman's weight. They may mean well, but these comments can make you feel bad and unsure about whether you have or haven't gained the right amount of weight for your baby.

To cope with comments, remember that your pregnancy and your weight are your private concerns. Also, remember that other people do not know how big or small you should be, how much weight you have gained or lost, or what your weight should be for your current stage of pregnancy. A well-timed reply, such as "Thank you for your concern" or "My doctor thinks I'm doing fine," can let your questioner know that his or her comments are off-limits.

See Table 3-1, "Weight Gain During Pregnancy," in Chapter 3, "Months 1 and 2 (Weeks 1 to 8)," for the recommended weight gain based on **body mass index (BMI)** before pregnancy. This chart shows the average weight gain by week of pregnancy.

MONTH 7 • 123

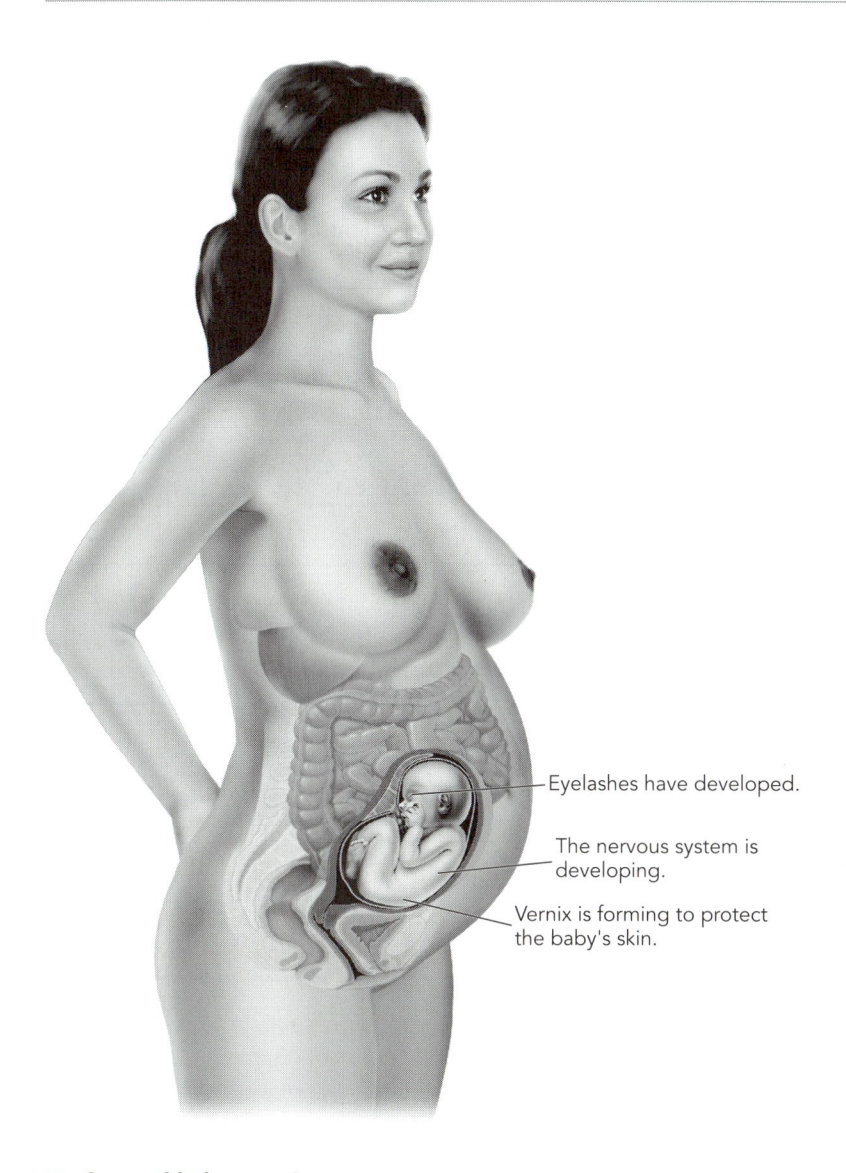

- Eyelashes have developed.
- The nervous system is developing.
- Vernix is forming to protect the baby's skin.

Mother and baby: Weeks 25 to 28
By the end of week 28, the baby is nearly 15 inches long and weighs about 2½ pounds.

If you're concerned about your weight, talk with your **obstetrician–gynecologist (ob-gyn)**. By this stage in your pregnancy, if you have been gaining weight too quickly or too slowly, your ob-gyn may have talked about it already. If not, bring up the issue yourself.

Discomforts and How to Manage Them

The third trimester is a time of rapid fetal growth, and you will probably start seeing—and feeling—the extra weight of your baby. The increasing size and weight of your **uterus** may trigger lower back pain and other pains as your body adjusts. Constipation may become a problem. You also may have "practice" contractions called **Braxton Hicks contractions**.

Lower Back Pain

Many pregnant women have lower back pain, especially during the later stages of pregnancy. Several things can cause this pain:

- The sacroiliac joints are the strong, weight-bearing joints in the pelvis. During pregnancy the **ligaments** in the sacroiliac get looser. A **hormone** called relaxin relaxes these ligaments to make your baby's passage through your pelvis easier. Looser joints may cause pain, especially when getting up from a chair, walking up a flight of stairs, or getting out of a car.

    If you have these symptoms, see your ob-gyn. He or she may suggest exercises that strengthen the muscles surrounding the joints. Usually, the problem goes away after the baby is born. But the more pregnancies a woman has, the greater the risk of sacroiliac joint problems.

- Another cause of lower back pain is sciatica. This condition is caused by the pressure of the growing uterus on the sciatic nerve. Sciatica causes pain in the lower back and hip that goes down the back of the leg. Sciatica

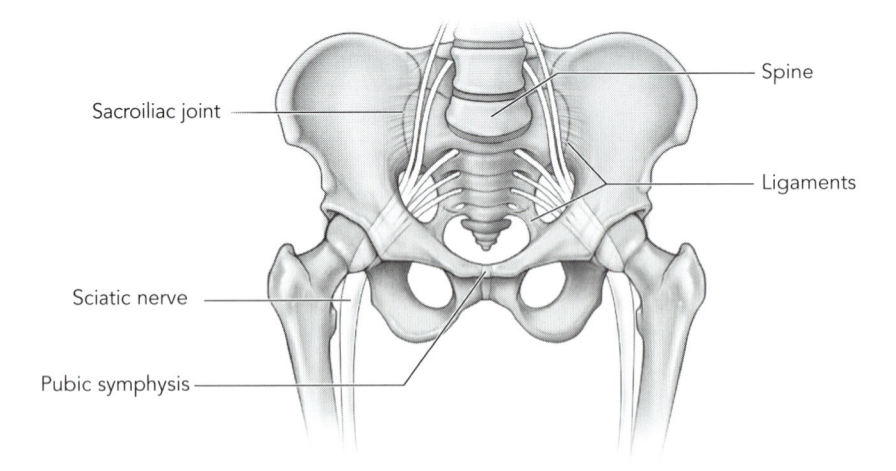

Causes of pain during pregnancy. Changes in the sacroiliac joint, the sciatic nerve, and the pubic symphysis all may cause pain during pregnancy.

often goes away after the baby is born. But if you have numbness in your feet or leg weakness with this pain, tell your ob-gyn. Also tell your ob-gyn if you have severe calf pain or tenderness, as these can be signs of **deep vein thrombosis (DVT)**.

Pelvic Bone Pain

The two halves of your pelvis are connected at the front by a joint called the pubic symphysis. This joint normally is stiff and hardly moves. The hormone relaxin also affects the pubic symphysis, making it more flexible during and just after pregnancy. Sometimes, the increased movement in this joint can cause pain in the pelvis. Avoid heavy lifting and standing for a long time. Exercises for abdominal and pelvic muscles also can help (see Chapter 23, "Exercise During Pregnancy").

Constipation

Even if you didn't have constipation early in your pregnancy, you most likely will have it now. Constipation is when you do not have bowel movements often and your stools are firm or hard to pass. It can happen for many reasons. High levels of **progesterone** may slow down digestion. Iron supplements can make constipation worse. Toward the end of pregnancy, the weight of the uterus puts pressure on your **rectum**, adding to the problem.

Although there is no miracle cure for constipation, the following tips may help:

- Drink plenty of liquids, especially water.
- Eat high-fiber foods, such as fruits, vegetables, beans, whole-grain bread, and bran cereal.
- Walk or do another safe exercise every day (see Chapter 23, "Exercise During Pregnancy").
- Eat several smaller meals each day instead of larger, less frequent meals. Smaller amounts of food eaten more often may be easier to digest.

You also can ask your ob-gyn about over-the-counter remedies for constipation:

- Bulk-forming agents absorb water in the intestines. This creates a more liquid-like stool that's easier to pass. If you take these agents, you need to drink plenty of water.

- Stool softeners add liquid to the stool to soften it.
- Stimulants trigger the intestines to contract and move stool through.

Talk with your ob-gyn before taking any over-the-counter remedy.

Braxton Hicks Contractions

As early as the second trimester, many women have "practice contractions" called Braxton Hicks contractions. Sometimes Braxton Hicks contractions are very mild. They can barely be felt or feel like a slight tightness in your belly. Other times, they can be painful. These contractions help your body get ready for birth but do not open the *cervix*. These contractions often happen

- in the afternoon or evening
- after physical activity
- after sex

They are more likely to happen when you are tired or dehydrated, so be sure to drink plenty of fluids. Braxton Hicks contractions tend to happen more often and get stronger as you get closer to your due date. See the section on "Preterm Labor" later in this chapter.

Mental Health During Pregnancy

Depression and anxiety are common during pregnancy. Some women have depression and anxiety for the first time in their lives during pregnancy or after delivery. It's important to know the signs and symptoms. Talk with your ob-gyn if you think you may be experiencing any of them.

Depression

The signs of depression can seem like the normal ups and downs of pregnancy. A blue mood now and then is normal. But you may have depression if you are sad most of the time or if you have any of these symptoms for at least 2 weeks:

- Depressed mood most of the day, nearly every day
- Loss of interest in work or other activities
- Feeling guilty, hopeless, or worthless
- Sleeping more than normal or lying awake at night
- Loss of appetite or losing weight (or eating much more than normal and gaining weight)

- Feeling very tired or without energy
- Having trouble paying attention and making decisions

Women who have severe depression during pregnancy may have trouble taking care of themselves. They may not eat well or get enough rest. For these reasons, it's important to tell your ob-gyn if you have any signs or symptoms of depression. Your ob-gyn also may ask you questions about your mood during **prenatal care** visits. See the box "Depression Screening Test" later in this chapter. Your answers will help your ob-gyn understand if you need help.

Treatment of depression may include medication and counseling. Support from your partner, family members, and friends also can be helpful. In addition to providing support, these people may be able to see if your symptoms are getting worse. You may not be the first to notice.

If your ob-gyn prescribes an **antidepressant**, you will discuss which drug is best for you. The benefits of taking an antidepressant during pregnancy need to be weighed against the risks. Studies suggest that **selective serotonin reuptake inhibitors (SSRIs)** do not increase the risk of **birth defects**. But researchers are still learning whether other antidepressants can cause certain birth defects. Your ob-gyn can recommend a medication that is best for you and your baby.

Keep in mind that not treating depression can have negative effects on your baby. Babies born to women with untreated depression are at risk of

- growth problems during pregnancy
- **preterm** birth
- low weight at birth
- **complications** after birth

If your ob-gyn prescribes an antidepressant, the type and the dosage should be specific for you.

Anxiety and Stress

Other problems that can affect pregnant women are anxiety and stress. Anxiety disorders are common—nearly 1 in 5 adults have one. Pregnancy also can trigger a specific anxiety disorder called obsessive–compulsive disorder. Anxiety and stress have been linked to some pregnancy problems and a more difficult delivery. If you have anxiety and stress, tell your ob-gyn so that you can get the help you need. Treatment may include therapy to help you learn coping strategies and relaxation techniques. Sometimes medication is prescribed.

Depression Screening Test

The following questionnaire is called the Edinburgh Postnatal Depression Scale. These questions can help identify signs and symptoms of depression during pregnancy or **postpartum depression**. It is not intended for self-diagnosis. Only a health care practitioner can diagnose depression. It is best to answer these questions with a health care practitioner.

In the past 7 days,

I have been able to laugh and see the funny side of things.
- ❑ 0 As much as I always could
- ❑ 1 Not quite so much now
- ❑ 2 Definitely not so much now
- ❑ 3 Not at all

I have looked forward to things.
- ❑ 0 As much as I always could
- ❑ 1 Not quite so much now
- ❑ 2 Definitely not so much now
- ❑ 3 Not at all

I have blamed myself unnecessarily when things go wrong.
- ❑ 3 Yes, most of the time
- ❑ 2 Yes, some of the time
- ❑ 1 Not very often
- ❑ 0 No, never

I have been anxious or worried for no good reason.
- ❑ 0 No, not at all
- ❑ 1 Hardly ever
- ❑ 2 Yes, sometimes
- ❑ 3 Yes, very often

I have felt scared or panicky for no very good reason.
- ❑ 3 Yes, quite a lot
- ❑ 2 Yes, sometimes
- ❑ 1 No, not much
- ❑ 0 No, not at all

Things have been getting the best of me.
- ❏ 3 Yes, most of the time I haven't been able to cope at all
- ❏ 2 Yes, sometimes I haven't been coping as well as usual
- ❏ 1 No, most of the time I have coped quite well
- ❏ 0 No, I have been coping as well as ever

I have been so unhappy that I have had difficulty sleeping.
- ❏ 3 Yes, most of the time
- ❏ 2 Yes, sometimes
- ❏ 1 Not very often
- ❏ 0 No, not at all

I have felt sad or miserable.
- ❏ 3 Yes, most of the time
- ❏ 2 Yes, quite often
- ❏ 1 Not very often
- ❏ 0 No, not at all

I have been so unhappy that I have been crying.
- ❏ 3 Yes, most of the time
- ❏ 2 Yes, quite often
- ❏ 1 Only occasionally
- ❏ 0 No, never

I have thought about harming myself.
- ❏ 3 Yes, quite often
- ❏ 2 Sometimes
- ❏ 1 Hardly ever
- ❏ 0 Never

Scoring: Add the numbers next to the items you have selected. A score of 10 or higher means that you should consult your ob-gyn to discuss your signs and symptoms.

Note: If you have thoughts of harming yourself, it is important to get help right away. Contact your ob-gyn or emergency medical services.

Cox J, Holden J, Sagovsky R. (1987) Detection of postnatal depression: development of the 10-item Edinburgh Postnatal Depression Scale. Brit J Psychiatry 1987;150:782–86.

Prenatal Care Visits

During this month's prenatal care visit, your ob-gyn likely will track the baby's growth by measuring the *fundal height*. It probably will measure between 25 and 28 centimeters. This is about equal to the number of weeks of your pregnancy.

Your ob-gyn should check your weight and blood pressure. You also may have a blood test to check for *anemia*, a condition in which there are too few red blood cells, which can cause fatigue. You also are likely to have the following tests and vaccinations:

- Glucose challenge—This test measures your body's response to sugar. The test is usually done between 24 and 28 weeks of pregnancy to see whether you have **gestational diabetes**. This is a type of **diabetes mellitus** that develops only during pregnancy. The test is done in two steps: 1) you drink a sugary solution, and 2) 1 hour later, a blood sample is taken to measure your blood sugar level. If the test result is positive, more testing is needed. Women at high risk of gestational diabetes are given this test earlier in pregnancy. If the earlier test result was negative, you may have a repeat test at 24 to 28 weeks (see Chapter 31, "Diabetes During Pregnancy").

- Rh antibody screening—In earlier prenatal care visits, your ob-gyn likely tested your blood to see if you are Rh negative or Rh positive. If you tested Rh negative then, you'll probably be tested for Rh *antibodies* this month. If the test result shows you are not producing antibodies, your ob-gyn may prescribe a shot of **Rh immunoglobulin (RhIg)**. This shot will prevent antibodies from forming during the rest of your pregnancy (see Chapter 36, "Blood Type Incompatibility").

- Tdap vaccination—The **tetanus toxoid, reduced diphtheria toxoid, and acellular pertussis (Tdap) vaccine** helps prevent **pertussis** (whooping cough). Whooping cough can be very serious in newborns. The Tdap vaccine creates antibodies in the woman that are passed to a baby. These antibodies give protection against whooping cough until a baby can get his or her first whooping cough shot at age 2 months. The shot is safe and recommended between 27 and 36 weeks of each pregnancy.

- ***Influenza*** (flu) vaccination—If you have not yet had a flu shot during your pregnancy, your ob-gyn may recommend one. It is best to get the flu shot early in the flu season, which is October through May. But you can get the shot any time during pregnancy. The flu shot is safe for you and your baby. It creates antibodies that are passed to the baby, which gives the baby protection against the flu until he or she can get the flu shot at age 6 months.

Discussions With Your Ob-Gyn

As your due date nears, you will need to make decisions about many different things. This month, you may want to focus on your birth experience and write a birth plan. Another issue to think about this month is whether you will want to save the baby's cord blood. You also may be starting to think about your **birth control** options after your baby is born.

Birth Plan

Some childbirth education classes will help you draft a birth plan, which is a written outline of what you would like to happen during labor and delivery. A birth plan might include

- where you want to deliver
- whether you plan to use pain medications
- the people you want to have with you

A birth plan is a way for you to share your wishes with those who will care for you during labor and delivery. This plan tells them what type of labor and birth you would like to have, what you want to happen, and what you would like to avoid.

Keep in mind, though, that having a birth plan does not guarantee that your labor and delivery will go according to that plan. Changes may need to be made based on how your labor progresses. Remember that you and your ob-gyn have a common goal: the safest possible delivery for you and your baby. A birth plan is a great starting point, but you should be prepared for the unexpected.

Review your birth plan with your ob-gyn well before your due date. Together, you can discuss how your plan fits with his or her policies and the hospital's policies. Not every hospital or birth center can accommodate every request. Still, a plan can help make your wishes clear. Talking about your expectations up front can help reduce surprises and disappointments later. See Chapter 12, "Preparing for Birth," for more on birth plans.

Cord Blood Banking

Cord blood is blood from the baby that is left in the **umbilical cord** and **placenta** after birth. This blood contains **stem cells** that can be used to treat some diseases, such as disorders of the blood, **metabolism,** and **immune system**. It's now possible to collect some of this cord blood after birth and store it.

If you plan to collect and store your baby's cord blood, let your ob-gyn know far in advance of your due date (at least 2 months). If you have chosen a private bank, arrange for the collection equipment to be sent to your ob-gyn. Also, there usually is a fee charged by your ob-gyn for collecting cord blood. This fee may not be covered by health insurance. There are other things to consider if you plan to store cord blood. See Chapter 12, "Preparing for Birth," for more details on cord blood banking.

Birth Control After Pregnancy

Women can get pregnant soon after having a baby if they have **sexual intercourse** and do not use **birth control**. Some women can get pregnant even before their **menstrual periods** return. If you have a male partner, it's important to use birth control after the baby is born. Starting a birth control method right after you have a baby can help you avoid an unintended pregnancy. Birth control also lets you control if or when you want to get pregnant again.

Using birth control also allows your body time to heal before having another baby. Ideally, pregnancies should be spaced at least 18 months apart. This offers the best health outcomes for you and your next baby. If you feel the need to attempt another pregnancy sooner, talk with your ob-gyn about the risk and benefits in your case.

You can talk with your ob-gyn about birth control options while you are still pregnant or right after giving birth. You also can talk with your ob-gyn before you go home from the hospital. See Chapter 21, "Birth Control After Pregnancy and Beyond," for a look at different birth control methods and how to choose one after pregnancy.

Special Concerns

Preterm labor is labor that starts before 37 weeks of pregnancy. It's important to watch for the signs of preterm labor so you can call your ob-gyn right away. You also should watch for vaginal bleeding.

Preterm Labor

Call your ob-gyn right away if you notice signs of preterm labor, including

- change in vaginal discharge (watery, mucus-like, or bloody)
- increase in amount of vaginal discharge
- pelvic or lower abdominal pressure
- constant, low, dull backache
- mild abdominal cramps, with or without diarrhea
- ruptured membranes (your water breaks—either a gush or a trickle)

Keep in mind that Braxton Hicks contractions may get stronger as your uterus grows. But if contractions come four times every 20 minutes or eight times an hour for more than 1 hour, call your ob-gyn.

Vaginal Bleeding

Vaginal bleeding can have many causes in the third trimester. Bleeding may be caused by something minor. Bleeding might happen if the *cervix* gets inflamed, for example. But some bleeding can signal a problem for you or the baby. To be safe, call your ob-gyn if you have any bleeding.

Month 7: When to Call Your Ob-Gyn

- You have vaginal bleeding, even a small amount.
- You have leg pain with numbness in your feet or leg weakness.
- You have pain or tenderness in one or both calves that does not go away.
- You have pain getting up from a chair, walking up stairs, or getting out of a car.
- You feel depressed, anxious, or stressed.
- You have signs of **preeclampsia**, such as swelling of the face or hands, headache that will not go away, and trouble breathing (see Chapter 30, "Hypertension and Preeclampsia," for more signs and symptoms).
- You have signs of preterm labor, including a change in vaginal discharge, constant low backache, and frequent contractions (see the "Preterm Labor" section in this chapter).

Heavy vaginal bleeding can mean there is a problem with the placenta. The most common problems are **placenta previa** and **placental abruption**. With placenta previa, the placenta lies low in the uterus and covers all or part of the cervix, blocking the baby's exit. This condition often causes painless vaginal bleeding.

With placental abruption, the placenta starts to separate from the wall of the uterus before the baby is born. This can be dangerous for you and your baby. Placental abruption often causes

- constant, severe pain in the belly
- contractions, which may be mild or severe
- heavy bleeding

Go to the emergency room right away if you have any of these symptoms.

With both placenta previa and placental abruption, the baby may need to be delivered preterm. If bleeding is severe, you may need a blood **transfusion**. **Cesarean birth** may be needed. In some cases, the bleeding may stop. If it does, the pregnancy may continue normally, but you will need to be monitored closely. See Chapter 37, "Placenta Problems."

Amniotic Fluid Problems

The amount of **amniotic fluid** in your uterus should increase until the beginning of your third trimester. After that, it gradually decreases until you give birth. But sometimes there may be too much fluid or too little fluid. Abnormal amounts of amniotic fluid could be a sign of problems with the baby or the placenta.

During your prenatal care visits, your ob-gyn should monitor the growth of your uterus. If he or she suspects a problem, you may have another **ultrasound exam** to check the baby's size and amount of amniotic fluid.

RESOURCES

Cord Blood: What You Need to Know
www.fda.gov/ForConsumers/ConsumerUpdates/ucm405558.htm
Information on storing and using cord blood from the U.S. Food and Drug Administration.

Depression During Pregnancy
www.marchofdimes.org/complications/depression-during-pregnancy.aspx
March of Dimes website that explains symptoms of depression during pregnancy and how you can get help.

Dietary Fiber
https://medlineplus.gov/dietaryfiber.html
Find the latest information related to dietary fiber from the U.S. National Library of Medicine.

National Cord Blood Program
www.nationalcordbloodprogram.org
Website from the largest public cord blood bank in the United States. Provides information about cord blood collection, storage, banking, and retrieval.

Postpartum Support International Helpline
www.postpartum.net
1-800-944-4773
Text 1-503-894-9453 (English) or 1-971-420-0294 (Spanish)
Non-emergency helpline for support, information, or referrals to postpartum mental health practitioners. The helpline is open 7 days per week. Leave a confidential message at any time, and a volunteer will return your call or text as soon as possible. PSI also offers online support group meetings to connect with other pregnant and postpartum women. You also can join PSI's weekly Chat with an Expert.

Your Pregnancy and Childbirth
www.acog.org/MyPregnancy
Website from the American College of Obstetricians and Gynecologists (ACOG) with information on pregnancy, labor, delivery, and postpartum care. Includes the latest information from the experts in women's health care, questions answered by ACOG ob-gyns, pregnancy stories from real women, and an A–Z directory of health topics covering pregnancy and beyond.

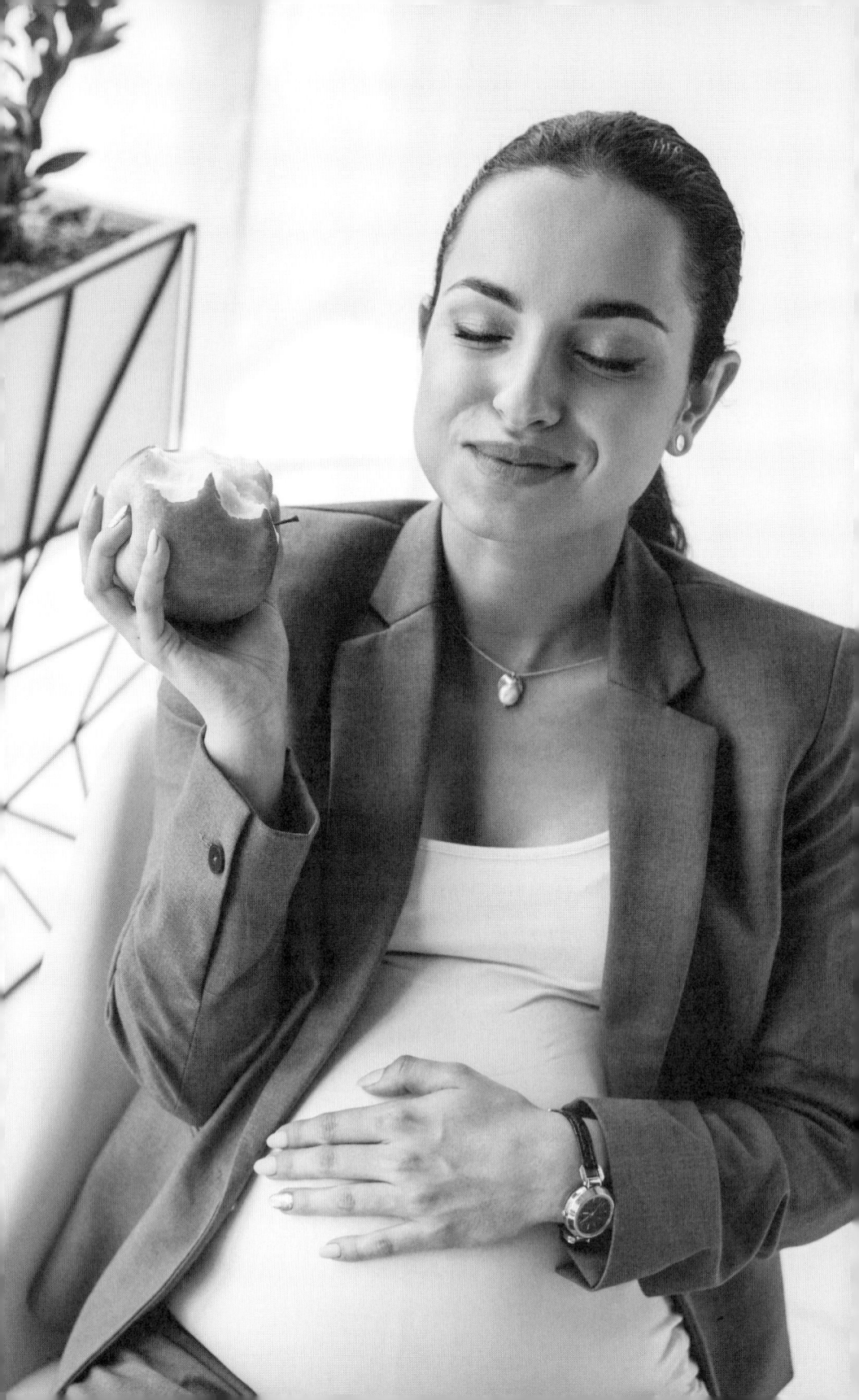

CHAPTER 9

Month 8
(Weeks 29 to 32)

YOUR BABY

➤ WEEK 29
The baby can stretch, kick, and make grasping motions. He or she reaches 2½ pounds this week.

> This week, your baby is about the size of a small butternut squash.

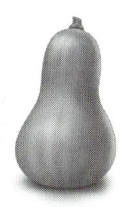

➤ WEEK 30
The eyes can open and close and sense changes in light. The baby's bone marrow is forming red blood cells. The baby also may have more hair on the head.

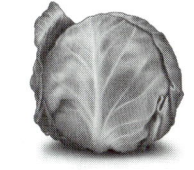

> This week, your baby is about the size of a cabbage.

➤ WEEK 31
Major development is finished, and the baby is gaining weight very quickly. He or she weighs almost 4 pounds. During the last 2½ months of pregnancy, the baby will grow another 3 to 4 inches in length and will double in weight. Your baby is going to need plenty of **nutrients** to finish growing.

> This week, your baby is about the size of a coconut.

➤ WEEK 32

The baby continues to form muscles. In boys, the **testicles** have begun to descend into the **scrotum**. This week, the fine hair that covered the baby's body (***lanugo***) begins to disappear. The baby is now almost 17 inches long.

> This week, your baby is about the size of a jicama, a potato-like vegetable.

YOUR PREGNANCY

Your Changing Body

You're reaching the homestretch of your pregnancy now. Most women find that they are more tired during the third ***trimester*** than they were during the second trimester. Feeling tired is normal at this stage of pregnancy. Your body is working hard to support a developing new life.

Your increasing size may make it difficult for you to find a comfortable sleeping position. Try to get as much rest as you can, even if it's a short nap during the day. Continue to exercise and eat well. Both will help boost your energy.

Discomforts and How to Manage Them

By this month, your **uterus** has expanded to midway between your belly button and your breasts. The size of your uterus may now be causing some unpleasant side effects.

Shortness of Breath

In these later weeks of pregnancy, you may have shortness of breath from time to time. Your uterus is now starting to take up more room in your belly, pressing the stomach and the diaphragm (a flat, strong muscle that aids in breathing) up toward the lungs. Although you may feel short of breath, your baby is still getting enough **oxygen**.

To help make breathing easier, move slowly and sit or stand up straight to give your lungs more room to expand. If there is a major change in your breathing or if you have a cough or chest pain, call your **obstetrician–gynecologist (ob-gyn)** right away.

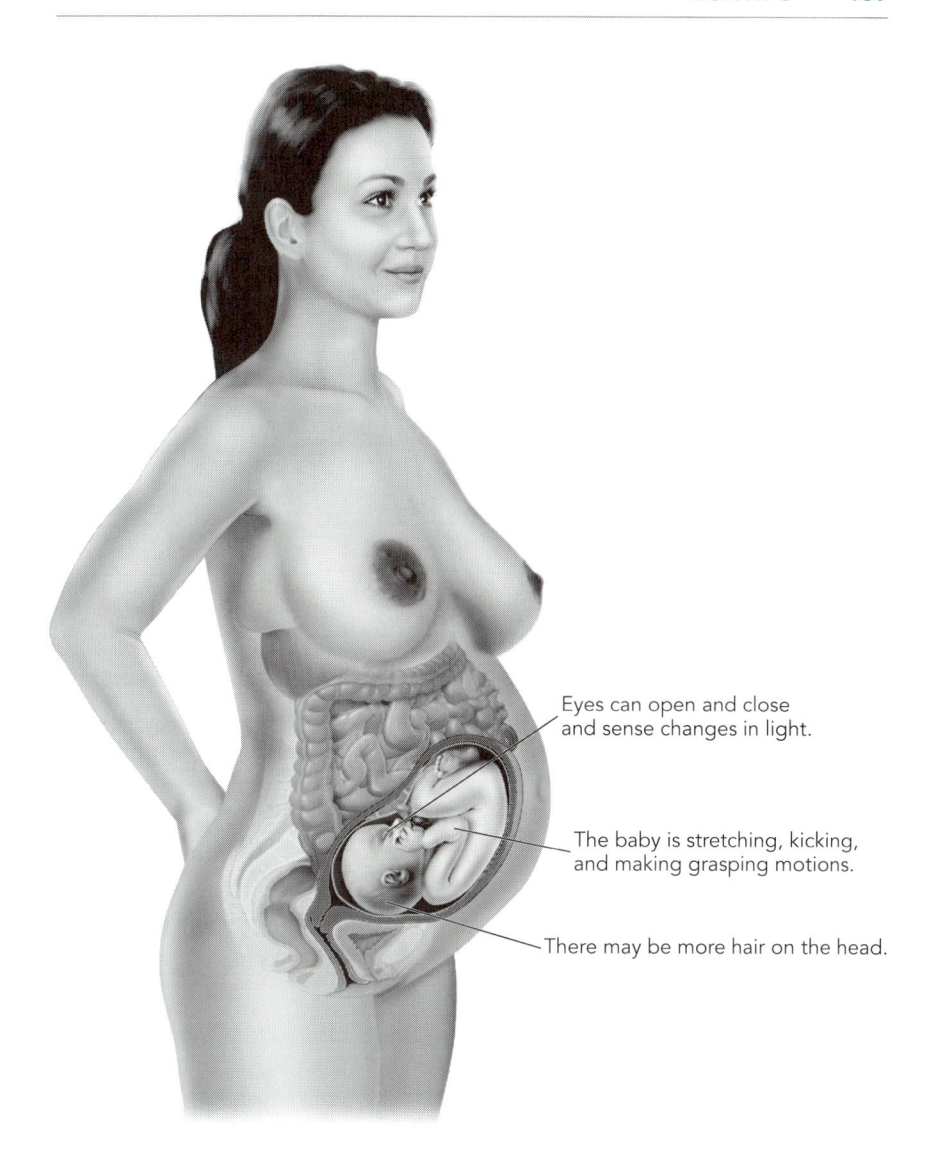

Eyes can open and close and sense changes in light.

The baby is stretching, kicking, and making grasping motions.

There may be more hair on the head.

Mother and baby: Weeks 29 to 32
By the end of week 32, the baby is almost 17 inches long and weighs a little more than 4 pounds.

Leg Cramps

Cramps in the lower legs are another common symptom in the second and third trimesters. You may experience sharp, painful cramps in your calves that can awaken you from a sound sleep. Experts are not sure what causes leg cramps late in pregnancy. The following tips may help:

- Stretch your legs before going to bed.

- If you get a cramp, flex your foot upward and then back down, which often brings immediate relief.

- Massage the calf in long downward strokes.

Varicose Veins and Leg Swelling

Many pregnant women develop *varicose veins*. They are caused by the weight of your uterus pressing down on a major vein. These veins also can appear near your *vagina*, *vulva*, and *rectum* (see the next section, "Hemorrhoids"). In most cases, varicose veins do not cause significant problems. They are more of a cosmetic issue.

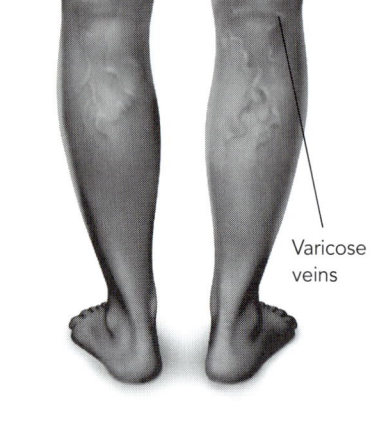

Varicose veins

Varicose veins are more likely to develop if you've been pregnant before. Varicose veins also tend to run in families. Although there is nothing you can do to prevent these sore and bulging veins, there are ways to relieve swelling and perhaps help stop them from getting worse:

Month 8: When to Call Your Ob-Gyn

- You have vaginal bleeding, a fever, severe abdominal pain, or a severe headache.

- You have a major change in your breathing, or you have a cough or chest pain.

- You have signs of **preeclampsia**, such as swelling of the face or hands, headache that will not go away, and trouble breathing (see Chapter 30, "Hypertension and Preeclampsia," for more signs and symptoms).

- You have signs of **preterm** labor, including a change in vaginal discharge, constant low backache, and frequent contractions (see the "Preterm Labor" section in this chapter).

- If you must sit or stand for long periods, be sure to move around often.
- Try to limit the time you sit with one leg crossed over another.
- Raise your legs and rest them on a couch, chair, or footstool as often as you can.
- Wear support hose that do not constrict at the thigh or knee.
- Do not wear stockings or socks that have a tight band of elastic around the legs.

Hemorrhoids

Pregnant women often have **hemorrhoids**—painful, itchy varicose veins in or around the **anus**. Hemorrhoids usually get worse right after delivery, then slowly get better during the **postpartum** period. Talk with your ob-gyn about using over-the-counter creams and suppositories. You also can try these tips for relief. Some of these tips may help you avoid the problem too:

- Eat a high-fiber diet and drink plenty of liquids to help avoid constipation.
- Keep your weight gain within the limits your ob-gyn suggests.
- Get up and move around to take weight off the veins of your pelvic area. Sitting for a long time puts pressure on these veins.
- Apply an ice pack or witch hazel pads to hemorrhoids. Witch hazel helps relieve pain and reduce swelling.
- Try soaking in a warm (not hot) tub a few times a day.

Itchy Skin

Some women find that their skin is very itchy during pregnancy, especially the skin over the belly and breasts. If you're bothered by itchy skin, try these tips:

- Drink plenty of fluids to stay hydrated.
- Apply a moisturizer to your skin in the morning and at night.
- Add cornstarch to your bath water.

If your itching is severe or you have a rash, talk with your ob-gyn. Some skin conditions that can happen during pregnancy should be treated.

Nutrition

It's important to stick to a healthy diet in these last weeks of pregnancy. Eating well will give you more energy and will ensure that your baby is getting the nutrients he or she needs. See Chapter 22, "Nutrition During Pregnancy."

Exercise

Even if you are feeling more tired, you should still try to keep up with your exercise routine (see Chapter 23, "Exercise During Pregnancy"). Monitor how you feel and stop if you are out of breath or feeling winded. Learning some relaxation techniques may be helpful as you count down these final weeks.

Relaxation Techniques

Relaxation techniques are a great way to help reduce the stress of pregnancy. These techniques also may help with anxiety you have about childbirth. Staying as calm as possible will help you conserve energy in the coming weeks. Learning some basic relaxation techniques can improve your health by

- slowing your heart rate
- lowering your blood pressure
- slowing your breathing rate
- increasing blood flow to major muscles
- reducing muscle tension

You may want to find a class in your neighborhood that teaches yoga or meditation. You also can find meditation DVDs to buy or rent from your library. Listening to music or getting a massage also are ways to relax. If you get a massage, be sure the massage therapist understands how to work with pregnant women. Whatever you do, make sure it calms you for some part of your day, especially when you're feeling most stressed.

Getting Ready for Delivery

Planning and making decisions may seem like all you are doing these days. But rest assured, planning can make your life less stressful. There is a lot you can do now to help labor and delivery go as smoothly as possible. This includes learning about the types of pain relief that are available and touring the hospital or birth center where you plan to give birth.

Checklist for Delivery

You should have the answers to the following questions well before your delivery day:

- Have I filled out all the paperwork needed to begin my maternity leave and collect disability pay?
- Do I need to register at the hospital before I check in for delivery? If so, have I done this?
- At what point in my labor should I leave for the hospital?
- Should I go straight to the hospital or call my ob-gyn's office first?
- What hospital number do I call if I have questions?
- Have I arranged for the care of my other children and pets while I'm in the hospital?
- When can family and guests visit me after I have the baby?
- What friends and family do we need to spread the news to once the baby arrives?
- Do I have their phone numbers or email addresses?
- Have I purchased a baby car seat, and do I know how to install it? Some hospitals offer a service to check that your car seat is installed correctly. Ask if this is available.

See Chapter 12, "Preparing for Birth," for a suggested packing list for the hospital.

Pain Relief During Labor

Now is a good time to think about whether you would like medications for pain relief during labor and delivery. You don't have to decide now, but it's good to know your options. Even if you do make a decision now, you may change your mind once you're in labor.

Each woman's labor experience is unique. No two women feel labor pain the same way. Also, if you've had a baby before, your pain may be different from the last time you were in labor. Pain depends on many factors, including

- the size and position of the baby
- the strength of contractions
- how you handle pain

Many women take classes to learn breathing and relaxation techniques to manage the pain of childbirth (see Chapter 13, "Pain Relief During Childbirth"). Some women use these techniques along with pain medications.

There are two types of pain-relieving drugs. An *analgesic* lessens pain. An *anesthetic* can block all feeling, including pain. Anesthesia can work in different ways:

- *Regional anesthesia* removes pain or sensation from certain parts of the body while you stay awake. **Epidural blocks** and **spinal blocks** are forms of *regional anesthesia*.

- *General anesthesia* creates a sleep-like state. You are not aware of your surroundings and feel no pain. General anesthesia usually is not used for vaginal births.

Not all hospitals and birth centers are able to offer all types of pain-relieving drugs. But at most facilities, an *anesthesiologist* will work with you and your health care team to choose the best method. See Chapter 13, "Pain Relief During Childbirth."

Childbirth Classes

Childbirth classes can teach you how to cope with pain and discomfort during labor and delivery. The most common classes—Lamaze, Bradley, and Read—are based on the theory that much of the pain of childbirth is caused by fear and tension. These childbirth classes focus on support, relaxation, paced breathing, and touch. See Chapter 13, "Pain Relief During Childbirth," for a description of childbirth preparation methods and tips on choosing a class.

You don't have to take childbirth classes. They are not a requirement for giving birth. Your labor nurses and ob-gyn will give you the instructions and information you need while you're at the hospital. If you do attend a childbirth class, you and your childbirth partner should practice the exercises you learn. This will help both of you remember them during labor.

Hospital Tour

Most hospitals offer tours of where you'll give birth. Take advantage of this opportunity if it's available. In fact, if you're taking childbirth classes at the hospital or birth center where you'll be giving birth, you may get a tour at some point during the course. If this will be your first time at the hospital, going for a tour also will give you a chance to learn the quickest route there and where to park the car when it's time for the birth. The tour also will give you a chance to ask the following:

- When your partner can be in the room during labor and delivery (even for **cesarean births**)
- Whether your partner can stay overnight in the room with you and the baby
- Whether your partner can take pictures or videos of the birth

See Chapter 13, "Pain Relief During Childbirth," for more information about making these decisions.

Prenatal Care Visits

During the third trimester, your ob-gyn should ask you to come in for more frequent checkups. These visits usually are

- every 2 weeks beginning at 32 weeks
- every week beginning at 36 weeks

Your ob-gyn should continue to check your weight and blood pressure and ask about any symptoms you may be experiencing.

Your ob-gyn also should check your baby's size and cardiac activity. A **pelvic exam** may be done to check whether your **cervix** has started preparing for birth.

Special Concerns

As in previous months, you should know the signs and symptoms of preterm labor. You also should be alert to the signs and symptoms of **prelabor rupture of membranes (PROM)**.

Preterm Labor

Preterm labor is still a problem to watch out for during this month of pregnancy. Babies born now usually have a better outcome than those who are born earlier. Call your ob-gyn right away if you notice signs of preterm labor, including

- change in vaginal discharge (watery, mucus-like, or bloody)
- increase in amount of vaginal discharge
- pelvic or lower abdominal pressure
- constant, low, dull backache
- mild abdominal cramps, with or without diarrhea
- ruptured membranes (your water breaks—either a gush or a trickle)

See Chapter 35, "When Labor Starts Too Soon: Preterm Labor, Prelabor Rupture of Membranes, and Preterm Birth."

Braxton Hicks contractions may intensify as you approach your due date. It's normal to have these contractions during the later stages of pregnancy. Be alert to how you are feeling and whether you have any of the symptoms above.

Prelabor Rupture of Membranes

In most cases, when your water breaks, it is followed by other signs of labor. When doctors talk about your water breaking, they are referring to the rupture of the **amniotic sac** that holds the amniotic fluid. When the sac ruptures at term but before labor begins, it is called prelabor rupture of membranes (PROM). When the sac ruptures before 37 weeks of pregnancy, it's called preterm PROM.

If you have any leakage of fluid from your vagina, you should contact your ob-gyn or go to the hospital. You will be examined to see if the amniotic sac has ruptured. PROM is confirmed when there is amniotic fluid in the vagina. Other reasons for fluid leakage may be cervical mucus, vaginal bleeding, or a vaginal infection.

Labor often starts after the amniotic sac ruptures. If the sac does not rupture and the pregnancy is at term, labor often is induced (see Chapter 14, "Labor Induction"). If the pregnancy is not at term, a decision needs to be made about whether to deliver the baby. See Chapter 35, "When Labor Starts Too Soon: Preterm Labor, Prelabor Rupture of Membranes, and Preterm Birth."

Activity Restriction and Bed Rest

Your ob-gyn may recommend that you be less active during the late stages of your pregnancy. He or she also may advise you to avoid certain activities, including sex. Activity restriction sometimes is recommended if you

- show signs of preterm labor
- are having a **multiple pregnancy**
- have **high blood pressure**

The American College of Obstetricians and Gynecologists (ACOG) cautions against bed rest in most cases. Sometimes bed rest is medically needed. But there is no scientific evidence that bed rest helps to prevent preterm birth. Also, bed rest can increase your risk of blood clots, bone weakening, and loss of muscle strength. It can mean you have to stop working earlier than you planned. If bed rest is recommended, talk with your ob-gyn about whether you need to stay in bed all the time or if you can do some forms of activity.

RESOURCES

Childbirth Education
www.icea.org
Website from the International Childbirth Education Association lets you search for childbirth classes or find educators or doulas in your area.

Hemorrhoids
https://medlineplus.gov/hemorrhoids.html
Webpage from the U.S. National Library of Medicine. Reviews the latest information on hemorrhoids and treatment.

Varicose Veins and Spider Veins
www.womenshealth.gov/a-z-topics/varicose-veins-and-spider-veins
Webpage from the U.S. Department of Health and Human Services. Explains what varicose veins are and how to manage them.

Your Pregnancy and Childbirth
www.acog.org/MyPregnancy
Website from the American College of Obstetricians and Gynecologists (ACOG) with information on pregnancy, labor, delivery, and postpartum care. Includes the latest information from the experts in women's health care, questions answered by ACOG ob-gyns, pregnancy stories from real women, and an A–Z directory of health topics covering pregnancy and beyond.

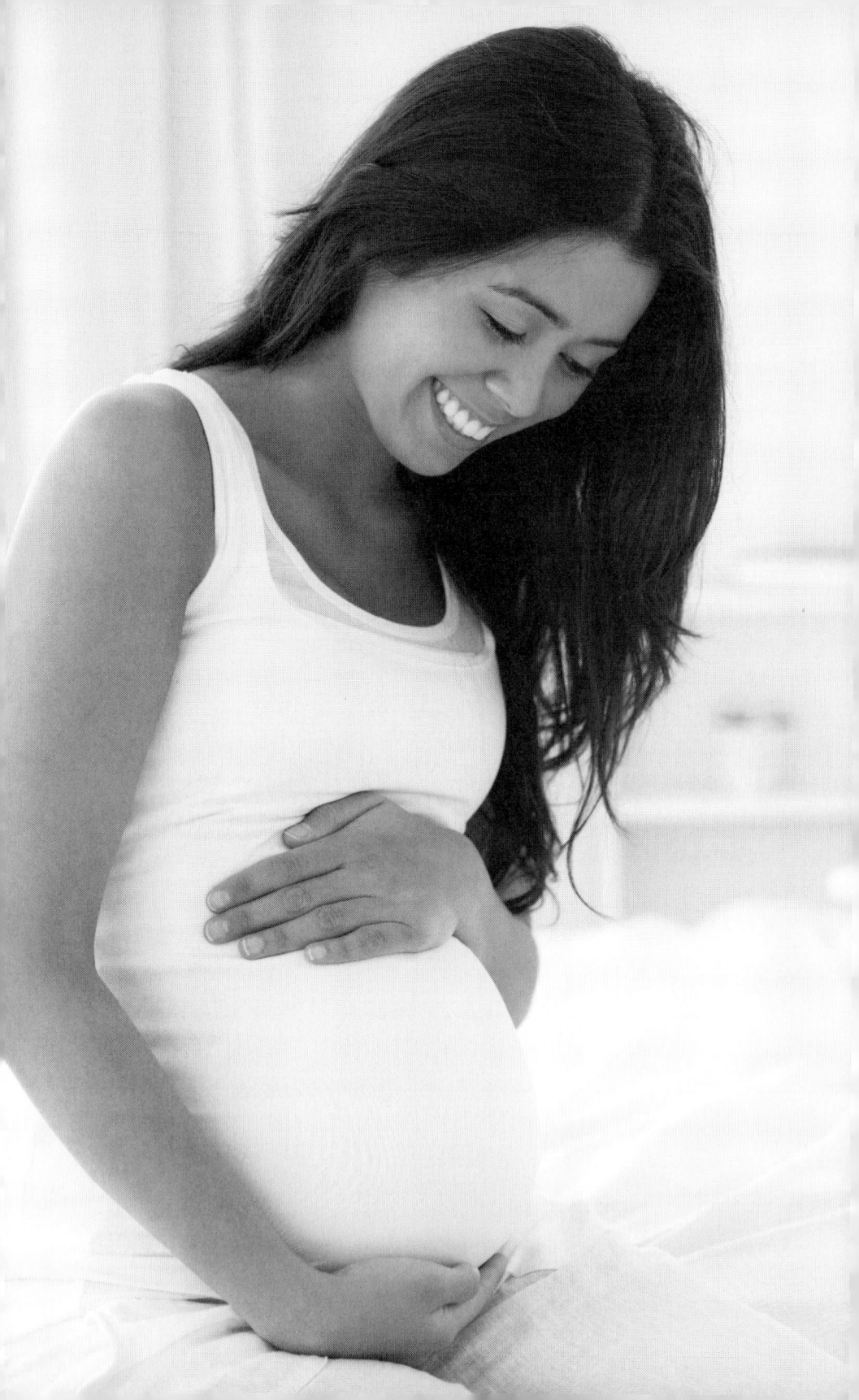

CHAPTER 10

Month 9
(Weeks 33 to 36)

YOUR BABY

▶ WEEK 33

The baby's brain is growing and developing rapidly. The bones harden, but the skull remains soft and flexible.

> This week, your baby is about the size of a small pineapple.

▶ WEEK 34

More fat is forming under the skin. The fingernails have grown to the end of the fingers. The baby weighs almost 5 pounds now.

> This week, your baby is about the size of a cantaloupe.

▶ WEEK 35

Your baby is now gaining about half a pound a week. Babies at this stage won't gain much more in length, but they will continue to put on weight. The limbs begin to look chubby.

> This week, your baby is about the size of a honeydew melon.

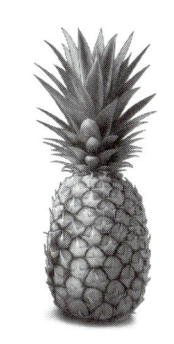

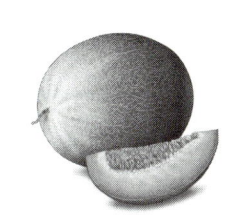

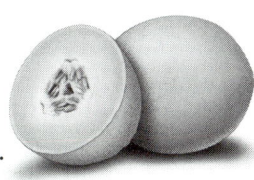

➤ WEEK 36

The skin is less wrinkled because of the fat that's been added underneath. During this week or the next, most babies turn to a head-down position for birth. The baby weighs about 6 pounds now.

> This week, your baby is about as long as a head of romaine lettuce.

YOUR PREGNANCY

Your Changing Body

During these weeks, you'll probably continue to feel tired and have trouble sleeping. Your **uterus** is putting more pressure on your lower body. You also may start to feel the baby "dropping" and settling into a deeper position in your pelvis this month. It's probably a busy time for you as you prepare your life, your home, and your family to welcome the new baby.

Discomforts and How to Manage Them

This month, the discomforts of pregnancy are likely at their peak. Remember to take care of yourself and get as much rest as you can during these last weeks.

Frequent Urination

In the final weeks of your pregnancy, you'll feel more pressure on your **bladder** as the baby moves deeper into your pelvis. You will urinate much more often during the day. You also may have to go several times during the night. Some women also leak urine during these later weeks, especially when laughing, coughing, sneezing, or even just with simple bending and lifting. This, too, is caused by the baby pressing on your bladder.

Braxton Hicks Contractions

As you near your due date, **Braxton Hicks contractions** may get stronger. You even may mistake them for labor contractions. It's easy to be fooled by these "practice" contractions. If you have contractions, time them. Note how long it is from the start of one contraction to the start of the next. Keep a record for an hour and jot down how your contractions feel. The time

MONTH 9 • 151

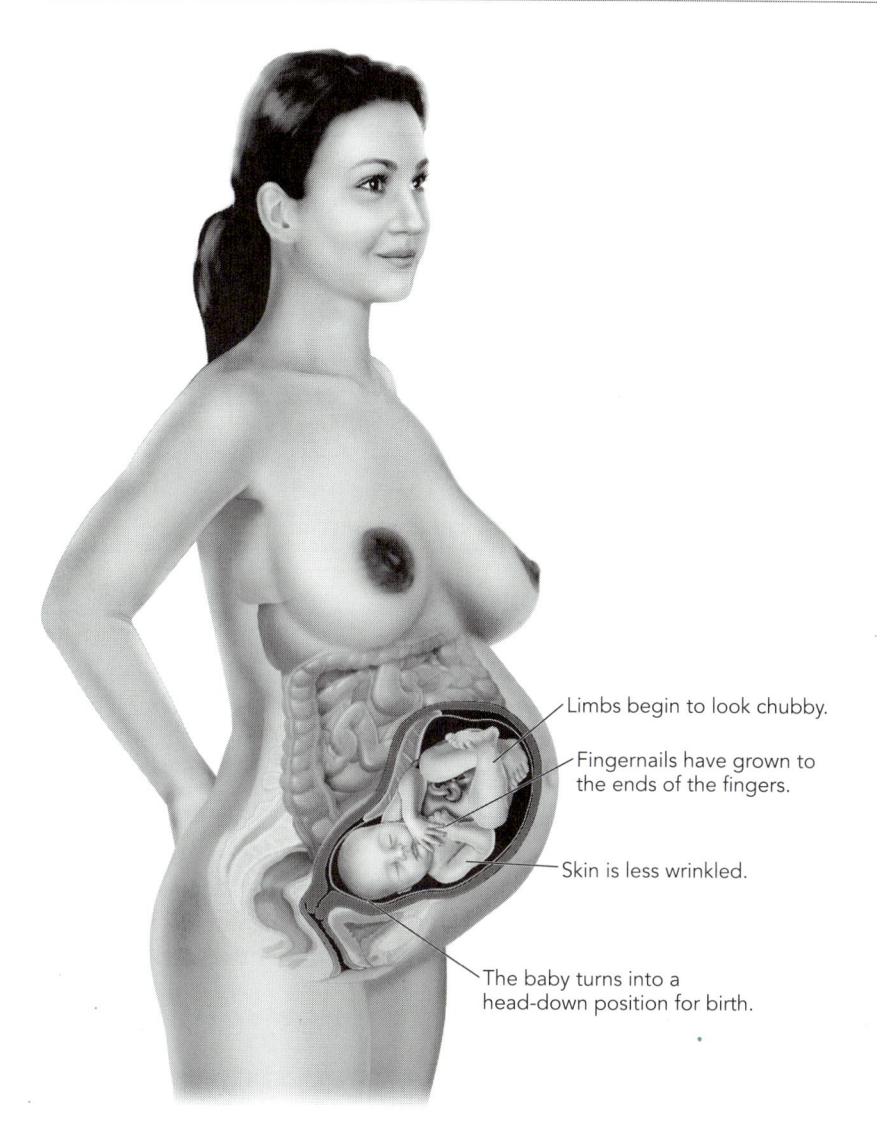

Limbs begin to look chubby.

Fingernails have grown to the ends of the fingers.

Skin is less wrinkled.

The baby turns into a head-down position for birth.

Mother and baby: Weeks 33 to 36
By the end of week 36, the baby is about 18 inches long and weighs a little more than 6 pounds.

between them will help tell you if you are truly in labor. When it's true labor, your contractions will

- come at regular intervals
- get closer together
- last 30 to 90 seconds

The intensity of the contractions also matters. It's more likely to be true labor if you have trouble walking and talking during a contraction.

No matter what your watch says about the timing of contractions, it's better to be safe. If you think you may be in labor, call your **obstetrician–gynecologist (ob-gyn)**. You may need to go to the office or hospital for a few hours for observation. A **pelvic exam** also may be done to see if your **cervix** is dilating (opening).

Trouble Sleeping

It's normal to have trouble sleeping again in the last few weeks of pregnancy. It's also normal for it to be almost impossible to find a comfortable position for sleep. Try not to worry about losing sleep. Make your bedroom as comfortable as possible. Use as many pillows as you need to prop yourself up to get support. Get a few hours of rest whenever you can.

Leg Swelling and Pain

Most pregnant women have some swelling in their legs and feet. Try not to stand for long periods of time. When sitting, prop up your legs on a pillow or use a footrest. Supportive shoes may help you feel more comfortable.

Pelvic Pressure

The baby will soon settle into a deeper position in your pelvis to get ready for birth. You may feel this settling as the baby "dropping" in your pelvis. When your baby drops, it can increase pressure in the pelvis, bladder, and hips. On the upside, you may feel less pressure against your diaphragm and lungs. There is not much you can do about the pressure other than try to stay off your feet when you are uncomfortable. Soaking in a warm bath may help. Bath water temperature should be no more than 100°F (37.8°C).

Numbness of Legs and Feet

Numbness and tingling in the hands and feet are normal in late pregnancy. Some women may develop **carpal tunnel syndrome**. This is discomfort in the hand caused by the compression of a nerve within the carpal tunnel, a passageway of bones and **ligaments** in the wrist. These symptoms usually go away after you give birth and the tissues return to normal. But if you have these symptoms, mention them to your ob-gyn. Wrist splints and resting the affected hand are often used to treat these symptoms during pregnancy.

Nutrition

Continue your healthy eating and make sure you are drinking plenty of water. Your baby needs lots of **nutrients** these last few weeks to fully mature and be ready for birth. You'll also need the energy that a healthy diet provides. See Chapter 22, "Nutrition During Pregnancy," for more on healthy eating in late pregnancy.

Exercise

Keep up with your exercise this month. Go for walks. Continue the strengthening and stretching exercises you learned early in your pregnancy. Avoid exercises where you will be flat on your back. Also avoid activities that increase your chance of falling and bumping your belly. See Chapter 23, "Exercise During Pregnancy," for more details on exercise.

You also can do yoga this month. Yoga will help with your breathing exercises once labor begins. Talk with a yoga instructor about which poses are safe for late pregnancy.

Getting Ready for Delivery

The last few weeks before delivery will be busy. Now is the time to shop for a car seat if you haven't done so already. You also should make sure that you have the clothes and supplies you'll need once the baby comes home. See Chapter 12, "Preparing for Birth," for checklists and tips that will help you prepare.

Packing for the Hospital

To help ease your transition from home to the hospital, pack a bag a few weeks before your due date. Leave the bag in a handy place, such as a hall closet or the trunk of your car. You can't pack everything ahead of time—you will need some things in the meantime, like glasses and slippers. Make a list of these last-minute items that need to be packed before you leave for the hospital. Put the list in a place that will trigger your memory, such as on top of the bag itself. Then you can grab the extra things on your way out.

Don't worry if you forget something. A friend or family member can bring you whatever you need. The hospital also may have some items, but you may be charged for them.

Preparing Your Home for the Baby

Wondering what you'll need when you bring your baby home? A trip to any baby supply retailer or a look at the many online baby supply websites will give you some ideas. Talk with other new moms to get an idea of what products they liked best. At a minimum, be sure you have:

- A crib for your baby to sleep in (see the "Safe Sleep" section in Chapter 12, "Preparing for Birth")
- A car seat (see "Buying a Car Seat" below)

This also is a great time to line up family and friends who can help when you and the baby are back at home. Don't be afraid to ask for help. You'll welcome an extra pair of hands once you're at home and spending some sleepless nights with the new baby. Make a list of some things you can use help with and ask family and friends to take their pick. Remember that you may need help for a few weeks, not just for a few days after the baby comes home.

Buying a Car Seat

You will not be able to take your newborn home from the hospital without a car seat secured in your car. All 50 states, the District of Columbia, and the Commonwealth of Puerto Rico have laws requiring child safety seats for babies and children at different ages.

All babies should ride in rear-facing car seats in the back seat starting with their first ride home from the hospital. In a rear-facing car seat, the baby is turned to face the back window of the car. There are several different types of car seats and many different manufacturers. Some communities and hospitals have programs for new parents to borrow an approved safety seat at no charge. But if your baby will routinely be in your car, you will need your own car seat.

Once you have the car seat, it's important to install it correctly. Even the best car seat won't protect your baby if it's not installed properly. Some fire departments will check the placement of your car seat. Some hospitals also will check to see if the car seat is installed correctly. Ask if your hospital has this service.

If your car seat is the type that detaches from a base that stays in the car, practice putting it in and out of the base to make sure you know how it is done before leaving the hospital. See Chapter 12, "Preparing for Birth," for information about choosing and installing a car seat.

Prenatal Care Visits

During this month, you'll have *prenatal care* appointments every 2 weeks. At these visits, your ob-gyn should

- check your weight, blood pressure, and urine
- measure the distance from your pubic bone to the top of your uterus (*fundal height*)
- check the baby's cardiac activity

Your ob-gyn also may

- estimate the baby's weight
- determine your baby's position in the uterus
- do a pelvic exam to see if your *cervix* is changing or opening in preparation for labor

Some women have extra tests at this point in their pregnancy to check on the health of the baby. These tests may be done if a problem develops during pregnancy or if you are at risk of *complications*. See Chapter 34, "Ultrasound Exams and Other Testing to Monitor Fetal Well-Being."

If you have not yet had the *tetanus toxoid, reduced diphtheria toxoid, and acellular pertussis (Tdap) vaccine*, you should get it between 27 and 36 weeks of pregnancy (see Chapter 25, "Protecting Yourself From Infections"). You also may need an *influenza* (flu) shot if you have not gotten one already.

Group B Streptococcus Screening

Group B streptococcus (GBS) is one of the many bacteria that live in the body. In women, GBS most often is found in the *vagina* and *rectum*. GBS usually does not cause problems in adults. But if GBS is passed from a woman to her baby during birth, the baby may get sick. This is rare and happens to 1 or 2 babies out of 100 when the mother does not receive treatment with *antibiotics* during labor. The chance of a newborn getting sick is much lower when the mother receives treatment.

Pregnant women have a screening test for GBS between 36 and 38 weeks of pregnancy as part of routine prenatal care. A swab is used to take a sample from the vagina and rectum. The sample is sent to a lab for testing.

If the results show that GBS is present, most women will receive antibiotics through an *intravenous (IV) line* once labor has started. The best time for treatment is during labor. This is done to help protect the baby from being infected.

You likely will have a GBS test during each pregnancy no matter what your test results were in a past pregnancy. In some cases, you automatically will be given antibiotics during labor without testing for GBS. Antibiotics may be given without testing if

- you had another child who had GBS disease
- you have GBS bacteria in your urine at any point during your pregnancy
- your GBS status is not known when you go into labor and you have a fever
- your GBS status is not known and you go into labor before 37 weeks
- your GBS status is not known and it has been 18 hours or more since your water broke
- your GBS status for this pregnancy is not known but you tested positive for GBS in a past pregnancy

Penicillin is the antibiotic that is most often given to prevent GBS disease in newborns. If you are allergic to penicillin, tell your ob-gyn before you are tested for GBS. You may have a skin test to determine the severity of your allergies. If needed, other antibiotics can be used.

If you are having a planned *cesarean delivery*, you do not need antibiotics for GBS during delivery as long as your labor has not started and your water has not broken. But you should still be tested for GBS because labor may happen before the planned delivery. If your test result is positive, your baby may need to be monitored for GBS disease after birth.

It's important for you to know your GBS test result. If you go into labor away from home, you can tell your caregivers if you need antibiotics during labor.

Other Screening Tests

You may have other screenings this month. Depending on your risk factors and state laws, your ob-gyn may repeat tests for

- *human immunodeficiency virus (HIV)*
- *syphilis*
- *chlamydia*
- *gonorrhea*

Discussions With Your Ob-Gyn

As you prepare for delivery, you may have questions for your ob-gyn about

- positions for labor and delivery
- where your baby will stay in the hospital
- feeding your baby

If you had a ***cesarean birth*** with another pregnancy, you may be interested in trying for a vaginal birth in this pregnancy. See Chapter 17, "Cesarean Delivery and Vaginal Birth After Cesarean Delivery," to learn about vaginal birth in women who have had cesarean births.

Positions for Labor and Childbirth

Thinking about what positions to use during labor and delivery? Discuss your ideas with your ob-gyn. He or she can help you learn what options are available at your hospital or birth center.

There are pros and cons with each type of birthing position. For example, birthing stools and chairs allow you to take advantage of gravity as the baby comes through the birth canal. But this position may make it hard for your ob-gyn to assist with the birth. Giving birth in a bed may make it easier for your ob-gyn to help you during delivery. But lying on your back or side doesn't allow gravity to do its work.

Think about all of your options and ask questions. In most cases, a labor nurse will be the one to help you into labor positions. You won't know which positions feel best to you until you are in labor. Don't get too attached to a specific method or position beforehand. Be open to changes once you get to the hospital or birth center. See Chapter 12, "Preparing for Birth," for a discussion of birthing positions.

Your Baby's Hospital Stay

Some hospitals and birth centers encourage "rooming-in." This means the baby stays in your room with you. Other hospitals and birth centers have a nursery that the baby can stay in for all or part of your hospital stay.

Rooming-in is a good way to get to know your new baby. It's also the best way to get started with breastfeeding. Having the baby nearby will help you learn his or her cues when it's time for feeding. But it's OK if the baby stays in the nursery so you can rest, especially if you have had a difficult labor. The baby will be brought to your room for feedings.

Be sure you know the options offered by your hospital. If you can room-in, you may want to have someone stay with you to help take care of the baby. See the "Your Baby's Hospital Stay" section in Chapter 12, "Preparing for Birth."

Feeding Your Baby

Deciding how to feed your new baby is a personal decision. Breastfeeding—feeding directly from the breast—works for some women. For others, feeding a baby pumped breast milk with a bottle is another very good option. Some women cannot or choose not to breastfeed or pump. These women feed their babies formula. Lastly, some women choose a combination of feeding methods.

Breast milk has the right amount of fat, sugar, water, protein, and minerals needed for a baby's growth and development. Breast milk also is easier to digest than formula. But not everyone is able to breastfeed or express milk, and some women choose not to breastfeed.

You may be unsure whether you can breastfeed, especially if you

- are taking medication
- have certain health conditions, such as **human immunodeficiency virus (HIV)** or another infectious disease
- are having more than one baby
- have had trouble breastfeeding in the past
- have had breast surgery
- have flat or inverted nipples
- are planning to go back to work soon after you give birth

In many situations, breastfeeding still is possible. Talk with your ob-gyn about your concerns. He or she can answer your questions and help you decide between breastfeeding, formula-feeding, or a combination of both. See Chapter 20, "Feeding Your Baby," for more detailed information about feeding options.

Many women wonder if there's anything they should do to get ready to breastfeed. Many hospitals offer breastfeeding classes taught by **international board-certified lactation consultants (IBCLCs)**. You also can ask how the hospital or birth center will support you while you and your baby learn to breastfeed. Your caregivers should show you how to breastfeed your baby. You should not be left on your own to learn the proper technique.

You also may look for a hospital or birth center with a Baby-Friendly® designation. Baby-Friendly designation means the facility has implemented specific steps to help women initiate breastfeeding. These facilities are audited to make sure they continue to meet the highest standards of education about breastfeeding.

You also can go online to the La Leche League International website. This organization aims to help mothers worldwide breastfeed. The American Academy of Pediatrics has a lot of information about breastfeeding, too. See the "Resources" section at the end of this chapter.

Finally, there are times when a woman cannot breastfeed, even with help and resources. If you can't breastfeed or you decide not to, it's OK. You will find the feeding method that is best for you, your baby, and your family.

Special Concerns

As you get closer to your due date, you should continue to be aware of the signs and symptoms that could indicate a problem, including **preterm** labor and **preeclampsia**.

Your baby should move to a head-down position about 3 or 4 weeks before your due date. If this does not happen and your baby's head is not pointing down, it is known as a **breech presentation**. If the baby does not turn, you will need to discuss a plan for delivery with your ob-gyn.

Preterm Labor

When labor starts before 37 weeks of pregnancy, it is called preterm labor. Preterm birth is a concern because babies who are born too early may not be fully developed. The risk of health problems is greatest for babies born before 34 weeks. But babies born between 34 and 37 weeks also are at risk of problems. The signs and symptoms of preterm labor include

- a change in vaginal discharge
- constant low backache
- frequent contractions

Call your ob-gyn right away if you think you are in preterm labor. See Chapter 35, "When Labor Starts Too Soon: Preterm Labor, Prelabor Rupture of Membranes, and Preterm Birth," for a longer list of the symptoms of preterm labor.

Preeclampsia

Preeclampsia is another concern that you should be aware of. It is most common in the third **trimester**, but it can happen any time after 20 weeks of pregnancy. It also can develop during the **postpartum** period.

> ### Month 9: When to Call Your Ob-Gyn
>
> - You have vaginal bleeding, a fever, severe abdominal pain, or a severe headache.
> - You have a major change in your breathing, or you have a cough or chest pain.
> - You have signs of preeclampsia, such as swelling of the face or hands, headache that will not go away, and trouble breathing (see Chapter 30, "Hypertension and Preeclampsia," for more signs and symptoms).
> - You have signs of preterm labor, such as a change in vaginal discharge, constant low backache, and frequent contractions (see Chapter 35, "When Labor Starts Too Soon: Preterm Labor, Prelabor Rupture of Membranes, and Preterm Birth," for more signs and symptoms).

It is important to know the signs and symptoms or preeclampsia (see the box "Month 9: When to Call Your Ob-Gyn"). If you have symptoms, call your ob-gyn right away. See Chapter 30, "Hypertension and Preeclampsia," for more details about preeclampsia symptoms and treatment.

Breech Presentation

Most babies move into a head-down position a few weeks before birth. This is called a ***cephalic presentation***. If the baby's buttocks, or buttocks and feet, are positioned to come out first, this is called a breech presentation.

During the last weeks of your pregnancy, you will have a physical exam to find out the baby's position. Your ob-gyn will place his or her hands on your belly to feel the outline of the baby. This exam will help locate the baby's head, back, and buttocks. If your ob-gyn thinks the baby is breech, an ***ultrasound exam*** may be done to be sure.

The baby's position can still change until the end of pregnancy. Your ob-gyn may not know for sure if your baby is still in a breech presentation until labor starts.

Sometimes a baby who is breech can be turned into a head-down position. This is done using a technique called ***external cephalic version (ECV)***. With ECV, your ob-gyn presses firmly on your belly to try to turn the baby inside the uterus. There is a risk of complications with ECV.

If there is only one baby and he or she is still breech by your due date, a planned cesarean delivery is the most common and safest option. But a vaginal delivery may be possible in certain situations. See Chapter 16, "Assisted Vaginal Delivery and Breech Presentation," for information about what to expect if your baby is breech.

RESOURCES

Baby-Friendly USA
www.babyfriendlyusa.org
Website that offers a "For Parents" page to help you find a facility with the Baby-Friendly designation.

Car Seats and Booster Seats
www.nhtsa.gov/equipment/car-seats-and-booster-seats
Webpage from the National Highway Traffic Safety Administration. Offers information on choosing the right car seat, installing it correctly, and keeping your child safe.

Group B Strep International
www.groupbstrepinternational.org
Group B Strep International promotes awareness and prevention of GBS infection in babies before birth through early infancy.

La Leche League International
www.llli.org
Provides information and support for breastfeeding women. Offers referrals to local support groups.

Where We Stand: Car Seats For Children
www.healthychildren.org/English/safety-prevention/on-the-go/Pages/Where-We-Stand-Car-Seats-For-Children.aspx
Information from the American Academy of Pediatrics. Provides the latest recommendations for car seat safety and gives tips about shopping for and installing car seats.

Your Pregnancy and Childbirth
www.acog.org/MyPregnancy
Website from the American College of Obstetricians and Gynecologists (ACOG) with information on pregnancy, labor, delivery, and postpartum care. Includes the latest information from the experts in women's health care, questions answered by ACOG ob-gyns, pregnancy stories from real women, and an A–Z directory of health topics covering pregnancy and beyond.

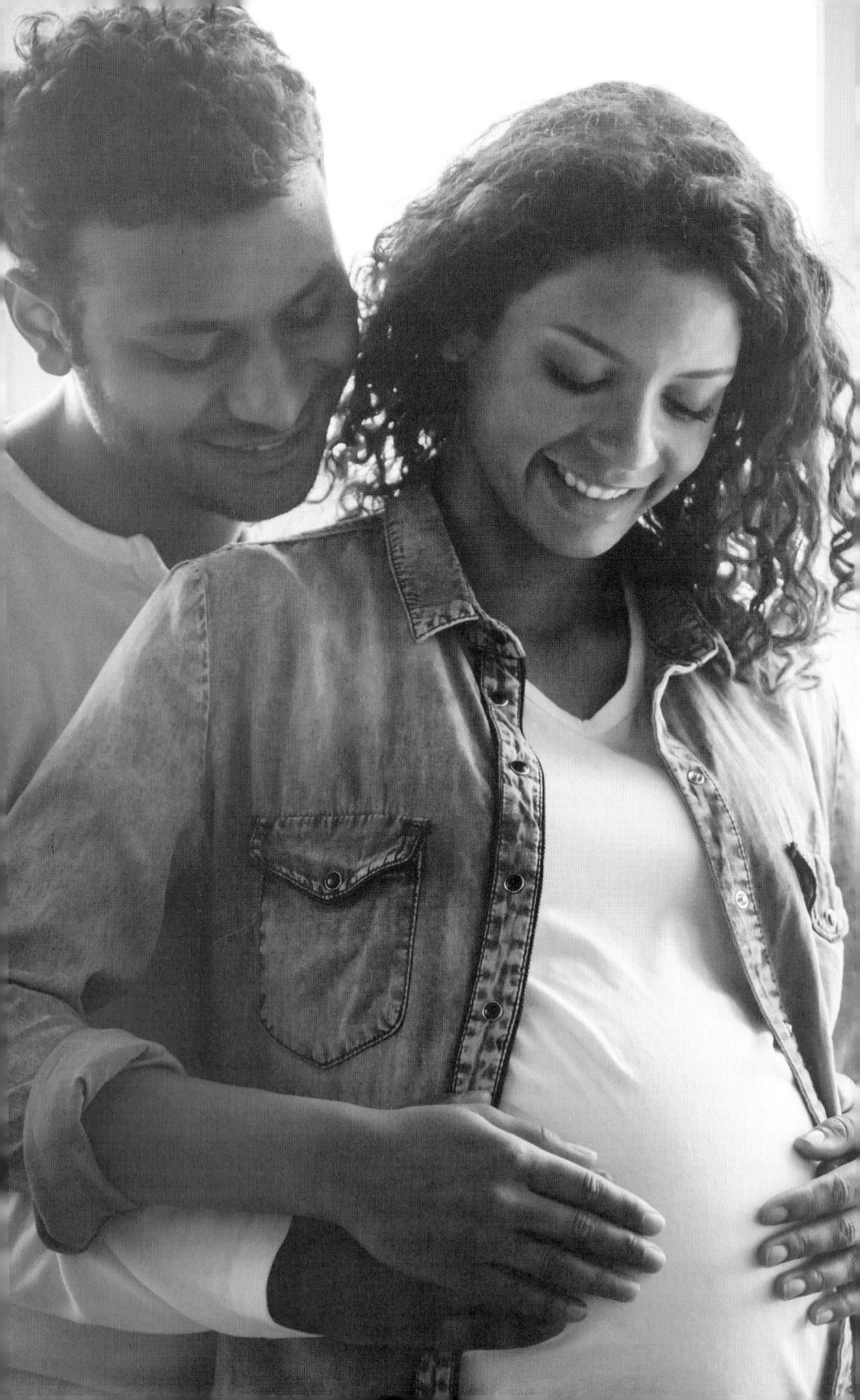

CHAPTER 11

Month 10
(Weeks 37 to 40)

YOUR BABY

▶ WEEK 37

The lungs continue to develop. So do the brain and nervous system. The circulatory system is complete, and so is the musculoskeletal system. At this stage, your pregnancy is considered to be **early term**. But babies who are born now have not yet finished developing and need more time.

> This week, your baby is about as long as a bunch of Swiss chard.

▶ WEEK 38

The baby may weigh 7 pounds now and may be nearly 20 inches long. The **lanugo** (body hair) that covered the baby has mostly been shed. Your baby is no longer growing much in length, but fat is still being added all over to keep your baby warm after birth. The baby is taking up a lot of space in the **amniotic sac**. There's not much room for rolling around and turning. You should continue to feel kicks and movement.

> This week, your baby is about as long as a leek.

➤ WEEK 39

At 39 weeks of pregnancy, your baby is considered to be *full term*. After birth, the lungs and brain continue to develop. The brain completes its growth when your child is about 2 years old.

> This week, your baby is about the size of a mini watermelon.

➤ WEEK 40

Now between 7½ and 8 pounds, the baby is ready to be born. By now, the baby's head may have dropped lower into position in your pelvis. Remember that your *estimated due date (EDD)* is only a rough idea for when your baby will be born. Only 1 in 20 women give birth on their EDD. Most women go into labor within about 2 weeks of their due dates—either before or after.

> This week, your baby is the size of a small pumpkin.

YOUR PREGNANCY

Your Changing Body

You've nearly reached the end of your pregnancy! This month, your *uterus* will finish expanding. The uterus has grown from about 2 ounces before you were pregnant to about 2½ pounds now.

You may be getting bored with just waiting for the baby to come. Or you may be keyed up and anxious. Try to keep your mind off the waiting. Staying active will help the days pass more quickly. Now is also the time to do last-minute things that can help prepare you, your family, and your home for the new baby (see the box "Things to Do This Month to Get Ready").

Having Sex

Unless your *obstetrician–gynecologist (ob-gyn)* has told you otherwise, it may be OK to have sex right up to the time you give birth. Talk with your partner about sexual activity that is comfortable for you.

MONTH 10 • 165

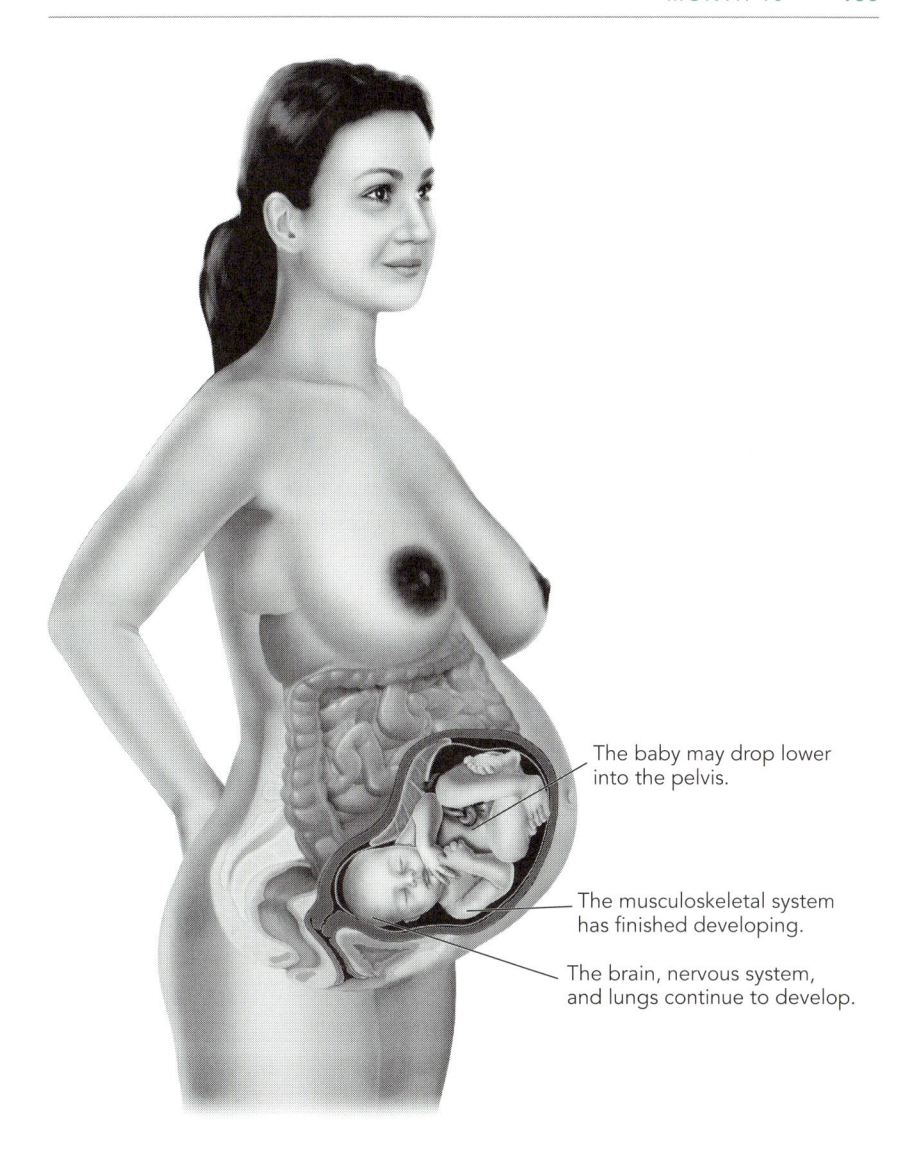

The baby may drop lower into the pelvis.

The musculoskeletal system has finished developing.

The brain, nervous system, and lungs continue to develop.

Mother and baby: Weeks 37 to 40
By the end of week 40, the baby is 20 inches long and may weigh 7½ to 8 pounds. The baby is now ready to be born.

Nesting

Many women approaching their due dates feel a strong urge to complete work projects and organize the house for the baby. This urge is known as the "nesting instinct." If the nesting urge strikes, go ahead and do what you need to do in order to satisfy your feelings. But remember not to overdo it, and don't exhaust yourself. Ask for help. Conserve your energy for labor, delivery, and caring for the baby.

Discomforts and How to Manage Them

At this stage, walking is an effort, and lying down is not much better. Many women report sleepless nights during the last few weeks. It may be difficult to get in and out of the car.

Frequent Urination

The uterus is bigger now than it has ever been and it is pressing much more on your **bladder**. This likely is causing many trips to the bathroom throughout the day. But don't cut back on drinking liquids during this time. Your body needs the fluids more than ever.

Things to Do This Month to Get Ready

- Put a waterproof sheet or mattress cover on your bed. This will protect it in case your water breaks during the night.
- Wash and organize the baby's clothes. Some people advise leaving the tags on and only washing them if you're sure your baby is going to need them. You may want to wait if you think you will be returning baby clothes to the store. You can always donate any clothes that you don't end up using.
- Line up family and friends who can help after the baby comes home. Make sure everyone knows what they should do and when they should do it. You may want to make a schedule to see on what days you may be short-handed. This also helps avoid an overload of people on any one day. Also, keep in mind that you still may need helpers a few weeks after the birth, not just in the first few days.
- Prepare meals that can be frozen and defrosted easily. Soups, stews, and casseroles are great to have on hand and easy to microwave when needed.
- Keep a journal. You may want to write down your thoughts and feelings as you get ready for the birth. Your child may enjoy reading your journal later, and you'll have a record of how you felt during this special time.

Snoring

If your partner says you've been snoring more than usual, blame it on normal changes in breathing during pregnancy. If your snoring is a real problem, try sleeping with nasal strips across the bridge of your nose. A humidifier in your bedroom also may help. But you should talk with your ob-gyn about snoring because it could be a sign of ***obstructive sleep apnea***.

Nausea

Sometimes mild nausea comes back in the final weeks of pregnancy. You may feel better eating four or five small meals during the day instead of three big ones. If mild nausea is a problem for you, try to eat bland foods, such as the BRATT diet (banana, rice, applesauce, tea, and toast). Remember to keep eating throughout the day. You and the baby will need the energy to cope with labor and birth. If nausea is severe or persistent, call your ob-gyn.

Vaginal Spotting

If you have light spotting between 37 and 40 weeks, it could be a sign that labor is starting. Pink or slightly bloody vaginal discharge may be caused by

- the ***cervix*** starting to dilate (open)
- the loosening of the thick mucus plug that seals off the cervix during pregnancy

If vaginal bleeding is heavy—as heavy as a normal ***menstrual period***—it could be a sign of a problem. Call your ob-gyn and go to the hospital right away if you have heavy bleeding.

Exercise

Exercise this month may be a challenge. Now is a good time for you and your partner to practice the breathing exercises you learned in childbirth class.

Preparing for Delivery

Telling real labor from false labor often is difficult. When do you go to the hospital? What can you eat if you think you're in labor? These are common questions many women ask during these final weeks. While you probably don't know exactly when you'll go into labor, you can make sure you're ready when it arrives.

Knowing When You're in Labor

Braxton Hicks contractions can happen for many weeks before real labor begins. These "practice" contractions can be very painful and can make you think you are in labor when you are not. There are certain changes in your body that signal real labor is near:

Month 10: When to Call Your Ob-Gyn

Call your ob-gyn if you notice any of these signs:

- You have vaginal discharge that is watery, bloody, or mucus-like.
- Your water breaks—either a gush or a trickle.
- You have pain or cramps in your back or pelvis, similar to menstrual cramps.
- You have contractions that happen in a regular pattern and get closer together over time.

Go to the hospital if you have any of these symptoms:

- You have a fever or a severe headache.
- There is a major change in your breathing, or you have a cough or chest pain.
- You have severe or persistent nausea.
- You are bleeding heavily from the vagina (other than bloody mucus or spotting).
- You have constant, severe pain. Contractions should have some relief between them.
- You notice the baby is moving less often.

Call your ob-gyn right away if you notice any signs of preeclampsia:

- Swelling of the face or hands
- A headache that will not go away
- Seeing spots or changes in eyesight
- Pain in the upper abdomen (near your ribs) or shoulder
- Nausea and vomiting (in the second half of pregnancy)
- Sudden weight gain
- Trouble breathing

- Lightening—You feel as if the baby has dropped lower. Because the baby isn't pressing on your diaphragm, you may feel "lighter." The baby's head settles deep into your pelvis. Lightening can happen anywhere from a few weeks to a few hours before labor begins.
- Loss of the mucus plug—A thick mucus plug forms at the cervix during pregnancy. When the cervix begins to dilate (open) several days before labor begins or at the start of labor, the plug is pushed into the **vagina**. You may notice an increase in vaginal discharge that's clear, pink, or slightly bloody. Some women expel the entire mucus plug.
- Rupture of membranes—The fluid-filled amniotic sac that surrounded the baby during pregnancy breaks (your "water breaks"). You may feel this as fluid that trickles or gushes from your **vagina**. Call your ob-gyn if your water breaks and follow his or her instructions. Once your water breaks, your ob-gyn will want to make sure labor begins soon if it hasn't already.
- Contractions—As your uterus contracts, you may feel pain in your back or pelvis. This pain may be similar to menstrual cramps. Labor contractions happen in a regular pattern and get closer together over time.

How can you tell the difference between "real" labor contractions and Braxton Hicks contractions? Time the contractions and note whether they go away when you move around. See Table 11-1, "Differences Between False Labor and True Labor."

If you think you are in labor, call your ob-gyn. You should go to the hospital if you have any of these signs:

- Your water has broken and you are not having contractions.
- You are bleeding heavily from the vagina.
- You have constant, severe pain with no relief between contractions.
- You notice the baby is moving less often.

When to Go to the Hospital

During the final weeks, you and your partner will likely wonder when the time is right to go to the hospital. It will depend mostly on the timing and intensity of your contractions or whether your water breaks. Your ob-gyn should give you clear instructions as you get close to your due date. Follow these instructions exactly.

When signs of labor start, you may be able to call your ob-gyn's office to talk about what you are feeling. This may help you decide when to head for the hospital.

TABLE 11-1 **Differences Between False Labor and True Labor**

Symptom	False Labor	True Labor
Timing of contractions	Contractions are not regular. They do not get closer together. These are called Braxton Hicks contractions.	Contractions come at regular intervals. As time goes on, they get closer together. Each lasts about 60 to 90 seconds.
Change with movement	Contractions may stop when you walk or rest. They also may stop with a change of position.	Contractions continue even when you rest or move around.
Strength of contractions	Contractions are weak and do not get much stronger. They may start strong and then weaken.	Contractions steadily get stronger.
Frequency of contractions	Contractions are irregular and do not have a pattern.	Contractions have a pattern.
Location of pain	Pain usually is felt only in the front.	Pain usually starts in the back and moves to the front.

Eating During Labor

Your ob-gyn or the hospital may have rules about eating and drinking during labor. You need to know these policies before your labor starts. Be sure to ask at one of your prenatal visits. Here are the latest guidelines from the American College of Obstetricians and Gynecologists (ACOG):

- Women with a healthy pregnancy can have small amounts of clear liquids during labor. Clear liquids include water, fruit juices without pulp, carbonated beverages, tea, and low-sugar sports drinks.

- Eating solid foods at the hospital will not be allowed. Solid food is restricted in case the situation changes and you need to have a **cesarean birth**. Cesarean birth often requires **anesthesia**, and you cannot eat before having anesthesia.

- Women with a planned cesarean birth should not eat any solid food for 6 to 8 hours before surgery. Your ob-gyn or hospital may allow some clear liquids up to 2 hours before surgery.

Prenatal Care Visits

You likely will see your ob-gyn once a week this month until you go into labor. Your weight, blood pressure, and uterus size will be measured just as they were last month. The baby's position will be checked. You will be asked about the baby's movements. Your cervix may be checked to see if it has started preparing for labor.

Also, if you were not screened for **group B streptococcus (GBS)** last month, you will be this month. Pregnant women have a screening test for GBS between 36 and 38 weeks of pregnancy as part of routine **prenatal care**. See the "Group B Streptococcus Screening" section of Chapter 10, "Month 9 (Weeks 33 to 36)," for more information about GBS.

Discussions With Your Ob-Gyn

A ***full term*** pregnancy is one that is 39 weeks and 0 days through 40 weeks and 6 days. If problems develop during pregnancy, delivery before 39 weeks may be needed. This may be done with **labor induction** or cesarean birth. Some medical reasons for delivery before 39 weeks include

- health problems, such as **gestational diabetes** or **high blood pressure**
- **placenta** problems, such as **placenta previa** or **placental abruption**
- problems with the baby, such as poor growth or certain **birth defects**
- a lack of **amniotic fluid**
- **preeclampsia** or **eclampsia**
- **prelabor rupture of membranes (PROM)**
- infection of the uterus
- scarring of the uterus from a past surgery, such as caesarean birth or surgery to remove **fibroids**

Women carrying more than one baby also may need to deliver before 39 weeks.

Babies born before 39 weeks are at risk of health problems. If an early delivery is recommended, it usually means that the risks of continuing the pregnancy are greater than the risks of an early birth. See Chapter 14, "Labor Induction," and Chapter 17, "Cesarean Delivery and Vaginal Birth After Cesarean Delivery."

Elective Delivery

An **elective delivery** is done for a nonmedical reason. Women have different reasons for choosing an elective delivery. These reasons might include

- wanting to schedule the birth on a specific date
- living far from the hospital and wanting to be certain when to go there
- discomfort in the last weeks of pregnancy

What Do the Terms Mean?

When ob-gyns talk about the length of pregnancy, they refer to weeks and days.

- **Early term:** The period from 37 weeks and 0 days through 38 weeks and 6 days.
- **Full term:** The period from 39 weeks and 0 days through 40 weeks and 6 days.
- **Late term:** The period from 41 weeks and 0 days through 41 weeks and 6 days.
- **Postterm:** The period greater than or equal to 42 weeks and 0 days.

If you are having a healthy pregnancy, you should wait to deliver your baby until at least 39 weeks of pregnancy (see the box "Why Wait Until 39 Weeks?"). If you decide to have an elective delivery, your ob-gyn should carefully review your records to be reasonably sure that you have reached 39 weeks. Keep in mind that some facilities do not have the resources to support labor induction or cesarean birth.

New research suggests that for some healthy women, inducing labor at 39 weeks may reduce the risk of

- cesarean birth
- preeclampsia
- *gestational hypertension*

These findings apply only if

- this is your first pregnancy
- you are carrying only one baby
- you and your baby are both healthy

If you aren't sure whether you want an elective delivery but you foresee problems with waiting for your labor to start naturally, it may help to think about your other options. If you live far away from the hospital, you might want to stay with someone who lives closer. You also may be able to travel to the hospital when you are in very early labor. Talk with your ob-gyn about your options.

Why Wait Until 39 Weeks?

If you are having a healthy pregnancy and there are no **complications**, you should wait to deliver your baby until your pregnancy has reached full term—39 weeks and 0 days or later.

- As you know, babies grow and develop throughout the entire 40 weeks of pregnancy. For example, the brain, liver, and lungs are among the last organs to mature. They aren't fully developed before 39 weeks of pregnancy.

- Babies who are born even a little before 39 weeks may not be as fully developed as those who are born after 39 weeks of pregnancy. These babies may have an increased risk of short-term and long-term health problems. Some of these problems can be serious and lifelong.

- Babies who are not fully developed may need extra care. They may have problems breathing or eating. They may have **anemia** or **jaundice**. These babies may need to spend time in a neonatal intensive care unit (NICU).

- The earlier a baby is born, the higher the risks of health problems and the more severe they are likely to be.

Cesarean Delivery on Request

Some women ask for a **cesarean delivery** even though there is no medical reason it must be done. This type of delivery is known as cesarean delivery on request.

If you are thinking about requesting a cesarean delivery, you and your ob-gyn should discuss whether it is right for you. A cesarean delivery is major surgery. Like all surgeries, it has risks, including

- heavy bleeding
- infection
- injury to the bowel or bladder
- problems with **anesthesia**
- longer recovery time than vaginal delivery

Cesarean delivery also increases risks for future pregnancies, including

- placenta problems
- rupture of the uterus
- **hysterectomy**

For these reasons, cesarean delivery on request is not recommended for women who plan to have more children.

Having a cesarean delivery before 39 weeks of pregnancy increases health risks for newborns. Babies who are born even a few weeks early may not be as developed as those who are born after 39 weeks of pregnancy. Babies born before 39 weeks may have an increased risk of short-term and long-term health problems, including

- *anemia*
- *jaundice*
- breathing problems
- feeding difficulties
- hearing and vision problems
- learning and behavioral issues in childhood

Babies born before 39 weeks also are more likely to spend time in a **neonatal intensive care unit (NICU).** When there is no medical reason to do so, having a planned cesarean delivery before 39 weeks of pregnancy is not recommended and may not be offered at certain hospitals. See Chapter 17, "Cesarean Delivery and Vaginal Birth After Cesarean Delivery."

Late Term and Postterm Pregnancy

A *late term* pregnancy is one that is 41 weeks and 0 days through 41 weeks and 6 days. A *postterm* pregnancy is one that is 42 weeks or longer. Postterm pregnancy is more likely when

- this is a woman's first pregnancy
- the woman has had a postterm pregnancy before
- the baby is a boy
- the woman is overweight

Another reason for a postterm pregnancy is an inaccurate due date. But this is less likely if you have an *ultrasound exam* that confirms your due date.

One technique that reduces the chances of having a postterm pregnancy is "stripping the membranes." To do this, your ob-gyn sweeps a gloved finger over the thin membranes that connect the *amniotic sac* to the wall of your uterus. This also is called "sweeping the membranes." This action is done when the cervix is partially dilated. It may cause your body to release natural *prostaglandins*, which soften the cervix more and may start contractions.

If your due date has come and gone, your ob-gyn should check your baby's health. If labor doesn't start on its own by 41 or 42 weeks, you and your ob-gyn may talk about labor induction.

Risks of Late Term and Postterm Pregnancy

When a pregnancy goes longer than 40 weeks, it can increase health risks for a woman and her baby. These risks include the following:

- After 42 weeks, the *placenta* may not work as well as it did earlier in pregnancy.
- As the baby grows, the amount of amniotic fluid may begin to decrease. Less fluid may cause the *umbilical cord* to be pinched as the baby moves or as the uterus contracts.
- The baby can grow larger than normal, which can complicate a vaginal delivery.
- Postterm pregnancy doubles the pregnant woman's risk of needing a cesarean delivery.

Despite these risks, most women who give birth after their due dates have healthy babies. When a baby is not born by the due date, certain tests can help monitor the baby's health. Some tests, such as a *kick count*, can be done on your own at home. Others are done in the ob-gyn's office or in the hospital. These tests include

- *nonstress test*
- *biophysical profile (BPP)*
- checking the level of amniotic fluid
- *contraction stress test*

See Chapter 34, "Ultrasound Exams and Other Testing to Monitor Fetal Well-Being," for descriptions of these tests.

Deciding to Induce Labor

Labor induction is the use of medication or other methods to start labor. Whether your labor will be induced depends on

- your health and your baby's health
- how far you are in your pregnancy
- whether your cervix has begun to soften and open
- results of tests to check your baby's health

To prepare for labor and delivery, the cervix begins to soften, thin out (*effacement*), and open (*dilation*). Your ob-gyn should do a *pelvic exam* in the last few weeks of pregnancy to see if your cervix has started these changes. There are several methods to start labor if it has not started naturally. These methods include

- ripening the cervix
- stripping or sweeping the membranes
- taking *oxytocin*
- rupturing the *amniotic sac*

See Chapter 14, "Labor Induction," for details on these ways of starting labor.

RESOURCES

40 Reasons to Go to the Full 40
www.health4mom.org/zones/go-the-full-40
Website from the Association of Women's Health, Obstetric and Neonatal Nurses explains why babies need a full 40 weeks of pregnancy to grow and develop.

Why at Least 39 Weeks Is Best for Your Baby
www.marchofdimes.com/pregnancy/why-at-least-39-weeks-is-best-for-your-baby.aspx
Website from the March of Dimes that explains why healthy babies need at least 39 weeks of development.

Your Pregnancy and Childbirth
www.acog.org/MyPregnancy
Website from the American College of Obstetricians and Gynecologists (ACOG) with information on pregnancy, labor, delivery, and postpartum care. Includes the latest information from the experts in women's health care, questions answered by ACOG ob-gyns, pregnancy stories from real women, and an A–Z directory of health topics covering pregnancy and beyond.

Month 10

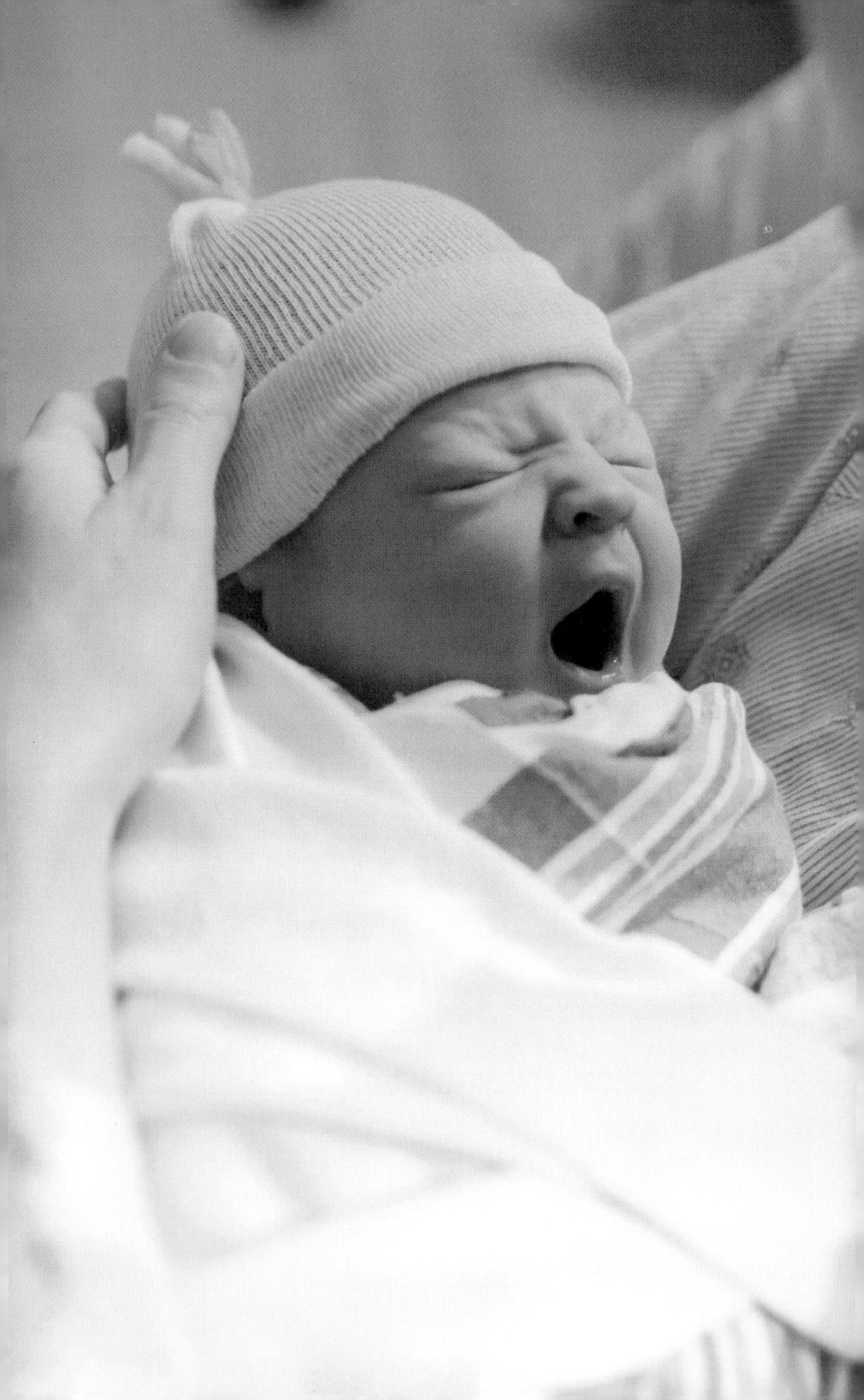

PART 2

Getting Ready for Labor and Delivery

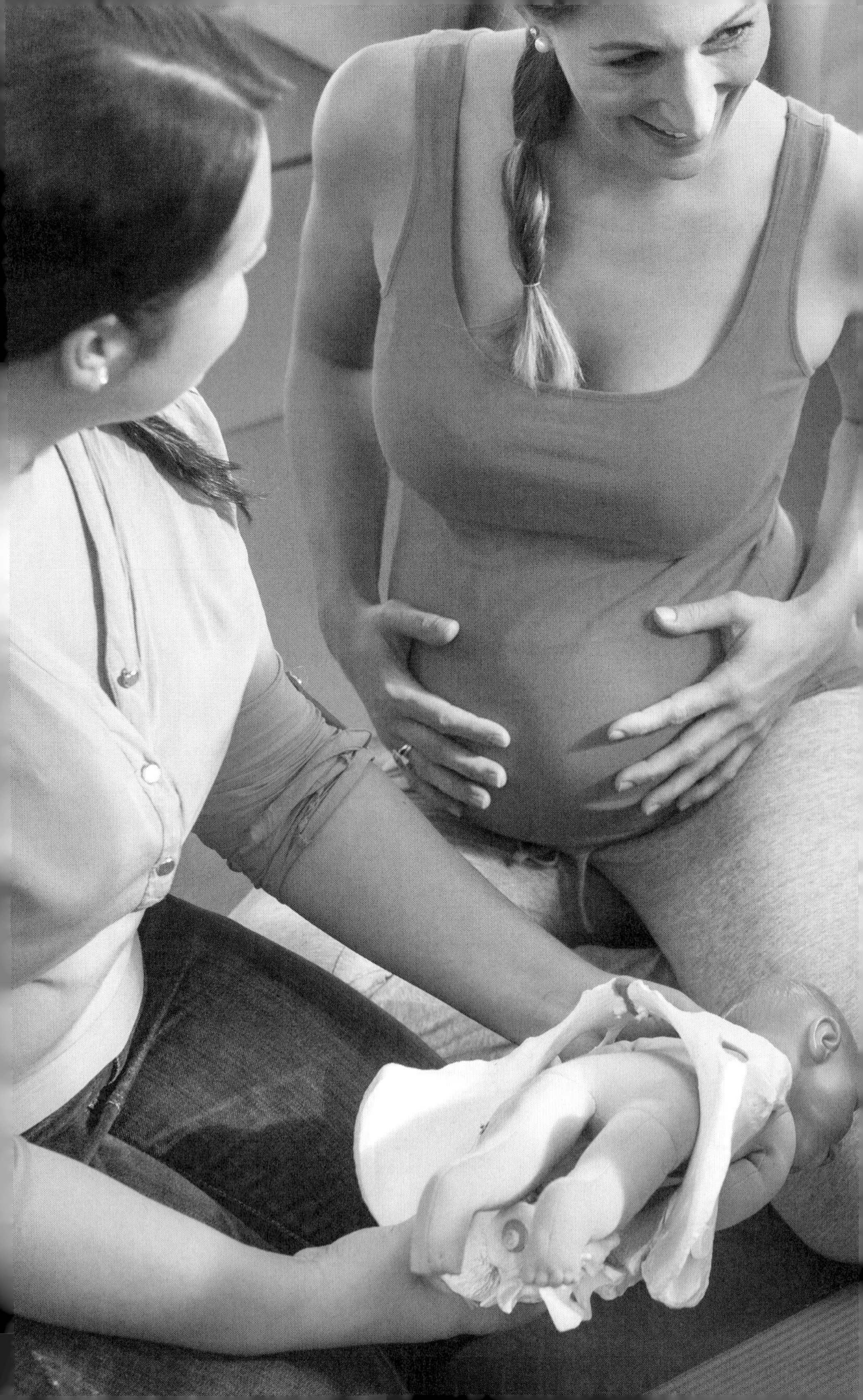

CHAPTER 12

Preparing for Birth

It's best to think about your childbirth options well before you give birth. You may want to write down your decisions in a birth plan. You also should make choices about your baby's care after delivery. Some options you may want to think about ahead of time include the following:

- Where do you want to give birth?

- What kind of childbirth preparation do you want? What classes are offered nearby?

- Do you want pain relief during labor, or will you try natural childbirth?

- If you have a boy, do you want him circumcised?

- Will you breastfeed your baby? Are there **lactation** classes in your area?

As your due date gets closer, think about preparing your home for the baby, buying a car seat, and finding reliable child care if you plan to return to work. You may want to discuss your future **birth control** options with your **obstetrician–gynecologist (ob-gyn)**. And starting around the ninth month of your pregnancy, you'll need to pack a bag for the hospital. Finally, this is a good time to choose the doctor who will care for your newborn.

This chapter discusses some of these decisions. Talk about your wishes with your partner and your ob-gyn.

Your Birth Plan

A birth plan is a written outline of what you would like to happen during labor and delivery. A birth plan might include

- the setting you want to deliver in
- the people you want to have with you
- whether you plan to use pain medications

A birth plan lets your ob-gyn and other health care practitioners know your wishes for your labor and delivery.

Go over your plan with your ob-gyn well before your due date. He or she can explain how your plan fits with his or her policies and the hospital's resources and policies. Not every hospital or birth center can accommodate every request. Still, a plan can help you make your wishes clear. Discussion about your expectations up front can help reduce surprises and disappointments later.

When writing your birth plan, think about how you would like labor and delivery to proceed. What things do you want during labor and delivery? What would enhance the experience for you? What would make you more comfortable? At the back of this book there is a Sample Birth Plan that you can use to write your own plan. A section of the sample plan also lists things that you want for your baby's care.

Here are some extra pointers for your birth plan:

- Keep it short.
- Bring two or three copies to the hospital or birth center.
- Give yourself permission to change your plan.

Keep in mind that having a birth plan does not guarantee that your labor and delivery will go according to that plan. Unexpected things can happen. Remember that you and your ob-gyn have a common goal: the safest possible delivery for you and your baby. A birth plan is a great starting point, but you should be prepared for changes as the situation dictates.

Finally, don't think that you must have a birth plan before you have your baby. It's not a requirement. If the idea of writing a plan doesn't appeal to you, that's perfectly OK.

Birth Places

The setting in which you give birth can have a major effect on your experience. Many hospitals offer a range of settings. In others, choice may be limited. There also are freestanding birth centers that are not in a hospital. The safest places to give birth are thought to be

- a hospital that offers various levels of care, depending on your situation
- a birth center within a hospital complex that meets the standards outlined by the American Academy of Pediatrics and the American College of Obstetricians and Gynecologists (ACOG)
- an accredited freestanding birth center that meets the standards of the Accreditation Association for Ambulatory Health Care, the Joint Commission, or the American Association of Birth Centers

Your choice of where you deliver will depend on

- what your area offers
- where your ob-gyn performs deliveries
- whether your pregnancy has any *complications*
- what your health insurance will cover

Your ob-gyn will let you know about the choices available. You can tour the hospitals and birth centers in your area to see which settings appeal to you.

If your pregnancy is healthy and you are delivering at term, you can deliver at a birth center or a local hospital that offers a basic level of care. But if your pregnancy has complications or if you have certain medical conditions, you may need to deliver at a hospital that offers higher levels of care. Discuss the options with your ob-gyn well in advance.

Hospital Tour

Most hospitals and birth centers offer tours. Take advantage of this opportunity if it's available. If you're taking childbirth classes at the hospital where you'll be giving birth, you'll probably get a tour at some point. If it will be your first time at the hospital, going for a tour also will give you a chance to learn the quickest route there and where to park the car when you arrive in labor.

Home Birth

What about giving birth at home? Although some women choose this option, you should be aware that even the healthiest pregnancies could have complications that arise with little or no warning during labor and delivery. If problems happen, a hospital setting offers the expert staff and equipment to give you and the baby the best care in a hurry. For this reason, ACOG believes that the safest place for you and your baby during labor, delivery, and the days after is a hospital, hospital-based birth center, or accredited freestanding birth center.

Your Labor Partner

Studies have shown that women have a better birthing experience if they have a support person from the start of labor until the baby is born. Choose someone who will help you stay relaxed and calm. A labor partner can be a partner, relative, or close friend. A growing trend is the use of a **doula**, a layperson with special training in labor support and childbirth.

If possible, your labor partner should come with you to **prenatal care** visits and tests. Your labor partner also needs to attend childbirth classes with you because this person has almost as much to learn as you do. Your labor partner will help you practice breathing and relaxation exercises. When you're in labor, your labor partner will coach you through contractions and help you carry out what you learned in class.

Doulas

You may want to consider hiring a professional labor assistant, or doula. The main role of these trained labor coaches is to help you during childbirth and the **postpartum** period. Doulas also provide you and your labor partner with emotional support. Doulas don't have medical training, and they don't replace the ob-gyn, nurses, and other trained health care practitioners caring for you in the hospital.

If you're interested in hiring a doula, ask your ob-gyn or the instructor of your childbirth class for recommendations. Ask friends and family members as well. You also can try the association of doulas, DONA International, which has an online locator service (see the "Resources" section at the end of this chapter). Most health insurance plans do not cover doula expenses. Doulas charge different rates for their services, so be sure to ask about their fees.

Pain Management During Labor

To cope with the pain of childbirth, many women take classes that teach breathing and relaxation techniques (see the "Childbirth Classes" section in this chapter). Others find it helps to use these techniques along with pain medication.

While you are pregnant, start thinking about the types of pain relief you would like to use during labor and delivery. Talk with your ob-gyn about your options. Not all types of pain relief are available at every hospital or birth center. Remember, there is no single "correct" choice. Think about the pain-relief options that are right for you. Also, give yourself permission to change your mind once you're in labor.

Pain Medication

There are two main types of pain-relief medications. An ***analgesic*** drug relieves pain without total loss of feeling or muscle movement. These drugs lessen pain but usually do not stop pain completely. An ***anesthetic*** drug relieves pain by blocking it. Anesthetic drugs may still let you feel pressure or touch. Pain relief medications may be given as a gas, as an injection, or in an ***intravenous (IV) line***. Medications may act on a single area of the body or on the whole body.

Keep in mind that in most hospitals and birth centers, women who get any type of pain relief medication need to stay in bed and cannot walk around. Discuss the timing of pain relief medication with your ob-gyn. See Chapter 13, "Pain Relief During Childbirth," for a discussion of pain-relief medications.

Other Pain-Relief Techniques

Non-medication options also can help during labor. Some of them may not relieve labor pain directly, but they can help you cope with pain better. These options include

- walking during the early stages of labor
- warm showers or baths during the early stages of labor (but note that water birth is not recommended)
- positions like squatting, standing, kneeling, or sitting, which allow gravity to help move the baby downward in the birth canal
- changing positions to get more comfortable, as long as this does not interfere with monitoring and treatment
- equipment such as adjustable birthing beds, chairs, stools, or balls (see Chapter 13, "Pain Relief During Childbirth")
- music and massage during labor
- breathing and relaxation techniques (see the "Childbirth Classes" section in this chapter)

Think about your options and ask questions. Some of these options require special equipment, so find out what your hospital or birth center offers. You also should remember that you won't know which positions feel best to you until you are in labor. Be open to alternatives once you get to the hospital or birth center.

Labor and Delivery in Water

Labor in water has become more popular in recent years. Many hospitals and birth centers offer this service. Some studies have shown that sitting in water during the first stage of labor may lessen pain and shorten labor. There is no scientific evidence that laboring in water has any benefits for the baby.

It is usually safe to go through the first stage of labor in a pool of water, but only if you do not have medical complications and your ob-gyn is able to monitor you and your baby as needed. Giving birth underwater is not recommended. There have been reports of serious harm to babies born underwater, including breathing problems, seizures, and near drowning. ACOG recommends that sitting in water be limited to the first stage of labor.

Other People in the Delivery Room

Some women want to have several friends or family members with them in the delivery room. Some women prefer more privacy, with just their labor partner and the health care team. If you want to have more than one person with you, talk with your ob-gyn and check your hospital's policy on how many people are allowed in a room at one time.

Some hospitals have medical students and residents who are learning how to care for pregnant and laboring women. You can consent to them being in the room while you are in labor, or not. It is your choice.

Some families invite their older children into the delivery room to see the baby's birth. Only you know if this is right for your child or for you. If you would like to make your baby's birth a family affair, talk with your ob-gyn first. Find out what the hospital policy is about children in the delivery room. Many hospitals and birth centers won't allow young children to be present.

If your other children are going to be in the room, each needs to have their own adult support person. Even if your child isn't with you during delivery, he or she can meet the new baby soon after birth.

Childbirth Classes

Childbirth preparation helps you cope with the pain of labor and delivery. Childbirth preparation classes are available that teach various techniques. The most common methods of preparation—Lamaze, Bradley, and Read— are based on the theory that much of the pain of childbirth is caused by fear and tension. Although specific techniques vary, these childbirth preparation methods seek to relieve discomfort through the general principles of education, support, relaxation, paced breathing, and touch. See Chapter 13, "Pain Relief During Childbirth," for descriptions of childbirth preparation methods and tips on choosing a class.

You don't have to select a particular childbirth method. It's not a requirement for giving birth. Your nurses and ob-gyn will give you the instructions and information you need while you're at the hospital or birth center. If you do opt to go to childbirth preparation classes, you and your labor partner should practice the exercises you learn so that you can more easily remember them when you are in labor.

Decisions About Your Baby's Health

In addition to your preferences for labor and delivery, you'll want to make some decisions ahead of time about various aspects of your baby's care. Think about *circumcision* (if it's a boy) and how you plan to feed your baby. Your hospital or birth center also may offer a choice of whether your baby stays in your room or in a nursery. The Sample Birth Plan at the back of this book has sections where you can specify your decisions. And you can think about **umbilical cord blood** banking.

Circumcision for Boys

Circumcision means removing the *foreskin*—a layer of skin that covers the tip of the *penis*. It is your choice whether to have your son circumcised. It is not required by law or by hospital policy. Because circumcision is an *elective procedure*, it may not be covered by your health insurance plan. Check with your health insurance plan.

It's important to have all of the information about the possible benefits and risks of the procedure before making a decision. You may think about future health benefits, religious or cultural beliefs, and personal preferences or social concerns. If you have questions or concerns, talk with your ob-gyn so you have enough time to make an informed decision.

- For some parents, circumcision is done for cultural or religious reasons, or it can be a matter of family tradition. There also can be medical benefits to circumcision, including a lower risk of **urinary tract infections (UTIs)** during the first year of life and a lower risk of getting some **sexually transmitted infections (STIs)** later in life, including **human immunodeficiency virus (HIV)**.

- Some parents choose not to circumcise their sons because they are worried about the pain the baby feels or the risks involved. Others believe it is a decision a boy should make himself when he is older. Keep in mind that recovery may take longer and the risk of complications is higher when circumcision is done later in life. Some parents also may worry that circumcision harms a man's sexual function, sensitivity, or satisfaction. But current evidence shows that it does not.

Complications from a circumcision are rare, but they can happen. Possible complications include bleeding, infection, or scarring. In rare cases, too much of the foreskin is removed, or not enough. Complications usually are minor, and they generally are less likely if the circumcision is done by someone well trained in the procedure. Complications also are less likely to happen if the circumcision is done in a hospital.

If you want your son circumcised, tell your ob-gyn ahead of time. Circumcision usually is done before the baby leaves the hospital. Circumcision should be done only when your baby is healthy. Before the procedure, ask what type of pain relief will be used and how to care for your son's penis as it heals.

In some cases, a circumcision may be done in a nonmedical setting for religious or cultural reasons. If this is the case, the person doing the circumcision should be well trained in how to do the procedure, how to relieve pain, and how to prevent infection.

Feeding Your Baby

Deciding how to feed your new baby is a personal decision. Breastfeeding—feeding directly from the breast—works for some women. For others, feeding a baby pumped breast milk with a bottle is another very good option. Some women cannot or choose not to breastfeed or pump. These women feed their babies formula. Lastly, some women choose a combination of feeding methods. These options are discussed in detail in Chapter 20, "Feeding Your Baby." If you have questions or need help making a decision, talk with your ob-gyn.

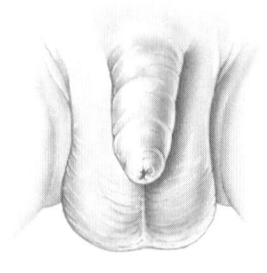

Uncircumcised penis

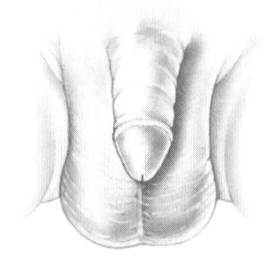

Circumcised penis

Circumcision. In this procedure, the foreskin of the penis is removed.

Many women wonder if there's anything they should do to get ready to breastfeed. There is very little you need to do to prepare your breasts for breastfeeding other than purchasing a good nursing bra. If you feel up to it, you can start breastfeeding as soon as the baby is born. A healthy baby is able to breastfeed in the first hour after birth. Keeping your baby on your chest (called skin-to-skin contact) is the best way to get breastfeeding started. Your labor nurses can help you and your baby get into the right position. See Chapter 18, "After the Baby Is Born."

If you have questions about breastfeeding before the baby arrives, contact the lactation specialist at your hospital or your local La Leche League chapter (see the "Resources" section at the end of this chapter). Keep in mind that the nurses at the hospital will show you how to breastfeed after you give birth, so you won't be left on your own to learn the proper technique. If you have decided that formula-feeding is a better option for you, you will need to buy formula, bottles, and nipples before the baby arrives.

Your Baby's Hospital Stay

The hospital or birth center where you give birth may offer several options for your baby's stay. Some hospitals and birth centers now encourage the option of "rooming-in." This means the baby stays with you at all times in your room. Others have a nursery that the baby can stay in for all or part of your hospital stay.

Rooming-in is a good way to get to know your new baby. It's also the best way to get started with breastfeeding. But having the baby stay in the nursery may be a good choice too, especially if you are exhausted or had a difficult labor. The baby will be brought to your room for feedings.

Be sure you know the options offered by your hospital or birth center. If rooming-in is encouraged, you may want to have someone stay with you to help take care of the baby. The Sample Birth Plan at the back of this book has a section for you to specify where you would like your baby to stay.

Delayed Cord Clamping

Delayed cord clamping is the practice of waiting a short time before cutting the umbilical cord. This allows blood from the umbilical cord, along with extra iron, **stem cells**, and **antibodies**, to flow back into the baby. Delayed cord clamping appears to be helpful for both full-term and **preterm** babies. For this reason, ACOG recommends delayed cord clamping for at least 30 to 60 seconds after birth for most babies.

- In full-term babies, one benefit of delayed cord clamping is a lower risk of *anemia* during the first year of life. There is a slightly higher risk of newborn *jaundice*, so your baby will be watched carefully and treated if signs of jaundice appear.

- In preterm babies (those born between 24 and 36 weeks of pregnancy), delayed cord clamping has several benefits, including less need for blood *transfusion*.

If you are planning to store your baby's cord blood in a cord blood bank, delayed cord clamping may interfere with this process, and there may not be enough cord blood left for storage.

Cord Blood Banking

Cord blood is blood from the baby that is left in the umbilical cord and *placenta* after birth. It contains stem cells that can be used to treat some diseases, such as disorders of the blood, *immune system*, and *metabolism*. For some of these diseases, stem cells are the only treatment. For other diseases, treatment with stem cells is considered when other treatments have not worked. Other uses are being studied.

It's possible to collect some cord blood after birth and store it. In some states, physicians must inform their patients about umbilical cord blood banking options. Before you make a decision about banking your baby's cord blood, it's important to get the facts.

Cord blood is kept in one of two types of banks: public or private. Public cord blood banks operate like regular blood banks. Cord blood is collected for later use by anyone who needs it. The stem cells in the donated cord blood can be used by any person who "matches."

There is no fee for storing cord blood in a public bank. Donors to public cord blood banks must be screened before birth. A limited number of hospitals participate in the public cord blood banking option. To find out more about public banks, visit the National Cord Blood Program website (see the "Resources" section at the end of this chapter).

The other storage choice is a private bank, which charges a yearly fee. Private banks store cord blood for use in treating only your baby and possibly your immediate family members, if you allow it. One thing to keep in mind is that the chances that your child will need to use his or her own cord blood are very low.

Also, if your baby is born with a genetic disorder, the stem cells from the baby's cord blood cannot be used for treatment because they will have the same *genes* that cause the disorder. The same is true if your child has leukemia (cancer of the blood). But stem cells from a healthy child can be used to treat another child's leukemia.

Whether to donate or store cord blood is your decision. If you decide to donate or store cord blood, you will need to choose a cord blood bank. Here are some questions to ask yourself when deciding on a bank:

- What will happen to the cord blood if a private bank goes out of business?
- Can you afford the yearly fee for a private bank?
- What are your options if a public bank's screening tests show that you cannot donate?

You must let your ob-gyn know far in advance of your due date (at least 2 months) if you want to collect and store your baby's cord blood. If you have chosen a private bank, you will need to arrange for the collection equipment to be sent to your ob-gyn. Also, there usually is a fee charged by your ob-gyn for collecting cord blood. Often, this fee is not covered by health insurance.

If you have planned to donate or store cord blood, it may not be possible to collect the blood after delivery. For example, if the baby is born preterm, there may not be enough cord blood for this purpose. **Delayed cord clamping** also reduces the amount of blood in the cord. If you have an infection, the cord blood may not be usable.

Packing for the Hospital

The last thing you want to be doing once labor starts is tossing items into a suitcase in a panic. To avoid this, pack your bag a few weeks before your due date. Leave it in a handy place, such as a hall closet or the trunk of your car. Of course, you can't pack everything ahead of time—you will need some things in the meantime, such as your glasses and slippers (see the box "Things You May Want to Pack"). Make a list of these last-minute items that need to be packed before you leave for the hospital or birth center. Put the list in a place that will trigger your memory, such as on the refrigerator.

Don't worry if you forget something. A friend or family member can bring you whatever you need. The hospital or birth center also may have some items, but you may be charged for them.

Choosing Your Baby's Doctor

Now is a good time to decide who will care for your baby after birth. Most parents choose a ***pediatrician***—a doctor who specializes in the health care of children from birth until young adulthood. Other parents choose a family medicine doctor who treats the entire family.

Things You May Want to Pack

For labor
- ❏ Your health insurance card, photo ID, and hospital registration forms
- ❏ Two or three copies of your birth plan
- ❏ Lotion or oil for massage
- ❏ Lip balm
- ❏ Hair elastics
- ❏ A nightgown or nightshirt (if you don't want to wear a hospital gown)
- ❏ A bathrobe, slippers, and socks
- ❏ Glasses, if you wear them (you may not be allowed to wear contact lenses)
- ❏ Camera
- ❏ Music to play during labor

For your stay
- ❏ Two or three nightgowns (be sure the gowns open at the front if you plan to breastfeed)
- ❏ Two or three nursing bras
- ❏ A few pairs of socks and panties
- ❏ Toiletries, such as toothbrush, toothpaste, and deodorant
- ❏ Contact lenses, if you wear them
- ❏ Phone numbers of people you want to call after the birth
- ❏ Reading material

For discharge
- ❏ A blanket, clothes, and diapers for your newborn to wear home
- ❏ Loose-fitting clothes for you to wear home
- ❏ Car seat for your baby

What not to bring

Many hospitals do not allow the following things
- ❏ Portable TVs, DVD players, or CD players
- ❏ Cell phones—You may be asked to turn off your cell phone in certain areas because cell phones can interfere with medical equipment.
- ❏ Valuables, such as jewelry—Leave your jewelry at home. If it is stolen, the hospital is not responsible for replacing it.
- ❏ Cigarettes, alcohol, and illegal drugs

Not sure how to find a doctor for your baby? Here are some ideas:

- Talk with friends and family members who are parents.
- Ask your ob-gyn for a referral.
- Check the website of the American Academy of Pediatrics (see the "Resources" section for website details).
- Search your health insurance plan's network of practitioners.

Make sure the doctor you want is accepting new patients, has an office near your home, and accepts your current health insurance. See Chapter 6, "Month 5 (Weeks 17 to 20)," for more on choosing your baby's doctor.

Preparing Your Home for the Baby

At least a few weeks before your due date, you'll need to shop for a car seat and make sure that you have the clothes and supplies you'll need once the baby comes home. A trip to any baby supply retailer or a look at the many online baby supply websites will give you plenty of ideas about what you'll need at home to get ready. Talk to other new moms as well to get an idea of what products they used and liked best.

Once your baby is home, it's important to keep him or her safe. You and anyone who will care for your baby should learn how to install and use your car seat and how to safely put your baby to sleep.

Car Seats

You will not be able to take the baby home from the hospital or birth center without a car seat already secured in your car. All 50 states, the District of Columbia, and the Commonwealth of Puerto Rico have laws requiring child safety seats for babies and children at different ages.

All babies should ride in rear-facing car seats in the back seat starting with their first ride home. In a rear-facing car seat, the baby is turned to face the back window. This means that the car seat supports the baby's neck, spine, and head. If there is a crash, a rear-facing car seat gives the most protection.

Babies and toddlers should ride in a rear-facing car seat for as long as possible, until they reach the highest weight or height allowed by the car seat's manufacturer. They then can sit facing the front. But they still must ride in the back seat of a car until they are 13 years old.

There are three types of rear-facing car seats:

1. An infant-only seat is for babies weighing up to 35 pounds. Most infant-only seats are made to pop out of a base. That way you can carry the seat by its handle or place it in a special stroller. An infant-only seat must be replaced when your baby reaches 35 pounds or the specific weight listed by the car seat maker.

2. A convertible seat isn't as portable as an infant-only seat, but it can be converted to a forward-facing seat when your child reaches the height and weight limit for riding in a rear-facing seat.

3. A 3-in-1 seat can be used as a rear-facing seat and a forward-facing seat as well as a booster seat when your child outgrows the forward-facing seat.

Many parents pass on baby supplies to new parents once their own children no longer use them. Be careful, though, with used car seats. If you borrow or reuse a car seat, make sure you know its history, such as whether it's been in an accident. Check the seat carefully for missing parts and defects. If you find any problems, do not use the car seat. The label with the car seat's model number should still be attached, and the instructions should be included with the car seat.

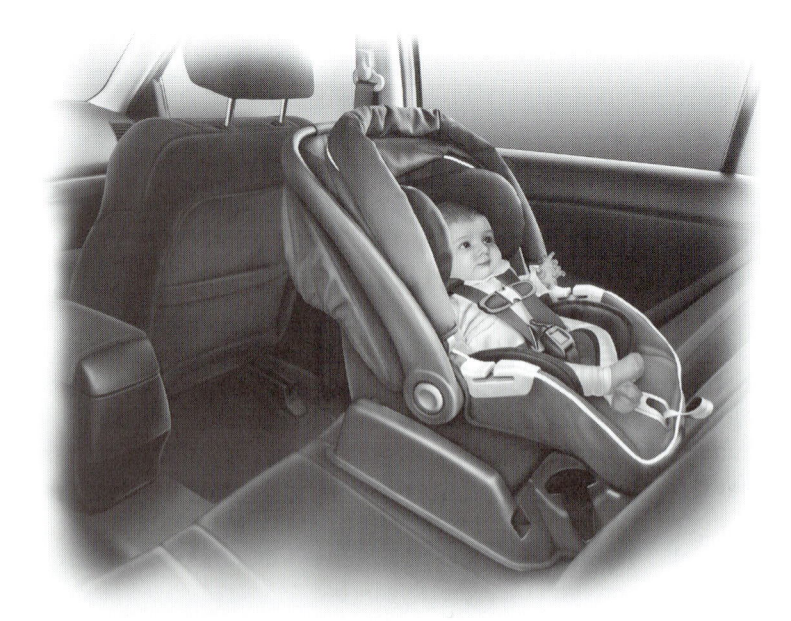

Car safety for a baby. A baby should ride in a rear-facing car seat as long as possible, until he or she reaches the top height and weight limit set by the rear-facing car seat maker.

Keep in mind that car seats have expiration dates. Check the expiration date for any car seat on the manufacturer's website. If you can't afford to buy a seat, some communities and hospitals have programs for new parents to borrow an approved safety seat at no charge.

Once you have the car seat, it's important to install it correctly (see the box "Tips for Buying and Installing a Car Seat"). Even the best car seat won't protect your baby if it's not installed properly. Some fire departments will check the placement of your car seat. Some hospitals also will check to see if the car seat is installed correctly. Ask if your hospital has this service. If your car seat is the type that detaches from a base that stays in the car, practice putting it in and out of the base to make sure you know how it is done before leaving the hospital.

Safe Sleep

Before you bring your newborn home, you and anyone who will care for your baby should learn about how to safely put your baby to sleep. Studies have shown that the risk of **sudden infant death syndrome (SIDS)** can be reduced by following certain guidelines.

Important Sleep Dos:

- Always place the baby on his or her back to sleep or nap or whenever the baby is left alone in a room.
- Place the baby on a firm sleep surface, such as a mattress covered with a fitted sheet.
- Remove soft toys and loose bedding from your baby's sleeping area.
- Dress your baby in light clothes for sleeping.
- Make sure nothing is covering the baby's head.

Use of a pacifier may reduce the risk of SIDS. It's recommended, though, that breastfeeding babies not use a pacifier until they are about 1 month of age to ensure that breastfeeding gets off to a good start.

Important Sleep Don'ts:

- Do not let your baby sleep in an adult bed, couch, or chair, either alone or with you or another person.
- Do not let your baby sleep in slings, carriers, strollers, or car seats outside the car.
- Do not use blankets, quilts, or bumper pads in the baby's sleeping area.
- Do not cover your baby with anything.
- Do not smoke or let anyone else smoke around the baby.

Tips for Buying and Installing a Car Seat

Some safety seats will fit in your car better than others. A well-designed seat that is easy to use is the best for you and your child. When buying a seat, keep these tips in mind:

- Know whether your car has the LATCH system. LATCH stands for *l*ower *a*nchors and *t*ethers for *ch*ildren. Special anchors, instead of safety belts, hold the seat in place. Newer cars and trucks will have the LATCH system. If either your car or your safety seat is not fitted with LATCH, you will need to use safety belts to install the car safety seat.

- Try locking and unlocking the buckle while you are in the store. Try changing the lengths of the straps.

- Not all car seats fit in all vehicles. Try the seat in your car to make sure it fits.

- Read the labels to check weight limits.

- Do not decide just based on price. Seats that cost more are not always better.

When installing the seat, follow these tips:

- Decide whether to place the seat in the middle of the rear seat or in one of the side seats. Some experts think that placing the car seat in the middle is best. But some cars do not have a middle seat or have a middle seat that is too narrow or uneven. Some LATCH systems do not work in the middle seat. The safest option is to place the car seat in the rear seat location where it can be tightly anchored with the seat belt or LATCH system.

- Lock the seat into its base, if it has one. The base should not move more than 1 inch when pushed front to back or side to side. If you are using the safety belts, make sure the lap part of the belt is tightly fastened to the car seat frame.

If you have questions about installing a car seat, contact your local fire department or other local agency, which may be able to check your seat's placement and make sure it's properly installed.

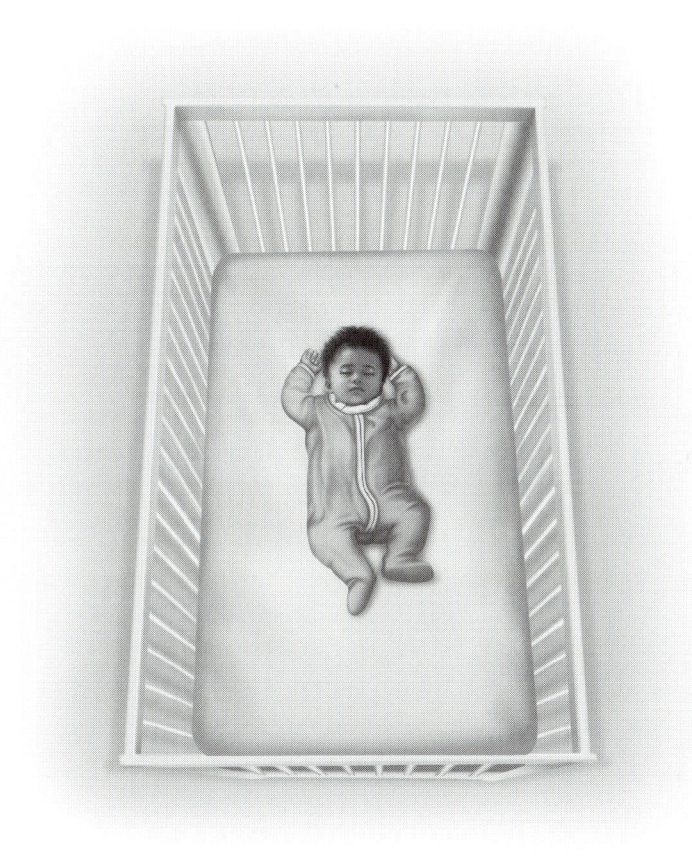

Safe sleep position for a baby. Always place the baby on his or her back on a firm sleep surface for nap time, sleep time, and whenever the baby is left alone in a room. Do not use bumper pads, stuffed animals, blankets, or other soft objects in the crib.

Child Care

If you plan to go back to work after the baby comes home, good child care will be a top priority. Give yourself some time to figure out which option is best for your family. Ask around for recommendations for child care. Your friends, neighbors, and coworkers are all good sources of information. The box "Finding Good Child Care" in this chapter can help direct your search.

There are three basic child care options:

1. Care in your home
2. Care in a caregiver's home
3. Care in a child care center

Finding Good Child Care

Getting answers to the following questions can help you find a child care provider who is right for you and your baby:

1. **Gather the facts.** Make a list of child care providers, family child care homes, and child care centers in your area. Then find out the following about each of them:
   - Where are they located?
   - Do they care for newborns or babies up to 1 year of age?
   - What hours are they available?
   - Do they provide year-round care (do they work during holidays)?
   - What's the cost for care (are there extra charges for some circumstances)?

2. **Check them out.** If you are thinking about family home or center care, visit more than once. Make an appointment the first time. If you like what you see during this visit, drop in the next time. (If drop-in visits aren't allowed, keep looking.) During your tour, find out the following:
   - Is the facility clean, safe, and well equipped?
   - Are there enough care providers (one adult per three to four babies, four to five toddlers, or six to nine preschoolers)?
   - Are the caregivers attentive and loving?
   - Do the children seem happy and well cared for?
   - What's a normal day like?
   - What's served at meal and snack times?

If you want to hire someone to care for your baby in your home (such as a nanny), contact agencies that focus on child care placements. Keep in mind that this type of care can be costly. To cut costs, some parents share a caregiver with another family. The caregiver in these "share-care" setups is paid to watch two babies in one family's home.

A less costly option is having a relative or a licensed provider care for your baby in their home. In most cases, licensed caregivers watch more than one child.

3. **Set up an interview.** Schedule a chat with a family child care provider, nanny, or center director. Have your baby with you and note how the caregiver responds to him or her. Ask the following:
   - What experience and training do the care providers have?
   - For an individual caregiver, why did he or she leave their last job?
   - For a center, what's the staff turnover rate?
   - Do the child care providers have training in first aid and CPR?
   - Are they willing to give your child prescribed medications?
   - What plans are in place in case of a medical emergency?
   - Is the home or center licensed, or is the caregiver certified?
   - Can you visit during the day to breastfeed?

4. **Check credentials.** Never leave your baby with someone until you have checked out his or her background. Ask for the following:
   - The document showing that the home or center is licensed or registered, or that the caregiver is certified. Call the licensing agency to ask if there have been any complaints.
   - Written policies on philosophy, procedures, and discipline
   - At least three references from other parents who have used the caregiver, home, or center

5. **Try them out.** Once you have chosen a caregiver, do a few "practice" runs before you go back to work. This way, if anything strikes you as being "off," you have time to keep looking. It also will help you and your baby get used to the setup before your maternity leave ends.

Child care centers may take care of many children of all different ages. Some accept babies as young as 6 weeks, but some do not take babies until they are out of diapers. Be sure to ask questions while you're doing your research.

RESOURCES

Car Seats and Booster Seats
www.nhtsa.gov/equipment/car-seats-and-booster-seats
Webpage from the National Highway Traffic Safety Administration. Offers information on choosing the right car seat, installing it correctly, and keeping your child safe.

Circumcision
www.healthychildren.org/English/ages-stages/prenatal/decisions-to-make/Pages/Circumcision.aspx
Webpage from the American Academy of Pediatrics (AAP) that describes the risks and benefits of male circumcision, how it is done, and what to expect after the procedure.

Cord Blood and Transplants
https://bethematch.org/transplant-basics/cord-blood-and-transplants/
Webpage from the National Bone Marrow Donor Program that offers information, maintains a donor registry, and facilitates donor–recipient matching of donated bone marrow and cord blood.

DONA International
www.dona.org
International association for training and certifying doulas. Includes an online locator service.

Find a Pediatrician or Pediatric Specialist
www.healthychildren.org/english/tips-tools/find-pediatrician/Pages/Pediatrician-Referral-Service.aspx
Use this tool to search for an AAP member pediatrician, pediatric sub-specialist, or pediatric surgical specialist.

Get Help Paying for Child Care
www.childcare.gov/consumer-education/get-help-paying-for-child-care
Tips for finding and paying for child care from the Administration for Children and Families division of the U.S. Department of Health and Human Services.

La Leche League International
www.llli.org
Provides information and support for breastfeeding moms. Offers referrals to local support groups.

National Cord Blood Program
www.nationalcordbloodprogram.org
Website for the largest public cord blood bank in the United States. Provides information about cord blood collection, storage, banking, and retrieval.

Safe Kids Worldwide
www.safekids.org
Information about child and teen safety in and around cars. Website maintains a list of child safety seat inspection events and keeps track of car seat safety recalls.

Safe to Sleep
https://safetosleep.nichd.nih.gov/
Information from the *Eunice Kennedy Shriver* National Institute of Child Health and Human Development on safe sleep for babies and preventing SIDS.

Where We Stand: Car Seats For Children
www.healthychildren.org/English/safety-prevention/on-the-go/Pages/Where-We-Stand-Car-Seats-For-Children.aspx
The latest recommendations for car seat safety from the AAP. Gives tips about shopping for and installing car seats.

Your Pregnancy and Childbirth
www.acog.org/MyPregnancy
Website from the American College of Obstetricians and Gynecologists (ACOG) with information on pregnancy, labor, delivery, and postpartum care. Includes the latest information from the experts in women's health care, questions answered by ACOG ob-gyns, pregnancy stories from real women, and an A–Z directory of health topics covering pregnancy and beyond.

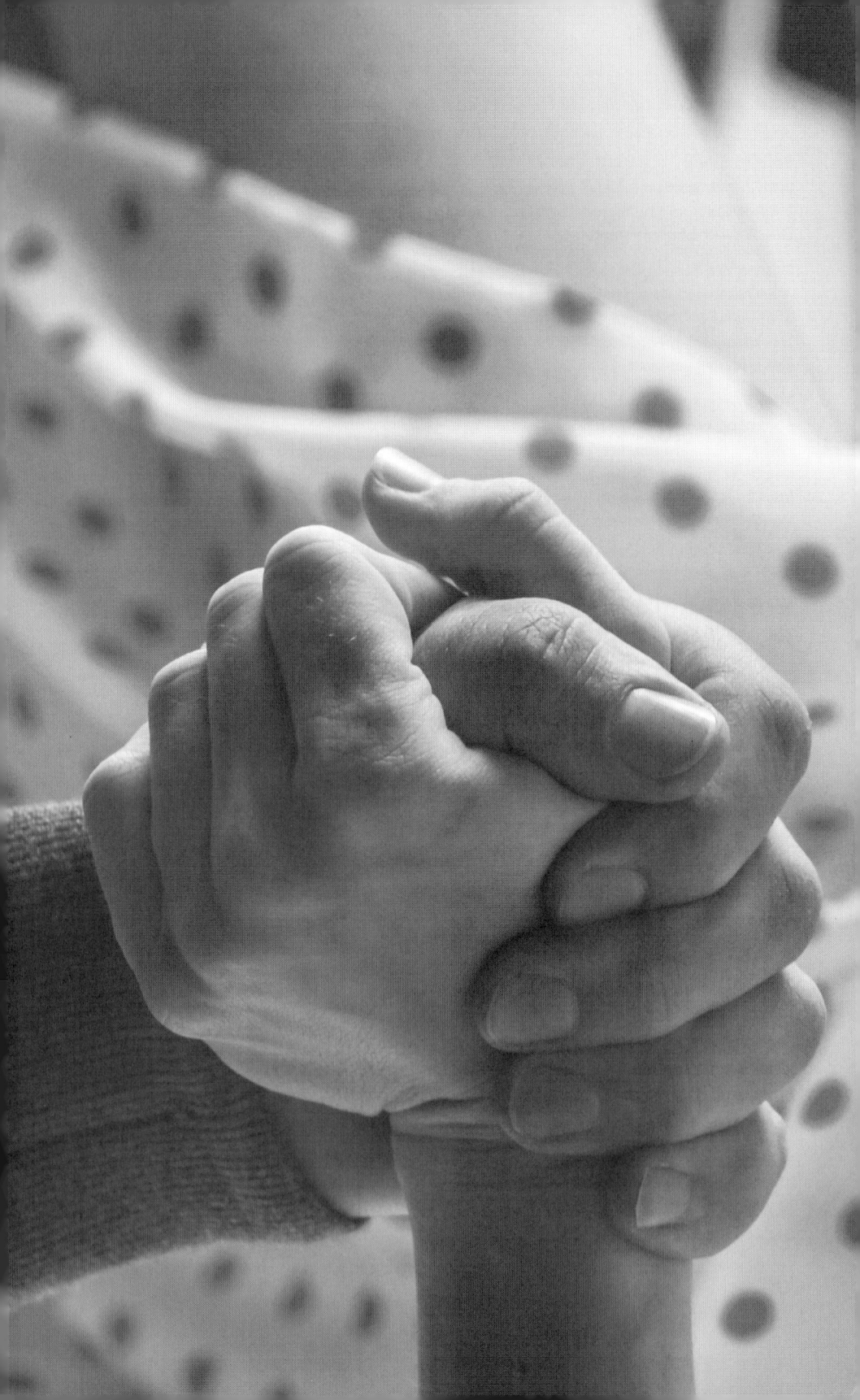

CHAPTER 13

Pain Relief During Childbirth

The pain felt during childbirth is different for every woman. It also can be different from your past deliveries if you have had other children. How you perceive the pain depends on

- the strength of your contractions
- the position of the baby
- how you recognize pain

To cope with the pain of childbirth, many women take classes that teach breathing and relaxation methods. Others find it helps to use these methods along with pain medication. Some women think that getting pain-relief medication will make the childbirth experience less natural. But other women find that pain-relief medications help them participate more fully in childbirth and give them better control.

Remember, there is no "correct" choice about whether to use pain medications during labor and delivery. You can decide what options are right for you.

Start thinking about pain relief before you are close to labor and delivery. Talk with your **obstetrician–gynecologist (ob-gyn)** about your options. Your options may be affected by

- back problems or past back surgery
- medical conditions affecting your pregnancy
- where you deliver

Not all types of pain relief are available at every hospital or birth center.

Medications for Pain Relief

There are two main types of pain-relief medication:

- An *analgesic* relieves pain without total loss of feeling or muscle movement. Analgesics lessen pain but usually do not stop it completely.

- An *anesthetic* blocks pain. Anesthetics may still let you feel pressure or touch. In most cases, anesthetic blocks are given by an *anesthesiologist*, a doctor who is trained to manage pain.

In most hospitals and birth centers, women who receive analgesics or anesthetics will need to stay in bed. These medications increase the risk of dizziness, weakness, and falls. Talk with your ob-gyn about the timing of pain medication during labor.

Systemic Analgesics

Systemic analgesics act on the body's entire nervous system, rather than a specific area, to lessen pain. They do not cause you to lose consciousness. The types of drugs used include

- *opioids*, which block the feeling of pain
- *sedatives*, which make you drowsy

These medications often are used during early labor to help you rest with less pain.

Systemic analgesics usually are given as a shot. The shot is given into a muscle or a vein. In some cases, the woman can control the amount of medication she receives through an *intravenous (IV) line*. This is called patient-controlled *analgesia*.

Systemic pain medications may have side effects:

- Minor side effects can include drowsiness, nausea, and trouble concentrating. Sometimes another medication is given at the same time to relieve nausea.

- High doses of systemic pain medications can cause breathing problems.

- Your baby may be drowsy after birth. Your baby may need help breathing at first, especially if an analgesic medicine is given just before delivery.

- Drowsiness also can make it harder for your baby to breastfeed in the first few hours after birth.

You and the baby should be monitored closely while you are getting this medication and for some time after.

Nitrous Oxide

Nitrous oxide ("laughing gas") is a tasteless and odorless gas that is used in some hospitals. It can reduce anxiety. It also can increase feelings of well-being so that pain is easier to deal with.

Nitrous oxide is mixed with **oxygen** and inhaled through a mask. A woman holds the mask herself and decides when she will inhale. It works best when a woman begins inhaling 30 seconds before the start of a contraction.

Nitrous oxide is safe for you and your baby. Some women have dizziness or nausea while inhaling nitrous oxide. But these sensations go away within a few minutes.

Local Anesthesia

Local anesthesia relieves pain in a small area of the body. You may have had local anesthesia if you've had a cavity filled at the dentist's office. Local anesthesia during labor may be injected into the tissues of the **vagina**, **vulva,** or **perineum**. This shot can be given to block pain

- in the perineum at delivery
- if an *episiotomy* is needed
- if a tear or episiotomy needs to be repaired

Local anesthesia does not lessen the pain of contractions.

Local anesthesia rarely affects the baby. There usually are no side effects for the woman once the medication wears off. Rarely, a woman may have an allergic reaction to a local anesthetic. Other risks, such as heart problems, are very rare but may occur if the medicine goes directly into a vein.

Regional Analgesia and Anesthesia

Regional analgesia and *regional anesthesia* act on a larger part of the body than a local anesthetic. For labor and delivery, including **cesarean birth**, these types of medication lessen or block pain below the waist. The most common types are an *epidural block* and a *spinal block*.

Epidural Block. An epidural block is the most common type of anesthesia used during childbirth in the United States. For this type of pain relief, medication is given through a **catheter** (a thin, soft tube) that is placed into the lower back through a needle. The medication that is given is usually a combination of an anesthetic and an analgesic.

With an epidural you will have some loss of feeling in the lower areas of your body, but the medicine will not make you drowsy. You should still be able to bear down and push your baby through the birth canal.

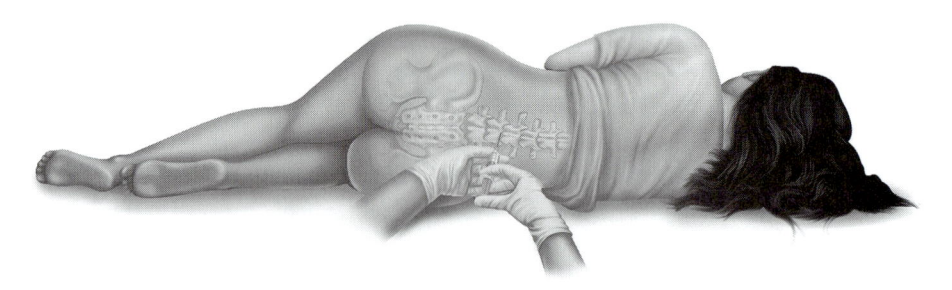

Epidural block and spinal block. In laboring women, regional pain relief reduces or blocks pain below the waist. Pain medication is injected into an area near the spine, in the small of the back.

An epidural may be started soon after your contractions start or later as your labor progresses. An anesthesiologist usually gives an epidural. The risk of side effects from an epidural is low (see the box "Side Effects of Epidural Block or Spinal Block").

To get ready for an epidural, your skin will be cleaned. Local anesthesia will be used to numb an area of your lower back. As you sit or lie on your side, a needle is inserted between the vertebrae (the bones of your spine) into the epidural space. This is a small area below the spinal cord and near the nerves that pass to your torso and lower limbs.

It's important to sit or lie very still while this is being done. After the epidural needle is inserted, a soft catheter usually is inserted and the needle is removed. The catheter remains in place so that medication can be given as needed.

It may take about 10 to 20 minutes for you to feel pain relief after the epidural block is placed. Depending on your level of pain, your anesthesiologist can adjust the amount of medication as needed throughout labor and delivery. Patient-controlled epidural analgesia also may be an option. With this option, you can give yourself a dose of medication by pushing a button. The device is programmed so that you can't give yourself too much medication.

With an epidural, you usually will be able to move, but you may not be able to walk around once the medication starts to work. You still may feel your contractions, but you will be more comfortable. Sometimes there will be an area where there is still pain, called a "window." If this happens, more medication may need to be given. Sometimes the epidural catheter will need to be adjusted or replaced.

If you are given an epidural during labor and then need to have a cesarean delivery, your anesthesiologist may be able to inject medication through the same catheter to increase your pain relief.

Side Effects of Epidural Block or Spinal Block

The risk of side effects from an epidural block or a spinal block is low. Side effects may include

- fever
- nausea and vomiting
- shivering
- trouble passing urine
- slowed breathing (when opioid medication is used)

Another possible side effect is a drop in the woman's blood pressure. This can reduce blood flow to the baby. This may require treatments such as position changes, intravenous (IV) fluids, or additional medications.

About 1 in 100 women will have a severe headache within a day to a week after receiving an epidural. This headache may happen if the needle pierces the covering of the spinal cord and causes spinal fluid to leak. Standard headache medications are tried first to relieve the headache. If these don't work, a simple procedure called a blood patch may be done. In this procedure, some of your own blood is injected into the epidural space, near the site where the needle went in. As this blood clots, it stops the spinal fluid from leaking out.

Rarely, the anesthesia medication might be injected into one of the veins in the epidural space. This can cause dizziness, heart-rate problems, or a funny taste in your mouth. To reduce the chance of these problems, you will be monitored closely while you are receiving epidural medication. Tell your anesthesia provider or a nurse if you have any of these symptoms.

Spinal Block. With a spinal block, a thin needle is used to inject a small amount of medication into the spinal fluid, below the level of the spinal cord. The medication starts to relieve pain quickly, but it lasts for only an hour or two. A spinal block usually is given only once. This is different from an epidural, which gives medication continuously. A spinal block can have the same side effects as an epidural (see the box "Side Effects of Epidural Block or Spinal Block").

Depending on the medications used, a spinal block can be used for analgesia or anesthesia. A combination of analgesics and anesthetics can be injected to provide short-term pain relief during labor. Higher doses of anesthetics can give more complete loss of feeling for cesarean delivery. Analgesics given during surgery also can lessen pain after cesarean delivery.

Combined Spinal–Epidural Block. A ***combined spinal–epidural (CSE) block*** has the benefits of both a spinal block and an epidural block. A spinal block is given first to relieve pain right away. An epidural catheter then is placed to provide pain medication throughout labor.

The CSE block sometimes is called a "walking epidural." Depending on your hospital's policy and your condition, you may be able to walk for a short distance after the CSE is in place, such as to the bathroom. But the medications may cause muscle weakness or loss of balance, so you may not be allowed to walk the hallways.

General Anesthesia

With *general anesthesia*, you are not awake. You feel no pain. General anesthesia can be started quickly and makes you unconscious quickly. This type of anesthesia most often is used in emergency situations. It may not be offered as an option that you can choose.

The medications that put you to sleep are given through an IV line or through a mask. After you are asleep, your anesthesiologist will place a breathing tube into your mouth and windpipe to help you breathe while you are unconscious. One risk of general anesthesia is difficulty placing the breathing tube.

Another rare risk of anesthesia is aspiration. While you are unconscious, food and drink from your stomach can come back into the mouth and go into the lungs when you inhale. Pregnancy and labor make it easier for food and liquids to pass back from your stomach to your esophagus (the tube that leads from your throat to your stomach). Labor also can cause undigested food to stay in the stomach longer than usual, so there is more undigested food and liquid in your stomach. If this food and liquid is breathed into the lungs ("aspirated"), it can cause serious lung irritation and infection.

The medicines used during general anesthesia can pass to the baby. This can make a newborn drowsy and cause the baby to have difficulty breathing. In rare cases, the baby may need help breathing after birth.

The effects of general anesthesia usually wear off quickly. There are no permanent effects from general anesthesia for you or for the baby's brain or development.

Opioid Use Disorder and Pain Relief During Labor

Opioid use disorder is a treatable disease that can be caused by using opioids in ways that were not prescribed for you. This disorder is sometimes called "opioid addiction." Opioids include drugs called oxycodone, hydromorphone, hydrocodone, fentanyl, and codeine. Symptoms of opioid use disorder include

- feeling a strong desire to take opioids
- feeling unable to stop or reduce opioid use
- having work, school, or family problems caused by your opioid use
- needing more opioids to get the same effect
- spending a lot of time trying to find and use opioids
- feeling unwell after stopping or reducing opioid use

If you have an opioid use disorder during pregnancy, it is important to tell your ob-gyn early in your pregnancy, especially if you are receiving treatment for the disorder. Together, you can plan for appropriate pain relief during labor and recovery. Also, before you go into labor it may be helpful to talk with an anesthesiologist.

Here are some things you should know:

- If you are taking methadone or buprenorphine to manage an opioid use disorder, you should continue taking your regular dose while you are in labor. Splitting up your regular daily dose into three or four smaller doses every 6 to 8 hours may help with pain relief.

- You also should have other pain relief available to you like women without opioid use disorder do. Women who are taking methadone or buprenorphine often need higher doses of opioids to get enough pain relief.

- If you do not want to take any opioids during labor, let your ob-gyn know.

- Some drugs that are used for pain relief during labor can reverse the effects of methadone or buprenorphine and cause sudden withdrawal symptoms. Your care team should know not to give you these drugs. Let your ob-gyn know all the medications you are taking.

- Effective non-opioid pain medications are available and can be part of your pain management plan during labor and after you go home.

- The pain-relief techniques described later in this chapter also may be helpful.

If you have used opioids during pregnancy, it's also important to tell your baby's care team. The baby will no longer be getting the drug after you give birth. As a result, the baby may have withdrawal symptoms that need to be treated. This is called **neonatal abstinence syndrome (NAS)**. NAS can last days or weeks. Swaddling, breastfeeding, and skin-to-skin contact can help babies with NAS feel better, but sometimes medications are needed.

The American College of Obstetricians and Gynecologists (ACOG) believes that pregnant women who have an opioid use disorder should receive medical care and counseling services, not punishment. Seeking help is the first step in recovering from addiction and making a better life for you and your family. Remember, opioid use disorder is a treatable disease. It also is important to know that states have different laws and policies about opioid use during pregnancy. It may be helpful to learn about your state's laws and policies. You can visit this site for more information: www.guttmacher.org/state-policy/explore/substance-use-during-pregnancy.

Pain Relief Techniques

Long before epidurals were invented, women used different methods to ease the pain of labor. If you are interested in using some of these techniques, check to make sure they are available or allowed at the hospital or birth center where you will give birth.

Walking

During the early stages of labor, walking may help you stay relaxed and ease some of the pain. If your ob-gyn says it's OK, take short walks down the hall with your labor partner. You likely will not be able to walk after receiving systemic analgesics or if you have an epidural or spinal block (see "Epidural Block" and "Spinal Block" earlier in this chapter).

If you are hooked up for **electronic fetal monitoring**, you still can walk or pace close to your bed. Some hospitals and birth centers have wireless monitoring devices to help you move around more freely.

Positions

Many women are more comfortable changing position regularly during labor. Moving from side to side can help. Other positions also may be tried if your ob-gyn says it's OK. More upright positions—like squatting, standing, kneeling, or sitting—allow gravity to help move the baby down in the birth canal. Being upright instead of lying down also may reduce the pressure of the baby on your spine. Squatting positions stretch the birth canal to its widest diameter, possibly making it easier for the baby to come out.

Consider all your options and ask plenty of questions. You may want to make a plan before labor begins. But be aware that not all birthing positions or equipment may be available at your facility. And remember that labor does not always go as planned. You may need to adjust your plan if circumstances change during your labor.

Warm Showers

Water has been used for pain relief for centuries. Many women report that taking a warm shower is helpful during labor. Having warm water flow on your back and belly may

- relax tense muscles
- help with overall relaxation
- help ease pain

For safety, you should have someone standing nearby to support you.

Sitting in Water

Labor in water has become more popular in recent years. More hospitals and birth centers have started offering this service. Some studies have shown that sitting in water during the first stage of labor can lessen pain and shorten labor, but results are not consistent. There is no evidence that laboring in water has any benefits for the baby.

It is usually safe to go through the first stage of labor in a pool of water, but only if you do not have medical **complications** and your health care team can monitor you and your baby as needed.

Giving birth underwater is not recommended. There have been reports of serious harm to babies born underwater, including breathing problems, seizures, and near drowning. ACOG recommends that sitting in water be limited to the first stage of labor.

If you want to try laboring in water, remember these precautions:

- Your hospital or birth center should have very high standards for cleaning and maintaining the birthing pool and preventing infection. If you aren't sure, ask.

- There should be a process in place to quickly and safely move you out of the tub if problems arise.

- You should move out of the tub when you start to push the baby out (the second stage of labor). This will help to avoid the chance that the baby will be born underwater by accident.

Music and Massage

Music and massage therapy can both help with pain relief during labor.

- Listening to music during labor has been shown to reduce pain for some women. Soft, relaxing music may help during early labor. For the later stages of labor, music with a steady beat may be better.

- A gentle, firm massage on the lower back and shoulders can relieve some of the pressure from contractions. Your labor partner's knuckles or a tennis ball can give the right amount of pressure.

Equipment for Labor and Delivery

Most women in the United States give birth while lying on their backs with their feet supported in stirrups or by a labor partner. Giving birth in this position may make it easier for your ob-gyn to help during the delivery. It also provides support for your back and legs.

Many hospitals and birth centers offer beds, chairs, and other special equipment to help with positions for labor and delivery. These are some of the options:

- Birthing bed—A birthing bed can be adjusted for squatting, sitting on the end of the bed with your feet supported, or lying on your side. A squatting bar that you can hang on to can be attached over the bed.

- Birthing stool—Birthing stools stabilize and support you while you squat.

- Birthing ball—You cannot give birth on one, but sitting on a birthing ball can provide some relief from labor pains. You can rock back and forth on the ball to help ease the pain of contractions. Or you can lean your upper body on the birthing ball if it is placed on the bed. You can bring a birthing ball from home if the hospital does not have one.

- Birthing chair—Birthing chairs are specially designed to let you give birth in a seated position.

Continuous Labor Support

When a woman has someone with her throughout labor and delivery, it's known as continuous labor support. Studies have shown that women have a better birthing experience if they have a support person from the start of labor until the baby is born. The women with support people

- had shorter labor times
- needed less pain medication
- were less likely to need a cesarean delivery
- were less likely to need the use of **forceps** or a **vacuum device** to guide the baby's head out of the vagina

   Your support person can be someone familiar to you, such as a partner, family member, or friend. He or she can assist by

- offering comfort and encouragement
- timing your contractions
- massaging your back and shoulders
- allowing you to lean on him or her while walking or swaying
- acting as a focal point during contractions

Hearing that you're doing a good job and that things are going well can be a big help.

Continuous labor support also can come from a trained professional, such as a nurse, midwife, or **doula**. Doulas are professional labor coaches who can be hired to help during childbirth. They don't have any medical training, but many doulas have training in relaxation methods, such as breathing techniques and massage. See the "Resources" section at the end of this chapter if you'd like to find a doula in your area.

Childbirth Classes

Childbirth classes teach pregnant women various techniques for coping with pain and reducing discomfort during labor and delivery. Childbirth classes all share the principles of education, support, relaxation, paced breathing, and touch. Here is a description of some childbirth preparation approaches:

- Lamaze method—This method of childbirth preparation was developed in the 1950s by a French obstetrician, Dr. Fernand Lamaze. This method is based on the idea that a woman's inner wisdom guides her through childbirth. Lamaze childbirth education helps women gain confidence in their bodies and learn to make informed decisions about pregnancy, birth, breastfeeding, and parenting. To learn more about this method, go to the Lamaze International website (see the "Resources" section at the end of this chapter).

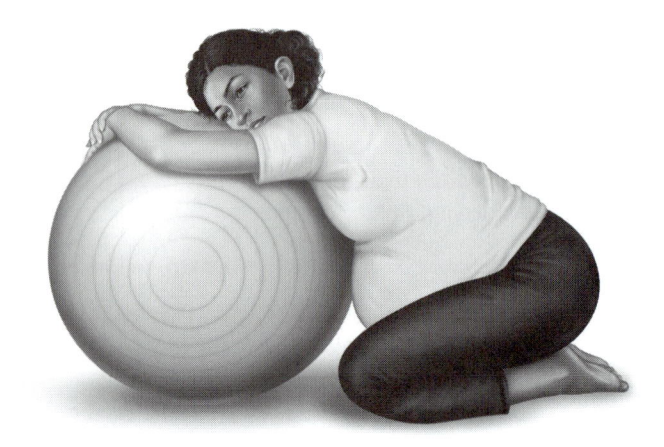

Birthing ball

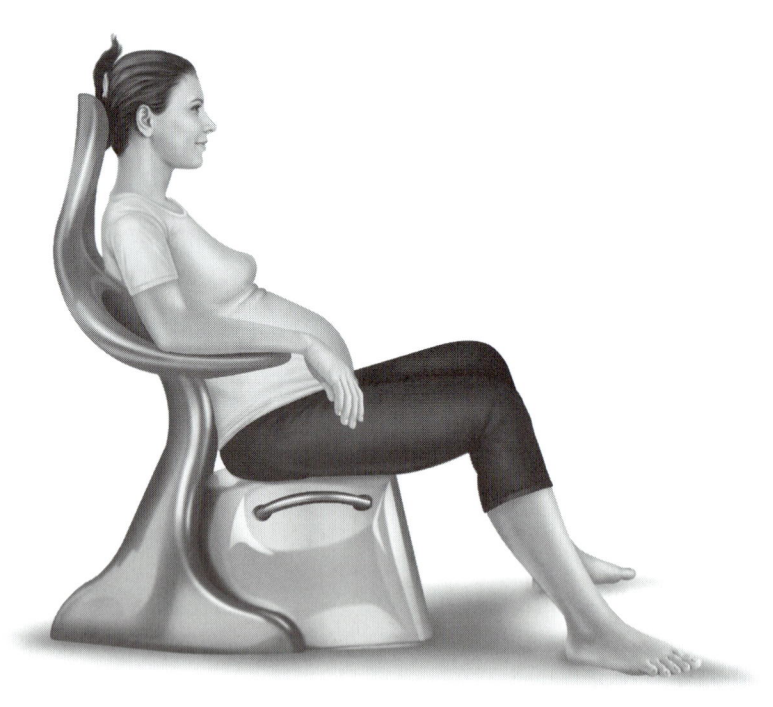

Birthing stool

Positions for labor and delivery. Many hospitals and birth centers offer special chairs and other equipment to help you get into comfortable positions for labor and delivery.

PAIN RELIEF DURING CHILDBIRTH • 215

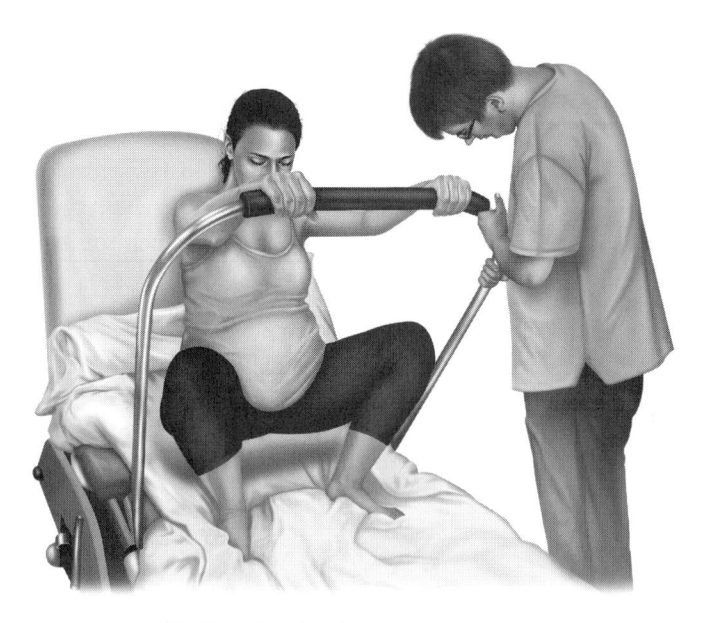

Birthing bed with squatting bar

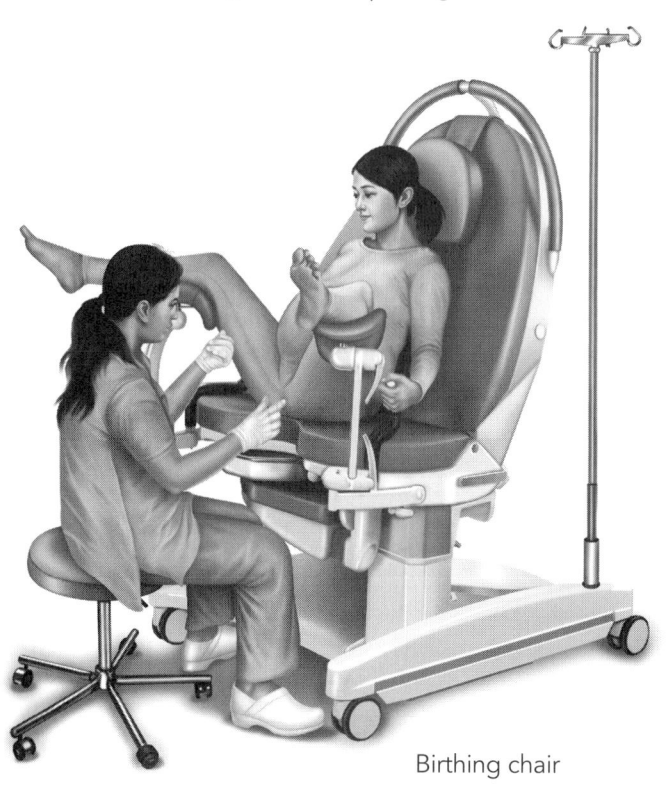

Birthing chair

- Bradley method—This method is based on the belief that a healthy pregnancy and birth can happen with education, preparation, and support from a labor partner. This method involves the active participation of the pregnant woman and her labor partner during the labor process. It also teaches a variety of relaxation techniques. Information about the Bradley method is available online (see the "Resources" section at the end of this chapter).

- Read method—This method seeks to manage fear and anxiety by educating pregnant women and labor partners about labor and delivery. The Read method is explained in the book *Childbirth Without Fear*, written by its founder, Dr. Grantly Dick-Read.

- Hypnosis—"Hypnobirthing" uses relaxation and self-hypnosis techniques to teach women how to achieve a natural and fear-free childbirth. Information about this method is available online (see the "Resources" section at the end of this chapter).

- Yoga and Sophrology—These methods come from Indian culture and teach control of the body and mind. Through relaxation, concentration, and meditation, these techniques can lessen the pain of labor. Ask your ob-gyn about prenatal yoga classes offered in your area.

With all the choices available, you're likely to find something that appeals to your own beliefs and preferences. As you consider your options, keep the following tips in mind:

- Contact the class instructor—The instructor's approach and knowledge are important factors in determining whether the class is right for you. Ask questions to get a sense of how the class is taught.

- Find out the location and schedule—Is the class offered nearby? How many weeks does it meet? You want to find a class that is convenient for you.

- Figure in the cost—Find out how much the class costs and what's included in the fee. Also, check whether your health insurance plan will cover any of these costs.

- Ask how many people are in the class—Some classes are small and offer personal attention. Others are larger. Talk with your labor partner about whether a small or large class is better for you.

Childbirth classes are discussed in more detail in Chapter 12, "Preparing for Birth." If you do not want to take classes to prepare for labor, that's OK. It's not a requirement for giving birth. Your ob-gyn and labor nurses will give you the instructions and information you need while you're at the hospital or birth center.

RESOURCES

Childbirth Classes
These websites offer three popular options for childbirth preparation. There are many more out there. Ask your ob-gyn for his or her recommendations as well.

Lamaze International
www.lamaze.org

Bradley Method of Natural Childbirth
www.bradleybirth.com

HypnoBirthing
www.hypnobirthing.com

DONA International
www.dona.org
International association for training and certifying doulas. Includes an online locator service.

International Childbirth Education Association
www.icea.org
Search for childbirth classes or find educators or doulas in your area.

Your Pregnancy and Childbirth
www.acog.org/MyPregnancy
Website from the American College of Obstetricians and Gynecologists (ACOG) with information on pregnancy, labor, delivery, and postpartum care. Includes the latest information from the experts in women's health care, questions answered by ACOG ob-gyns, pregnancy stories from real women, and an A–Z directory of health topics covering pregnancy and beyond.

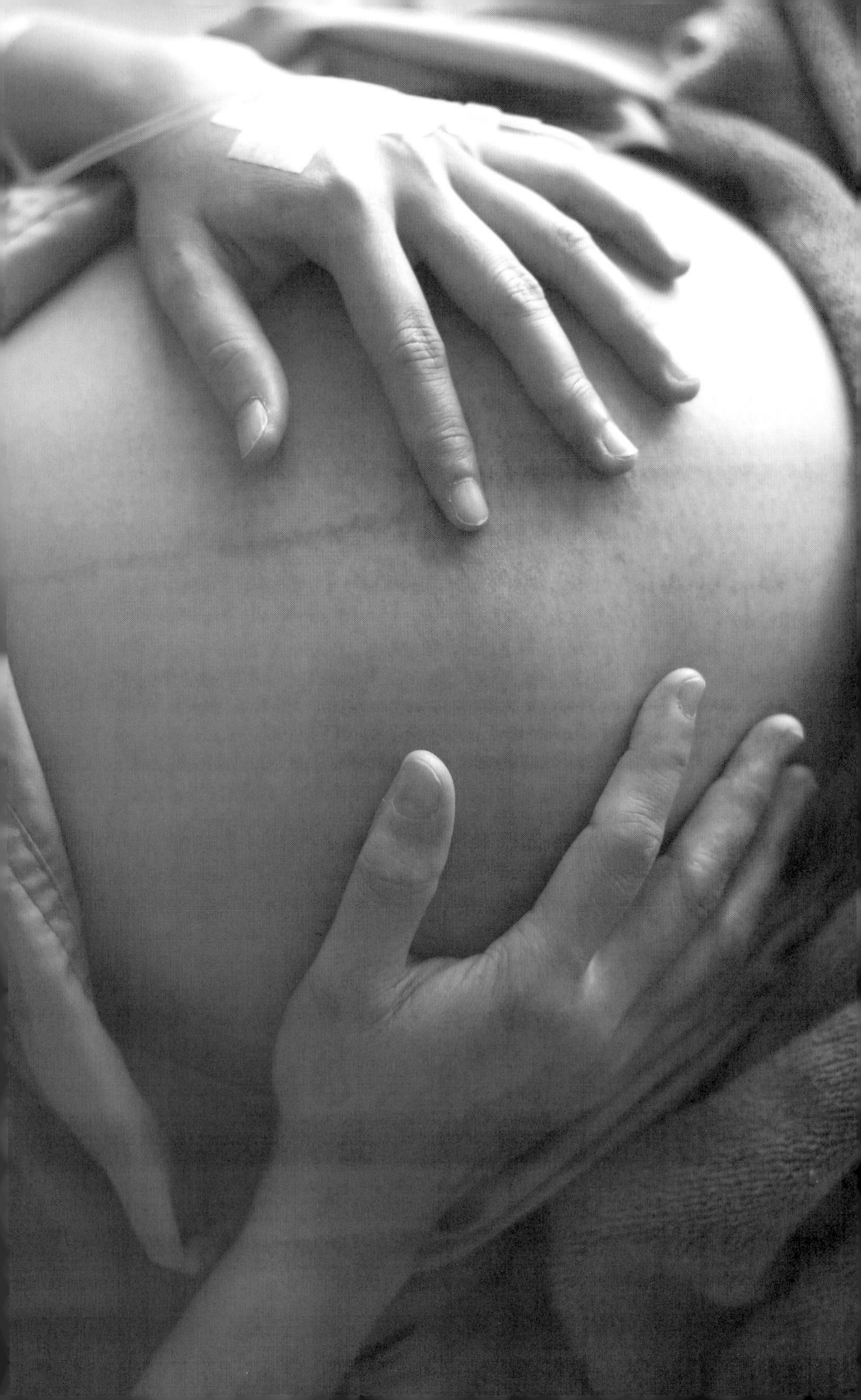

CHAPTER 14

Labor Induction

Sometimes continuing a pregnancy becomes too risky for a woman's health or the health of her baby. If this happens, you and your **obstetrician–gynecologist (ob-gyn)** may discuss starting labor early so that you can try to have a vaginal birth. This is called **labor induction**.

More than 1 in 5 women in the United States have labor induction each year. In general, labor is induced when the benefits of having the baby soon outweigh the risks of continuing the pregnancy. But labor induction also can increase the risk of certain **complications**. If you and your ob-gyn are thinking about inducing your labor, you will talk together about the benefits and risks for you and your baby.

Medical Reasons for Labor Induction

There are many reasons why your ob-gyn may recommend labor induction. Here are a few of the most common reasons:

- Your pregnancy has lasted more than 41 to 42 weeks.

- You have health problems, such as problems with your heart, lungs, or **kidneys.**

- There are problems with the **placenta**.

- There are problems with the baby, such as poor growth.

- There is a decrease in **amniotic fluid.**

- You have an infection of the **uterus**.

- You have **gestational diabetes** or had **diabetes mellitus** before pregnancy.
- You have chronic **hypertension**, **preeclampsia**, or **eclampsia**.
- You have **prelabor rupture of membranes (PROM)**.

Before labor is induced, your ob-gyn should check your health and the baby's health. This is done to assess the possible risks for either of you.

In very high-risk pregnancies, labor induction may be needed even if it means the baby will be born **preterm**. If preterm delivery is recommended, it usually means that continuing the pregnancy has more risks than a preterm birth.

Late Term and Postterm Pregnancy

A **late term** pregnancy is one that goes from 41 weeks and 0 days to 41 weeks and 6 days. A **postterm pregnancy** is one that is 42 weeks or longer. When a pregnancy goes longer than 40 weeks, it can increase health risks for a woman and her baby. These risks include the following:

- After 42 weeks, the placenta may not work as well as it did earlier in pregnancy.
- As the baby grows, the amount of amniotic fluid may begin to decrease. Less fluid may cause the **umbilical cord** to be pinched as the baby moves or as the uterus contracts.
- The baby can grow larger than normal, which can complicate a vaginal delivery.
- Postterm pregnancy doubles the pregnant woman's risk of needing a **cesarean delivery**.

Despite these risks, most women who give birth after their due dates have healthy babies.

If your due date has come and gone, your ob-gyn most likely will do an evaluation to check your baby's health. If you don't start labor on your own by 41 to 42 weeks, you and your ob-gyn should talk about the option of inducing labor.

Elective Reasons for Labor Induction

Sometimes, labor is induced at a woman's request for nonmedical reasons, such as physical discomfort, a history of quick labor, or living far away from the hospital. This is called an elective induction.

Induction at 39 Weeks

New research suggests that induction for healthy women at 39 weeks may reduce the chance of **cesarean birth**. It also may reduce the risk of preeclampsia or gestational hypertension. These findings apply only if:

- This is your first pregnancy.
- You are carrying only one baby.
- You and your baby are both healthy.

Early labor is the time when a woman's contractions start and her **cervix** begins to open. Women who have induction at 39 weeks should be allowed up to 24 hours or longer for the early phase of labor. They also should be given **oxytocin** at least 12 to 18 hours after stripping or sweeping of the membranes. If a woman's labor does not progress, it may be considered a failed attempt at induction. In most cases, a cesarean delivery is needed when induction fails.

When a woman and her baby are healthy, induction should not be done before 39 weeks. Babies born at or after 39 weeks have the best chance at healthy outcomes compared with babies born before 39 weeks. But when the health of the woman, her baby, or both is at risk, induction before 39 weeks may be recommended.

If you are thinking about elective induction, your ob-gyn should review your records to be reasonably sure that you have reached 39 weeks of pregnancy. Most hospitals also require documentation showing you have reached 39 weeks. This is done by confirming one of the following:

- You had an **ultrasound exam** at less than 20 weeks of pregnancy that supports a **gestational age** of 39 weeks or greater.
- The baby's cardiac activity has been present for at least 30 weeks.
- It has been at least 36 weeks since a positive pregnancy test result.

When Is Labor Not Induced?

There are some situations that make labor induction or vaginal delivery unsafe for you and the baby. These may include the following:

- The placenta is covering part or all of the opening of the uterus. This is called **placenta previa**.

- The baby is lying sideways in the uterus or is in a **breech presentation**.
- The umbilical cord has dropped down into the **vagina** ahead of the baby. This is called **umbilical cord prolapse**.
- You have an active **genital herpes** infection.
- You had a past surgery of your uterus, such as certain types of cesarean birth or surgery to remove *fibroids*.

In these situations, you may need a cesarean birth to protect the health of you and your baby (see Chapter 17, "Cesarean Delivery and Vaginal Birth After Cesarean Delivery").

How Induction Is Done

There are several ways to start labor if it hasn't started naturally. The method used depends on several factors, including your health and how

> ### Why Wait Until 39 Weeks?
>
> If you are having a healthy pregnancy and there are no complications, you should wait to deliver your baby until your pregnancy has reached full term—39 weeks and 0 days or later.
>
> - As you know, babies grow and develop throughout the entire 40 weeks of pregnancy. For example, the brain, liver, and lungs are among the last organs to mature. They aren't fully developed before 39 weeks of pregnancy.
> - Babies who are born even a little before 39 weeks may not be as fully developed as those who are born after 39 weeks of pregnancy. These babies may have an increased risk of short-term and long-term health problems. Some of these problems can be serious and lifelong.
> - Babies who are not fully developed may need extra care. They may have problems breathing or eating. They may have **anemia** or **jaundice**. These babies may need to spend time in a **neonatal intensive care unit (NICU)**.
> - The earlier a baby is born, the higher the risks of health problems and the more severe they are likely to be.

your ob-gyn prefers to induce labor. Sometimes, several of these methods are used together. Some of the methods used to induce labor also are used for women in spontaneous labor that is not progressing as it should.

If you are having labor induction, *electronic fetal monitoring* may be done at first. This measures the baby's heart rate and your contractions. If you have a medical condition or a pregnancy complication, you may have electronic fetal monitoring continuously during labor.

Getting the Cervix Ready for Labor

"Ripening the cervix" is a procedure that helps the cervix soften and thin out so that it will dilate (open) during labor. If labor is going to be induced but the cervix is not yet soft, labor may not be able to progress.

Before inducing labor, your ob-gyn should check to see if your cervix has started this change. Ob-gyns may use the Bishop score to rate the readiness of the cervix for labor. With this scoring system, a number ranging from 0 to 13 is given. A score of 6 or less means that your cervix is not yet ready for labor. In this case, your ob-gyn may recommend starting your induction by ripening the cervix.

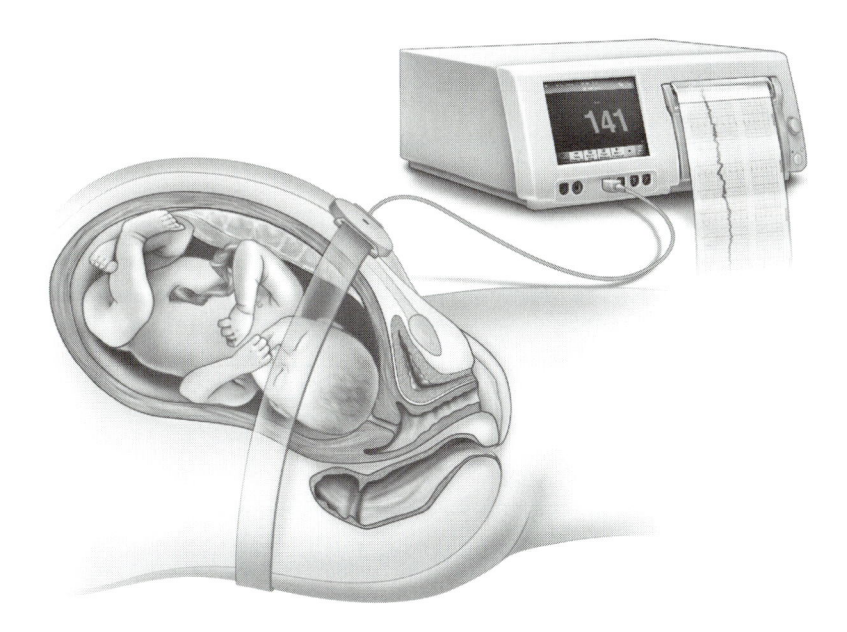

Electronic fetal heart rate monitoring. This type of monitoring checks the baby's heart rate during labor.

Ripening of the cervix may be done with medications or without medications. When done with medications, ripening includes:

- Using medications that contain **prostaglandins**. These medications can be inserted into the vagina or taken by mouth.

When done without medications, ripening includes:

- Using a thin tube **catheter** that has an inflatable balloon on the end. The tube is inserted through the vagina and into the opening of the cervix. Then the balloon is expanded, which helps open the cervix.
- Using **laminaria.** These are slender rods inserted into the cervix to dilate it. They are made of a natural or artificial substance that expands when it absorbs water.

These ways of ripening the cervix may be used together or one after another. You and your ob-gyn should talk about which approaches may work best for you and your cervix.

Stripping or Sweeping the Amniotic Membranes

To "strip or sweep the membranes," your ob-gyn sweeps a gloved finger between the **amniotic sac** and the wall of your uterus, separating the fetal membranes. This action is done when the cervix is partially dilated. It may cause your body to release natural prostaglandins, which soften the cervix more and may start contractions.

Oxytocin

Oxytocin is a **hormone** that causes contractions of the uterus. It can be used to start labor or to speed up labor that started on its own. Contractions may start soon after oxytocin is given. Oxytocin is given through an **intravenous (IV) line** in the arm.

Amniotomy

When your water breaks, the fluid-filled amniotic sac that surrounds the baby has ruptured (burst). Most women go into labor within hours after their water breaks. If the sac hasn't burst already, breaking it can start contractions. Or, if the contractions have already started, breaking the sac can make them stronger and more frequent.

To rupture the amniotic sac, an ob-gyn makes a hole in the sac with a special device. This procedure, called an **amniotomy,** may be done before or after a woman has been given oxytocin. Amniotomy can be performed to

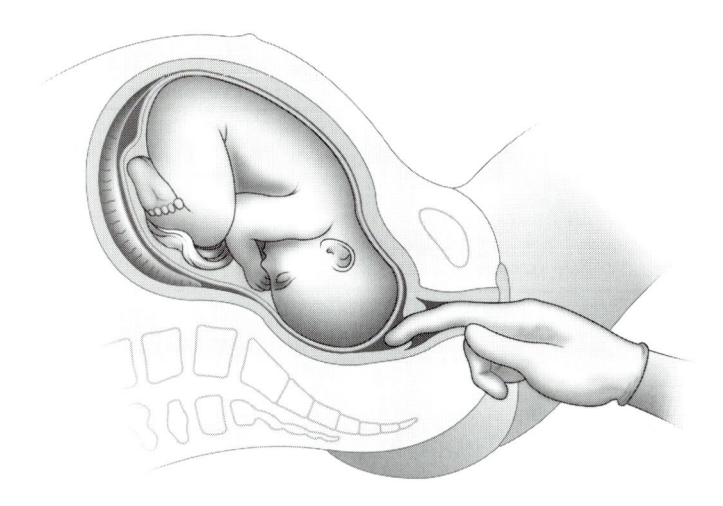

Stripping or sweeping the amniotic membranes. Your ob-gyn may sweep a gloved finger over the amniotic membranes to separate them from the cervix. This action may help start your labor.

start labor when the cervix is dilated and the baby's head has moved down into the pelvis. Most women go into labor within a few hours after the amniotic sac breaks, but sometimes oxytocin may be needed.

Risks of Labor Induction

There are risks with labor induction. One risk is that when oxytocin is used, the uterus may be overstimulated. This may cause the uterus to contract too often. Too many contractions may lead to changes in the baby's heart rate. If there are problems with the baby's heart rate, oxytocin may be reduced or stopped. Other treatments also may be needed to steady the baby's heart rate.

Other risks of labor induction may include

- ***chorioamnionitis,*** an infection of the ***amniotic fluid***, placenta, or membranes
- infection in the baby
- rupture of the uterus (rare)

Sometimes labor induction doesn't work. If you and your baby are doing well and the amniotic sac has not ruptured, you may be given the option to go home. You can schedule another appointment to try induction again. If your labor starts, you should go back to the hospital.

If you or your baby are not doing well during or after attempting induction, a cesarean delivery may be needed. Although most cesarean deliveries are safe, there may be additional risks for you, including

- infection
- **hemorrhage** (heavy bleeding)
- complications from **anesthesia**

The recovery time after a cesarean delivery usually is longer than for a vaginal delivery.

There also are considerations for future pregnancies. With each cesarean delivery, the risk of serious placenta problems in future pregnancies goes up. In addition, the number of cesarean deliveries you have had is a major factor in how you will give birth to any future babies. See Chapter 17, "Cesarean Delivery and Vaginal Birth After Cesarean Delivery," for a detailed discussion of cesarean delivery.

If Your Labor Is Going to Be Induced

If your ob-gyn recommends labor induction, make sure that you understand

- why the induction is recommended
- the method or methods that will be used
- what you can reasonably expect to happen during your induction

The first stage of labor typically lasts longer when labor is induced than when it starts on its own. Pain relief during an induced labor can be given in just the same way as in a spontaneous labor. This pain relief may include an **epidural block, spinal block,** or medications given through an IV line. Discuss your pain-relief options with your ob-gyn before labor.

RESOURCES

Inducing Labor
www.nlm.nih.gov/medlineplus/ency/patientinstructions/000625.htm
Webpage from the U.S. National Library of Medicine. Provides a basic overview of the ways labor can be induced.

Your Pregnancy and Childbirth
www.acog.org/MyPregnancy
Website from the American College of Obstetricians and Gynecologists (ACOG) with information on pregnancy, labor, delivery, and postpartum care. Includes the latest information from the experts in women's health care, questions answered by ACOG ob-gyns, pregnancy stories from real women, and an A–Z directory of health topics covering pregnancy and beyond.

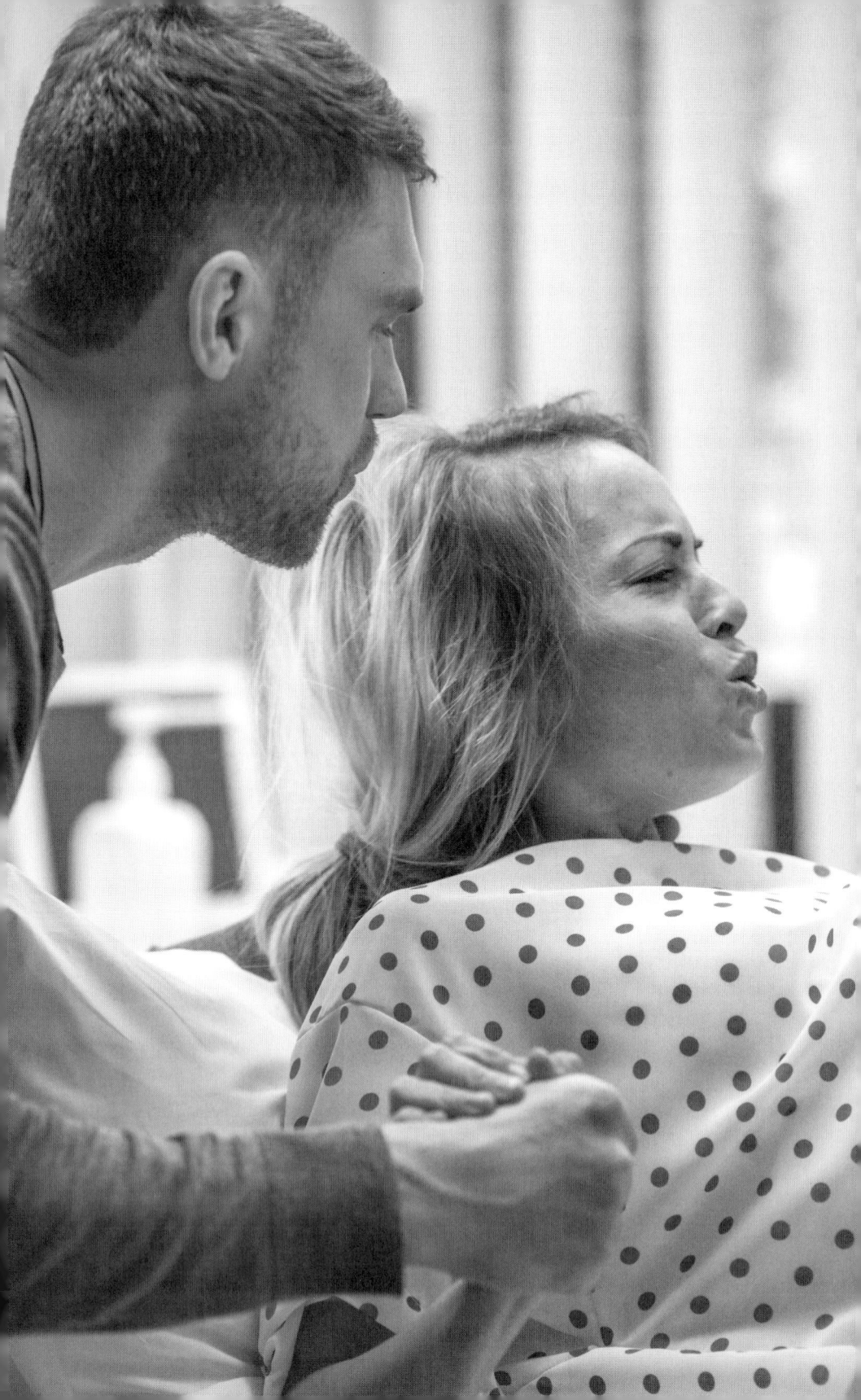

CHAPTER 15

Labor and Delivery

Labor is the process that gets your body ready to deliver your baby. As labor begins, the **cervix** starts to dilate (open). The **uterus** contracts at regular intervals, with contractions getting stronger and closer together.

For a woman having her first baby, labor typically lasts 12 to 18 hours. For women who have given birth before, it typically lasts 8 to 10 hours. But every woman is different. Your labor may not be like your mother's, your sister's, or your friend's labor. It may even be different with each child you have. Even so, labor and delivery usually follow a pattern. The more you know about what to expect during labor, the better prepared you will be once it begins.

Knowing When You're in Labor

It sometimes can be hard to tell when you're in labor. ***Braxton Hicks contractions*** can happen for many weeks before real labor begins. These "practice" contractions can be very painful and can make you think you are in labor when you are not. There are certain changes in your body that signal real labor is near:

- Lightening—You feel as if the baby has dropped lower. Because the baby isn't pressing on your diaphragm, you may feel "lighter." The baby's head settles deep into your pelvis. Lightening can happen anywhere from a few weeks to a few hours before labor begins.

- Loss of the mucus plug—A thick mucus plug forms at the cervix during pregnancy. When the cervix begins to dilate (open) several days before

Common Labor Terms

You may hear your **obstetrician–gynecologist (ob-gyn)** and labor nurses use specific terms to describe how your labor is progressing:

- **Effacement**—Shortening and thinning of the cervix. When not in labor, your cervix is a strong, thick tube that connects the top of the vagina to the bottom of the uterus. As your labor progresses, the cervix will soften and thin out until it is right up against the uterine wall. Effacement is estimated in percentages, from zero percent (no effacement) to 100 percent (complete effacement). Effacement makes it possible for your cervix to dilate (open) and for the baby to pass through the opening.

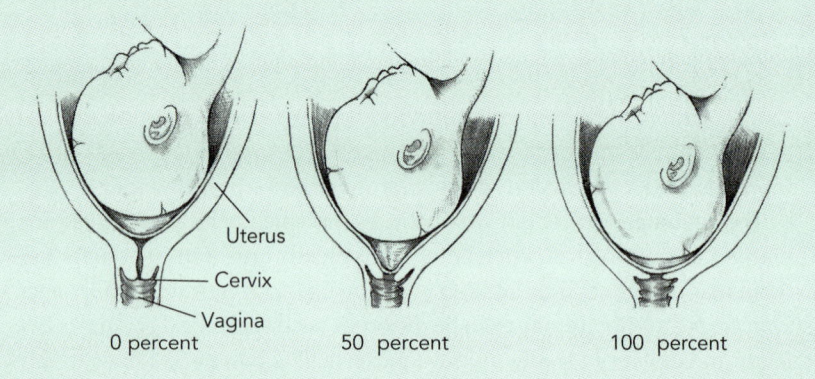

- **Dilation**—The amount that the cervix has opened. It is measured in centimeters (cm), from 0 cm (no dilation) to 10 cm (fully dilated).

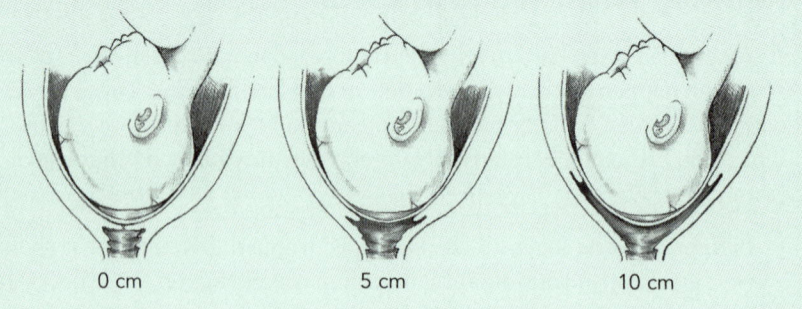

- **Cervical ripening**—The process of softening, thinning, and dilation of the cervix in preparation for birth.

- **Presentation**—The part of the baby that is lowest in the vagina. Normally, the baby's head is the presenting part. This is called a **cephalic presentation.**

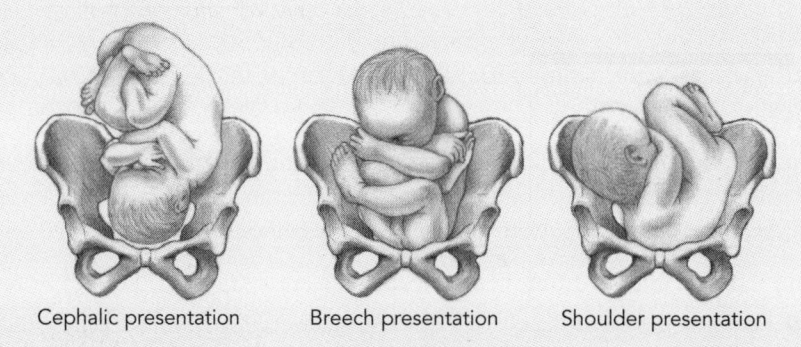

Cephalic presentation   Breech presentation   Shoulder presentation

- **Station**—The location of the presenting part of the baby (usually the head) in the vagina. The ischial spines, which are the bony parts of the pelvis that stick out into the birth canal, are used as a reference point. Station is measured in numbers, describing where the presenting part is relative to the ischial spines. A negative station (from −1 to −5) means that the presenting part is above the spines. A positive station (from +1 to +5) describes a presenting part that has progressed down the birth canal. At +5, the baby is **crowning**, and the head is visible just at the opening of a woman's vagina during a pelvic exam.

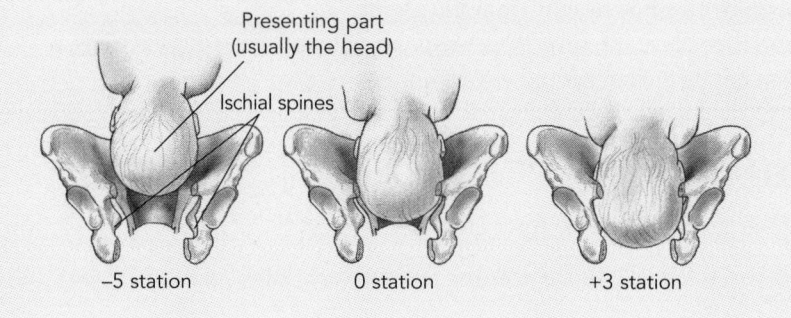

Presenting part (usually the head)
Ischial spines

−5 station   0 station   +3 station

labor begins or at the start of labor, the plug passes into the **vagina**. You may notice an increase in vaginal discharge that's clear, pink, or slightly bloody. Some women expel the entire mucus plug.

- Rupture of membranes—The fluid-filled **amniotic sac** that surrounds the baby during pregnancy breaks (your "water breaks"). You may feel this as fluid that trickles or gushes from your vagina. Call your ob-gyn's office and go directly to the hospital if your water breaks. Once your water breaks, your ob-gyn will want to make sure labor begins soon if it hasn't already. A delayed labor after the water breaks increases the chance of an infection in the uterus (**chorioamnionitis**) that is dangerous for the woman and her baby.

- Contractions—As your uterus contracts, you may feel pain in your back or pelvis. This pain may be similar to menstrual cramps. Labor contractions happen in a regular pattern and get closer together over time.

How can you tell the difference between true labor contractions and Braxton Hicks contractions? Time the contractions and note whether they continue when you are resting and drinking water. If rest and hydration make the contractions go away, they are not true labor contractions. Table 15-1, "Differences Between False Labor and True Labor," shows other differences.

If you think you are in labor (or are not sure), call your ob-gyn. Sometimes the only way to tell the difference is by having a vaginal exam to look for changes in your cervix. You should go to the hospital if you have any of these signs:

- Your water has broken and you are not having contractions.
- You are bleeding heavily from the vagina.
- You have constant, severe pain with no relief between contractions.
- You notice the baby is moving less often.

Stages of Childbirth

Childbirth is divided into three stages:

- Stage 1 is labor. This stage is divided into early labor and active labor.
- Stage 2 is the pushing and delivery phase, when you push out the baby.
- Stage 3 is the delivery of the **placenta**.

TABLE 15-1 **Differences Between False Labor and True Labor**

Symptom	False Labor	True Labor
Timing of contractions	Contractions are not regular. They do not get closer together. These are called Braxton Hicks contractions.	Contractions come at regular intervals. As time goes on, they get closer together. Each lasts about 60 to 90 seconds.
Change with movement	Contractions may stop when you walk or rest. They also may stop with a change of position.	Contractions continue even when you rest or move around.
Strength of contractions	Contractions are weak and do not get much stronger. They may start strong and then weaken.	Contractions steadily get stronger.
Frequency of contractions	Contractions are irregular and do not have a pattern.	Contractions have a pattern.
Location of pain	Pain usually is felt only in the front.	Pain usually starts in the back and moves to the front.

When reading this chapter, remember that every woman's labor is unique to her. The descriptions of the typical labor below may not describe exactly what you will experience.

Stage 1: Early Labor

Stage 1 is divided into two phases: early labor and active labor. The beginning of early labor can be difficult to define, but it usually means that you are having regular contractions until the cervix dilates to 6 cm. You may hear this stage described as "latent labor."

What Happens During Early Labor. During early labor, you may feel mild contractions that happen 5 to 15 minutes apart and last about 60 to 90 seconds. The contractions gradually will get closer together. Toward the end of early labor, they will be less than 5 minutes apart.

During these contractions, you may feel pain or pressure that starts in your back and moves around to your lower belly. When this happens, your belly will tighten and feel hard. Between contractions, the uterus relaxes, and your belly softens. These contractions are doing important work. They help dilate the cervix and push the baby lower into the pelvis.

The first stage of labor is almost always the longest. How long it lasts is different for every woman and every pregnancy. For first-time moms, the average is from 6 to 12 hours, but it can last up to 20 hours for some women. For repeat moms, the first stage of labor can last up to 14 hours.

STAGE 1
Early labor — Active labor

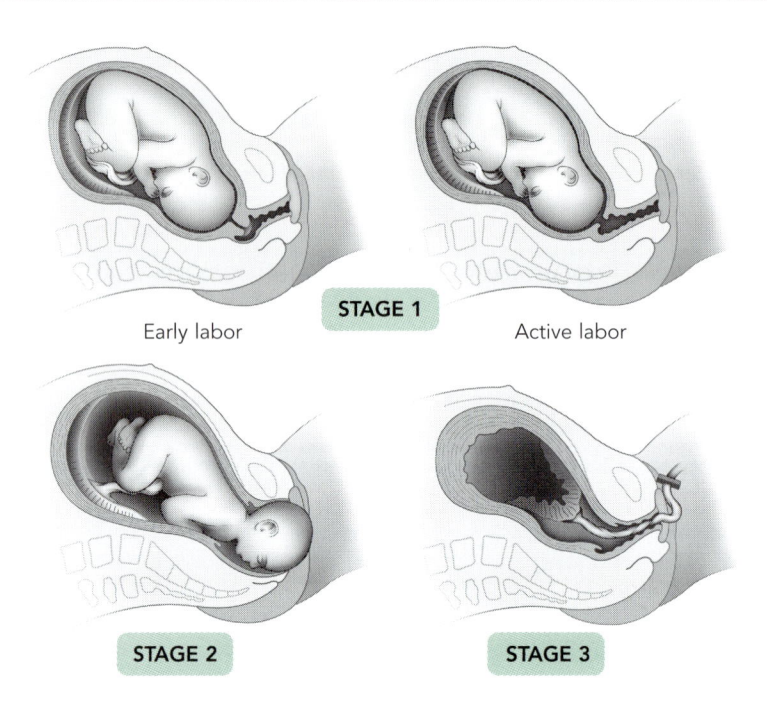

STAGE 2

STAGE 3

The three stages of childbirth. In Stage 1, the cervix dilates. In Stage 2, the cervix completely dilates, and the woman pushes the baby out of the vagina. In Stage 3, the placenta comes away from the uterus and is delivered.

The intensity of early labor also varies. Some women do not feel any contractions in very early labor. For others, contractions are more intense but usually are manageable.

If you are having a low-risk pregnancy, you probably will spend most of early labor at home, waiting for the contractions to get closer together. Your ob-gyn most likely will have given you instructions for when to leave for the hospital. Follow these instructions exactly. If your water breaks or if you have significant bleeding, call your ob-gyn and go to the hospital right away.

What You Can Do. During early labor, try to stay as relaxed as possible. Staying relaxed will help your cervix thin out and dilate. You may want to alternate active movements with rest. Here are some things you can do during early labor:

- Go for a walk.
- Take a shower or bath.
- Play some relaxing music.

- Do the relaxation and breathing techniques you learned in childbirth class.
- Change positions often.
- Make sure you have everything you need for the hospital.
- Make sure you have arranged for child care and pet care, if needed.

Slow, relaxed breathing may be helpful during this stage:
- Take a deep, cleansing breath at the beginning of a contraction.
- Breathe out slowly during the contraction, focusing on the in-and-out movement of your breath.
- Try counting during the contraction.
- At the end of the contraction, take a deep, cleansing breath.

How Your Labor Partner Can Help. Your labor partner can be a big help to you during the early stage of labor. Now is the time for your labor partner to help you with the strategies you learned in childbirth class about how to relax and cope with the pain. Other ways your labor partner can help include

- keeping you distracted by playing cards or other games
- massaging your back and shoulders
- timing your contractions (how long they last and how far apart they are)
- placing a heating pad or ice pack on your lower back
- making phone calls with you

Stage 1: Active Labor

As active labor begins, your contractions get stronger and come closer together. It is during this stage that the cervix dilates fastest. Active labor starts when a woman is having regular contractions and her cervix is dilated to 6 cm. It's hard to know exactly when this happens, so when your contractions are stronger, closer together, and regular, it's time to go to the hospital.

What Happens When You Go to the Hospital. Before you are checked in to the hospital or birth center, the staff will determine whether you are in labor. You may be taken to a special room or the hospital's emergency room. The health care team will check

- your vital signs (temperature, blood pressure, pulse)
- the baby's heart rate
- how often you have contractions and how long they are

- the position of the baby
- the estimated weight of the baby

You may have a **pelvic exam** to check cervical dilation and ***effacement.*** You may be checked for vaginal bleeding or to see if your water has broken. The health care team also may ask if you have a high-risk medical or pregnancy-specific condition.

The only way to diagnose labor is for your ob-gyn to see changes taking place in the cervix. If your cervix is changing, you may be checked in to the hospital or birth center. If your cervix is not changing, and you and the baby are doing well, you may be given some time to see if the changes start. Some hospitals and birth centers allow women to walk around to see if labor progresses. Or you may be sent home until your contractions are more regular.

If you are checked in, the following things usually happen:

- You'll be taken to a room. In some hospitals and birth centers, you will stay in the same room for both labor and delivery. Others have a separate delivery room.
- You'll be asked to put on a hospital gown.
- An ***intravenous (IV) line*** or "hep-lock" may be placed in your arm so that medications and fluids can be given if you need them.
- Depending on your hospital's policy and the health of you and your baby, you may be connected to a fetal monitor. ***Electronic fetal monitoring*** lets your care team monitor your baby's heart rate and the frequency of your contractions.

After you have been examined and your condition is assessed, you may be asked to sign consent forms. These forms vary, but most spell out

- who will be taking care of you
- why a procedure is being done
- the risks that are involved

Read any forms you are given and ask about anything that's not clear. Signing a consent form means that you understand your medical condition and agree to the care described. You may need to sign separate consent forms if you need ***anesthesia*** or a ***cesarean birth.***

Once you're in your room, a labor and delivery nurse will check on you from the time you arrive until after your baby is born. Labor nurses are trained to help women through the physical and emotional demands of labor.

In teaching hospitals, a resident doctor, student nurse, or medical student also may be a part of your birth team.

Your own ob-gyn may be there from start to finish, or he or she may arrive shortly before you give birth. If your ob-gyn works in a group practice, the "on call" ob-gyn may be there instead. During your prenatal visits, ask your ob-gyn about who you can expect to be there for your delivery.

During active labor, the health care team will closely monitor

- your heart rate and blood pressure
- the time between and length of your contractions
- how much your cervix has dilated
- the baby's heartbeat, either continuously with an electronic fetal monitor or periodically with a **Doppler ultrasound exam** or a special stethoscope

What Happens During Active Labor. During active labor the cervix dilates from 6 cm to 10 cm. Contractions get stronger and may come 2 to 3 minutes apart. Each contraction lasts about 45 seconds, but they can be as short as 30 seconds or as long as 70 seconds. Active labor can last about 4 to 8 hours. During this time, you may experience the following:

- Your water may break if it hasn't already.
- Your contractions will get stronger.
- You may have back pain if the baby's head presses on your backbone during contractions.
- Your legs may cramp.
- You may feel the urge to push.
- You may feel nauseated.

What You Can Do. Your contractions will get more intense, so focus on your breathing and take each contraction one at a time. Let your labor partner and nurse help you through your breathing and relaxation exercises. When each contraction passes, try to relax, and don't think about the next one. It may help to move around to find a position that is most comfortable for you. Medications for pain relief also can be given. See Chapter 13, "Pain Relief During Childbirth," for a discussion of pain-relief techniques.

There are some other things you can do now to cope with the contractions:

- If you feel like it and your ob-gyn says it's OK, walk the halls.

- If you want to, your ob-gyn agrees, and the hospital has the proper equipment, sit in a water bath. You also may be able to take a shower.

- Urinate often, because an empty **bladder** gives the baby's head more room to move down.

- If you feel the urge to push, tell your ob-gyn. Don't give in to the urge just yet—pant or blow out air to keep yourself from bearing down. Pushing too soon can cause swelling and pain in the **vulva** and can lead to tears of the tissues.

Eating solid food during active labor is not recommended. If circumstances change and you need to have a cesarean birth, having food in your stomach can lead to serious **complications**. Women with a healthy pregnancy can have small amounts of clear liquids during labor. Clear liquids include water, fruit juices without pulp, carbonated beverages, tea, and sports drinks. Your hospital or birth center may have some of these drinks on hand, or you can bring your own liquids from home.

How Your Labor Partner Can Help. You'll depend on your labor partner more and more as the labor pains intensify. Let your labor partner help you through the pain-management methods you learned in childbirth class. Your labor partner also can help by

- applying firm pressure on your lower back
- massaging your lower back with knuckles or a tennis ball
- flexing your feet to help relieve your leg cramps
- acting as a focal point during contractions
- offering comfort and support
- giving you small amounts of clear liquids if you want them

If labor isn't progressing the way it should, your ob-gyn may recommend **labor augmentation**. This means doing things to help your labor along, including

- rupturing the membranes (if your water hasn't already broken)
- giving **oxytocin** to increase the frequency and length of contractions

Labor may be augmented if the woman is in active labor but her contractions are so infrequent or mild that they won't cause the cervix to dilate. See Chapter 14, "Labor Induction," for details on how labor induction is done.

Transition to Stage 2

Toward the end of the active phase of labor, it is common for labor to intensify. For many women, this will be the toughest stage and the most painful. If you've been given an **epidural block** or other pain medication, the pain may not be as intense. Contractions will come closer together and can last 60 to 90 seconds. With each contraction, you may feel an urge to bear down or push. You'll feel a lot of pressure in your lower back and **rectum**. This can feel like the urge to have a bowel movement but much stronger.

Tell your ob-gyn or nurse as soon as you feel like pushing. He or she will check your cervix to see how much it has dilated. Until your cervix is fully dilated and your ob-gyn or nurse gives you the go-ahead, you should try not to push. Pushing before your cervix is fully dilated can exhaust you. It also can cause some swelling of the cervix, which may stop it from fully dilating. Controlling your breathing or blowing air out in short puffs can help you resist the urge to push.

Stage 2: Pushing and Delivery

At this stage, you actively participate in pushing out your baby. Stage 2 is different for every woman and for every pregnancy. The second stage of labor often is shorter than the first stage, but it usually involves the most work for the laboring woman. During Stage 2, you'll notice a change in the way your contractions feel. They usually are stronger and more painful, come 2 to 5 minutes apart, and last about 60 to 90 seconds.

The second stage of labor can last anywhere from minutes to 2 to 3 hours. If you have had an epidural, it may take longer to push out the baby. If the second stage lasts longer than 2 hours (for a woman who has given birth before) or 3 hours (for a first-time mom) and you have not had anesthesia, you may need help to get the baby out if you are not making progress. This may mean any of the following:

- An **assisted vaginal delivery** using **forceps** or a **vacuum device** (see Chapter 16, "Assisted Vaginal Delivery and Breech Presentation")
- Turning the baby so that it is in a better position for birth
- A **cesarean delivery** (see Chapter 17, "Cesarean Delivery and Vaginal Birth After Cesarean Delivery")

If you have had an epidural, a longer time may be allowed for the second stage, especially if you are making progress.

What You Can Do. If you have labored in a room that also is equipped for delivery, your ob-gyn and nurse will help you get into a good delivery position. If you have labored in a room that is not equipped for delivery, you will be moved to a delivery room before you are helped into a good delivery position.

Many women give birth to their babies while propped up in bed, with their legs in stirrups or braced by their labor partner. There are other birth positions you can try if your ob-gyn approves. See Chapter 13, "Pain Relief During Childbirth," for more on labor and delivery positions.

Once your ob-gyn gives you the go-ahead, bear down with each contraction or when you are told to push. When the baby's head appears at the opening of your vagina, you may feel a burning or stinging sensation as the *perineum* stretches and bulges. This feeling is normal.

After the head emerges from the birth canal, one shoulder delivers and then the other. After the shoulders are delivered, the rest of the baby's body follows quickly. Your ob-gyn or your labor partner will cut the **umbilical cord**. Some of the blood in the umbilical cord may be taken for newborn blood tests, such as blood typing.

How Your Labor Partner Can Help. Your labor partner can make a real difference during this stage of labor. For some birth positions, your labor partner is needed to give you physical support. For squatting positions, you may need to lean on or hold onto your labor partner for balance. If you are lying on your back, your labor partner can support one of your legs.

Offering words of support also can be a big help. Tell your labor partner what kind of support you need. If you need your labor partner to be hands off, that's OK too.

Stage 3: Delivery of the Placenta

After your baby is delivered, the placenta is still in the uterus and will need to be delivered. This last stage of labor is the shortest of all, but it can last 30 minutes or more.

During this stage, you still will have contractions. They will be closer together and less painful. These contractions help the placenta separate from the wall of the uterus. Then the contractions will move the placenta down into the birth canal. Once the placenta is in the vagina, you will need to bear down to push it out. Some ob-gyns help by applying gentle traction to the umbilical cord or reaching inside the vagina to grasp the placenta.

If you had an *episiotomy* or tear, it will be repaired now. If you have chosen to store cord blood, it will be collected either before or after delivery of the placenta. See Chapter 12, "Preparing for Birth," for a discussion of cord blood banking.

After the placenta is delivered, your uterus will continue to contract. These contractions help your uterus return to its smaller size. Medication may be given (either before or after the placenta is delivered) to help the uterus contract and prevent too much bleeding. A nurse may press on your belly to massage the uterus, which helps it contract and helps decrease bleeding. As the uterus shrinks, the body naturally seals the blood vessels that led to the placenta. This also helps control blood loss.

After the Baby Is Born

If you had an uncomplicated labor and delivery, your baby will be placed on your belly or chest, against your skin, right after he or she is born. If you had any problems during labor or delivery or if the baby is **preterm**, he or she may need to be evaluated by medical staff first or placed under a warming light.

If all is well, you most likely will be able to spend as much time as you want with your baby. The staff will check on you and your baby often to make sure you are both doing well. A physical exam and tests of your newborn can be done about an hour after birth, when you and your baby are ready (see Chapter 18, "After the Baby Is Born").

Your blood pressure, pulse, and temperature will be measured often for the next few hours. This is done to monitor you for signs of infection or heavy bleeding. If you had an epidural block or a **spinal block**, you will be observed for a few hours. If you were moved to a delivery room for the birth, you will be returned to a regular room when your condition is stable.

RESOURCES

Childbirth
https://medlineplus.gov/childbirth.html
Webpage from the U.S. National Library of Medicine. A starting point with links to detailed resources on many childbirth topics.

Your Pregnancy and Childbirth
www.acog.org/MyPregnancy
Website from the American College of Obstetricians and Gynecologists (ACOG) with information on pregnancy, labor, delivery, and postpartum care. Includes the latest information from the experts in women's health care, questions answered by ACOG ob-gyns, pregnancy stories from real women, and an A–Z directory of health topics covering pregnancy and beyond.

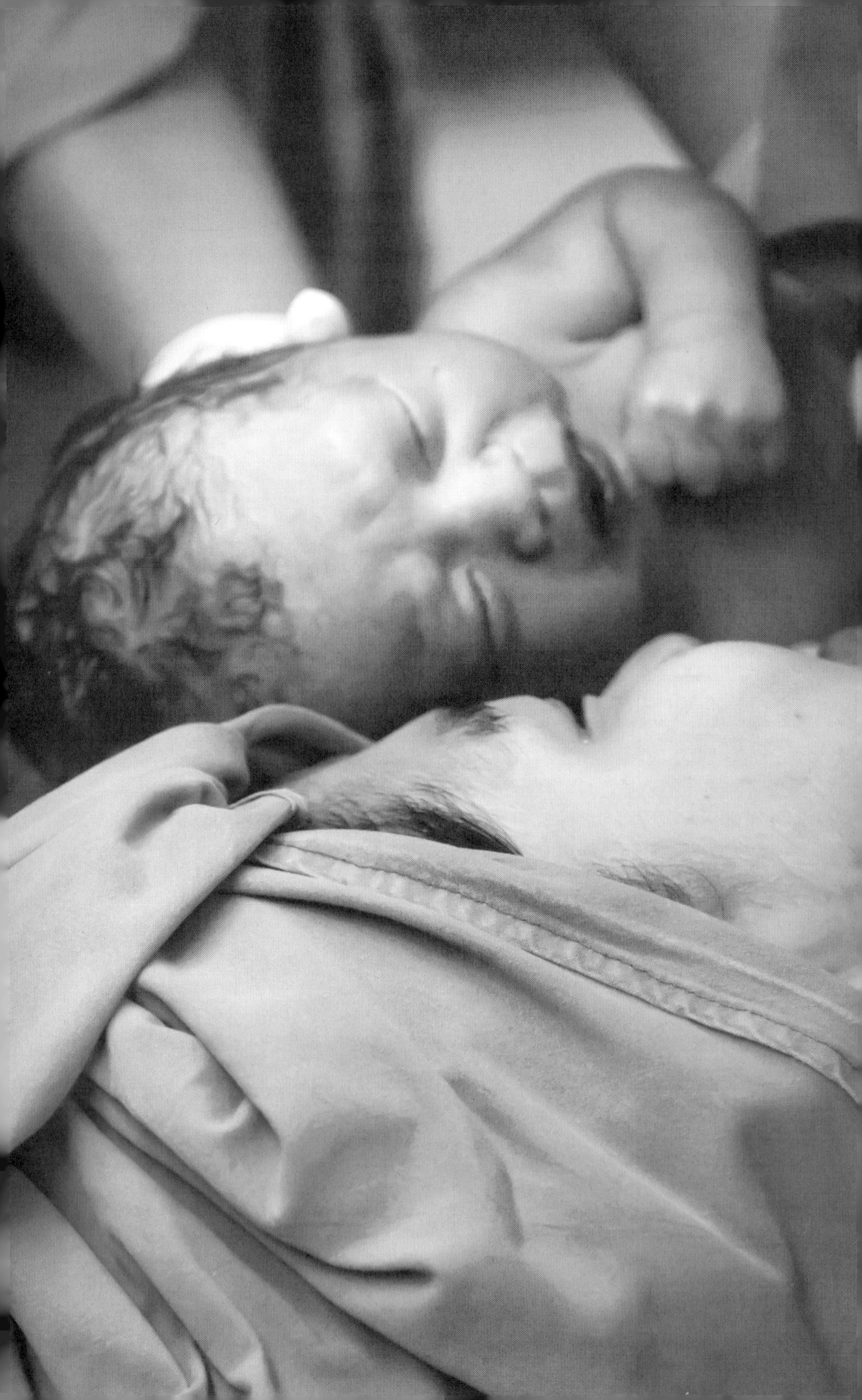

CHAPTER 16

Assisted Vaginal Delivery and Breech Presentation

Sometimes labor doesn't go as planned. Labor can slow down or stop. Problems with the baby or with labor may arise. If your **obstetrician–gynecologist (ob-gyn)** thinks that continuing labor or a vaginal delivery would be unsafe for you or your baby, he or she may recommend **assisted vaginal delivery** or **cesarean delivery**. This chapter covers assisted vaginal delivery. Cesarean delivery is discussed in a separate chapter (see Chapter 17, "Cesarean Delivery and Vaginal Birth After Cesarean Delivery").

A **breech presentation** is when a baby is positioned to come out feet or bottom first. This is often detected a few weeks before labor starts. But sometimes a breech presentation is not detected until you are in labor. In rare cases, babies have been known to turn from head down to breech during labor. If your baby is in a breech position, it may be possible to turn the baby before delivery. If the baby does not turn, you will need to discuss a plan for delivery with your ob-gyn.

Assisted Vaginal Delivery

Once labor starts, it usually progresses steadily. No one can predict just how the birth of a baby will happen. Some births happen quickly and there are no problems. With others, the woman may push for hours and not make much progress, or problems may happen during labor. In some cases, your ob-gyn may recommend an assisted delivery with **forceps** or a **vacuum device**. This type of delivery is called assisted vaginal delivery.

Assisted vaginal delivery is done in about 3 in 100 vaginal deliveries in the United States. If your ob-gyn recommends an assisted vaginal delivery, you should talk together about why it may be needed. Some of the reasons why an assisted vaginal delivery may be done include the following:

- There are concerns about your baby's well-being during labor (for example, your baby's heart rate becomes slow or erratic).
- You have pushed for a long time, but the baby's head has stopped moving down the birth canal.
- You are very tired from a long labor.
- A medical condition limits your ability to push safely and effectively.

Before recommending assisted vaginal delivery, your ob-gyn will consider a number of factors, including

- your baby's estimated weight
- where your baby is in the birth canal
- the size and shape of your pelvis and if it seems there is enough room for the baby to pass through
- whether your *cervix* is fully dilated (opened)

One of the main advantages of assisted vaginal delivery is that it may help avoid a cesarean delivery. Cesarean delivery is major surgery. Although rare, risks of cesarean delivery include

- heavy bleeding
- infection
- injury to the bowel or *bladder*
- problems related to the *anesthesia* used
- longer recovery time than vaginal delivery

Cesarean delivery also increases risks for future pregnancies, including

- *placenta* problems
- rupture of the *uterus*
- *hysterectomy*

Recovery from a vaginal delivery generally is shorter than recovery from a cesarean delivery. Often, assisted vaginal delivery can be done more quickly than a cesarean delivery.

Types of Assisted Vaginal Delivery

There are two types of assisted vaginal delivery:

- Forceps-assisted delivery—Forceps look like two large spoons. They are inserted into the *vagina* and placed around the baby's cheekbones and jaw. The forceps then are used to gently guide the baby's head out of the birth canal while you continue to push.

- Vacuum-assisted delivery—A vacuum device has a suction cup with a handle attached. The suction cup is inserted into the vagina and is pressed to the baby's head. Suction holds the cup in place. Your ob-gyn uses the handle to gently guide the baby's head out through the birth canal while you continue to push.

Both types of delivery are safe. The choice depends on several factors, including the experience of your ob-gyn and your labor situation.

Risks of Assisted Vaginal Delivery

In most cases, using these devices to help with delivery causes no major problems. But as with most medical procedures, there are some risks associated with assisted vaginal delivery, for both you and the baby. Discuss these risks with your ob-gyn before assisted vaginal delivery is done.

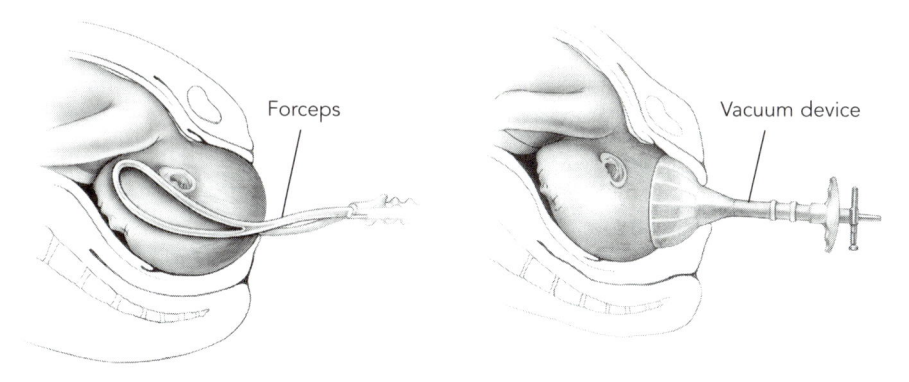

Forceps-assisted delivery

Vacuum-assisted delivery

Types of assisted vaginal delivery. Assisted vaginal delivery involves the use of forceps or a vacuum device. Using one of these devices, your ob-gyn can help gently guide the baby's head while you continue to push.

Risks for the Baby. Although the overall rate of injury to the baby is low, there still is a risk of certain **complications**. The risks of assisted vaginal delivery include

- injuries to the baby's scalp, head, and eyes
- seizures and bleeding inside the skull (rare)
- problems with the nerves located in the arm and face

Jaundice happens more often in newborns delivered by vacuum assistance. There is no evidence that an uncomplicated assisted vaginal delivery has any effect on a child's development.

Risks for You. Both forceps-assisted delivery and vacuum-assisted delivery may cause injury to the vagina, **perineum**, and **anus**. But keep in mind that any vaginal delivery might cause these injuries. If you have had a tear, it may require repair with stitches. After spontaneous or assisted vaginal delivery, you may have perineal swelling, pain, and bruising. You likely will have a few weeks of swelling and pain as the perineum heals. It may be hard to walk or sit for a time.

Injuries after spontaneous or assisted vaginal deliveries can lead to problems after delivery, including

- **anal incontinence**
- **urinary incontinence**
- **pelvic organ prolapse (POP)**

Some women with these problems may need surgery later in life to help fix them.

If you have had one assisted vaginal delivery, you are more likely to have one in a later pregnancy. But the chances are good that you will have a normal, spontaneous vaginal delivery the next time. Some of the factors that increase the risk of another assisted vaginal delivery include

- a long interval between pregnancies (more than 3 years)
- a baby that is estimated to be larger than average

Breech Presentation

By 3 or 4 weeks before the due date, most babies change position so their heads are down near the birth canal. This is called a **cephalic presentation**. If the baby does not change position, he or she may be in a breech presentation.

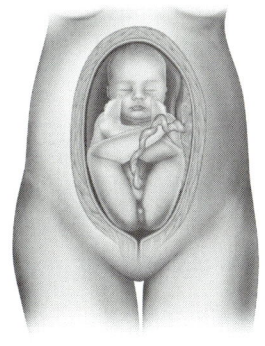

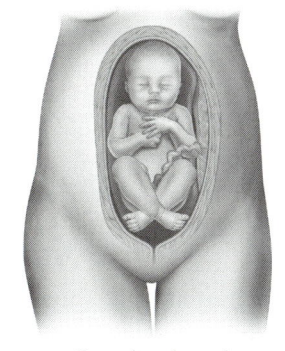

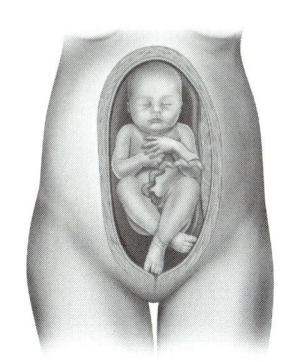

Frank breech　　　　Complete breech　　　　Footling breech

Breech presentations. In a breech presentation, the baby's bottom, both feet, or one foot may be in place to come out first during birth.

This happens in 3 to 4 in 100 pregnancies that are carried to *full term*. It happens more often in *preterm* babies.

The reasons why a baby goes into a breech position are not well known. But it is more common in one or more of the following situations:

- You have had more than one pregnancy.
- You are having twins.
- The uterus has too much or too little *amniotic fluid*.
- The uterus is abnormal in shape or has abnormal growths (*fibroids*, for example).
- The *placenta* covers all or part of the opening of the uterus (*placenta previa*).

Occasionally, babies with certain *birth defects* also will stay in a breech position at term. But most babies who are breech are otherwise normal.

The Baby's Position

During the last weeks of your pregnancy, your ob-gyn should do a physical exam to find out the baby's position. Your ob-gyn will place his or her hands on your belly and try to feel the outline of the baby. By locating the baby's head, back, and bottom, your ob-gyn can tell what position the baby is in. If a breech presentation is suspected, an *ultrasound exam* may be done to confirm the position.

The baby's position can change until the end of pregnancy. As the time of delivery nears, some babies turn on their own. Your ob-gyn may not know for sure if your baby has settled in a breech position until labor starts. Sometimes a breech position is first found during a pelvic exam of a woman in labor.

Turning the Baby

If the baby is breech—and depending on the condition of you and the baby—your ob-gyn may try to turn the baby head down so that you can deliver vaginally without complications. This procedure is known as **external cephalic version (ECV)**. The chances that ECV will be successful are about 50-50. ECV won't be tried in any of the following situations:

- You are carrying more than one baby.
- There are possible fetal heart rate problems.
- You have certain abnormalities of the reproductive system.
- The placenta is in the wrong place (placenta previa).
- The placenta has detached from the wall of the uterus (**placental abruption**).

ECV may be considered if you had a **cesarean birth** with another pregnancy. This depends on the reason why the cesarean delivery was done and the type of uterine scar that you have. You and your ob-gyn should discuss the risks and benefits of ECV in this situation so that you can make an informed decision.

ECV usually is not done until you are at least 37 weeks pregnant. If it is done before this time, the baby may go back to a breech position. If that happens, ECV may be tried again. But it may be harder because the baby is bigger and there is less room for him or her to move.

How ECV Is Done. ECV usually is done near a delivery room so that if a problem happens, the baby can be delivered quickly by cesarean.

- The baby's heart rate is checked before and after ECV.
- Sometimes a medicine is given to relax the uterus. This may make it easier to turn the baby.
- Pain-relieving medication may be given. This may include an **epidural block** or medicine given through an **intravenous (IV) line**.
- To turn the baby, the ob-gyn places his or her hands on your belly.
- Firm pressure is applied to your belly to try to turn your baby.
- In some cases, a second health care practitioner may be asked to help turn the baby or do an ultrasound exam to monitor the baby.

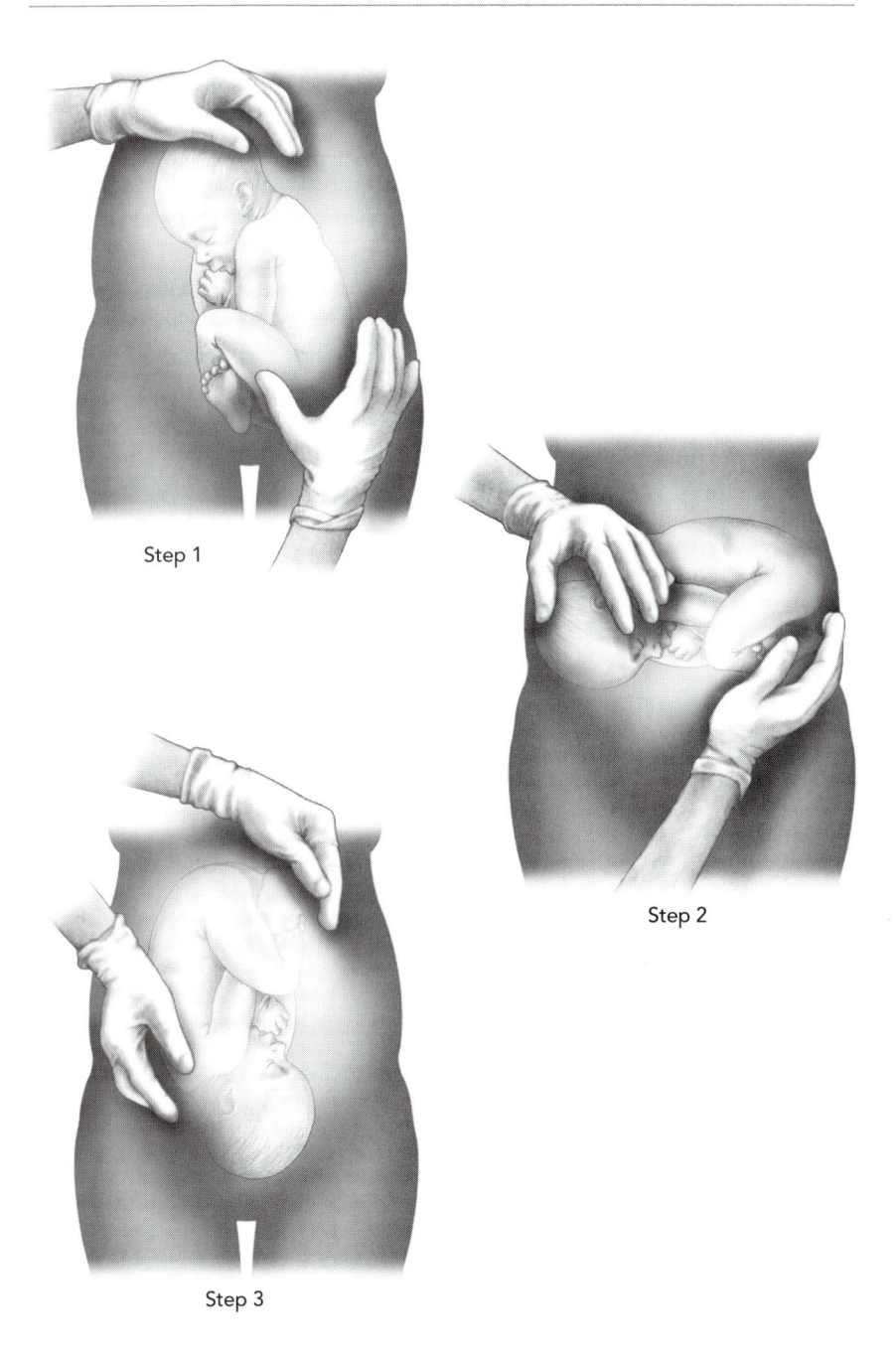

ASSISTED VAGINAL DELIVERY AND BREECH PRESENTATION • 249

Step 1

Step 2

Step 3

External cephalic version (ECV). In this procedure, the ob-gyn tries to move the baby from a breech position to a cephalic (head down) position. Firm pressure is applied to the belly to try to turn the baby.

The chance of complications with ECV is low. These complications may include

- ***prelabor rupture of membranes (PROM)***
- problems with the baby's heart rate
- placental abruption

After the procedure, you will be monitored for some time to make sure your condition and the baby's condition are stable.

Options for Delivery

If your baby is breech, you and your ob-gyn should talk about the best type of birth for you and your baby. If the baby can be turned with ECV, vaginal birth may be an option. But if the baby still is breech as the time of delivery nears, cesarean delivery may be best. Your ob-gyn should review the risks and benefits of both types of birth in detail. Together you will decide on the best plan for you and your baby.

Cesarean Delivery. Most breech babies are born by planned cesarean delivery. But it is not always possible to plan for cesarean delivery. The baby may move into the breech position just before labor begins. Some babies even move from head down to breech during labor, although this is very rare.

Vaginal Birth. Vaginal birth may be more difficult when a baby is breech. At birth, the head is the largest and firmest part of the baby's body. In the head-down position, the head comes out first, and the rest of the body follows. When a baby is breech, the baby's bottom or feet come out first, leaving the largest part of the body (the head) to be delivered last. This can increase complications for you and the baby:

- A breech baby's body may not stretch the ***cervix*** enough to allow room for the baby's head to come out easily. The head or shoulders may get stuck. You and the baby can be injured if this happens.

- The ***umbilical cord*** may slip through the cervix into the birth canal before the baby does. This is called an ***umbilical cord prolapse***. If the cord gets pinched, it can stop the flow of blood through the cord to the baby. This is an emergency. See Chapter 39, "Problems During Labor and Delivery," for information on how umbilical cord prolapse is managed.

Vaginal birth may be possible in certain situations. You and your ob-gyn should discuss the possible risks of a vaginal birth with a breech presentation. Keep in mind that these risks are higher than if a cesarean birth is planned.

An important factor is the experience of your ob-gyn in delivering breech babies vaginally. You also may need to meet certain guidelines before planning to deliver your breech baby vaginally. Lastly, the hospital or birth center's policies may dictate how you can deliver a breech baby.

RESOURCES

Breech Babies: What Can I Do if My Baby Is Breech?
https://familydoctor.org/breech-babies-what-can-i-do-if-my-baby-is-breech/
Information from the American Academy of Family Physicians. Provides a detailed explanation of all aspects of breech presentation.

Breech Birth
https://medlineplus.gov/ency/patientinstructions/000623.htm
Webpage from the U.S. National Library of Medicine. Gives an overview of breech presentation and external cephalic version (ECV).

Your Pregnancy and Childbirth
www.acog.org/MyPregnancy
Website from the American College of Obstetricians and Gynecologists (ACOG) with information on pregnancy, labor, delivery, and postpartum care. Includes the latest information from the experts in women's health care, questions answered by ACOG ob-gyns, pregnancy stories from real women, and an A–Z directory of health topics covering pregnancy and beyond.

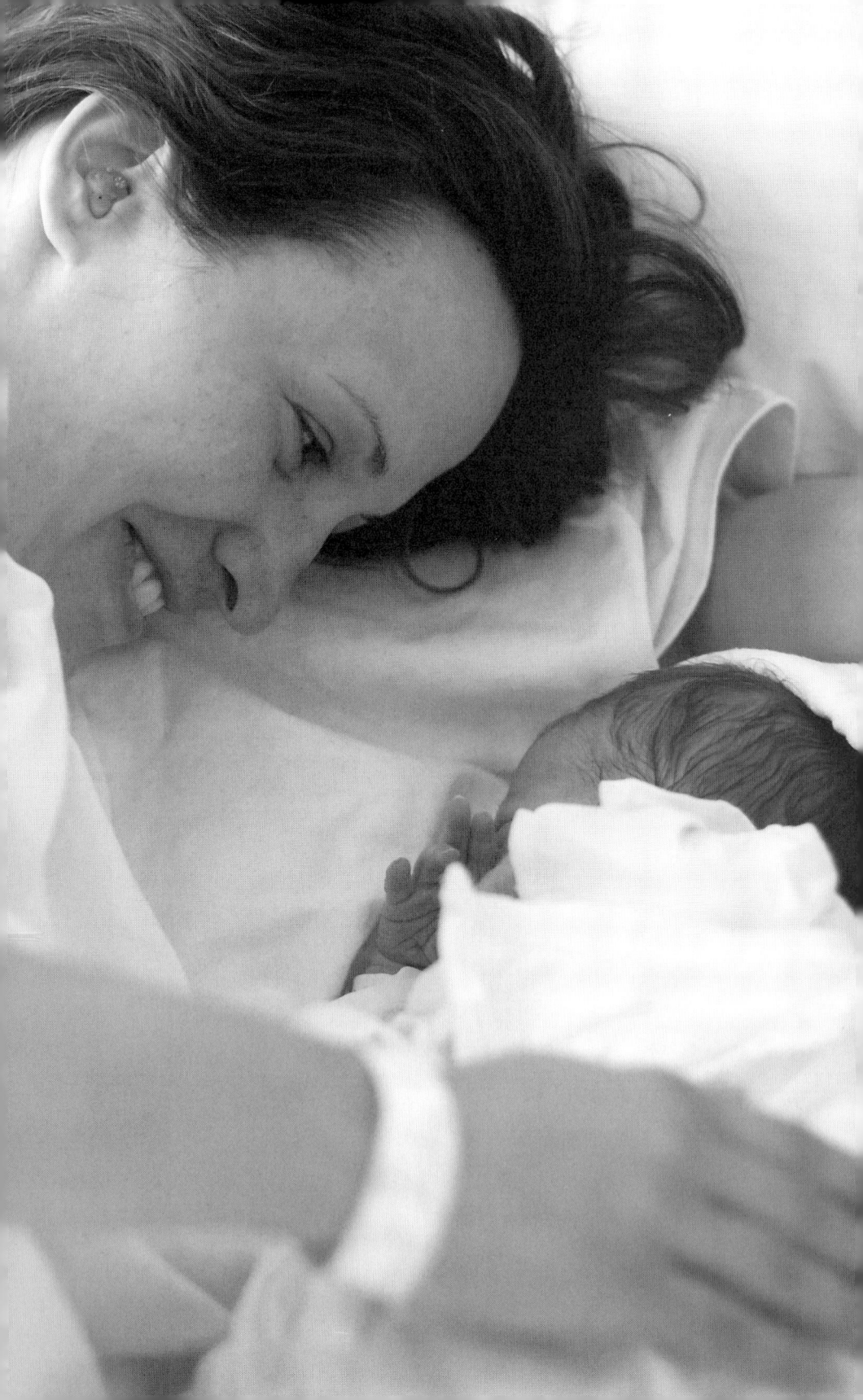

CHAPTER 17

Cesarean Delivery and Vaginal Birth After Cesarean Delivery

Most babies are born through the *vagina*. But in many pregnancies, a baby is delivered through *incisions* (surgical cuts) in the woman's belly and *uterus*. This is known as a *cesarean delivery*. Cesarean deliveries are common. In the United States, 1 in 3 babies is delivered this way.

It once was thought that if a woman had one *cesarean birth*, she would need to have all her other babies by cesarean delivery as well. Today, it is known that many women can attempt a *trial of labor after cesarean delivery (TOLAC)*. If a TOLAC is successful, a woman may be able to give birth through the vagina. This is called a *vaginal birth after cesarean (VBAC) delivery*.

Cesarean Delivery

Things can happen during labor that make a cesarean birth a safer choice—for either the woman or the baby—than a vaginal delivery.

Reasons for Cesarean Delivery

- Labor fails to progress—One of the most common reasons for a cesarean delivery is that labor slows down or stops. For example, contractions may be too weak or too far apart to dilate (open) the *cervix* wide enough for the baby. Sometimes the baby may be too big for the pelvis. Or the baby may be in the wrong position for safe passage.

- The baby's heart rate is abnormal—A heart rate outside the range of normal (110 to 160 beats per minute) could mean the labor is too stressful for the baby.

- There is a problem with the **umbilical cord**—If the umbilical cord gets pinched, the baby may not get enough **oxygen**. A fetal heart rate monitor is usually what tells the health care team this is happening.

A cesarean delivery also may need to be scheduled before a woman goes into labor because of certain problems or conditions. These may include the following:

- You had a certain type of incision for your last cesarean birth—Depending on the way the incision in your uterus was made, a previous cesarean birth may mean that you'll need to have a cesarean birth again.

- You're having multiple babies—If you are carrying two or more babies, you may need to have a cesarean birth. Many women having twins can have a vaginal delivery. But if the babies are born too early, you may need a cesarean delivery. This also may be needed if the "presenting twin" (the twin who is in position to be born first) is not in a head-down position. The chance of having a cesarean delivery goes up with the number of babies (see Chapter 28, "Multiples: When It's Twins, Triplets, or More").

- You have a large baby (**macrosomia**) or a small pelvis—Sometimes a baby is too big to pass safely through a woman's pelvis and vagina.

- Your baby is in a **breech presentation** or abnormal position—If your baby is breech, a planned cesarean delivery is the safest and most common method of delivery (see Chapter 16, "Assisted Vaginal Delivery and Breech Presentation"). If the baby is lying transverse (sideways) in the uterus rather than head down, a cesarean delivery is the only choice for delivery.

- There are problems with the **placenta**—**Placenta previa** means the placenta is below the baby and covers the opening of the uterus. This blocks the baby's exit. It also increases the risk of heavy bleeding if a vaginal delivery is attempted (see Chapter 37, "Placenta Problems").

- You have a medical condition that may make vaginal birth risky—A cesarean delivery may be done if a woman has an active **genital herpes** infection during labor. It also may be done if a woman has certain heart conditions or certain brain problems, such as an aneurysm.

Cesarean Delivery on Request

Some women ask to have a cesarean delivery even though there is no medical reason for it. This is known as cesarean delivery on maternal request. Some women ask for a cesarean delivery because they are anxious about labor and delivery. Other women ask for cesarean delivery because they fear the pain of vaginal delivery.

If you are thinking about asking for a cesarean delivery, you and your **obstetrician–gynecologist (ob-gyn)** should discuss whether it is right for you. Your discussion will focus on the risks and benefits of each type of delivery. Some of these risks and benefits depend on

- your age
- your **body mass index (BMI)**
- whether you want to have more children

If you are considering cesarean delivery on request because you are afraid of the pain of childbirth, talk with your ob-gyn about pain-relief options (see Chapter 13, "Pain Relief During Childbirth"). It also may help to learn all you can about the birth process (see Chapter 15, "Labor and Delivery"). If you had a difficult birth experience in the past, talk with your ob-gyn about your concerns.

A cesarean delivery is a major surgical procedure. Like all surgeries, it has risks. These risks include, but are not limited to

- heavy bleeding
- infection
- injury to the bowel, **bladder**, or other organs
- problems with **anesthesia**
- longer recovery time than vaginal delivery

Cesarean delivery also increases risks for future pregnancies. These risks may include

- placenta problems with heavy bleeding
- rupture of the uterus
- **hysterectomy**

For these reasons, cesarean delivery on request is not recommended for women who plan to have more children.

Having a cesarean delivery before 39 weeks of pregnancy increases health risks for newborns. Babies who are born even a few weeks or even days early may not be as developed as those who are born after 39 weeks. Babies born before 39 weeks may have an increased risk of short-term and long-term health problems, including

- *anemia*
- *jaundice*
- breathing problems
- feeding difficulties
- hearing and vision problems
- learning and behavioral issues in childhood

Babies born before 39 weeks also are more likely to spend time in a **neonatal intensive care unit (NICU).** When there is no medical reason to do so, having a planned cesarean delivery before 39 weeks is not recommended.

What Happens During a Cesarean Delivery

The way a cesarean delivery is done may depend on why it is being done. In most cases, cesarean deliveries follow a similar procedure.

Anesthesia

Different types of **anesthesia** are used for pain relief during a cesarean delivery. They include

- *epidural block*
- *spinal block*
- *combined spinal–epidural block*
- *general anesthesia*

The type of anesthesia used depends on several factors, including your health, the health of your baby, and the reason for the cesarean delivery. An **anesthesiologist** will talk with you about the benefits and risks of each type of anesthesia and suggest the best option for you (see Chapter 13, "Pain Relief During Childbirth").

If you are given an epidural during labor and then need to have a cesarean birth, your anesthesiologist may be able to inject more medication or a different medication through the same **catheter** to increase your pain relief. The **anesthetic** will numb you completely for the surgery. Although you will not feel any pain, there may be a feeling of pressure.

Preparing for Surgery

Before the cesarean delivery starts, a few steps are taken to prepare you for surgery:

- Your blood pressure, heart rate, and breathing will be monitored. An **oxygen** mask will be placed over your nose and mouth or an oxygen tube will be placed under your nose. This will help make sure you and your baby get plenty of oxygen.

- You will receive **antibiotics** through an **intravenous (IV) line**. This is done to prevent infection.

- Your belly will be washed and then swabbed with an antiseptic. If needed, pubic hair may be trimmed with clippers before washing the belly. (If your cesarean delivery is planned, do not shave your pubic hair the night before or morning of surgery. Using a razor can cause small cuts and increase the risk of infection of the incision.)

- Sometimes the vagina is also swabbed with antiseptic solution to reduce risk of infection.

- Sterile cloths will be placed around the area of the incision.

- A **catheter** will be inserted through your **urethra** and into your bladder. The catheter keeps the bladder empty to reduce the risk of bladder injury during surgery.

- Massaging sleeves will be put around your legs to reduce the risk of **deep vein thrombosis (DVT)** during surgery. These sleeves periodically fill with air to encourage blood circulation in your veins. If you have risk factors for blood clots, you also may receive medication to help prevent clots.

In cesarean deliveries that are not being done for an emergency, most hospitals allow you to have a support person with you in the operating room if you do not have general anesthesia. Your support person will be given a surgical gown, mask, hat, and gloves to wear. This person may be able to stay with you throughout the surgery.

Making the Incisions

There are many layers between your baby and the outside world, including your skin, the muscles of the abdominal wall, the lining of the abdominal cavity (**peritoneum**), your uterus, and the placenta. Once your belly is cleaned and you are numb from the anesthetic, your ob-gyn will make an incision.

- The skin incision usually goes from side to side, just above the pubic hairline (transverse). In some cases, the incision is up and down (vertical). The incision is made through the skin of the belly and the tissue just below the skin.
- The abdominal muscles are separated, and an incision is made through the lining of the abdominal cavity. The abdominal muscles usually are not cut.
- Another cut is made in the uterus. This incision also can be side to side or up and down. In most cases, a side-to-side incision is made. This type of cut is done in the lower, thinner part of the uterus. It causes less bleeding and heals with a stronger scar. A vertical incision may need to be done if you have *placenta previa*, if the baby is in an unusual position, or if your baby is extremely *preterm*, larger than average, or smaller than average.

The incision made in your skin may be different from the incision made in your uterus. This information should be entered into your medical record. Make sure that you know the type of incision that was made in your uterus. This is a major factor in determining whether you can have a vaginal birth in the future. A low transverse incision is best for a future TOLAC.

Delivering the Baby

The baby is delivered through the incisions. The umbilical cord is cut. The baby may be passed to a nurse, your partner, or your labor coach. Talk with your ob-gyn about these options (see Chapter 18, "After the Baby Is Born").

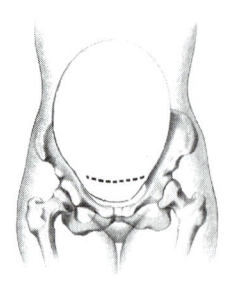

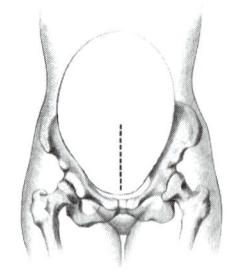

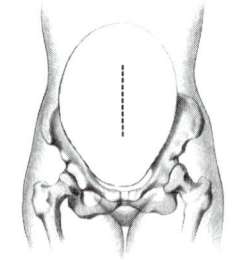

Low transverse   Low vertical   High vertical (classical)

Types of uterine incisions for a cesarean delivery. The scar from a low transverse incision is the least likely to rupture (break open) during a trial of labor after cesarean delivery (TOLAC). Keep in mind that the incision made in the skin for a cesarean delivery may not match the incision made in the uterus.

Delivering the Placenta and Closing the Incisions

After the baby is delivered, the placenta is removed from the uterus. The incisions in the uterus and abdominal wall are closed with stitches.

Surgical thread, staples, surgical glue, or a combination may be used to close the abdominal incision. Staples and some types of stitches must be removed a few days later. Most closures are absorbed by the body and do not need to be removed.

Risks of Cesarean Delivery

Like any major surgery, cesarean delivery has risks. Problems happen in a small number of surgeries. These problems usually can be treated. But in very rare cases, **complications** can be serious or even fatal:

- The uterus, nearby pelvic organs, or skin incision can get infected.

- You may bleed too much. This is called a **hemorrhage**. In some cases, a blood **transfusion** may be needed. In very rare cases, a hysterectomy may need to be done if bleeding cannot be controlled.

- You may develop blood clots in the legs that can travel to the lungs. For this reason, it's routine practice to put massaging sleeves around your legs to reduce the risk of blood clots during surgery. These devices periodically fill with air to encourage blood circulation in your veins.

- Your bowel or bladder may be injured.

- You may have an allergic reaction to the medications or anesthetics that are used.

Cesarean birth also increases risks for future pregnancies. These risks include placenta problems, rupture of the uterus, and hysterectomy. Some placenta problems can cause serious complications (see Chapter 37, "Placenta Problems").

Because of these risks, cesarean delivery usually is done only when the benefits of the surgery outweigh the risks. In some situations, cesarean delivery is the best option. In other situations, vaginal birth is best. Talk with your ob-gyn about the risks and benefits for your situation.

Recovery After Cesarean Delivery

After your cesarean delivery you will be taken from the operating room to a recovery room or directly to your room. If you are awake for the cesarean delivery, you may be able to hold your baby in the recovery room after the surgery. A nurse will watch you and check your

- blood pressure
- pulse rate
- breathing rate
- amount of bleeding
- abdominal incision

You will receive fluids through your IV line after your delivery until you are able to eat and drink. You should be able to eat and drink as soon as you would like.

You may need to stay in bed for a while. The first few times you get out of bed, a nurse or other adult should help you.

The catheter may be removed within a few hours of surgery or the next day. A nurse will help you get out of bed and sit in a chair. Walking soon after a cesarean delivery helps to lower the risk of developing blood clots. You will be encouraged to walk a short distance as soon as you feel able to do so. If you want to shower, check with a nurse to be sure you are stable on your feet.

The abdominal incision will be sore for the first few days. You may be given pain medication through your epidural catheter or your IV line for the first day. After the anesthesia wears off, you will be given pain medication by mouth. There are many ways to control pain. Talk with your ob-gyn about your options.

Most women can walk on their own, eat, and drink within 24 hours of surgery. The average stay after a cesarean birth is 3 days. How many days you stay will depend on why you needed a cesarean birth and how long it takes for your body to recover.

If you plan to breastfeed, tell your ob-gyn before the surgery. If all is going well for you and your baby, you should be able to start breastfeeding soon after delivery.

Back at Home

When you are at home, take care of yourself and limit your activities. Ask for help from your partner, family, and friends. If you are having difficulty moving after your delivery, also ask for help when lifting or carrying your baby. Your ob-gyn should give you specific instructions about what you can and can't do.

The bottom line is that you need to take it easy. You just had major surgery, and it will take a few weeks for your body to heal. During the weeks you are recovering from surgery, you may experience

- mild cramping, especially when you are breastfeeding
- vaginal bleeding or discharge for about 4 to 6 weeks
- bleeding with clots and cramps
- pain, numbness, or both in the incision

To prevent infection, do not to place anything in your vagina (such as tampons) or have sex for a few weeks. Give yourself time to heal before doing any strenuous activity. See Chapter 19, "Your Postpartum Care," for more on adjusting after the birth of your baby.

Vaginal Birth After Cesarean Delivery

It once was thought that if a woman had one cesarean delivery, she should give birth to all her other babies the same way in the future. Now many women can try to give birth through the vagina (vaginally) after a cesarean delivery. This is known as having a trial of labor after cesarean delivery (TOLAC). Some women attempting a trial of labor will be able to give birth through the vagina—known as a vaginal birth after cesarean (VBAC) delivery.

As many as 8 in 10 women who attempt a TOLAC go on to give birth vaginally. But sometimes there are problems. One of the most serious is **uterine rupture**. This happens when the scar on the uterus from a past cesarean birth breaks open. When this happens, a woman needs an emergency cesarean delivery.

The decision of whether to try a vaginal delivery or to have a repeat cesarean delivery can be complex. There are a few factors that can help determine if TOLAC is a good choice for your delivery.

When to Call Your Ob-Gyn

After a cesarean birth, call your ob-gyn right away if you have

- fever
- chills
- leg pain
- draining or leakage from your incision
- heavy bleeding
- worsening pain
- shortness of breath

Factors to Consider

TOLAC is considered a safe option for many women, but not for every woman. You and your ob-gyn should talk about the following factors:

- Type of uterine incision—The incision made in your uterus (not the one in your skin) for your previous cesarean birth is a key factor in deciding whether you should try to have a VBAC. This information should be in your medical records. A low transverse (side to side) incision is the most common type used in cesarean delivery. It also is the least likely to rupture.

- Past deliveries—A VBAC is more likely to be successful if you have had at least one vaginal delivery as well as your previous cesarean delivery. Also, a VBAC may be considered in women who have had up to two previous cesarean deliveries.

- Future deliveries—Multiple cesarean deliveries are associated with more risks. If you know that you want more children, you should keep these risks in mind when making your decision.

- A pregnancy problem or medical condition—Vaginal delivery is riskier if there is a problem with the placenta, problems with the baby, or certain medical conditions during pregnancy.

- Type of hospital— TOLAC should take place in a hospital that can manage situations that threaten the life of the woman or her baby. Some hospitals may not offer TOLAC because hospital staff do not feel they can provide this type of emergency care. You and your ob-gyn should consider the resources available at the hospital you have chosen.

Your ob-gyn cannot know for sure whether TOLAC will be successful, but some factors are known to affect the chances. You are more likely to have a successful TOLAC if:

- You have given birth vaginally before.
- You had a cesarean birth because of a specific problem, such as breech presentation, that you do not have this time.
- Your labor starts naturally without needing to be induced (started with drugs or other methods).

You are less likely to have a successful TOLAC if:

- Your baby weighs more than 9 pounds.
- Your pregnancy has lasted more than 40 weeks.

- You gave birth to another baby 18 months ago or less.
- You have *preeclampsia*.
- You are older.
- You have a higher BMI.

The decision should be made only after a detailed discussion with your ob-gyn. Every pregnancy is unique.

Let your ob-gyn know early in your pregnancy if you're interested in trying to have a VBAC. Together, you and your ob-gyn can consider this option. Many of the factors that go into the decision are known early in pregnancy. You may need to get your medical records from your last pregnancy to know what type of incision was used. Talking about VBAC early in pregnancy lets you consider all the benefits and risks.

Benefits of a VBAC

The benefits of a successful VBAC compared with a cesarean delivery include

- no abdominal surgery
- shorter recovery period
- lower risk of infection
- less blood loss

Many women would like to have the experience of vaginal birth, and when successful, VBAC allows this to happen. For women planning to have more children, VBAC may help them avoid certain health problems linked to multiple cesarean deliveries. These problems may include

- bowel or bladder injury
- problems with the placenta in future pregnancies
- hysterectomy

If you know that you want more children, this may figure into your decision.

Risks of a TOLAC

TOLAC is not the right choice for every woman. There are risks, including infection, injury, and blood loss. One rare but serious TOLAC risk is that the cesarean scar on the uterus may rupture. Although a rupture of the uterus is rare, it is very serious and may be life-threatening for you and your baby. If you are at high risk of uterine rupture, TOLAC should not be tried.

Your risk of rupture may depend on the type of incision you had for your last cesarean birth. After a cesarean, you will have a scar on your skin and a scar on your uterus. Some uterine scars are more likely than others to cause a rupture during a TOLAC. The type of scar depends on the type of cut in the uterus:

1. Low transverse—A side-to-side cut made across the lower, thinner part of the uterus. This is the most common type of incision and carries the least chance of future rupture.
2. Low vertical—An up-and-down cut made in the lower, thinner part of the uterus. This type of incision carries a higher risk of rupture than a low transverse incision.
3. High vertical (also called "classical")—An up-and-down cut made in the upper part of the uterus. This is sometimes done for very preterm cesarean births. It has the highest risk of rupture.

You cannot tell what kind of cut was made in the uterus by looking at the scar on the skin. Medical records from the previous delivery should include this information. Get the medical records of your prior cesarean delivery so your ob-gyn can review them.

Be Prepared for Changes

You and your ob-gyn may have a plan for your delivery, but things can change during your pregnancy and labor. It's important to be flexible and ready to change your plan.

If you have chosen to try a TOLAC, things can happen that change the balance of risks and benefits. For example, you may need to have your labor induced (started with drugs or other methods). This can reduce the chances of a successful vaginal delivery. Labor induction also may increase the chance of complications during labor. If circumstances change, you and your ob-gyn may want to reconsider your decision.

The reverse also may be true. For example, if you have planned a cesarean delivery but go into labor before your scheduled surgery, it may be best to consider VBAC if you are far enough along in your labor and your baby is healthy.

RESOURCES

Cesarean Section
https://medlineplus.gov/cesareansection.html
Webpage from the U.S. National Library of Medicine that reviews all things related to cesarean birth.

Your Pregnancy and Childbirth
www.acog.org/MyPregnancy
Website from the American College of Obstetricians and Gynecologists (ACOG) with information on pregnancy, labor, delivery, and postpartum care. Includes the latest information from the experts in women's health care, questions answered by ACOG ob-gyns, pregnancy stories from real women, and an A–Z directory of health topics covering pregnancy and beyond.

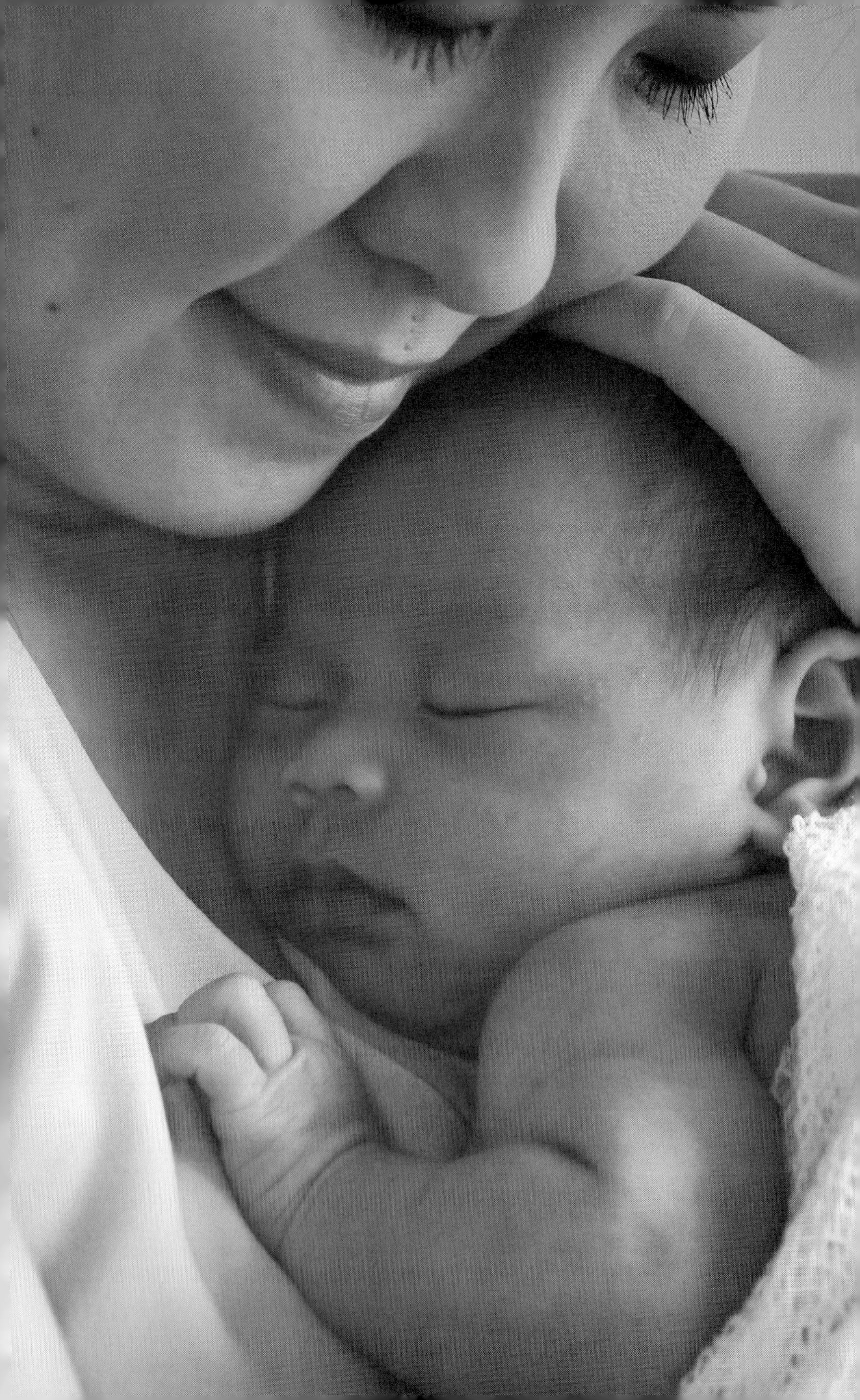

PART 3

Postpartum Care

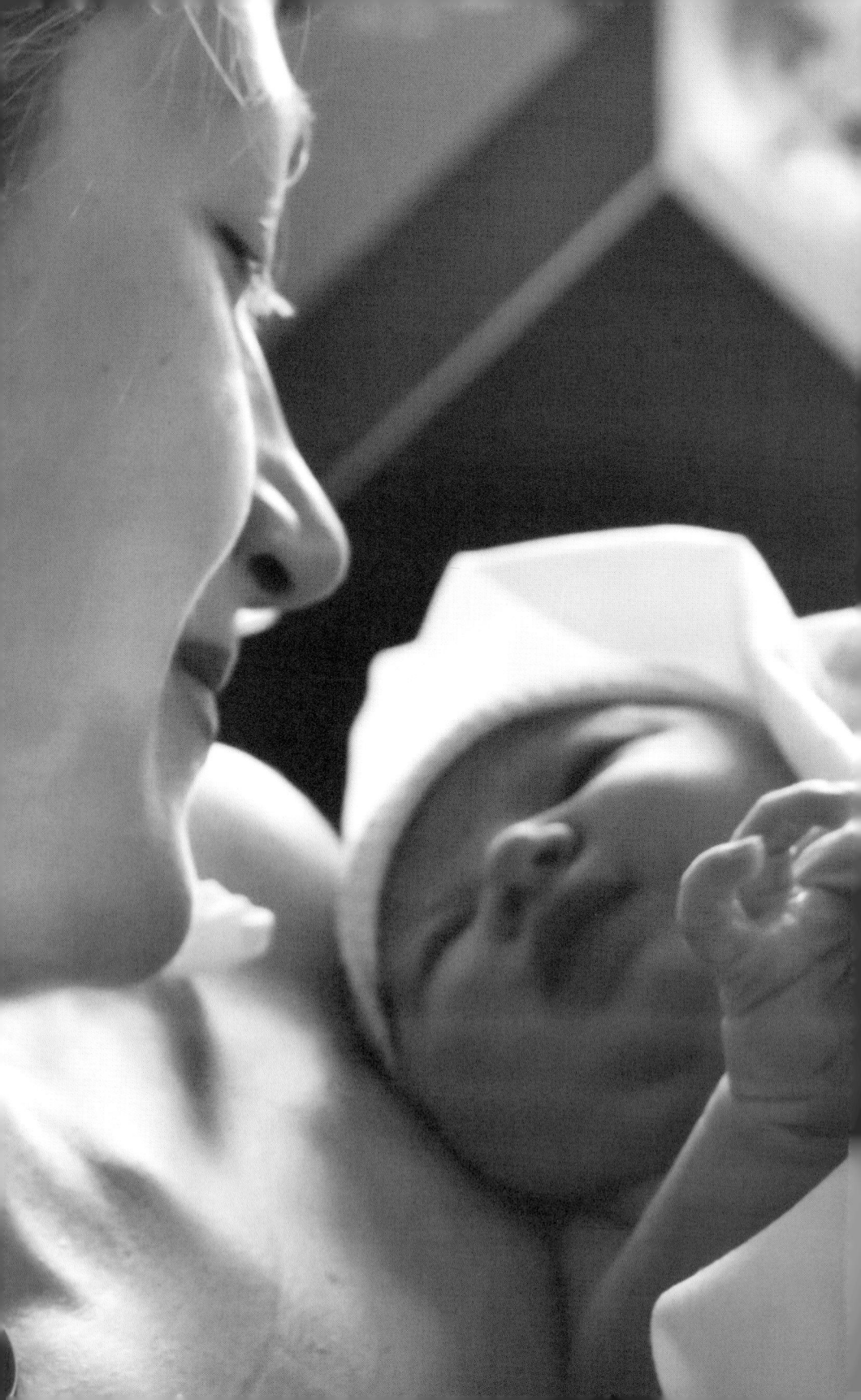

CHAPTER 18

After the Baby Is Born

In the moments after birth, you should be able to hold your baby if you both are doing well. Over the next few hours, your caregivers will be busy checking your health and the health of your newborn. They also will be checking your condition as you recover.

If you had a normal vaginal delivery and you are doing well, you may be sent home from the hospital or birth center 1 to 2 days after the baby is born. If you had a **cesarean delivery**, you may stay longer. How long you stay may depend on why the surgery was done.

Before you go home with your baby, it's important to know

- who is on your **postpartum** care team
- how to take care of yourself and your baby
- what will happen next

This will be a time of adjustment and change. Being prepared will make the transition easier.

The First Few Hours

If you had a normal labor and delivery, your baby should be placed on your chest and belly right after birth. If you had any problems or if the baby is **preterm**, your baby may need to be checked by medical staff first or placed under a warming light.

If all is well, you most likely will be able to spend as much time as you want with your baby. The staff should check on you and your baby often. A physical exam and tests of your newborn can be done about an hour after birth, when you and your baby are ready.

Skin-to-Skin Care

A healthy baby should be placed skin-to-skin on your chest and belly right after birth. Your baby should stay there for at least the first hour of life, sometimes called the "golden hour" or the "sacred hour." Skin-to-skin contact can

- keep the baby warm
- encourage breastfeeding, which may reduce the need to supplement with formula
- help the baby be less stressed by painful procedures, such as a vitamin K shot
- help stabilize the breathing and heartbeat, especially if your baby is late preterm (born between 34 weeks and 0 days and 36 weeks and 6 days)

Skin-to-skin contact also may be possible after a **cesarean birth**. Check with your **obstetrician–gynecologist (ob-gyn)**.

Breastfeeding Your Baby

Breastfeeding—feeding a baby directly from your breast—is the recommended way to feed. If you've decided to breastfeed, you probably can start now.

Most healthy newborns are ready to breastfeed within the first hour after birth. Those who are breastfed soon after birth may have an easier time breastfeeding than babies who are not. Babies who have skin-to-skin contact may seek out your breast and latch on by themselves. There are many things your care team can do to help you and your baby get off to a good start with breastfeeding (see Chapter 20, "Feeding Your Baby").

Your Baby's Health

In the first few minutes after birth, the staff will make sure your baby looks healthy and is breathing well. They also will make sure your baby is warm enough.

Your Baby's First Breath

During pregnancy, your baby received **oxygen** through the **umbilical cord** and **placenta**. In the moments after birth, your newborn takes the first breath of air. It's not just the lungs that must be working and able to fill with air seconds after delivery. All the related body parts, such as muscles around the lungs and airways leading from the mouth and nose, also must be ready to start working.

After birth, there's more pressure outside the lungs than there is inside them. This pressure causes the lungs to expand and fill with air. As a result, the baby may start crying. Many babies cry on their own at birth. Others don't cry right away. Instead, they simply start breathing.

After birth, your baby's breathing should be monitored closely. If the baby isn't breathing well, steps should be taken to help. Often, this simply means rubbing the baby's body. Sometimes the baby may be given oxygen.

Your Baby's Apgar Score

Your baby's health should be assessed with the Apgar test 1 minute after birth and then again 5 minutes after birth. The ***Apgar score***, developed by Dr. Virginia Apgar in 1952, rates the newborn's

- heart rate
- breathing
- muscle tone
- reflexes
- skin color

Each of these features is given a score of 0, 1, or 2. The scores are added up, with a maximum possible score of 10. Most babies have an Apgar score of 7 or more at 5 minutes after birth. Few babies score a perfect 10.

The Apgar score is used to check the baby's condition right after delivery. It is a good way to measure how well the baby adjusts to the outside world in the first few minutes after birth. The Apgar score does not show how healthy

TABLE 18–1 The Apgar* Score

Component	Score 0	Score 1	Score 2
Heart rate	No heartbeats	Fewer than 100 beats per minute	More than 100 beats per minute
Respiration	No breathing	Weak cry or hyperventilation	Good, strong cry
Muscle tone	Limp	Some flexing of arms and legs	Active motion
Reflexes (response to airway being suctioned)	No response	Grimace	Cries or withdraws; coughs; sneezes
Color†	Blue or pale	Body is pink; hands and feet are blue	Pink all over

* Using Dr. Apgar's name, APGAR stands for **a**ppearance, **p**ulse, **g**rimace, **a**ctivity, and **r**espiration.
† In babies with dark skin, the mouth, lips, palms, and soles of the feet are examined.

your baby was before birth. It also does not tell you how healthy your baby will be in the future.

Keeping the Baby Warm

Before birth, your baby was kept warm inside your body. After the baby is born, the body needs to adjust to an environment that's much cooler. The baby's skin is wet with **amniotic fluid**, and a lot of heat can be lost as the moisture on the skin evaporates. Holding your baby on your bare chest and belly right after birth can help keep the baby warm. The staff may cover your baby with a blanket as well.

In the coming days, it also will be important to monitor the baby's environment and make sure that the baby is dressed appropriately. As a rule, the baby should be dressed in one more layer than what you are wearing.

Getting to Know Your Baby

You'll never forget the first time you see your new baby. If you're a first-time mom, you may have questions about the way your newborn looks and acts. Knowing what's normal and what to expect at this time in your baby's life will help you relax and enjoy watching your baby grow.

Your Baby's Weight

One of the first questions people ask after birth is how much the baby weighs. In fact, that's one of the first things your ob-gyn wants to know, too. Most full-term babies weigh between 5½ and 9½ pounds. The average weight is 7½ pounds. In the first 3 days after birth, it is normal for a baby to lose a small amount of weight before beginning to gain weight.

How Your Baby Looks

If you have seen babies on television, you may be surprised to know that most "newborns" on TV are already a few months old. Real newborns look very different in the first few days after birth:

- The body may seem scrunched up. A new baby draws arms and legs up close, into the so-called fetal position. This is the way babies fit in the **uterus**. Even though there's more room now, it'll take a few weeks for the baby to stretch out a bit.

- The face may be slightly swollen. The area around the eyes may be a little puffy for a few days.

- The head may be long and swollen for a few days or weeks. Babies have two soft spots on the top of their heads where the skull bones haven't joined yet. These soft spots make the head flexible enough to fit through the birth canal.
- The **genitals** may be swollen. The swelling usually is caused by extra fluid that has built up in the baby's body. In girls, the **labia** may be swollen because of the **hormones** they were exposed to in the uterus. Boys may have extra fluid around their **testicles** that may make the **scrotum** appear swollen. This swelling usually goes down within days.

How Your Baby Acts

Most newborns have the same responses to being in the outside world. Even so, each baby has a unique personality right from the start. The way one baby behaves and interacts with people can be very different from the way another baby acts. Some babies are quiet and calm. Other babies are bundles of energy from the start.

After the stress of birth, most newborns are very alert for the first hour or so. This is a good time to attempt to breastfeed, talk to, or just hold your new baby.

When this alertness fades, the baby will get sleepy. Don't worry if your newborn seems very drowsy or sleeps a lot for the next few hours or even days. After all, you're not the only one who needs to recover. The birth process is hard for the baby, too. Many babies do little else besides sleep at first. Most newborns spend 14 to 18 hours a day sleeping, although not all at once. It's normal to see short stretches of sleep broken up by brief periods of alertness.

But again, it depends on the baby. Some newborns sleep less and are fussy when they wake up. Others sleep for long stretches and are quiet and calm when they are awake.

What Happens Next for Your Baby

When you are ready, nurses should weigh and measure the baby, give a bath, slip identification bands around the baby's ankle and wrist, and perhaps take handprints and footprints. For the next few hours, both you and your baby should be monitored very closely to make sure you're doing well.

Many hospitals and birth centers encourage "rooming-in," which means your baby stays in your room with you instead of in the nursery. Rooming-in makes it easier for you to breastfeed and allows you and your family to bond with the baby. In most hospitals and birth centers, you can room-in even if you have had a cesarean birth. You may need to have someone with you throughout your stay to help you take care of the baby.

In some hospitals and birth centers, the baby also can stay in the nursery. The baby does not have to stay there all the time. As long as your baby is healthy, you can have your baby with you whenever you want.

Medical Care

Your baby should receive a complete physical exam in the hospital. A health care professional should

- examine your baby from head to toe, including feeling the belly and looking for normal newborn reflexes
- listen to the breathing and heartbeat
- check the pulse

Other steps should be taken to help prevent health problems:

- Vitamin K shot—A newborn's body can't make vitamin K on its own for a few days, so vitamin K routinely is given by an injection. Vitamin K is needed for the blood to clot after a cut. The vitamin K shot also helps protect against a rare but severe bleeding disorder that can cause permanent brain injury.
- **Antibiotic** ointment or solution in the baby's eyes—This treatment protects against a serious infection from **bacteria** that can get into the eyes during birth. It can be done after you've had time to hold and breastfeed your baby.
- **Hepatitis B vaccination**—The hepatitis B **vaccine** is a series of three shots. Babies get the first dose of vaccine before leaving the hospital or birth center. The second dose should be given at 1 to 2 months of age. The third dose should be given by 6 to 18 months of age.

Newborn Screening Tests

By law, all babies must have newborn screening tests. Most babies are born healthy, but some may have health problems that are not easy to see. Screening tests can find these problems. If problems are found early, treatment can help prevent serious medical conditions or death.

Before you leave the hospital, a nurse or technician will take a few drops of blood from your baby's heel. The hospital will send the blood sample to a newborn screening lab. Your baby's hearing also will be tested. Testing may be done with a small earphone, microphone, or both. And the oxygen level in your baby's blood will be measured. This test is done with painless skin sensors (called pulse oximetry). Low blood oxygen levels can be a sign of a heart problem.

The results of some tests (hearing and pulse oximetry) may be available before you leave the hospital or birth center. Blood test results will take longer. Your baby's doctor (**pediatrician** or family medicine doctor) should get the results and share them with you. In some cases, your state health department will give you the results. Ask about the results when you see your baby's doctor. Make sure that your hospital and your baby's doctor have your correct address and phone number.

If your baby has an abnormal test result for any condition, further testing may be recommended. Retesting does not necessarily mean that your child will have a health problem. Your baby's doctor or the state health department should contact you if your baby needs to have another test. They will tell you why your baby needs to be retested and what to do next. Talk with your baby's doctor so you understand your options and reasons for retesting.

Circumcision

Circumcision means removing the foreskin, a layer of skin that covers the tip of the ***penis***. If you have decided to have your baby boy circumcised, it may be done by an obstetrician, your baby's doctor, or your family medicine doctor before the baby leaves the hospital. The procedure is done with ***local anesthesia***. Circumcision for religious reasons can be done outside the hospital.

If you are not sure about having your baby boy circumcised, talk with your ob-gyn or the doctor you have chosen for your baby's care. See Chapter 12, "Preparing for Birth," for more discussion.

Your Recovery After Delivery

Your blood pressure, pulse, and temperature will be measured often for the first few hours after delivery. This is done to monitor you for ***hemorrhage*** (heavy bleeding) or other ***complications***. If you have had an ***epidural block*** or a ***spinal block***, you will be observed for a few hours. If you were moved to a delivery room for the birth, you will be returned to a regular room once your condition is stable.

While you are in the hospital or birth center, it is important to sleep, get your strength back, and recover from the effects of any ***anesthesia*** you had. If you have no complications, you may start eating normally very soon. Check with your ob-gyn and nurse for the best timing for you. Everyone's recovery is different.

You should try to urinate soon after delivery, if possible. It's common to have trouble with this right after giving birth, so your care team should make sure you are urinating properly during the first 24 hours after birth.

Walking reduces the risk of **deep vein thrombosis (DVT)**. But you should check with your nurse first if you want to get out of bed and walk around. Make sure you have someone to help you the first time you get out of bed. You also should ask your nurse if you want to shower. Your nurse will want to make sure you are stable on your feet.

During this time, your care team should help you learn how to care for your baby. They also will teach you how to care for any tears or incisions, including

- tears in the **vulva** or **perineum** (the area between your **vagina** and **anus**)
- an **episiotomy**, if you had one
- your abdominal incision, if you had a cesarean birth

Ask your caregivers if you have any questions.

Vaccinations

Vaccinations are a simple, safe, and effective way to protect you and your baby from infections. If you did not get certain vaccinations before or during your pregnancy, you should get them now. This will help to protect your baby from infections. Recommended vaccines for women in the postpartum period may include

- *measles–mumps–rubella (MMR) vaccine*
- *influenza (flu) vaccine*
- *tetanus toxoid, reduced diphtheria toxoid, and acellular pertussis (Tdap) vaccine*
- *varicella (chickenpox) vaccine*

If you have family members who will be in close contact with your baby, and they have not been vaccinated with Tdap, they also should get a single dose of Tdap. This dose should be given at least 2 weeks before they have any close contact with the baby.

If you are Rh negative and your baby is Rh positive, you should be given a dose of **Rh immunoglobulin (RhIg)** within 72 hours after giving birth, even if you received RhIg while you were pregnant. You do not need RhIg if your baby is Rh negative (see Chapter 36, "Blood Type Incompatibility").

Pain Relief

In the first few days after birth, it is common to have pain from

- swollen, engorged breasts as your breasts fill with milk
- uterine contractions as your uterus starts to go back to its normal size

- pain in the perineum, if you had a vaginal delivery
- pain from your incision, if you had a cesarean birth

Let your care team know if you have pain. Some pain can be managed without medication. See Chapter 19, "Your Postpartum Care," for information about managing specific issues. But if these methods do not relieve your pain, medication is available that is safe for you and your breastfeeding baby. Your ob-gyn may recommend one or more of the following while you are in the hospital:

- A ***nonsteroidal anti-inflammatory drug (NSAID),*** such as ibuprofen
- Acetaminophen
- An ***opioid*** medication. Opioids can cause constipation and drowsiness, so they should be used only if your pain is not well controlled with other methods.

A combination of an NSAID and acetaminophen, taken on a regular schedule, can give good pain relief and reduce the need for opioids. Talk with your ob-gyn about the best method for you.

If you had a cesarean birth, you may be given pain medication through your spinal or epidural ***catheter*** or through your ***intravenous (IV) line*** for the first day. After the anesthesia wears off, you may be given pain medication by mouth. A heating pad also may be helpful.

When it is time to go home, your ob-gyn may give you a prescription for pain medication. Make sure you know how and when to use this medication. Everyone is different. Your pain may go away faster than expected, and you may not need to use all the pills in the prescription.

When you are at home, it is important to take your medication only as prescribed. Let your nurse, ob-gyn, or pharmacist know if you have any questions.

Going Home With Your Baby

If you had a normal vaginal delivery, you will go home from the hospital or birth center when your condition is stable and the baby is doing well. How long you stay in the hospital may depend on your health. How long you stay after a cesarean birth may depend on why the ***cesarean delivery*** was done and how much time you need to recover (see Chapter 17, "Cesarean Delivery and Vaginal Birth After Cesarean Delivery").

Before you and your baby go home, you should

- be comfortable feeding your baby (see Chapter 20, "Feeding Your Baby")
- feel prepared to care for yourself and your baby

- know when and where your baby will be seen for ongoing care
- be able to recognize problems or an emergency and know what to do
- review and update your postpartum care plan with the help of your ob-gyn (see Chapter 19, "Your Postpartum Care")
- know who is on your postpartum care team, including the health care practitioners, friends, and family who will support you and your baby in your first months together (see Chapter 19, "Your Postpartum Care")
- have an approved car seat secured in your car (see Chapter 12, "Preparing for Birth")

For your follow-up care, it is best if you schedule

- a checkup with your ob-gyn within 3 weeks of giving birth by phone, video chat, or in person
- ongoing care as needed, especially if you have a chronic condition, had health problems during pregnancy, or had complications during labor, delivery, or postpartum
- a full, in-person health care visit within 12 weeks of giving birth

What You Should Know Before You Go Home

- Normal moods and feelings to expect over the next few weeks, including the **baby blues**
- Symptoms of **postpartum depression**
- Normal changes in vaginal bleeding (**lochia**)
- How to take care of your breasts, perineum, and **bladder**
- Warning signs to watch for, including fever, chills, leg pains, drainage from your incision or tear, or increased vaginal bleeding
- What kinds of physical activity you can do, and how much
- Your nutrition needs, especially if you are breastfeeding
- Contact information for breastfeeding support in your community
- Contact information for everyone on your postpartum care team
- The date of your next postpartum checkup and information about any ongoing follow-up care you may need

For more information, see Chapter 19, "Your Postpartum Care."

Talk with your ob-gyn about what schedule makes sense for you. You can schedule your visits based on your health needs, health insurance, work schedule, transportation to the office, and other personal factors.

Your baby should be seen by a pediatrician or family medicine doctor within 3 to 5 days of birth, unless there are issues that need to be addressed sooner. After that, your baby usually will be seen by a doctor at 1, 2, and 4 months of age.

Welcome to motherhood! Remember that your postpartum care team is there to support you in this new stage of your life. You don't have to do it all on your own. The next stage in your journey is described in Chapter 19, "Your Postpartum Care."

RESOURCES

About Skin-to-Skin Care
www.healthychildren.org/English/ages-stages/baby/preemie/Pages/About-Skin-to-Skin-Care.aspx
Webpage from the American Academy of Pediatrics that explains the benefits of skin-to-skin care right after birth.

Newborn Screening Tests
https://medlineplus.gov/ency/article/007257.htm
Webpage from the U.S. National Library of Medicine that provides a general description of newborn screening tests, how they are done, and what the results may mean.

Postpartum Support International Helpline
www.postpartum.net
1-800-944-4773
Text 1-503-894-9453 (English) or 1-971-420-0294 (Spanish)
Non-emergency helpline for support, information, or referrals to postpartum mental health practitioners. The helpline is open 7 days per week. Leave a confidential message at any time, and a volunteer will return your call or text as soon as possible. PSI also offers online support group meetings to connect with other pregnant and postpartum women. You also can join PSI's weekly Chat with an Expert.

Your Pregnancy and Childbirth
www.acog.org/MyPregnancy
Website from the American College of Obstetricians and Gynecologists (ACOG) with information on pregnancy, labor, delivery, and postpartum care. Includes the latest information from the experts in women's health care, questions answered by ACOG ob-gyns, pregnancy stories from real women, and an A–Z directory of health topics covering pregnancy and beyond.

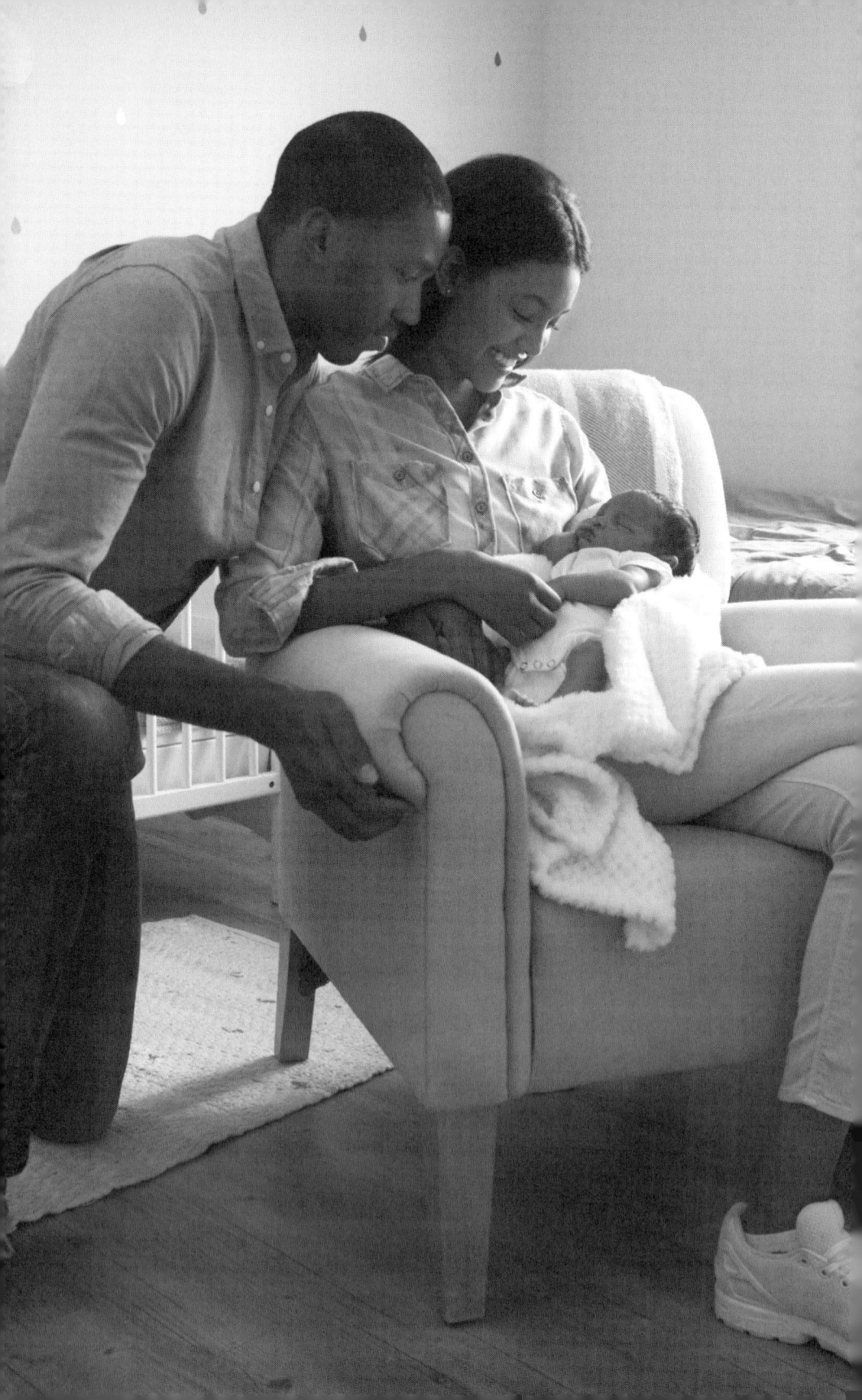

CHAPTER 19

Your Postpartum Care

After you have a baby, you begin what's called the "fourth trimester." Also known as the **postpartum** period, this is the time of recovery after the birth of a child. The postpartum period lasts up to 12 weeks. It can be a time of mixed emotions—joy, excitement, anxiety, and sometimes sadness—and a time of physical changes.

Your health is important during this time. If you know what to expect and plan for the care you need, you can have a healthy fourth trimester. You also can set the stage for your long-term health.

Planning Your Postpartum Care

Before your baby is born, you and your **obstetrician–gynecologist (ob-gyn)** should develop a postpartum care plan. Your care plan should include a care team and postpartum checkups. Your checkups can help make sure you are

- healing physically, mentally, and emotionally
- feeling good about your health
- feeling that you can ask for help if you need it

Before you and your baby go home from the hospital or birth center, you should be given instructions to follow in case of problems or an emergency (see the box "When to Call Your Doctor" on the next page).

When to Call Your Doctor

Postpartum discomforts are normal. But some discomforts may be a sign that there is a problem. Call your ob-gyn if you have

- fever more than 100.4°F
- nausea and vomiting
- pain or burning during urination
- bleeding that's heavier than a normal **menstrual period** or that increases
- severe pain in your lower belly
- pain, swelling, and tenderness in your legs
- chest pain and coughing or gasping for air
- headache that does not go away
- changes in eyesight
- difficulty breathing
- swelling of the face or hands
- red streaks on your breasts or painful new lumps in your breasts
- redness, discharge, or pain that doesn't go away or that gets worse from an **episiotomy**, perineal tear, or abdominal incision
- vaginal discharge that smells bad
- feelings of hopelessness that last more than 10 days after delivery

Postpartum Visit Schedule

For many years, postpartum care in the United States has been one office visit between 4 and 6 weeks after childbirth. The American College of Obstetricians and Gynecologists (ACOG) now recommends that women have earlier and more frequent postpartum checkups. It is best if you schedule

- a checkup with your ob-gyn within 3 weeks of giving birth by phone, video chat, or in person
- ongoing care as needed, especially if you have a chronic condition, had health problems during pregnancy, or had **complications** during labor, delivery, or postpartum
- a full, in-person health care visit within 12 weeks of giving birth

Postpartum Visit Schedule

Birth

3 weeks

First checkup within 3 weeks of giving birth.
Checkup can be done by phone, video chat, or in person.

More checkups as needed.
Especially if you have a chronic condition or had health problems during pregnancy.

Full, in-person checkup within 12 weeks of giving birth.
Full check of physical, mental, and emotional well-being.

12 weeks

Talk with your ob-gyn about what schedule makes sense for you. You can schedule your visits based on your health needs, health insurance, work schedule, transportation to the office, and other personal factors.

Many women have concerns right after childbirth. They may wonder if they are healing well or they may have questions about breastfeeding. As time goes on, other concerns may come up, such as questions about when exercise and sexual activity are safe again. Use the "My Postpartum Care Checklist" at the back of this book to keep track of concerns you want to discuss with your ob-gyn.

Having contact with your care team gives you the best chance to be sure you are healing well. It gives you time to talk about your concerns. These visits also can help you prepare for your future health care.

Postpartum Care Team

When you plan your postpartum care, you should think about who you want on your care team. This is a group of family, friends, and health care professionals who can help with medical care, emotional support, child care, pet care, and household tasks. Members of your postpartum care team may include the following people:

- Your partner, family and friends. They may be able to offer emotional support and help with child care, chores, meals, breastfeeding support, and transportation.

- Your maternal care practitioner. This is the ob-gyn who is in charge of your care during the postpartum period. This is the first person you should call if you have questions about your health or recovery after delivery.

- Your baby's doctor. This is the *pediatrician* or family medicine doctor who is in charge of your baby's care. You should call this person if you have questions about your baby's health.

- Other professionals. These may include other doctors to help with medical conditions, counselors to help with breastfeeding, nurses, social workers, and other trained professionals.

Talk with your ob-gyn about your postpartum care team before you give birth (see Chapter 12, "Preparing for Birth"). After you give birth, review and update your plan as needed. Use the "My Postpartum Care Team Chart" at the back of this book to write down the names and contact information of everyone on your care team.

Physical Health After Childbirth

After you give birth—no matter how your labor and delivery went—your body will need time to heal. You may experience symptoms that you have never felt before. Some of these problems may last a few days. Others may last several weeks. It may be helpful to learn

- which symptoms are typical for the postpartum period
- how to take care of yourself
- when to call your ob-gyn

Postpartum Bleeding

After your baby is born, your body sheds the blood and tissue that lined your *uterus*. This vaginal discharge is called *lochia*. For the first few days after delivery, lochia is heavy and bright red. It may have a few small clots. You should use sanitary pads during this time. Do not use tampons.

As time goes on, the flow gets lighter. A week or so after birth, lochia often is pink or brown. Bright red discharge can come back, though. You may feel a gush of blood from your *vagina* during breastfeeding, when your uterus contracts. By 2 weeks postpartum, lochia often is light brown or yellow. Typically, lochia slowly goes away by 6 to 8 weeks postpartum. You may want to use sanitary pads until lochia has stopped for several days.

Discharge is different for each woman. Some women have discharge for just a couple of weeks after their babies are born. Others have it for a month or longer. If bleeding is heavy, call your ob-gyn. Heavy bleeding is soaking through two sanitary pads an hour for more than an hour or two.

Bladder Problems

Painful Urination. During vaginal childbirth, the baby's head puts a lot of pressure on your **bladder**, **urethra**, and the muscles that control **urine** flow. This pressure can cause swelling and stretching. In the first days after delivery, you may feel the urge to urinate but not be able to pass any urine. You may feel pain and burning when you do urinate.

To lessen swelling or pain, try a warm sitz bath (sitting in warm water that's just deep enough to cover your bottom and hips). There are special basins that can be filled with clean, warm water from the faucet and then placed on a toilet seat for this purpose. When you are on the toilet, spray warm water over your **genitals** with a squeeze bottle. This can help trigger the flow of urine. Drink plenty of fluids as well.

Painful urination usually goes away within days of delivery. If the pain continues or is severe, contact your ob-gyn.

Urinary Incontinence. Many new mothers have another problem: involuntary leakage of urine. This is called **urinary incontinence**. With time, your pelvic muscles will return to normal, and the incontinence will go away in most cases.

You may feel more comfortable wearing a sanitary pad until urine leakage goes away. Doing **Kegel exercises** also will help tighten pelvic muscles sooner (see the box "Kegel Exercises" on the next page). If you are leaking large amounts of urine, see your ob-gyn. You also may see a pelvic floor physical therapist to help you strengthen your muscles.

Bowel Problems

Constipation and Painful Gas. It may be hard to have bowel movements for a few days after delivery. There may be several reasons for this, including

- stretched abdominal muscles
- sluggish bowels caused by surgery or pain medication
- an empty stomach after not eating during labor

You also may be afraid to move your bowels because of pain from **hemorrhoids** or a tear in your **perineum**, the area between your vagina and **anus**.

If you have constipation or painful gas after giving birth, try these tips:

- Take short walks as soon as you can.
- Eat foods high in fiber and drink plenty of fluids.
- Ask your ob-gyn about taking a stool softener. This is an over-the-counter medication that makes it easier to have a bowel movement.

Accidental Bowel Leakage. The urge to have a bowel movement may not feel the way it used to. In some cases, you may not be able to control your bowel movements. You also may pass gas when you do not mean to or do not expect it. Loss of normal control of the bowels is called **accidental bowel leakage**. It also is called *fecal incontinence*. It can be caused by damage to the muscles and nerves of the **rectum** and **anus** during childbirth.

Kegel Exercises

If you are not already doing Kegel exercises, the postpartum period is a good time to start. Kegel exercises help tone the muscles that support your urethra, bladder, uterus, and rectum. Strengthening these muscles may help improve bladder control and tighten vaginal muscles that are stretched from childbirth. Here is how they are done:

- Squeeze the muscles that you use to stop the flow of urine. This contraction pulls the vagina and rectum up and back.
- Hold for 3 seconds, then relax for 3 seconds.
- Do 10 contractions three times a day.
- Increase your hold by 1 second each week. Work your way up to holds of 10 seconds.

Make sure you are not squeezing your stomach, thigh, or buttock muscles. You also should breathe normally. Do not hold your breath as you do these exercises.

You can do Kegel exercises anywhere—while working, driving in your car, or watching television. But you should not do these exercises when you are urinating.

If you have lost normal control of your bowels, tell your ob-gyn about your symptoms. Several treatments are available, including lifestyle changes, physical therapy, medications, and in some cases, surgery.

Hemorrhoids

If you had **varicose veins** in your **vulva** or hemorrhoids in or around the anus during pregnancy, they may get worse after delivery. These sore, swollen veins also can show up for the first time now because of the intense straining you did during labor. In time, hemorrhoids and varicose veins usually get smaller or go away.

If you have hemorrhoids, some things you can try include

- medicated sprays or ointments
- dry heat (such as from a hair dryer turned on low)
- sitz baths
- cold witch-hazel compresses

Also, straining when you have a bowel movement can make hemorrhoids worse. Ask your ob-gyn about taking a stool softener.

Vaginal Birth: Perineal Pain

Your perineum is the area between your vagina and anus. During vaginal childbirth, the skin of the perineum stretches to accommodate the baby's head. Sometimes, the skin and tissues in this area tear.

There are different kinds of perineal tears. Minor tears may heal on their own without stitches. Some tears can be repaired with a few stitches in the delivery room right after birth. A tear that involves the **sphincter muscle** of the anus or muscles of the rectum may require repair in the operating room.

Perineal tears are different than an **episiotomy**. An episiotomy is a surgical cut made in the perineum to widen the vaginal opening for delivery.

If you have a tear or you had an episiotomy, you'll likely have a few weeks of swelling and pain as the perineum heals. The more severe the tear, the longer it may take to heal. To help ease the pain and heal quickly, try these tips:

- Apply cold packs or chilled witch-hazel pads to the area.
- Take ibuprofen, an over-the-counter pain reliever, to reduce pain and swelling.
- If sitting is uncomfortable, sit on a pillow. There also are special cushions that may be helpful.
- Try a sitz bath. Special basins that can be filled with clean, warm water from the faucet and then placed on a toilet seat are made for this purpose.

- When you are on the toilet, clean your genitals by spraying warm water with a squeeze bottle. This also can help trigger the flow of urine. Pat dry when you're finished.
- Try breastfeeding while lying on your side. Your ob-gyn can show you how. This position doesn't put pressure on your perineum.

You also can ask your ob-gyn about

- using a numbing spray or cream to ease pain
- taking a stool softener

Stool softeners may make it easier for you to have a bowel movement.

Cesarean Birth: Incision Pain

If you had a **cesarean birth**, your abdominal incision (surgical cut) will be sore for the first few weeks. Your ob-gyn may prescribe pain medication for you. A heating pad or an abdominal binder (compression belt) may be helpful. For breastfeeding, ask your ob-gyn for advice about the "football" or side-lying positions, which put less pressure on your incision. There are many ways to control pain, including medications you can take even if you are breastfeeding. Talk with your ob-gyn about your options.

Your Changing Body

In the weeks after childbirth, your body will change as it adjusts to not being pregnant. Some of these changes will happen right away. Other changes will take a little longer. Give your body time to get back to normal.

Return of Periods

If you are not breastfeeding, your menstrual period may return about 6 to 8 weeks after giving birth. It could start even sooner. If you are breastfeeding, your periods may not start again for months. Some breastfeeding women don't have a period until their babies are fully weaned.

Once your period returns, it may not be the same as before you were pregnant. Periods may be shorter or longer. In most cases, periods slowly return to what is normal for you. Some women notice that menstrual cramps are less painful than they were before they got pregnant.

After giving birth, your **ovaries** may release an **egg** before you have your first period. This means you can get pregnant sooner than you may think. If you and your partner don't want another baby right away, talk with your ob-gyn about what **birth control** is right for you. See the "Birth Control" section in this chapter.

Swollen Breasts

Your breasts fill with milk about 2 to 4 days after delivery. When this happens, your breasts may feel very full, hard, and tender. This is called engorgement. The best relief for engorgement is breastfeeding. Once you and your baby settle into a regular nursing pattern, the discomfort usually goes away. Severe engorgement should not last more than about 36 hours. If your breasts are so hard that your baby can't attach or "latch on" to your breast, ask your ob-gyn for help right away.

If you are formula-feeding instead of breastfeeding, your breasts will not be stimulated to produce more milk. Engorgement will go away gradually, in about 7 to 10 days. In the meantime, if engorgement causes discomfort, try the following:

- Wear a well-fitting support bra or sports bra. Do not bind your breasts, which can make your pain worse.
- Apply ice packs to your breasts to reduce swelling.
- Do not express (squeeze out) any milk. This sends a signal to your breasts to make more.
- Take over-the-counter pain medication, such as ibuprofen, if you need it.

Abdomen and Uterus

After delivery, you still will look like you are pregnant. During pregnancy, the abdominal muscles stretched out little by little. It will take time for these muscles to return to normal. Exercise will help. See the "Exercise" section in this chapter.

Over the coming days, your uterus also will get smaller and firmer. It will lower from the level of your belly button to back behind the bladder. You will feel your uterus contract and then relax as it shrinks back to its normal size. These cramps sometimes are called afterbirth pains. By about 10 days after birth, you will no longer be able to feel your uterus in your abdomen.

Your Feelings After Childbirth

Your recovery after childbirth is not just about physical healing. Your mood and emotional well-being are just as important as how your body feels. Watch for changes in your moods and talk with your ob-gyn about your emotions.

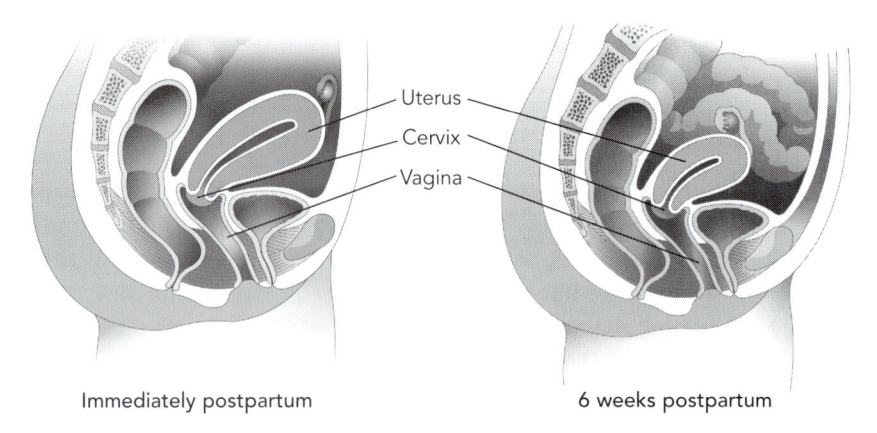

The uterus after birth. Just after birth, the uterus measures about 7 inches long and weighs about 2 pounds (*left*). In 6 weeks, it has returned to normal size (*right*). The normal size is about 3 inches long and about 2 ounces.

Postpartum Mood Disorders

Feeling sad or overwhelmed after having a baby is common. As many as 8 in 10 new mothers have feelings of sadness after giving birth. For some women, these feelings are more intense and don't go away in a few weeks. This can signal a more serious condition called ***postpartum depression***.

Baby Blues. The ***baby blues*** are caused by changes in hormones after birth. The baby blues usually start within a few days of giving birth. Many women feel anxious, sad, or upset after the birth of a child. These emotions are normal. Most often, the baby blues go away on their own within 1 or 2 weeks.

If you feel down, remind yourself that you have just taken on a huge job. Feeling sad, anxious, or even angry is very common. It means that your body is adjusting to the normal changes that follow the birth of a child.

It can be helpful to talk with your ob-gyn about your feelings. The following also may help you feel better:

- Talk with your partner or a good friend about how you feel.
- Take time to nap during the day when the baby is sleeping.
- Ask your partner, friends, and family for help.
- Take time for yourself. Get out of the house each day, even if it's only for a short time.

Postpartum Depression. Women with postpartum depression feel despair, severe anxiety, or hopelessness that gets in the way of daily life. Postpartum depression can occur up to 1 year after having a baby, but it most commonly happens about 1 to 3 weeks after childbirth.

Some women are more likely to have postpartum depression than others. Risk factors for postpartum depression include

- a history of ***depression*** or anxiety before, after, or during pregnancy
- a history of ***premenstrual syndrome (PMS)*** or ***premenstrual dysphoric disorder (PMDD)***
- recent stress, such as losing a loved one, a family illness, or moving to a new city
- lack of support from family and friends
- a ***preterm*** birth or traumatic birth experience
- having a baby stay in the ***neonatal intensive care unit (NICU)***
- problems with breastfeeding

If you think you might have postpartum depression, review the statements in the box "Warning Signs of Postpartum Depression". See your ob-gyn right away if you agree with any of these statements.

If your ob-gyn finds that you have postpartum depression, you should work together to find the best treatment to relieve your symptoms. Depression can be treated with medications called ***antidepressants***. Talk therapy also is used to treat depression, often in combination with medication.

Warning Signs of Postpartum Depression

Ask yourself whether any of these statements have been true for you in the past 7 days:

- I've felt anxious or worried for no clear reason.
- I've felt sad, scared, or panicky.
- I've felt so unhappy that I can't sleep.
- I've been crying a lot.
- I've had thoughts of harming myself or my baby.

See your ob-gyn right away if you agree with any of these statements. Do not wait until your next checkup to ask for help. The sooner you get help, the sooner you can feel better.

Antidepressants can be passed to babies during breastfeeding, although the amounts generally are very low. Breastfeeding has many benefits for both you and your baby. Many women find that the benefits of antidepressants help them better care for their baby. Deciding whether to take an antidepressant while breastfeeding involves weighing these benefits against the potential risks of your baby being exposed to the medication in your breast milk. Discuss this decision with your ob-gyn and your baby's doctor.

Lifestyle Habits

The healthy lifestyle habits you followed while you were pregnant should continue after your baby is born. For example, if you stopped smoking during pregnancy, it's important not to start again. You also should try to get enough rest, exercise, and healthy food.

Sleep and Fatigue

Pregnancy and childbirth are physically challenging. You are going to be tired. Your new baby will cause you many sleepless nights until your baby gets into a regular sleeping schedule. Here are some things you can do to adjust:

- Ask for help—Your partner, family, and friends are more than likely eager to pitch in. Let them. Be specific when others want to know what they can do. Ask a friend to bring something for dinner, stop at the grocery store, start a load of laundry, or watch the baby or an older child for a couple of hours so you can take a nap.

- Sleep when your baby sleeps—Use your baby's nap time to rest, not to tackle household chores. Try to sleep for 4 to 6 hours at night while another caregiver looks after your baby. The caregiver can bring your baby to you to nurse while you are in bed, and then they can change, settle, and soothe your baby while you sleep.

- Suggest quiet play—Set up your older children with a few puzzles, picture books, or other quiet activities so you and the baby can rest.

- Take it easy—Only do what must be done and keep trips out of the house short.

- Limit visitors—If you are feeling tired, it's perfectly fine to say no to family and friends who want to stop by. There will be plenty of time for people to meet your new baby when you are feeling rested.

- Eat a healthy diet—It may be hard to find time to eat when you are caring for a new baby. Even so, it's vital that you do. Stock up on foods rich in protein and iron, such as chicken, beans, and leafy greens. Eating well will help fight fatigue.

Nutrition and Weight Loss

Keep up the good eating habits you began in pregnancy (see Chapter 22, "Nutrition During Pregnancy"). A balanced, healthy diet can help your body heal, give you energy, and help with breastfeeding. Getting to a healthy weight may take some time. Be patient with weight loss. Combining healthy eating with exercise will help the process.

The U.S. Department of Agriculture's website MyPlate can help you plan healthy meals (see the "Resources" section at the end of this chapter). One half of your plate should be fruits and vegetables. The other half should be grains and protein foods. Try to make at least half of the grains you eat whole grains (for example, whole-wheat bread, brown rice, and oatmeal). Eat more foods that are naturally low in sugar and fat, such as many types of fish and vegetables. Cut down on sugary drinks, such as soft drinks and sweetened tea.

Exercise

When you are caring for a newborn, finding time for exercise can be a challenge. Hormonal changes can affect you emotionally, and sleepless nights can be exhausting. Although you may feel too tired to exercise, being active can give you more energy. Even exercising for a few minutes each day has benefits.

If you had a healthy pregnancy and a normal vaginal delivery, you should be able to start exercising again soon after the baby is born. Usually, it is safe to exercise a few days after giving birth. But if you had a cesarean birth or other complications, ask your ob-gyn when it is safe to begin exercising again. See Chapter 23, "Exercise During Pregnancy," for a section on postpartum exercises.

Sex and Family Planning

If you plan to have sex again after childbirth, you can take these steps to prepare:

- Learn how to manage discomfort you may feel with sexual activity.
- Choose a birth control option that is right for you.
- Think about your plans for having more children.

There is no set time for when you can resume having sex after childbirth. After about 2 weeks postpartum, bleeding and infection are not likely to occur. Many ob-gyns recommend waiting until 6 weeks after childbirth. Start a reliable birth control method before having sex again. Talk with your ob-gyn about birth control options.

After childbirth, it is common to feel discomfort during sex. The following suggestions may help ease dryness or pain:

- Use a water-based lubricant to help with vaginal dryness.
- Avoid oil-based lubricants, which include petroleum jelly, baby oil, and mineral oil. Oil-based lubricants should not be used with latex condoms. You also should avoid "warming" lubricants, which can make inflamed vaginal tissues feel worse.
- Try different positions to take pressure off a sore area and to control **penetration**. Being on top may be more comfortable for you.

If painful sex continues to be a problem, talk with your ob-gyn. **Estrogen** cream may be prescribed for vaginal dryness or to help heal a perineal tear. This cream is placed in the vagina. It is safe to use if you are breastfeeding. If **sexual intercourse** or penetration is not comfortable, explore other ways to be intimate until you are ready to have sex again.

Lack of Interest in Sex

It's normal to not have much interest in sex, even several months after childbirth. Reasons for this may include

- fatigue
- stress
- fear of pain
- lack of desire from decreased **hormone** levels
- lack of time, energy, or focus
- feeling "touched out" from caring for your baby

During the weeks that you may not feel up to sexual activity, you can be intimate with your partner in other ways, such as hugging and kissing. When you do feel comfortable and ready to have sex again, it's a good idea to keep the following things in mind:

- Find a time for sex when you are not rushed. Wait until the baby is sound asleep or you can drop the baby off with a friend or a relative for a couple of hours.

- Spend private time with your partner when you talk only about each other—not the baby or household problems.
- If sex or penetration isn't comfortable yet, there are many other ways to give and receive sexual pleasure, such as mutual masturbation or oral sex.

If you have concerns about your sex life, it may help to discuss your feelings with your partner. You also can talk with your ob-gyn:

- "I have some concerns about my sex life."
- "I do not enjoy sex like I used to."
- "I have been having trouble with physical intimacy. What can I do?"
- "I am just not interested in sex. Do you have any advice?"

Birth Control

It's possible to get pregnant very soon after having a baby if you have sexual intercourse and do not use birth control. Some women can get pregnant even before their periods come back. Starting a birth control method right after you have a baby can help you avoid an unintended pregnancy. It also lets you plan and control when you try to get pregnant again, if you want more children in the future.

It is possible to get pregnant while you are breastfeeding. But the risk of pregnancy is low if all of these are true:

- You are breastfeeding your baby every few hours.
- Your baby is less than 6 months old.
- Your period has not come back.

If any of these three things are not true, you should use birth control to prevent pregnancy.

You can talk with your ob-gyn about birth control options while you are still pregnant. You also can have this discussion after giving birth, before you go home from the hospital. When choosing a birth control method to use after you have a baby, think about the following:

- Timing—Some birth control methods can be started right after childbirth. With other methods, you need to wait a few weeks to start.
- Breastfeeding—All methods are safe to use while breastfeeding. But there are a few methods that are not recommended during the first weeks of breastfeeding because they might affect your milk supply.

- Effectiveness—The method you used before pregnancy may not be the best choice after pregnancy. For example, the sponge and cervical cap are much less effective in women who have given birth.

See Chapter 21, "Birth Control After Pregnancy and Beyond," for details on birth control methods.

Having Another Baby

The timing of your next pregnancy is your decision. Only you can decide what you are ready to handle physically, emotionally, and financially. But ideally, pregnancies should be spaced at least 18 months apart. This offers the best health outcomes for both mom and baby. If you feel the need to try for another pregnancy sooner, talk with your ob-gyn about the risks and benefits in your case. See Chapter 42, "Having Another Baby: What to Expect the Next Time Around," for more on planning your next pregnancy.

Your Future Health

Even after you have healed from childbirth and finished your postpartum checkups, you still need to keep your health top of mind. You can do this by

- focusing on any ongoing medical issues
- staying up to date with your vaccinations
- continuing to see your health care practitioners

Health Problems During Pregnancy

Some pregnancy complications, such as **high blood pressure** or **diabetes mellitus** during pregnancy, may get better after childbirth. But this is not always true. If you had health problems before or during pregnancy, you may need to see your ob-gyn earlier or more often after childbirth so he or she can keep a close eye on your health.

If you had certain problems during pregnancy, it may mean you are more likely to have other problems in the future. For example, if you had high blood pressure during pregnancy, you may have a higher risk of heart disease later in life.

This does not mean that you definitely will have health problems in the future. But it is good to understand your risk so that you can take extra steps to prevent future health conditions (see Table 19-1, "Future Health Risks").

If you saw health care practitioners for any chronic health problems before you were pregnant, make sure you keep seeing those practitioners

TABLE 19-1 Future Health Risks

If you had certain health conditions before or during pregnancy, you may be at risk for future health problems. Use this table to understand these possible risks and what they may mean for your postpartum care.

Condition	Possible Future Health Risks	Postpartum Health Care
Gestational diabetes	Type 2 diabetes	• Breastfeeding is encouraged • Blood sugar screening 4 to 12 weeks after giving birth; then every 3 years • If initial test shows prediabetes, then yearly screening for diabetes is recommended • Possible referral to a specialist
Diabetes mellitus	If poorly controlled: **kidney disease**, nerve damage, eye damage, heart disease, birth defects in future pregnancies	• Blood sugar screening • Maintain healthy weight • Thyroid screening for women with type 1 diabetes • Possible prescription of low-dose aspirin for future pregnancies
Preeclampsia and high blood pressure during pregnancy	Preeclampsia in future pregnancies, heart disease	• Blood pressure monitoring for 72 hours after giving birth, and then for 7 to 10 days • Possible prescription of low-dose aspirin for future pregnancies • Maintain healthy weight
Chronic high blood pressure	If poorly controlled: **stroke**, organ damage, kidney disease, heart disease	• Blood pressure monitoring for 72 hours postpartum, and then for 1 to 2 weeks • Possible prescription of low-dose aspirin for future pregnancies • Maintain healthy weight
Excessive weight gain during pregnancy	More weight gain and **obesity**	• Measure **body mass index (BMI)** • Screening for diabetes and high blood pressure • Reach prepregnancy weight by 6 to 12 months postpartum; aim for near-normal BMI
Obesity	Type 2 diabetes, high blood pressure, certain types of cancer, arthritis, heart disease	• Measure BMI • Screening for diabetes, high blood pressure, high **cholesterol** and **triglycerides** • Reach prepregnancy weight by 6 to 12 months after giving birth; aim for near-normal BMI
Preterm birth or small infant size	Heart disease (the highest risk is linked to delivery at less than 32 weeks of pregnancy)	• Screening for certain risk factors of heart disease, such as high blood pressure

after childbirth. These practitioners should be a part of your postpartum care team. Use the "My Postpartum Care Team Chart" at the back of this book to note names and contact information.

If you were taking medications before or during pregnancy, talk with your health care practitioners about taking these medications after childbirth. Some medications may not be safe to take while you are breastfeeding.

Vaccinations

Vaccinations are a simple, safe, and effective way to protect you and your baby from infections. If you did not get certain vaccinations before or during pregnancy or before going home from the hospital, you should get them now. This will help protect your baby from infections. Recommended vaccines for women in the postpartum period may include

- *measles–mumps–rubella (MMR) vaccine*
- *influenza (flu) vaccine*
- *tetanus toxoid, reduced diphtheria toxoid, and acellular pertussis (Tdap) vaccine*
- *varicella (chickenpox) vaccine*

Talk with your ob-gyn about the vaccines you may need after pregnancy. It also is a good idea to ask your family, caregivers, and anyone else who will be near your baby to be up to date with their vaccines.

Ongoing Well-Woman Care

After you finish your postpartum health care visits, you should switch to regular well-woman health care visits. These are checkups with a health care practitioner where you discuss your overall health and have routine screenings. This ongoing care is important to help you stay healthy for the rest of your life.

Talk with your ob-gyn about who should continue your care after the postpartum period. The main person responsible for your health care is called your primary care practitioner (PCP). This person may be your ob-gyn or it may be someone else.

Taking care of yourself during the postpartum period is important for your long-term health. Remember that postpartum care should be an ongoing process, designed just for you and your needs. Talk with your ob-gyn to make sure you are getting the health care that you need to be healthy—now and in the future.

RESOURCES

International Lactation Consultant Association
www.ilca.org
Provides a directory of *certified lactation consultants* and *international board-certified lactation consultants (IBCLCs)* as well as information about breastfeeding.

La Leche League International
www.llli.org
Provides information and support for breastfeeding women and offers referrals to local support groups.

MyPlate
www.ChooseMyPlate.gov
Website from the U.S. Department of Agriculture. The customized MyPlate Plan lets you enter your information for tips on what and how much to eat.

Postpartum Depression
https://medlineplus.gov/postpartumdepression.html
Webpage from the U.S. National Library of Medicine. A starting place to find more information about postpartum depression.

Postpartum Support International Helpline
www.postpartum.net
1-800-944-4773
Text 1-503-894-9453 (English) or 1-971-420-0294 (Spanish)
Non-emergency helpline for support, information, or referrals to postpartum mental health practitioners. The helpline is open 7 days per week. Leave a confidential message at any time, and a volunteer will return your call or text as soon as possible. PSI also offers online support group meetings to connect with other pregnant and postpartum women. You also can join PSI's weekly Chat with an Expert.

Your Pregnancy and Childbirth
www.acog.org/MyPregnancy
Website from the American College of Obstetricians and Gynecologists (ACOG) with information on pregnancy, labor, delivery, and postpartum care. Includes the latest information from the experts in women's health care, questions answered by ACOG ob-gyns, pregnancy stories from real women, and an A–Z directory of health topics covering pregnancy and beyond.

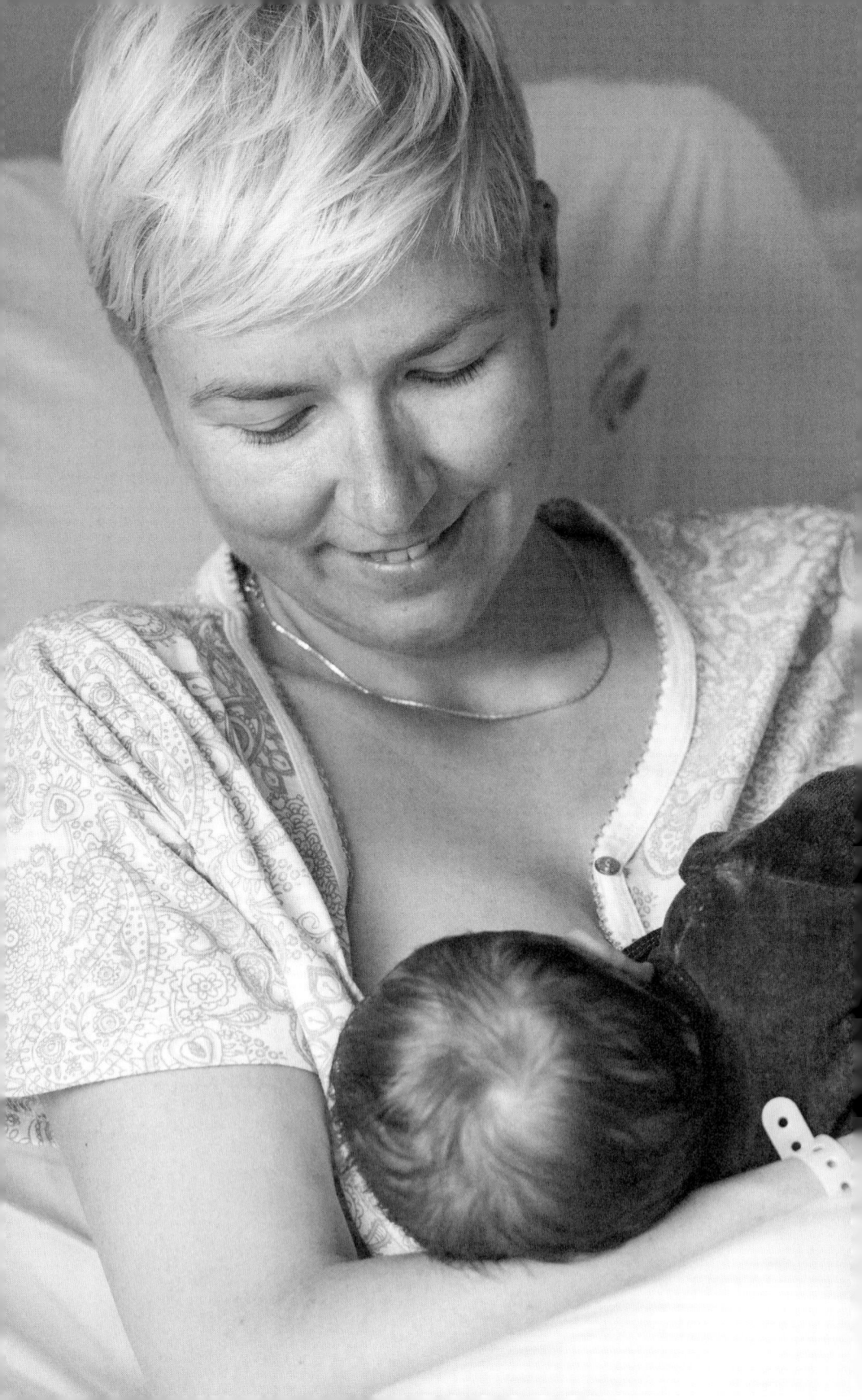

CHAPTER 20

Feeding Your Baby

How you will feed your newborn is an important decision that is best to make by the time you deliver. Breastfeeding—feeding directly from the breast—works for some women. For others, feeding a baby pumped breast milk with a bottle is another very good option. Some women cannot or choose not to breastfeed or pump. These women feed their babies formula. Lastly, some women choose a combination of feeding methods.

If you need help deciding which way is best for you, talk with your ***obstetrician–gynecologist (ob-gyn)*** or your baby's doctor. Learn about each of the options to help you make the best decision for you and your baby (see the "Resources" section at the end of this chapter).

Remember that the decision is a personal one. Feeding your baby should be enjoyable and comfortable for both of you. Whichever option you choose, you should have support from your ob-gyn, your partner, and your family.

Benefits of Breastfeeding

Breastfeeding is good for your baby and good for you. The benefits for your baby include the following:

- Human milk is the most complete form of ***nutrition*** for babies. It has the right amount of fats, sugars, water, and protein needed for growth and development. As your baby grows, your breast milk changes to meet the baby's changing nutritional needs.

- Human milk is easier than formula for babies to digest. Breastfed babies have less gas and fewer feeding problems. They often have less constipation than babies given formula.

- Human milk contains **antibodies** that protect babies from infections. Studies show that breastfed babies have a reduced risk of infections of the ears, lungs, and digestive system. Babies who are breastfed also tend to get sick less often overall and recover from certain illnesses more quickly than babies who are not breastfed.

- Breastfed babies have a lower risk of **sudden infant death syndrome (SIDS)**. Any amount of breastfeeding appears to help lower this risk. Using a pacifier also lowers the risk of SIDS. But pacifiers should be introduced only after breastfeeding is well established, ideally about 3 to 4 weeks after you start breastfeeding.

- For **preterm** babies, breast milk can be especially helpful. Preterm babies who are fed human milk are less likely to develop some of the health problems of being born too early. Breastfeeding also may improve the development of thinking and reasoning skills later in life.

Breastfeeding also has benefits for mothers:

- Breastfeeding triggers the release of a hormone called **oxytocin**. This hormone makes the **uterus** contract and return to its original size. These contractions also reduce the amount of bleeding you may have after giving birth.

- Breastfeeding burns **calories**, which may make it easier to lose the weight you gained during pregnancy.

- Breastfeeding delays the return of **ovulation** and **menstrual cycles**. This may help prevent pregnancy in the first 6 months after delivery. But you should talk with your ob-gyn about **birth control** options before you start having sex again.

- Breastfeeding has been shown to reduce the risk of **ovarian cancer** and some types of breast cancer. More research is needed to understand how breastfeeding helps reduce cancer risk.

- Women who breastfeed longer have lower rates of **diabetes mellitus** and **high blood pressure**.

When You Should Not Breastfeed

As healthy as breastfeeding can be, it is not the best choice for every woman. There are some situations in which a woman should not breastfeed.

Infections

Certain infections can be passed to your baby through breastfeeding. But not all infections prevent you from breastfeeding—only some (see the box "You Can Breastfeed If You Have…"). Women with **human immunodeficiency virus (HIV)** should not breastfeed. Women with certain other infections may need to express (squeeze out) and throw away their milk until there's no longer a risk of infecting the baby. These infections include

- active *tuberculosis (TB)*
- *chickenpox* contracted 5 days before delivery through 2 days after delivery
- a *herpes* outbreak that affects the breast

If you have TB that is being treated and you are no longer contagious, you can pump and feed the baby breast milk even during treatment. If you have herpes sores on the breast, you can breastfeed once the sores heal.

Wash your hands with soap and water before and after breastfeeding. Keep any active herpes sores or chickenpox sores covered while breastfeeding. If you have chickenpox, you can express your milk and give it to your baby and then go back to breastfeeding when you are well.

As this book went to press, many women had questions about breastfeeding when a woman has coronavirus (COVID-19). Most information shows that it is safe to feed breast milk to your baby if you have COVID-19. Remember that breast milk is the best source of nutrition for most babies. For this reason, having COVID-19 should not stop you from giving your baby breast milk.

Women with COVID-19 should wear a face mask or covering while breastfeeding or bottle-feeding. They also should wash their hands before touching the baby, a breast pump, or bottle parts. And they should wash their hands and all pump and bottle parts after use.

As time goes on, researchers are learning more about COVID-19. If you have COVID-19 during pregnancy, ask your ob-gyn for the most up-to-date information for you and your baby.

Prescription and Illegal Drug Use

Using some substances while breastfeeding can harm your baby. These substances include

- illegal drugs, such as cocaine, heroin, and methamphetamines
- prescription drugs taken for nonmedical reasons

> **You Can Breastfeed If You Have . . .**
>
> - **Hepatitis B** infection, as long as your baby was given the hepatitis B vaccine and **hepatitis B immune globulin** within the first few hours after birth
> - **Hepatitis C** infection
> - Cold sores or **genital herpes**, as long as the breast or nipple is not affected and any active sores are covered
> - **Chorioamnionitis** before delivery or **endometritis** after delivery
> - **Cytomegalovirus (CMV)** infection, but if your baby is preterm, talk with your ob-gyn and the baby's doctor

Recreational and medical marijuana are legal in many states, but neither should be used when you are breastfeeding. If you need help stopping drug use, talk with your ob-gyn. Until you are able to stop using these substances, formula feeding is best for your baby.

Medications

Most medications are safe to use when you are breastfeeding. Some medications that are unsafe to take during pregnancy may be OK to take while breastfeeding. This is because of the ways medications may cross the **placenta** and enter breast milk. If there is concern about a medication you are taking, you may be able to switch to one that may be safer. See the "Medication" section later in this chapter and talk with your ob-gyn.

Breastfeeding

If you've decided to breastfeed, find information about it while you are still pregnant. **Lactation** is the term used for milk production. Many hospitals and parents' centers offer breastfeeding classes taught by lactation specialists. These specialists can teach you what you need to know to get started. Lactation specialists also can help you with some common problems many women face when they breastfeed.

You can find breastfeeding support near you through several organizations, including the

Is Your Hospital Baby-Friendly?

In 1991, a team of global experts developed 10 steps that hospitals can take to help mothers and babies get off to a good start with breastfeeding. Studies have shown that women who give birth in Baby-Friendly® hospitals are more likely to achieve their breastfeeding goals. Hospitals that adopt all 10 steps are certified as Baby-Friendly. These hospitals follow these practices:

1. They have a written breastfeeding policy that is shared with all health care staff.
2. They train all health care staff to implement this policy.
3. They tell all pregnant women about the benefits and management of breastfeeding.
4. They help mothers initiate breastfeeding within 1 hour of birth.
5. They show mothers how to breastfeed and how to maintain milk production, even if they are separated from their babies.
6. They give babies no food or drinks other than breast milk, unless medically indicated.
7. They practice rooming-in, which keeps mothers and babies together 24 hours a day.
8. They encourage breastfeeding on demand.
9. They give no pacifiers or artificial nipples to breastfeeding babies.
10. They help develop breastfeeding support groups and refer women to them when they leave the hospital.

Visit www.babyfriendlyusa.org to find out whether your hospital is certified as Baby-Friendly. If your hospital is not certified, it may just mean that the hospital has not met all of the criteria for certification yet. Or the hospital may use other ways to implement best practices. You can call your hospital to ask about its breastfeeding policies and whether they are working on Baby-Friendly certification.

- International Lactation Consultant Association
- La Leche League International
- Women, Infants, and Children (WIC) Breastfeeding Support Program from the U.S. Department of Agriculture (see the "Resources" section at the end of this chapter)

There are other support groups that vary by community and state. You also may want to check out whether your hospital has a Baby-Friendly® designation (see the box "Is Your Hospital Baby-Friendly?").

The American College of Obstetricians and Gynecologists (ACOG), the American Academy of Pediatrics, and many other organizations recommend ***exclusive breastfeeding.*** This means that human milk is the only food given for the first 6 months of the baby's life. Medicines and vitamin supplements can be given, but no other food, water, or juice are needed, unless your baby's doctor recommends otherwise. Breastfeeding should ideally continue as new foods are introduced up to the baby's first birthday or beyond, if both mother and baby want to continue.

Getting Started

Most healthy newborns are ready to breastfeed within the first hour after birth (see Chapter 18, "After the Baby Is Born"). Babies who breastfeed soon after birth may have an easier time breastfeeding than babies who do not. Tell your ob-gyn while you are pregnant that you want to breastfeed. When you get to the hospital or birth center to give birth, remind your health care team that you plan to breastfeed.

Holding your baby directly against your bare skin immediately after birth helps encourage your baby to start breastfeeding. Skin-to-skin contact also helps stabilize the baby's

- body temperature
- heart rate
- breathing
- blood sugar level

Skin-to-skin contact may be possible after a **cesarean delivery**. Ask your ob-gyn whether this is an option at your hospital or birth center. If it is not an option, ask to be united with your baby as soon as possible after the surgery is complete.

During the first few days after birth, your breasts make **colostrum**, a thick, yellowish fluid. It is the same fluid that leaks from some women's breasts during pregnancy. The colostrum that your breasts make after birth helps your newborn's digestive system grow and mature. The fluid is rich in protein and calories and is all your baby needs for the first few days of life, unless your baby's doctor recommends otherwise. Colostrum is especially high in antibodies that help protect your baby against illnesses.

About 40 to 72 hours after birth, your breasts begin to make a larger amount of milk. You may hear this referred to as your milk "coming in." You will probably notice a change in the size of your breasts 2 to 5 days after delivery.

Milk is made continuously in the breast and stored in breast tissue. When your baby starts to breastfeed, the nerves in your nipples send a message to your brain. In response, your brain releases hormones that signal the **milk lobules** to contract (squeeze) and push out milk so that it flows through your nipples. This is called the let-down reflex.

Some women barely notice let-down. Others have a "pins-and-needles" feeling or even sharp pain in their breasts 2 to 3 minutes after their babies start nursing. In the first week after birth, some women also have cramping as their uterus contracts. Called "afterpains," this pain may be relieved with ibuprofen. For most women, pain during let-down eases as their bodies adjust to breastfeeding. Let-down also can be triggered by

- looking at your baby
- thinking about your baby
- hearing your baby cry

In some women, hearing any baby cry will trigger the let-down reflex.

When your baby starts feeding from your breast, the milk that is released first is thin, watery, and sweet. It quenches the baby's thirst and provides sugar, proteins, and minerals. Once the baby gets this "foremilk," the milk then becomes thick and creamy. This milk will satisfy hunger and give your baby the **nutrients** needed to grow.

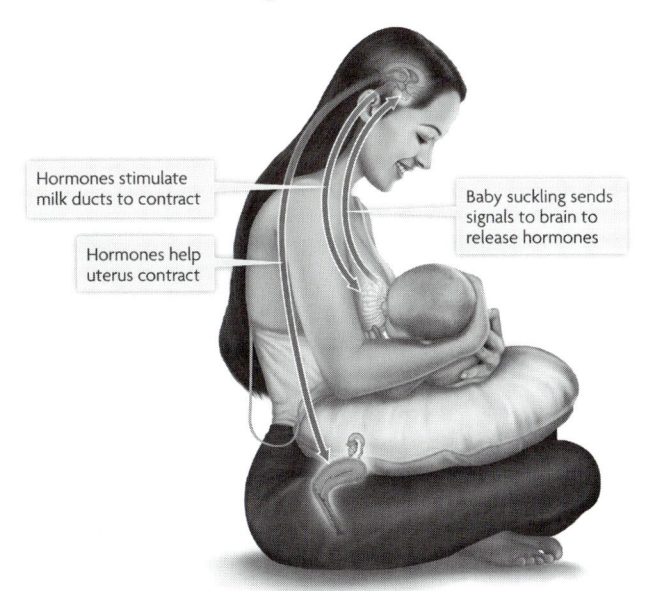

Let-down reflex. The baby's mouth on the mother's nipple signals the brain to release hormones. These hormones cause the milk ducts to contract and expel milk and stimulate the uterus to contract.

The more milk your baby removes from your breast, the more milk you will produce. This way your milk production will keep up with the baby's demand. If your baby needs more milk—during a growth spurt, for example—the baby's increased suckling leads to increased emptying of your breast. This in turn stimulates more milk production.

Latching On

To begin breastfeeding, the baby needs to attach to or "latch on" to your breast. Your ob-gyn, a nurse, or lactation specialist can help you find a good position (see the box "Breastfeeding Positions"). Cup your breast in your hand and stroke your baby's lower lip with your nipple. This stimulates the baby's rooting reflex. This is a baby's instinct to turn toward the nipple, open the mouth, and suck.

The baby will open the mouth wide (like a yawn). Pull the baby close to you, aiming the nipple toward the roof of the baby's mouth. Bring your baby to your breast—not your breast to your baby.

Babies are born with a set of reflexes that help guide them to the breast. Another way to get the baby to latch on is to use a technique called "baby-led latch." Lie back on a bed or couch with your back and shoulders supported. Place your baby belly-down onto your chest, with the baby's cheek close to your bare breast. Over a few minutes, most babies will explore the breast, find the nipple, and latch. Most women use one hand to support the breast and one hand to support the head and neck during this time. As babies get older, they usually need less support.

Baby's Breastfeeding Technique

The baby should have all of your nipple and most of the *areola* in the mouth. The baby's nose will be touching your breast. The goal is for the nipple to be as far back in the baby's mouth as possible. The baby's lips also will be curled out on your breast. The baby's sucking should be smooth and even. You should hear the baby swallow. You may feel a slight tugging.

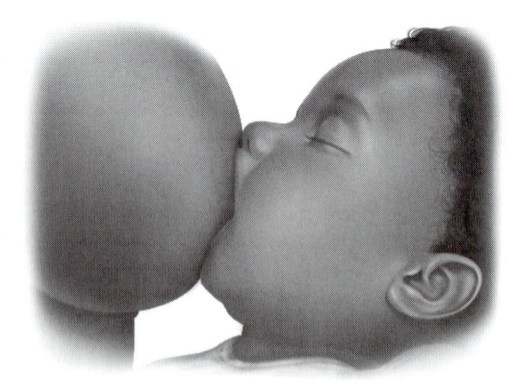

Correct latch. The baby should have all of your nipple and a good deal of the areola in the mouth. The baby's nose will be touching your breast. The baby's lips also will be curled against your breast.

Breastfeeding Positions

Finding a good position will help the baby latch on. It also will help you relax and be comfortable. Use pillows or folded blankets to help support the baby.

- **Cradle Hold**—Sit up as straight as you can and cradle your baby in the crook of your arm. The baby's body should be turned toward you and the belly should be against yours. Support the head in the bend of your elbow so the baby is facing your breast.

- **Cross-Cradle Hold**—As in the cradle hold, nuzzle your baby's belly against yours. Hold the baby in the arm opposite the breast you are using to nurse. For instance, if the baby is nursing from your right breast, hold him or her with your left arm. Place the baby's bottom in the crook of your left arm and support the baby's head and neck with your left hand. This position gives you more control of the baby's head. It's a good position for a newborn who is having trouble nursing.

- **Football Hold**—Tuck your baby under your arm like a football. Hold the baby at your side, level with your waist, so the baby is facing you. Support the baby's back with your upper arm and hold the head level with your breast.

- **Side-Lying Position**—Lie on your side and nestle your baby next to you. Place your fingers beneath your breast and lift it up to help your baby reach your nipple. Rest your head on your lower arm. You may want to tuck a pillow behind your back to help hold yourself up. This position is good for night feedings. It's also good for women who had a **cesarean birth** because it keeps the baby's weight off your belly and incision.

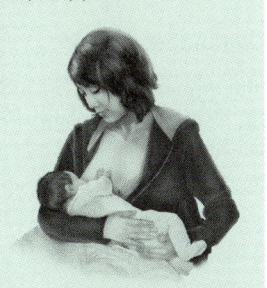

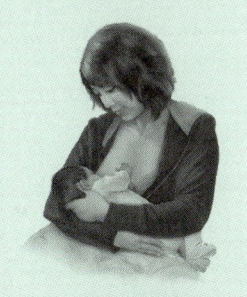

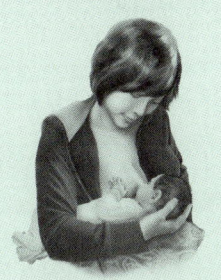

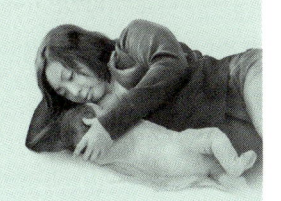

If you feel discomfort or notice that your baby's mouth is not wide open, gently break the suction by inserting a clean finger between your breast and your baby's gums. When you hear or feel a soft pop, pull your nipple out of the baby's mouth. If you have severe breast pain, or pain that continues through feeding, talk with your ob-gyn or a lactation specialist.

How Long to Feed

Let your baby set the nursing pattern. In the first few weeks, it's normal for newborns to feed up to 12 times a day (see the box "Is My Baby Getting Enough Milk?"). Newborns usually nurse for at least 10 to 15 minutes on each breast. They also can nurse for much longer periods. Long breastfeeding sessions, called cluster feeds, may happen during a growth spurt. They also happen most often toward the end of the day.

Some babies feed from one breast per feeding, while others feed from both breasts. When your baby releases one breast, offer the other. Plan to start on the other side for the next feeding. Some women wear an elastic band on the wrist of the side that the baby nursed on the last time. Others use an app on the phone to remind them.

Signs That Your Baby Wants to Feed

When babies are hungry, they will nuzzle against your breast, smack their lips, stick out their tongue, suck on their hands, or flex their fingers and arms. Crying usually is a late sign of hunger. When babies are full, they relax their arms and legs and close their eyes.

The baby's stomach is very small at first—it holds only a little more than half an ounce at birth. Also, human milk leaves a baby's stomach faster than formula. For these reasons, you will typically breastfeed at least 8 to 12 times in 24 hours. That's at least every 2 to 3 hours during the first weeks of your baby's life.

If it has been more than 4 hours since the last feeding, you may need to wake up your baby to feed. Some newborns are happy to go 3 hours between feedings (see the box "Is My Baby Getting Enough Milk?"). Others need to nurse once an hour for the first few weeks. That's a lot of work for you, so have your partner, family, and friends nearby to take care of you while you are taking care of your baby. Over time, you and your baby will set your own schedule.

Vitamin D and Iron Supplements

All babies need 400 international units (IU) of vitamin D each day. Vitamin D helps with bone growth. Breastfed or partially breastfed babies need supplementation starting in the first days after birth. Vitamin D is available in liquid form that you give your baby with a dropper. Note that the label may say 10 micrograms (mcg), which is the same as 400 IU.

Is My Baby Getting Enough Milk?

When feeding with a bottle, you can see how much the baby is eating by looking at the side of the bottle. Of course, breasts don't have ounces marked on the sides, but babies are smart, and they use cues to tell their mothers and caregivers when they are satisfied:

- Your baby uses body language. A full baby's arms are typically relaxed, with palms outstretched, and the baby is drowsy and content. When the baby is ready to eat again, arms will be flexed with hands in a fist, and the baby will try to suck on his or her fingers. Watch for these early feeding cues, not the clock, to know when to offer the breast.
- Your baby nurses often. Healthy newborns nurse at least 8 to 12 times in 24 hours. As babies grow, their stomachs are able to hold more at each feeding, and they will need to nurse less often. Even so, healthy newborns don't go more than about 3 to 4 hours without nursing, even at night.

Each nursing session should last 10 to 45 minutes. Babies may eat for a brief time and then want to eat again a short time later. Sometimes, a newborn may eat for an extended period (1 to 2 hours) and then fall into a deep sleep.

- Your baby goes through lots of diapers. Once your breasts transition from making colostrum to mature milk, your baby should soak at least six diapers per day. The baby's urine should be light in color rather than dark yellow. During the first month of life, your baby may have at least three bowel movements per day. The stool should be soft and yellow.
- Your baby is gaining weight. All newborns lose a little weight in the first few days of life—a loss of 8 to 10 percent of birth weight is normal. For example, a healthy 8-pound baby might lose up to 9 oz in the first few days of life. After 10 to 14 days, your baby should be back to his or her weight at birth.

The baby's doctor should weigh your baby at each visit and keep track of his or her weight. If you are worried that your baby isn't getting enough breast milk, call your ob-gyn or the baby's doctor.

Another option is for you to take 6,400 IU of vitamin D per day. This increases the amount of vitamin D in your breast milk. Formula has vitamin D, so babies who are formula-feeding usually do not need extra vitamin D.

Breastfed or partially breastfed babies also need an iron supplement starting at around 6 months of age. Formula-feeding babies should be on a formula that has iron. Ask your baby's doctor how much iron your baby needs.

Pacifiers

Many women wonder about giving their babies pacifiers for comfort. In the first few weeks, it's good for babies to suckle at the breast for comfort instead of using a pacifier. Suckling at the breast stimulates milk-making hormones and helps women to establish a milk supply.

There are a few instances when a pacifier may be OK. You may want to give a pacifier to help with pain relief (while getting a shot, for instance). Allowing your baby to suck on your clean pinky finger also can help with pain relief. Sometimes a pacifier can soothe a fussy baby. If your nipples are sore or cracked, a pacifier can comfort your baby while your nipples heal.

Note that pacifiers ideally should not be used until breastfeeding is well established, about 3 to 4 weeks after you've started. After breastfeeding is established, babies can be given pacifiers when lying on their backs before sleep. This may help reduce the risk of SIDS.

Food, Drinks, and Medication While Breastfeeding

When you are pregnant, your body stores extra nutrients and fat to prepare for breastfeeding. Even so, once your baby is born, you need more food and nutrients than normal to fuel milk production. You'll also need to drink lots of liquids, because breastfeeding uses up lots of fluid. You need at least eight glasses of liquid per day. **Dehydration** can reduce your milk supply.

Keep in mind that when you breastfeed, what you put into your body can still go to your baby, just like when you were pregnant. Most medications are safe to take while you are breastfeeding, but there are some exceptions. See the "Medication" section below. And as always, if you have any questions or concerns, talk with your ob-gyn.

Nutrition

Breastfeeding women need 1,000 milligrams (mg) of calcium per day. You can get this amount by eating plenty of dairy products like milk, yogurt, and cheese. If you don't eat or can't digest milk products, ask your ob-gyn about taking a calcium supplement.

Be sure to get at least 400 micrograms (mcg) of folic acid each day too. This will help you maintain good health and ensure that you have plenty of folic acid stores. Your ob-gyn may suggest that you keep taking a daily prenatal vitamin supplement until your baby is weaned (stops breastfeeding). If the vitamin label lists dietary folate equivalents (DFE) instead, it should have 667 mcg DFE.

Fish and shellfish are great sources of protein and provide vitamins and minerals for you and your baby. While you're breastfeeding, try to eat fish about 2 to 3 times a week (at least 8 ounces [oz] but no more than 12 oz total).

Medication

Most medications are safe to take while you are breastfeeding. When you take medication, sometimes it can pass to your breast milk. But the level of medication in your milk is usually lower than the level in your bloodstream. The latest information about medications and their effects on breastfed babies can be found at LactMed, a database of scientific information. LactMed also can be downloaded as a free app on your smartphone (see the "Resources" section at the end of this chapter).

If you need to take a prescription medication, talk with your ob-gyn and the baby's doctor. Your ob-gyn can help determine the safest drug while you are breastfeeding. Sometimes, the amount of the drug that reaches a breastfeeding baby can be reduced if a woman takes her medication after feedings.

If you need to take a medication that is known to pose a risk to a breastfeeding baby, the baby should be monitored. Your baby's doctor may do blood tests from time to time to measure how much of the drug is in your baby's system. Remember that taking medication you need may outweigh any risks of the medication for your breastfeeding baby.

Tobacco

If you smoke, quitting smoking is the best thing you can do for your health and your baby's health. Secondhand smoke increases the risk of SIDS. But it's better for your baby to breastfeed than to formula-feed, even if you continue to smoke.

Alcohol

No matter how much or how often you drink, alcohol passes into breast milk. You should wait about 2 hours per serving for the alcohol to leave your body. A serving is

- beer or wine cooler—12 oz
- table wine—5 oz

- malt liquor—8 to 9 oz
- 80-Proof spirits—1.5 oz

An occasional drink of alcohol is likely safe when you are breastfeeding. But moderate or heavy alcohol drinking can cause problems for your baby, including

- drowsiness
- weakness
- problems gaining weight

Heavy drinking is having more than three drinks per occasion or more than seven drinks per week.

Breastfeeding Challenges

Some new mothers breastfeed without any problems. For others, breastfeeding can be a challenge. You and your baby are both learning something new, so it's normal to have challenges at first. Many problems can be overcome with support. If you need help, or if you are concerned that your baby is not getting enough milk, call your ob-gyn or a lactation specialist.

Sore Nipples

Many women have nipple tenderness or pain in the first few weeks of breastfeeding. This tenderness usually goes away as you continue to breastfeed. If it doesn't, there are things that you can try to be more comfortable.

First, make sure that your baby is latched on well. Poor latch is the major cause of sore nipples. This is because the baby is not getting enough of the areola into the mouth and is sucking mostly on the nipple.

Check the positioning of your baby's body and the way the baby latches on and sucks. Make sure that your baby's mouth is open wide, with as much of the areola in the mouth as possible. If it hurts, break the baby's suction with a clean finger and try again. You may find that it feels better right away once the baby is positioned correctly.

After breastfeeding, you can apply a little expressed milk to your nipple, which may provide pain relief. A barrier ointment, such as coconut oil or vegetable shortening, may help your nipples heal and is safe for the baby. If the pain is severe, see your ob-gyn or a lactation specialist.

If you are having pain and using a breast pump to express milk, you may need to try a different size suction cup or lower the suction on your pump. The pump suction should feel like a gentle tugging. It should not be painful.

Some women describe shooting, burning pain that goes from the nipple out to the rest of the breast after feeding their babies. This pain may be caused by spasms of the blood vessels in the breast. A heating pad or warm gel pack applied after breastfeeding may be helpful. See your ob-gyn if the pain continues for more than a few days.

Engorgement

Engorgement can happen when your milk comes in a few days after delivery. Engorged breasts feel full and tender. You even may run a low fever. If the fever goes above 101°F or if you are in severe pain, call your ob-gyn. If your breasts are very engorged, it can be hard for your baby to latch on. Once your body figures out how much milk your baby needs, the problem should go away. This often takes a week or so. The following things may bring relief:

- Feed the baby more often to help drain your breasts.
- Express a little milk with a pump or by hand to soften your breasts before nursing (see the "Feeding Expressed or Pumped Breast Milk" section in this chapter).
- Before feedings, massage your breasts, take warm showers, or apply warm packs to your breasts.
- After feedings, apply cold packs to your breasts to relieve discomfort and reduce swelling.

If you still cannot express milk or the baby cannot latch on, ask your ob-gyn or a lactation specialist for help.

Delayed Milk Production

A woman's milk usually "comes in" within 72 hours of birth. For some women, milk production can be delayed. If it takes more than 3 days for milk to be produced, it is called "delayed lactogenesis." It's not known what causes this condition, but it can be related to

- hormonal factors
- a long or difficult labor
- having a cesarean birth
- breast injury or other problems
- medications

Whatever the cause, delayed lactogenesis can be hard for you and your baby. The more stressed and anxious you are, the more it can affect the natural let-down reflex. Delayed milk production is one reason why some women stop trying to breastfeed exclusively.

If milk production is delayed, work with a lactation specialist or a health care practitioner with expertise in breastfeeding. Increasing the number of breastfeeding sessions can be helpful. So can using a breast pump to express milk after breastfeeding.

In some situations, such as if your baby has lost more than 8 to 10 percent of birth weight, they may need small supplemental feedings with expressed breast milk, formula, or donor milk from a human milk bank. If your baby needs supplementation, a lactation specialist can help you.

Low Milk Supply

The most common cause of low milk supply is not removing milk effectively or often enough. Healthy newborns generally feed 8 to 12 times a day. For some women, less frequent feeding or pumping sends a signal to the breast to make less milk.

Another cause of not removing milk frequently enough is preterm birth. If the baby is born early, the baby may tire easily and not drink enough milk to stimulate milk production. To sort out these possibilities, work with a lactation specialist or a health care practitioner with breastfeeding expertise.

Even with frequent feedings and skilled support, some women are not able to make enough milk to feed their babies only breast milk. It is not true that "every mother can breastfeed." The fact is that breastfeeding, like any other body function, may not work for some women because of various circumstances. Supplemental feedings with expressed breast milk, formula, or donor milk may be recommended. That said, you can still nurture your baby at your breast no matter how much milk you make.

Inverted or Flat Nipples

Nipples normally stick out from the breast. But some women have flat nipples. Others have inverted nipples, which sink into the areola instead of sticking out.

In most cases, women with flat or inverted nipples can breastfeed. Flat or inverted nipples are most likely to cause problems during the first feedings after birth, when the baby is learning to latch on. It may be hard for the baby to latch on at first, but breastfeeding will be easier as the baby grows bigger and stronger.

Nipple shields can be helpful for flat nipples. A nipple shield is a nipple-shaped piece of plastic with holes in the end that can be placed over your nipple. When the baby latches directly onto the nipple shield, your nipple will be sucked into the shield while the baby nurses.

After using the shield for a while, your nipple may begin to stick out more and the baby can latch directly onto your nipple. Talk with a lactation specialist or a health care practitioner with breastfeeding expertise about whether a nipple shield might be helpful. They can show you and your baby how to latch with a shield in place. They also can work with you to wean from the shield as the baby gets used to breastfeeding.

Using a manual or electric breast pump just before feeding also may be helpful in getting flat nipples to stick out. If you have any concerns about the shape of your nipples, talk with your health care practitioner or a lactation specialist.

Breast Surgery

Some women have had surgery to remove cysts and other benign breast lumps. This rarely causes problems with future breastfeeding. If you have had breast surgery, talk with your ob-gyn before delivery to help plan for breastfeeding. Tell your baby's doctor, too, so that your baby's weight gain can be monitored in the first few weeks.

Most women who have had their breasts enlarged can nurse their babies, especially if the implant is placed behind the chest muscles. But if the implant is very large, it may limit the amount of milk that the breast can store. A large implant also may restrict blood flow in the breast. This can decrease the amount of milk that can be produced.

Women who have had surgery to reduce the size of their breasts and whose nipples have been repositioned may have breastfeeding problems. Breast-reduction surgery can cut into ***milk ducts*** and keep a nursing woman from making enough milk. It also can limit milk storage capacity. If you have had this surgery, talk with your surgeon about what type of surgery was done. Let your ob-gyn and the baby's doctor know if you had a breast reduction so they can monitor the baby's weight gain.

Lastly, some women have had breast surgery or radiation treatment due to breast cancer. Many of these women nurse effectively on the other breast. They may make some milk from the breast that had surgery. If you had breast cancer treatment, talk with a lactation specialist before the baby is born. Many women enjoy nursing their babies, even if they can't make 100 percent of the milk that their babies need.

Blocked Ducts

If a duct gets clogged with milk, a hard and tender lump can form in your breast. Call your ob-gyn if the lump doesn't go away within 1 to 2 days or if you run a fever. In the meantime, try these tips:

- Take a warm shower or apply a warm pack to the lump before nursing.
- Offer the breast with the blocked duct first.
- Let your baby nurse long and often on the breast that is blocked.
- Massage the lump while your baby nurses to help the milk drain.
- Pump or hand-express any milk left in your breast after a feeding.
- Use a handheld massager or the handle of an electric tooth brush to help loosen the blocked area.
- Try other nursing positions to see if that helps relieve the blocked area.

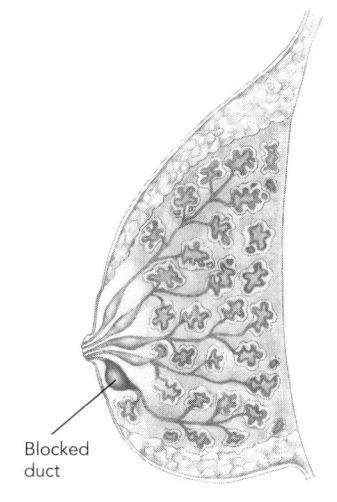

Blocked duct. A blocked milk duct can cause tenderness and lead to infection. Warm packs, massaging the area, and pumping after breastfeeding may help relieve the problem.

Mastitis

If a blocked duct doesn't drain, it may get inflamed and a breast infection (*mastitis*) can result. Mastitis can cause flu-like symptoms, including

- fever
- body aches
- fatigue

Your breasts also may be

- swollen
- painful
- hot to the touch
- streaked with red

If you think you have mastitis, call your ob-gyn right away. He or she may prescribe an **antibiotic** to treat the infection. The medication chosen will be safe to take while breastfeeding. You should feel better within a day or two of starting treatment. Take all of the medication. If you are not feeling better within a day or two, see your ob-gyn.

Until then, do the same things you'd do to treat a blocked duct. Get plenty of rest and drink lots of fluids. Your ob-gyn may suggest taking ibuprofen for pain. And continue breastfeeding or pumping—your baby will help drain your breast and unclog the blocked area. The baby won't get sick because it is the breast tissue, not the milk, that has the infection. If you do not empty the infected breast, your milk supply will go down, and recovery may take longer.

Breastfeeding Twins

Some sets of twins can breastfeed exclusively. But it is more common to need some supplementation with formula, especially if the twins are born preterm. Triplets often need supplementation too, but any breastfeeding you can do has benefits for the babies and you.

It's best to start out breastfeeding each baby individually. Multiples may not have the same sucking abilities, so feeding them one at a time at first can be less stressful for you. Later, when you have adjusted to breastfeeding multiple babies, you can learn how to feed them at the same time, which is called "tandem feeding" (see the box "Positions for Breastfeeding Twins").

Over time, you can adapt your schedule to your needs and the needs of your babies. Some women breastfeed exclusively, which means the babies receive only breast milk. Other women use a combination of breastfeeding and formula-feeding. Expressing milk into bottles allows your partner and others to help with feeding duties.

Feeding Expressed or Pumped Breast Milk

Some women express breast milk and feed their babies from a bottle. This option often is used when a baby is preterm or sick and in a **neonatal intensive care unit (NICU)**, or simply if the baby will not latch. Women who breastfeed their babies from birth also use this option when they go back to work or school, or if they are temporarily separated from their baby. Even if you are at home with your baby and exclusively breastfeeding, it can be useful to know how to express milk so that your partner or another caregiver can feed your baby when desired.

There are two ways to express milk from your breast: 1) by hand or 2) with a pump. Whichever method you choose, stimulating the let-down reflex is important so you can express the most milk possible. It may help to try things to help you relax, such as looking at a picture of your baby, or thinking about your baby. You also can try other things to stimulate the let-down reflex, including

- applying warm, moist compresses to the breasts
- gently massaging the breast

You will need a supply of bottles and nipples to store breast milk and feed your baby (see the box "Bottles and Nipples"). Store and use expressed breast milk safely, whether you are at work or home.

Expressing Milk by Hand

Expressing milk by hand can be a good solution if you are away from your baby for a short time. It also can help relieve engorgement. It can take up to 20 to 30 minutes to manually express milk from both breasts, but often it's much shorter once you learn how. This also is a great skill to have in case of an emergency, when you may not have access to electricity, your pump is not working, or you are unexpectedly separated from your baby.

To start, wash your hands with soap and water. Make sure the container you are using is clean. Use your fingers to form a "C" around the areola. Your fingers should be below the areola, and your thumb should be a little more than 1 inch above the nipple. Press inward toward your chest and then roll your thumb and fingers toward the nipple.

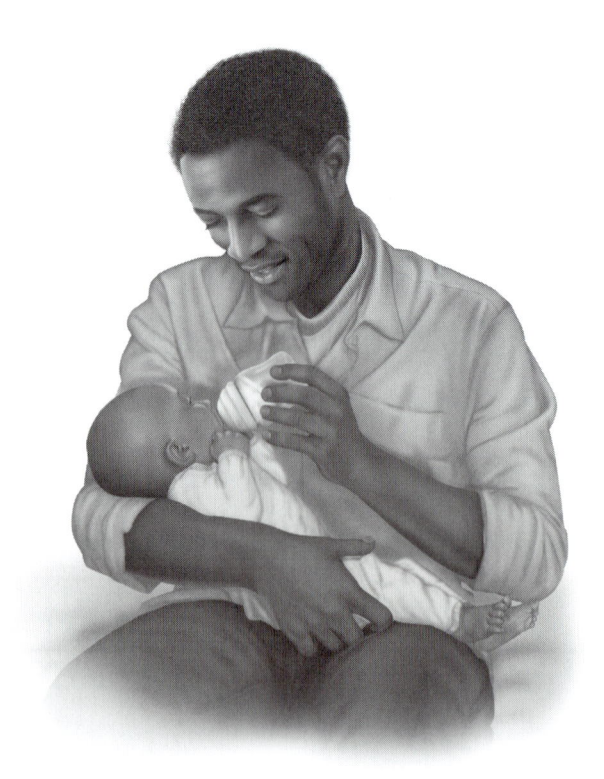

Bottle-feeding. Bottle-feeding, either with expressed breast milk or formula, allows your partner or other family members to help with feeding duties.

Positions for Breastfeeding Twins

- **Football or double-clutch hold**—Hold one baby under each arm, elbows bent, like you are holding two footballs. Hold the babies at your sides, level with your waist, so they are facing you. Support the babies' backs with your upper arms and hold their heads level with your breasts. Or, use a pillow or other support device on your lap to support the babies' backs and heads. This hold is good for newborns and for moms who have had a cesarean birth.

- **Parallel or "spoons" hold**—One baby is held in a cradle hold (head cradled in the crook of your arm). The second baby lies parallel to the first baby. The babies both face in the same direction on the same side. Pillows are helpful for this hold.

- **Criss-cross or double-cradle hold**—Sit up as straight as you can and cradle each baby in the crook of each arm. The babies' bodies should be turned toward you and their bellies should be against yours. The babies' legs should be criss-crossed in front of you. Support the babies' heads in the bends of your elbows so that they are facing your breasts.

- **Front V hold**—This position is useful when the babies are able to sit up and their heads don't require as much support. In this hold, you sit on a chair with the babies kneeling or sitting on your lap. Each baby faces you while you support their upper bodies in the bends of your elbows. The babies do not recline, so their legs do not criss-cross in front of you.

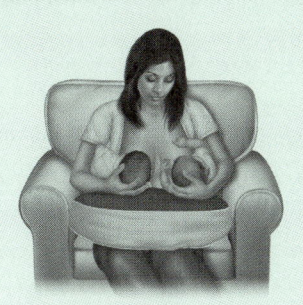

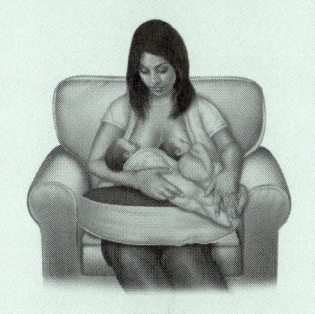

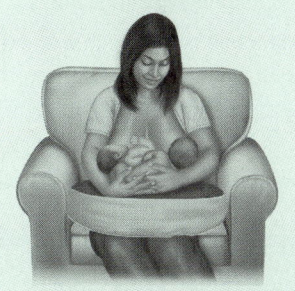

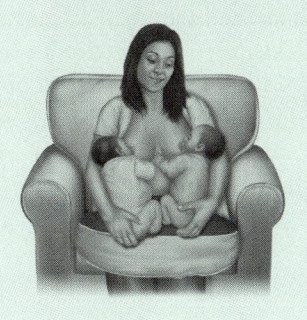

Reposition your hand periodically so you go all around the areola while you press and roll. Don't squeeze the nipple itself. To get the most milk, massage your breast with your other hand. Start from the outside and move inward.

Using a Breast Pump

Under the Affordable Care Act, health insurance providers are required to pay for a breast pump (or the cost to rent one) and breastfeeding counseling. Check with your insurance carrier for details about what kinds of pumps are covered and how to get one. You may need to have your ob-gyn write a prescription for a breast pump.

WIC also provides coverage for breast pumps. If you think you are eligible for WIC, ask about the rules in your state. See the "Resources" section at the end of this chapter.

Many types of breast pumps are available, but they fall into three broad categories:

1. Manual pumps—You provide the suction for these pumps by squeezing a lever or handle.

2. Battery-operated pumps—These pumps run on batteries. They also may have a plug to make them electrical if needed.

3. Electric pumps—These pumps are plugged into an electrical outlet. You can buy a single electric pump that pumps one breast at a time or a double pump that pumps both breasts at the same time. Double pumps can save you time and are especially useful if you need to pump milk during your workday. Electric pumps also can be operated by batteries if needed.

You also can rent a pump from a hospital, doctor's office, or breastfeeding center. Rental costs may be covered by your health insurance. If you rent a pump, you will need to purchase a new pump kit that includes the breast shield and tubing that only you will use.

No matter what type of pump you choose, you need to maintain a clean environment before, during, and after pumping:

1. Wash your hands before pumping your breast milk.

2. Make sure the table or area where you are pumping also is clean.

3. After pumping, wash your equipment with soap and water, or use a microwave-sterilization bag. This helps prevent germs from getting into the milk.

Manual pumping. With a manual breast pump, you provide the suction by squeezing a lever or handle. Manual pumps are small and can be carried anywhere, but they may not be as efficient as battery-operated or electric pumps.

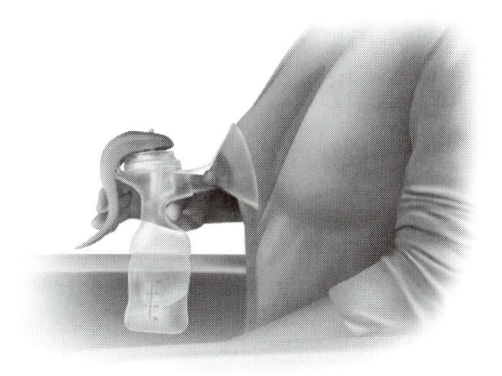

If there isn't an easy way to wash your pump equipment at work, pack several sets and wash them all when you get home.

Storing and Using Breast Milk

Store your breast milk in clean glass or plastic bottles or special milk-collection bags. Store it in small amounts (2 to 4 oz) to avoid wasting it. Mark the bottles or bags with the date the milk was pumped. If you are going to freeze it, leave a 1-inch space at the top of the container—milk may expand when frozen. You can add freshly expressed milk to breast milk that was pumped before.

Breast milk can be kept at a room temperature of 68°F to 72°F for 3 to 4 hours. You can keep your milk in the refrigerator (39°F or below) for up to 3 days. Store your breast milk in the back of the refrigerator or freezer where it is coldest.

Warm previously chilled breast milk by placing it in a bowl of very warm water. Don't heat bottles on the stove or in the microwave. This destroys breast milk's disease-fighting qualities and creates hot spots, which can burn your baby's mouth.

Breast milk can be kept frozen at 0°F or below for up to 6 months, or 12 months in a separate deep freezer. To thaw frozen milk, hold it under cool running water. Once it has begun to thaw, use warm running water to finish. You also can let frozen milk slowly thaw in the fridge. Never thaw frozen milk at room temperature. Also, never refreeze milk that has been thawed. Once milk is thawed, use it within 24 hours.

Expressed Milk as Your Baby's Primary Feeding Method

Some women choose to express breast milk and bottle-feed as the primary way to feed their babies. Women who choose this option have several reasons, including

- difficulty establishing breastfeeding, which can have a variety of causes
- breastfeeding problems, such as mastitis that keeps coming back
- concerns about feeding the baby in public
- ability to share feeding duties

Your baby will get the same antibodies and nutrients no matter how the breast milk is given.

There are some challenges that you may have if you express and bottle-feed. It may be more difficult for your body to regulate milk production. Milk is produced in response to the baby's suckling and how fast the baby empties the breast. A baby going through a growth spurt will empty the breast more quickly, and the woman's body responds by making more milk. A woman who expresses her milk will need to increase the number of pumping or hand-expressing sessions to keep up with these growth spurts.

Expressing and storing breast milk also may not be as convenient as breastfeeding. In addition to expressing your breast milk, you will need to maintain the pump (if you use one), get bottles ready, and store the milk at appropriate temperatures. But many women like the flexibility of sharing the feeding duties.

If you are interested in this option as the primary way of feeding your baby, talk with your ob-gyn or a lactation specialist. If you feel that this option is right for you, you should be supported in your decision.

Bottles and Nipples

A wide variety of bottle and nipple systems are available for feeding expressed breast milk or formula. Your baby may take to just about any bottle or be more particular. Start with the least expensive bottles and see if they work first before moving on to the deluxe models.

Bottles and nipples must be sanitized before they are used the first time, either in the dishwasher or microwave or on the stove. You then must wash them after each time you use them, either in the dishwasher or by hand. Bottles and nipples can transmit **bacteria** if they aren't cleaned properly, as can breast milk or formula if they aren't stored in sterile containers.

Expressing Milk at Work

If you will be breastfeeding when you return to work, it can be helpful to talk with your supervisor before you go on maternity leave. Discuss where you will be expressing your milk and how to store it. Before you go back to work, contact your supervisor and the human resources (HR) department and tell them that you will need to take breaks throughout the day to express your milk to give to your baby later.

Employers must provide break time and a safe, clean place that is not a bathroom for hourly workers and some salaried workers to express milk for a baby for up to 1 year after birth. Businesses with 50 employees or fewer may apply for an exemption from this law.

When you go back to work, make sure that the area where you will be expressing your milk is clean and private. You'll need a chair, a small table, and an outlet if you are using an electric pump. Make sure you have a place to store the milk.

You can plan to express your milk during lunch or other breaks. If you use a breast pump, you should be able to pump enough milk during morning, lunch, and afternoon breaks. Using a double breast pump—which pumps both breasts at the same time—is even quicker. By double pumping, you may be able to pump in 10 to 15 minutes rather than 20 to 30 minutes. A hands-free pumping bra makes double pumping easier. If your employer does not provide break time and a clean space, talk with your baby's doctor. He or she can write a letter of medical need to give to your HR department.

Feeding With Formula

If you choose not to or are unable to breastfeed or express your milk, formula-feeding is a good alternative. Some women also use formula to supplement breast milk if they cannot make enough breast milk. Mothers may choose formula-feeding for several reasons:

- Babies who are fed baby formula most likely are getting the recommended amount of vitamin D per day and do not need extra vitamin D supplements. Check the label on your baby's formula to make sure.

- Because formula digests more slowly than breast milk, formula-fed babies may need to eat less often than breastfed babies do.

- Women who formula-feed don't have to worry about any medications they take passing to the baby through breast milk.

- Anyone can feed the baby a bottle at any time. But keep in mind that babies also can be bottle-fed with expressed breast milk that you pump and store (see the "Feeding Expressed or Pumped Breast Milk" section).

Choosing a Formula

If you have decided that formula-feeding is a better option for you, formulas on the market today will give your baby the right nutrients needed to grow. There are three major types available:

1. Cow's milk formulas—Most baby formula is made with cow's milk that has been changed to give it the right balance of nutrients for a baby. Do not give regular cow's milk until a baby is 1 year old.

2. Soy formulas—Soy-based formulas are an option for babies who can't digest or are allergic to cow's milk formula or to *lactose*. But babies who are allergic to cow's milk also may be allergic to soy milk.

3. Protein hydrolysate formulas—These are meant for babies who have milk or soy allergies. Protein hydrolysate formulas are easier to digest and less likely to cause allergic reactions than are other types of formula.

Once you choose the type of formula to feed your baby, you'll have to decide which form to buy as well. Baby formulas come in three forms:

1. Powdered formula is the least expensive. Each scoop of powdered formula must be mixed with water. It does not need to be refrigerated until it is mixed with water.

2. Liquid concentrated formula also must be mixed with water and must be refrigerated once the container is opened.

3. Ready-to-use formulas are the most expensive, but often they are the most convenient. They do not need to be mixed with water, but they must be refrigerated once the container is opened.

Using Formula Safely

Families who formula-feed their babies may have a few challenges. Dealing with these challenges requires some time and planning.

You will need to have enough formula on hand at all times, and you must prepare the bottles. The powdered and condensed formulas must be prepared with sterile water until the baby is at least 6 months old. This means boiling the water you use. You also can purchase sterile water at most drugstores or baby supply stores, but even with sterile water, the Centers for Disease Control and Prevention (CDC) recommends heating water to at least 158°F when preparing powdered formula. You also will need a supply of bottles and nipples, which must be kept clean (see the box "Bottles and Nipples").

Some parents warm bottles before a feeding, although this often isn't necessary. Never microwave a baby's bottle because it can create dangerous hot spots that can burn a baby's mouth. Instead, run refrigerated bottles under warm water for a few minutes if the baby prefers a warm bottle to a cold one. Another option is to put the baby's bottles in a pan of hot water (away from the heat of the stove) or a product called a "bottle warmer" and test the temperature by squirting a drop or two of formula on the inside of your wrist.

How Long Should Breastfeeding Last?

Any amount of breastfeeding is good for you and your baby. The longer you breastfeed, the healthier you and your baby will be. Start out with short-term goals, like breastfeeding for the next week, and see how it goes. Congratulate yourself each time you reach a goal. Think about how the benefits of breastfeeding compare to any challenges you have. The bottom line: you're the best person to decide whether continuing to breastfeed is best for you and your baby.

Weaning

When you want to stop breastfeeding or pumping, there are a few ways to do it. Some moms and babies gradually reduce feedings as the baby eats more food and starts drinking from a cup. This can be a long process. It's a gradual change for both of you.

Other women decide to wean when their baby reaches a certain age. In this case, it's still best to take it slow. A sudden stop in breastfeeding or pumping can cause you physical pain, engorgement, clogged ducts, or even mastitis. It also can be emotionally hard for you, your baby, or both of you.

One approach is to replace one nursing session with a bottle or cup feeding every few days. Start by cutting out the feedings your baby seems to enjoy the least. Slowly work your way up to the longer or more important ones. Most often, the feeding before bedtime is the last to go and the hardest to give up. As you reduce the amount you nurse, your milk supply will decrease slowly.

Final Thoughts on Feeding Your Baby

If you decide to breastfeed your baby, there are plenty of resources and support available. But if you can't breastfeed or decide not to, it's OK. You will find the feeding method that is best for you, your baby, and your family.

RESOURCES

Affordable Care Act Breastfeeding Benefits
www.healthcare.gov/coverage/breast-feeding-benefits/
Government website that explains the benefits that breastfeeding women and babies are entitled to under the Affordable Care Act.

Baby-Friendly USA
www.babyfriendlyusa.org
Offers a "For Parents" page to help you find a facility with the Baby-Friendly designation.

Breastfeeding While Working
www.abetterbalance.org/our-campaigns/breastfeeding-while-working/
Explains patients' rights and offers resources related to nursing.

Drugs and Lactation Database (LactMed)
www.ncbi.nlm.nih.gov/books/NBK501922/
Provides a searchable database of drugs to which breastfeeding women may be exposed. Gives information about the possible effects on breastfed babies as well as alternative drugs to consider. There also is a free app that you can download onto a smartphone.

Human Milk Banking Association of North America
www.hmbana.org
Professional association for human milk banks. Issues safety guidelines for member banks on screening human milk donors and collecting, processing, handling, testing, and storing milk.

Infant Feeding
www.cdc.gov/healthywater/hygiene/healthychildcare/infantfeeding.html
Information from the Centers for Disease Control and Prevention on how to clean, sanitize, and store items such as bottles, nipples, and breast pumps.

International Lactation Consultant Association
www.ilca.org
Offers a directory of lactation consultants as well as information about breastfeeding.

La Leche League International
www.llli.org
Provides information and support for breastfeeding women. Offers referrals to local support groups.

MotherToBaby
www.mothertobaby.org
1-866-626-6847
1-855-999-3525 (text messages only)
Fact sheets on the safety of specific medications during pregnancy and breastfeeding, available in English and Spanish. The site, run by the Organization of Teratology Information Specialists (OTIS), also offers information by phone, email, or online chat.

National Conference of State Legislatures
www.ncsl.org/issues-research/health/breastfeeding-state-laws.aspx
Provides a list of U.S. breastfeeding laws by state and territory. Includes information about breastfeeding in public.

Women, Infants, and Children (WIC) Breastfeeding Support Program
https://wicbreastfeeding.fns.usda.gov
The WIC breastfeeding campaign from the U.S. Department of Agriculture offers women information, resources, and support for breastfeeding.

Your Pregnancy and Childbirth
www.acog.org/MyPregnancy
Website from the American College of Obstetricians and Gynecologists (ACOG) with information on pregnancy, labor, delivery, and postpartum care. Includes the latest information from the experts in women's health care, questions answered by ACOG ob-gyns, pregnancy stories from real women, and an A–Z directory of health topics covering pregnancy and beyond.

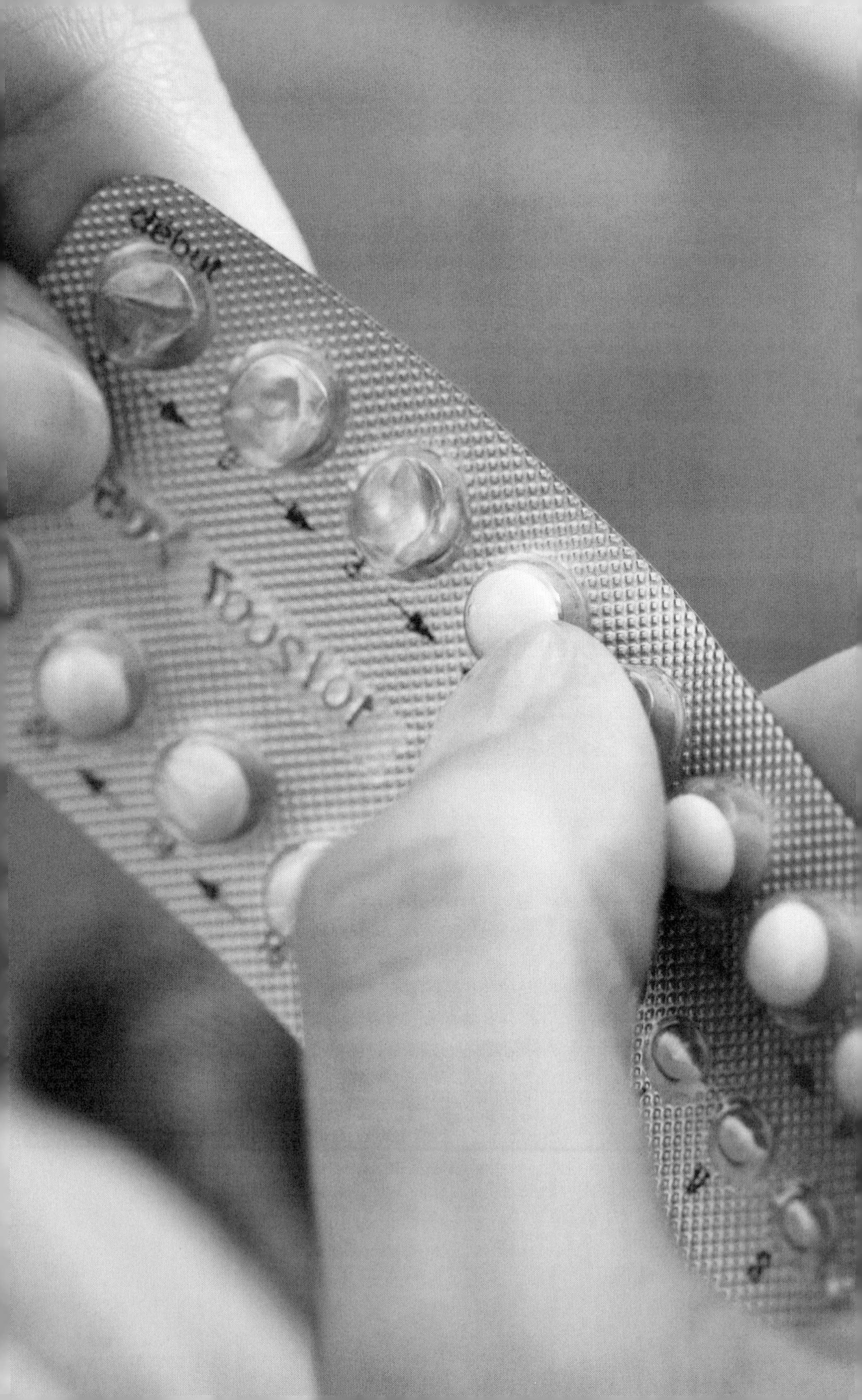

CHAPTER 21

Birth Control After Pregnancy and Beyond

Women can get pregnant soon after having a baby if they have **sexual intercourse** and do not use **birth control**. Some women can get pregnant even before their **menstrual period** returns. If you plan to have sex again after your pregnancy, it's important to use birth control. Starting a birth control method right after you have a baby can help you avoid an unintended pregnancy. Birth control also lets you plan and control when you try to get pregnant again, if you want more children in the future.

Using birth control allows your body time to heal before having another baby. Ideally, you should wait 18 months before another pregnancy. This offers the best health outcomes for both mom and baby. There may be a greater risk of certain **complications** when the time between pregnancies is less than 18 months, including **preterm** birth and **low birth weight**.

There are a few theories about why these problems may happen. Some experts believe having children too close together doesn't give your body enough time to build up your stores of folate and iron. Other theories suggest that a woman's body needs enough time to heal before another pregnancy. This is especially important after a **cesarean birth**. See Chapter 42, "Having Another Baby: What to Expect the Next Time Around," for more discussion.

Choosing a Birth Control Method

The birth control method you used before pregnancy may **not be the** best choice for you after childbirth. If you want to have more children, you can choose a method that is easily reversible. If you are sure that you don't want more children, **sterilization**—a permanent form of birth control—may be an option for you.

Some reversible birth control methods can be started right after childbirth. With others, you need to wait a few weeks to start. To prevent an unintended pregnancy, it's important to keep these waiting periods in mind. Also, some forms of birth control are not effective right away, so you need to use an extra method for a number of days. Table 21–1, "Birth Control After Childbirth," has information you may need to consider, including

- the effectiveness of each method
- when each method can be started after childbirth
- whether an extra method of birth control is needed
- whether you can breastfeed while using the method

You can talk with your **obstetrician–gynecologist (ob-gyn)** about birth control options while you are still pregnant or right after giving birth. You also can talk with your ob-gyn before you go home from the hospital.

Reversible Birth Control

Reversible birth control means that you can easily stop the method when you are ready to get pregnant again. Many different forms of reversible birth control are available.

The **intrauterine device (IUD)** and the **birth control implant** are called **long-acting reversible contraception (LARC)** methods. Once they are inserted, you don't need to do anything else to prevent pregnancy. LARC methods last for several years, and you can stop using them at any time. Both methods are safe to use while breastfeeding. Using the IUD or the implant does not decrease your ability to get pregnant in the future.

Other reversible birth control methods include hormonal methods and **barrier methods**. These methods take more work than LARC methods. You will need to take a pill every day or use a barrier method every time you have sex.

Intrauterine Device

The IUD is a small, T-shaped, plastic device that is inserted into and left inside the **uterus**. The IUD is a safe and effective form of birth control. There are two types of IUDs:

1. The hormonal IUD releases ***progestin*** in the uterus. Depending on the brand, hormonal IUDs are approved for up to 3 to 6 years of use.

2. The copper IUD releases copper in the uterus. This IUD does not contain ***hormones***. It is approved for up to 10 years of use.

The IUD works mainly by preventing ***fertilization*** of an ***egg*** by ***sperm***. The progestin in the hormonal IUD thickens mucus found in the ***cervix***.

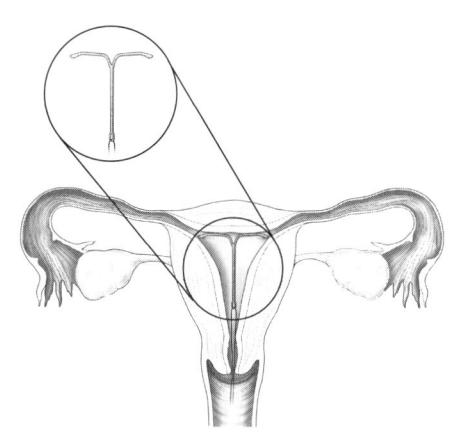

Intrauterine device

Thicker mucus makes it harder for sperm to enter the uterus. Progestin also thins the lining of the uterus. The copper in the copper IUD interferes with sperm's ability to move. When sperm stop acting normally, it is harder for them to enter the uterus and reach an egg.

The most common side effects of using an IUD are changes in menstrual bleeding. These changes are normal and not harmful. The IUD has the following benefits:

- If you wish to get pregnant again or if you want to stop using it, you can have the IUD removed at any time by an ob-gyn or other health care practitioner.

- Once the IUD is in place, you do not have to do anything else to prevent pregnancy.

- It does not interfere with sex or daily activities.

- There are few medical problems that prevent its use. Almost all teenagers and adult women are able to use an IUD.

- Over time, the hormonal IUDs may help decrease menstrual pain and heavy periods.

IUDs do not protect against ***sexually transmitted infections (STIs)***. Using a latex or polyurethane condom every time you have vaginal, oral, or anal sex may reduce the chance of getting an STI.

The IUD can be inserted in the uterus within 10 minutes of a vaginal birth or cesarean birth. Most women can have an IUD inserted after giving birth, but some should not, including those with infection or heavy bleeding. The IUD is safe for breastfeeding women to use.

TABLE 21-1 Birth Control After Childbirth

Effectiveness	Method	OK With Breastfeeding?
Less than 1 pregnancy per 100 women per year	Sterilization	Yes
	Intrauterine device (IUD)	Yes
	Implant	Yes
6 to 12 pregnancies per 100 women per year	Injection	Yes
	Combined hormonal methods (pills, patch, ring)	Yes, after breastfeeding is established (usually 4 to 6 weeks after childbirth)
	Progestin-only pills	Yes
	Diaphragm	Yes
18 or more pregnancies per 100 women per year	Condom (male and female)	Yes
	Cervical cap	Yes
	Sponge	Yes
	Spermicide	Yes

Implant

The birth control implant is a flexible, plastic rod that is inserted just under the skin in the upper arm. The implant is a safe and effective form of birth control. It releases progestin into the body and is approved for up to 3 years of use.

While you are using the implant, progestin prevents pregnancy mainly by stopping **ovulation**. The progestin in the implant also thickens the mucus of the cervix, which makes it harder for sperm to enter the uterus. And progestin thins the lining of the uterus.

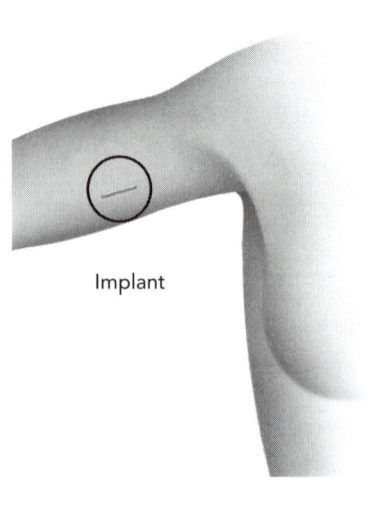

Implant

How Soon Can You Start It?
Postpartum sterilization: Can be done right after childbirth. *Laparoscopic sterilization:* Can be done as a separate procedure after childbirth.
Can be inserted right after childbirth.
Can be inserted right after childbirth.
Can be started right after childbirth.
Can be started 3 weeks after childbirth if you are not breastfeeding and have no additional risk factors for **deep vein thrombosis (DVT)**. Can be started 4 to 6 weeks after childbirth if you are breastfeeding and have no risk factors for DVT.
Can be started right after childbirth.
Wait 6 weeks after giving birth to use the diaphragm until the uterus and cervix return to normal size. If you used a diaphragm before, you must be refitted after giving birth.
Can be used at any time following childbirth.
Wait 6 weeks after giving birth to use the cervical cap until the uterus and cervix return to normal size. If you used a cervical cap before, it needs to be refitted after giving birth.
Wait 6 weeks after giving birth to use the sponge until the uterus and cervix return to normal size.
Can be used at any time following childbirth.

The most common side effect is unpredictable bleeding, especially in the first 3 months of use. The implant has the following benefits:

- If you wish to get pregnant again or if you want to stop using it, you can have the implant removed at any time by an ob-gyn or other health care practitioner.
- Once the implant is in place, you do not have to do anything else to prevent pregnancy.
- It does not interfere with sex or daily activities.
- There are few medical conditions that prevent its use. Almost all teenagers and adult women are able to use the implant.
- It may reduce pain during your period.

The implant does not protect against STIs. Using a latex or polyurethane condom every time you have vaginal, oral, or anal sex may reduce the chance of getting an STI.

The implant can be inserted in the delivery room or at any time before you leave the hospital after giving birth, even if you are breastfeeding. A health care practitioner inserts the implant into your arm. He or she will numb a small area on the inside of your upper arm with a pain medicine. The implant is placed under the skin with a special inserter. The procedure takes only a few minutes.

Injection

The birth control injection is an injection of the hormone depot medroxyprogesterone acetate (DMPA). It provides protection against pregnancy for 3 months. The injection has several effects that work together to prevent pregnancy:

- It stops ovulation.
- It thickens the amount of mucus in the cervix. This makes it difficult for sperm to enter the uterus.
- It thins the lining of the uterus.

Injection

The shot is given at an office visit. The first shot can be given at any time during your menstrual cycle as long as you and your practitioner are reasonably sure that you are not pregnant. You must return every 13 weeks for repeated injections.

The injection may cause irregular bleeding. Some women report weight gain while using progestin-only birth control methods. Among women who gained weight, the average amount of weight gained was less than 5 pounds.

Bone loss also may occur while using the birth control injection. When the injections are stopped, most if not all of the bone that was lost is regained.

Women who have multiple risk factors for heart disease may be at increased risk of heart disease while using the injection. This increased risk may last for some time after the method is stopped.

The birth control injection has several benefits:

- It does not need to be taken daily.
- It does not interfere with sex or daily activities.

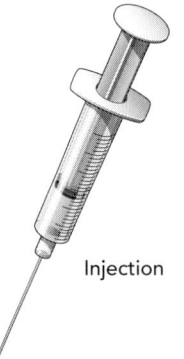

The injection does not protect against STIs. Using a latex or polyurethane condom every time you have vaginal, oral, or anal sex may reduce the chance of getting an STI.

It takes an average of 10 months for fertility to return after stopping the injection. The injections can be started right after childbirth, even if you are breastfeeding.

Combined Hormonal Methods

Birth control pills, the birth control patch, and the vaginal ring are combined hormonal birth control methods. They contain: *estrogen* and progestin. These *hormones* prevent pregnancy mainly by stopping *ovulation*. They also cause other changes in the body that help prevent pregnancy. The mucus in the cervix thickens, making it hard for sperm to enter the uterus. The lining of the uterus also thins.

Combined hormonal methods have several benefits in addition to protecting against pregnancy:

- They may make your period more regular, lighter, and shorter.
- They may help reduce menstrual cramps.
- They may decrease the risk of cancer of the uterus, *ovary*, and colon.
- They may improve acne and reduce unwanted hair growth.
- They can be used to treat certain disorders that cause heavy bleeding and menstrual pain, such as *fibroids* and *endometriosis*.
- They can be used to treat heavy bleeding and menstrual pain by stopping periods.
- Used continuously, they can reduce the frequency of migraines associated with *menstruation* (although they should not be used if you have migraines with *aura*).

Combined hormonal methods are safe for most women, but they are associated with a small increased risk of deep vein thrombosis (DVT), heart attack, and *stroke*. The risk is higher in some women, including women over 35 who smoke more than 15 cigarettes a day or women who have multiple risk factors for *cardiovascular disease*, including

- high cholesterol
- *high blood pressure*
- *diabetes mellitus*
- history of stroke, heart attack, or DVT

Possible side effects of combined hormonal methods include

- headache
- nausea

- breast tenderness
- ***breakthrough bleeding***

Breakthrough bleeding usually is a temporary side effect as the body adjusts to a change in hormone levels.

You should not use combined hormonal methods during the first 3 weeks after delivery. This is when the risk of DVT is highest after childbirth. If you have other risk factors for DVT, you should wait to use combined hormonal methods until after the first 4 to 6 weeks after delivery.

If you are breastfeeding, estrogen may affect your milk supply. You should wait until the fifth week after delivery to start using these methods, when breastfeeding has been well established.

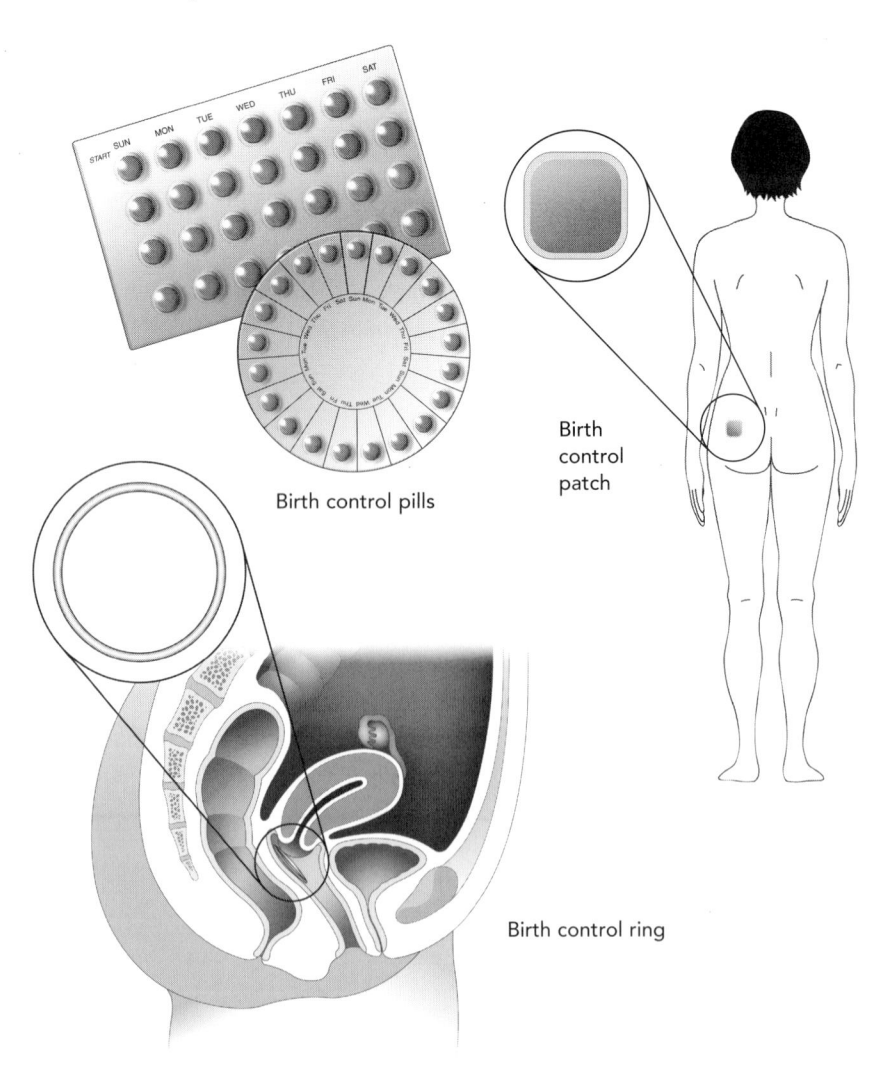

Birth control pills

Birth control patch

Birth control ring

Combined hormonal methods do not protect against STIs. Using a latex or polyurethane condom every time you have vaginal, oral, or anal sex may reduce the chance of getting an STI.

Progestin-Only Pills

Progestin-only birth control pills, sometimes called "mini-pills," have several effects in the body that help prevent pregnancy:

- They stop ovulation, but they do not do so consistently. About 2 in 5 women who use progestin-only pills will continue to ovulate.
- They thicken the mucus in the cervix, making it difficult for sperm to enter the uterus.
- They thin the lining of the uterus.

The benefits of progestin-only pills include the following:

- They may reduce menstrual bleeding or stop your period altogether.
- They are not associated with an increased risk of high blood pressure or cardiovascular disease and can be taken even if you have certain health conditions that prevent you from taking combination pills, such as a history of DVT or uncontrolled high blood pressure.
- They can be used immediately after childbirth, even if you are breastfeeding.

Progestin-only pills may not be a good choice for women who have certain medical conditions, such as **lupus** (systemic lupus erythematosus or SLE). Women with a history of breast cancer should not take progestin-only pills. Possible side effects include unpredictable bleeding, headaches, nausea, and breast tenderness.

Progestin-only pills should be taken within an hour of the same time each day. If you are not good at remembering to take a pill at the same time each day, this may not be the right choice for you.

Progestin-only pills do not protect against STIs. Using a latex or polyurethane condom every time you have vaginal, oral, or anal sex may reduce the chance of getting an STI.

Barrier Methods

Barrier methods work by keeping sperm from reaching the egg. If you choose a barrier method, it must be used each time you have sex to be effective. The following barrier methods are available:

Male condom

Female condom

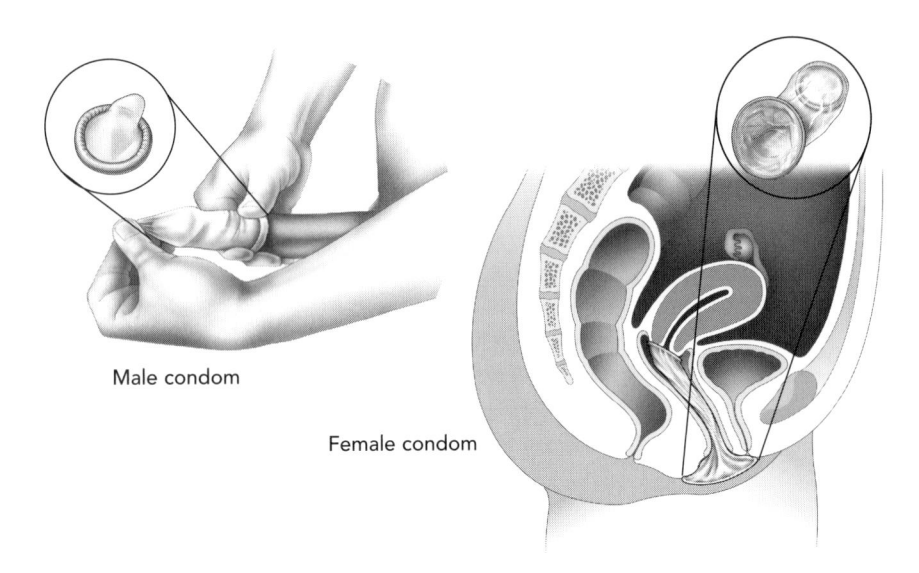

- Condom—The male condom is a thin latex sheath worn over a man's **penis.** The female condom is a plastic pouch that lines the vagina. It is held in place by a closed inner ring at the cervix and an open outer ring at the entrance of the vagina. The male condom provides the best protection against STIs. The female condom also provides some protection against STIs.
- Diaphragm—A diaphragm is a dome-shaped device that is inserted inside the vagina and covers the cervix. It can be inserted 1 to 2 hours before you have sex and is used with a spermicide. The diaphragm must be fitted by a health care practitioner. If you used a diaphragm before pregnancy, you must be refitted after childbirth. You should wait 6 weeks after giving birth to use a diaphragm, until the uterus and cervix return to normal size. The diaphragm does not protect against STIs.
- Cervical cap—The cervical cap is smaller than a diaphragm and fits more tightly over the cervix. It stays in place by suction and is used with spermicide. Like the diaphragm, it must be fitted by a health care practitioner. If you used a cervical cap before pregnancy, you must be refitted after childbirth. You should wait 6 weeks after giving birth to use the cervical cap, until the uterus and cervix return to normal size. The cervical cap does not protect against STIs.
- Sponge—The sponge is a doughnut-shaped device made of soft foam with spermicide. It is inserted into the vagina and covers the cervix. The sponge is convenient because it's available over the counter. But it is less effective in women who have given birth. The sponge does not protect against STIs.

BIRTH CONTROL AFTER PREGNANCY AND BEYOND • 341

Sponge

Spermicide

Diaphragm

Cervical cap

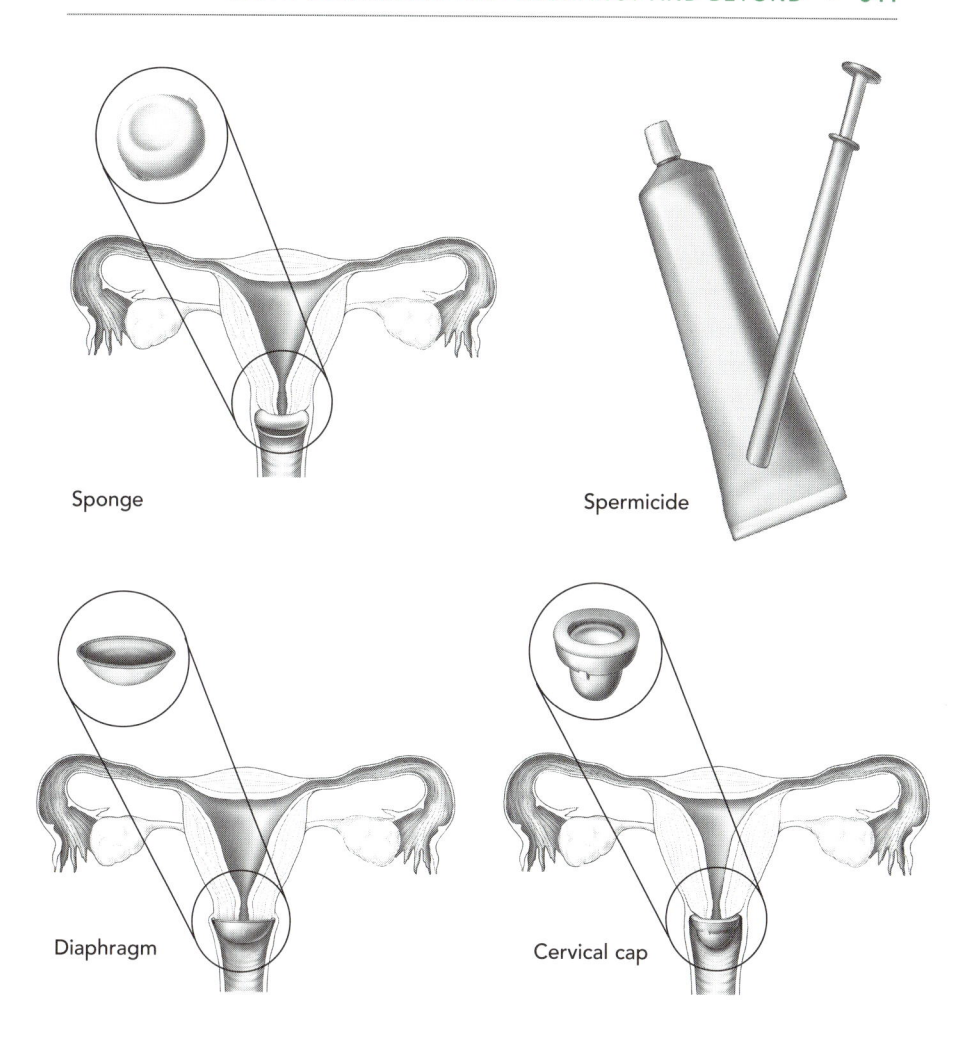

- Spermicides—Spermicides are chemicals that destroy sperm before they can fertilize the egg. Spermicides come in various forms, including creams, gels, foams, and vaginal suppositories. Spermicides are placed in the vagina, close to the cervix, before sex. Spermicides do not protect against STIs.

Lactational Amenorrhea Method

The *lactational amenorrhea method (LAM)* is a temporary method of birth control. It is based on the natural way the body prevents ovulation when a woman is breastfeeding. If a woman does not **ovulate**, she cannot get pregnant. The method is 98 percent effective if used correctly.

For this method to work, three conditions must be met:

1. Your menstrual period has not returned.
2. You are exclusively breastfeeding.
3. Your baby is 6 months or younger.

Exclusive breastfeeding means that the baby gets only breast milk and no other liquid or food, not even water. Also, you should breastfeed at least every 4 hours during the day and every 6 hours at night.

An important part of LAM is knowing when to start using another form of birth control to prevent pregnancy. To determine this time, you should ask yourself three questions:

1. Has my period started again?
2. Am I supplementing regularly with formula or other food or liquids or going long periods without breastfeeding, either during the day or at night?
3. Is my baby more than 6 months old?

If you answer yes to any of these questions, your risk of pregnancy is higher, and you should use another form of birth control. If you wish to use LAM as birth control, talk with your ob-gyn or a lactation consultant to be sure you understand how it works.

Fertility Awareness Methods

Fertility awareness is recognizing when the fertile time (when a woman can get pregnant) happens in the menstrual cycle. If you are practicing fertility awareness to prevent pregnancy, you should avoid having sex or use a barrier method of birth control, such as a condom, during the fertile period. The following methods are based on fertility awareness:

- Standard Days method
- Cervical mucus method
- ***Basal body temperature (BBT)*** method
- ***Symptothermal method***

If you are interested in using fertility awareness to prevent pregnancy, it may be best to learn the method from a qualified teacher or group. Your health care practitioner or local health department may be able to provide information about where to find a teacher. Tools such as smartphone apps and websites are available to help you record information about your menstrual cycle and calculate your fertile periods.

Fertility awareness is not the best choice for a woman who has just given birth. You may want to delay using fertility awareness-based methods until your menstrual periods are regular. If any of the following conditions apply to you, you may need extra training to make sure you are using fertility awareness correctly:

- You are approaching **menopause**.
- You have just started having menstrual periods.
- You have recently stopped using a hormonal birth control method or are using other medications that can affect the signs of fertility.

Fertility awareness–based methods cost very little to use. Many women like the fact that fertility awareness is a form of birth control that does not use medications or devices. Note that these methods do not protect against STIs.

The disadvantage of fertility awareness methods is that they only predict the days when you are likely to be fertile. They do not give exact days. Also, these methods are less effective than other methods. With typical use, 12 to 24 women in 100 will get pregnant in the first year, depending on the method.

Permanent Birth Control

If you or your partner are sure you don't want more children, sterilization is an option. Sterilization is more than 99 percent effective. Although there is surgery to reverse sterilization, many women still are not able to get pregnant afterwards. ***In vitro fertilization (IVF)*** may be an option, but there are no guarantees that it will be successful.

You should avoid making this choice during times of stress (such as during a divorce). You also should not make this choice under pressure from a partner or others. Research shows that women younger than 30 are more likely than older women to regret having the procedure.

Female Sterilization

Female sterilization closes off or removes the ***fallopian tubes***. This prevents the egg from moving down the fallopian tube to the uterus and keeps the sperm from reaching the egg. It can be done during abdominal surgery or **hysteroscopy**.

Postpartum Sterilization. ***Postpartum sterilization*** usually is done within a few hours or days after delivery. The surgery is easier to do then because the uterus still is enlarged and pushes the fallopian tubes up in the abdomen. It's also convenient because you don't have to return to the hospital to have it done and it is effective right away. How the surgery is done depends on whether you had a vaginal birth or a cesarean birth:

- If you had a vaginal delivery, a small incision is made in the abdomen. The fallopian tubes are brought up through the incision. The tubes are then closed off with clips or bands. Sometimes a small section of each tube or the entire tube is removed. If you had an **epidural block** for delivery, it often can be used for pain-relief during the procedure. If you did not have an epidural block, you may have **regional anesthesia** or **general anesthesia** for sterilization.

- If you had a cesarean birth, sterilization can be done right afterward through the same incision that was made for delivery of the baby.

Fallopian tube

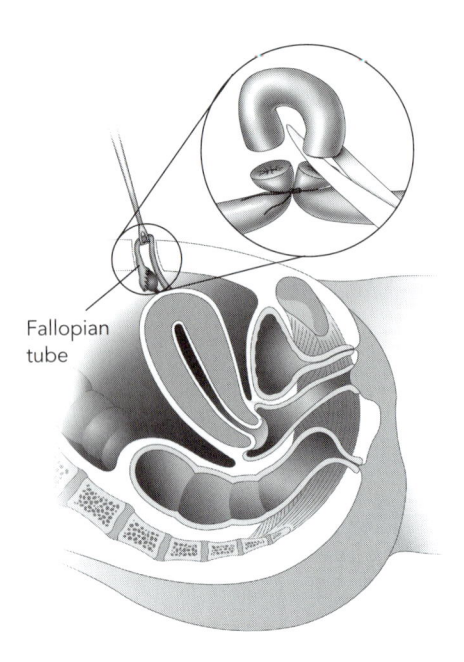

Postpartum sterilization. Right after childbirth, the uterus is still enlarged and the fallopian tubes are pushed up, making them more accessible. The tubes are brought up through an incision. The tubes are closed off with clips or bands, or a small section or the entire tube is removed.

As with any type of surgery, there is a risk of bleeding, problems with wound healing, infection, and complications from the anesthesia used.

If you are interested in postpartum sterilization, talk with your ob-gyn about it well before you have the baby. Check with the hospital where you plan to give birth to see if they offer sterilization. And check with your health insurance plan to see if the procedure is covered.

Laparoscopic Sterilization. You also can choose to have sterilization later as a separate procedure. The method used is called **laparoscopy**, which typically is done with general anesthesia. A device called a **laparoscope** is inserted through a small incision made in or near the belly button. The laparoscope allows your ob-gyn to see the pelvic organs.

In this procedure, the fallopian tubes are closed off using instruments passed through the laparoscope or with another instrument inserted through

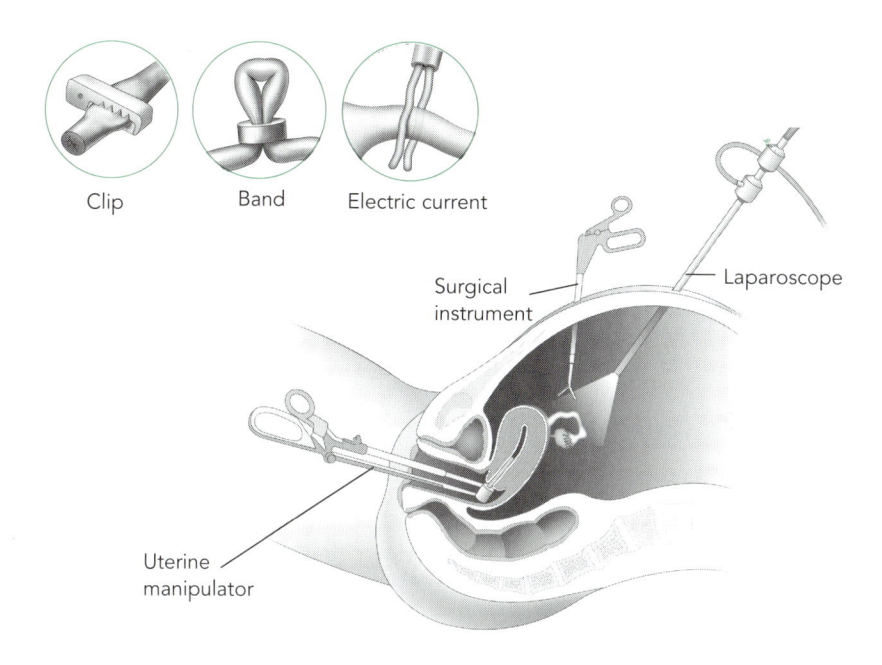

Laparoscopic sterilization. This method of sterilization requires a few small incisions in the abdomen.

a second small incision. The tubes can be closed with bands, clips, or an electric current. Sometimes a small section of each tube or the entire tubes are removed. Laparoscopy can be done as outpatient surgery, so you can go home the same day if there are no problems.

Male Sterilization

Male sterilization is called ***vasectomy***. It involves cutting or tying the ***vas deferens*** (tubes through which sperm travel) so that no sperm are released when a man ***ejaculates***. Vasectomy does not affect a man's ability to maintain an ***erection***, have an ***orgasm***, or ejaculate. It also does not decrease a man's sexual pleasure.

Unlike female sterilization, the majority of vasectomies can be done in a doctor's office or clinic. Rarely, it needs to be done at the hospital. The man can go home the same day if there are no complications. Vasectomy generally is considered safer than female sterilization and requires only local anesthesia.

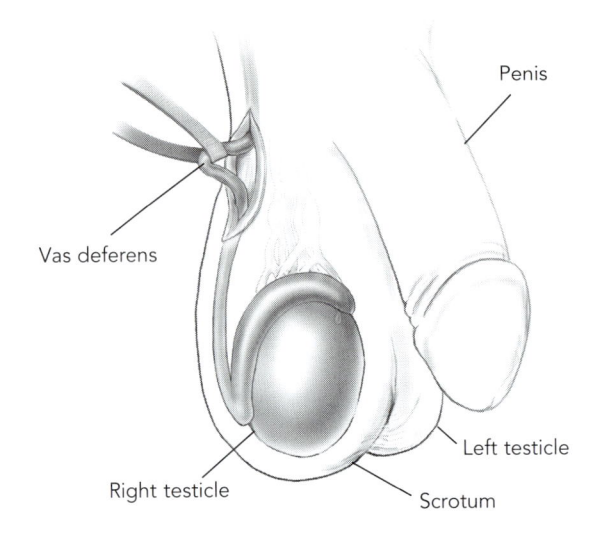

Vasectomy. The left or right vas deferens is tied, cut, or sealed to prevent the release of sperm. Then the other side is done.

A vasectomy is not effective right away because some sperm still may be in the vas deferens at the time of the procedure. It takes about 2 to 4 months for *semen* to become totally free of sperm. A couple must use another method of birth control or avoid sex until a sperm count confirms that no sperm are present.

Emergency Contraception

Emergency contraception (EC) reduces the chance of pregnancy after unprotected sexual intercourse. Common situations in which EC could be used include

- forgetting to take a progestin-only birth control pill within 3 hours of the usual time
- forgetting to take several combined hormonal birth control pills in a row
- having a condom break or slip off

EC also can be used after a woman has been raped.

EC prevents pregnancy from occurring. It must be used as soon as possible after unprotected sex to be effective. EC does not work if pregnancy has already occurred.

There are several types of emergency contraception:

1. Progestin-only pills—These pills must be taken as soon as possible within 3 days of unprotected sex. Some states sell EC pills over the counter and do not require a prescription. See the "Resources" section for information on how to buy these pills.

2. Ulipristal pill—This pill is available only by prescription. The pill must be taken as soon as possible within 5 days of unprotected sex.

3. Combined estrogen–progestin birth control pills—These pills must be taken within 5 days of unprotected sex. They require a prescription.

4. Copper IUD—This is the most effective form of emergency contraception. The IUD must be inserted by a health care practitioner within 5 days of unprotected sex. After insertion, the IUD is approved for birth control for up to 10 years.

RESOURCES

Birth Control
https://medlineplus.gov/birthcontrol.html
Overview of birth control and related information from the U.S. National Library of Medicine. Includes links to other resources.

Birth Control Methods
www.womenshealth.gov/a-z-topics/birth-control-methods
Detailed information about birth control from the Office on Women's Health.

Vasectomy
https://medlineplus.gov/vasectomy.html
Information about male sterilization from the U.S. National Library of Medicine.

Your Pregnancy and Childbirth
www.acog.org/MyPregnancy
Website from the American College of Obstetricians and Gynecologists (ACOG) with information on pregnancy, labor, delivery, and postpartum care. Includes the latest information from the experts in women's health care, questions answered by ACOG ob-gyns, pregnancy stories from real women, and an A–Z directory of health topics covering pregnancy and beyond.

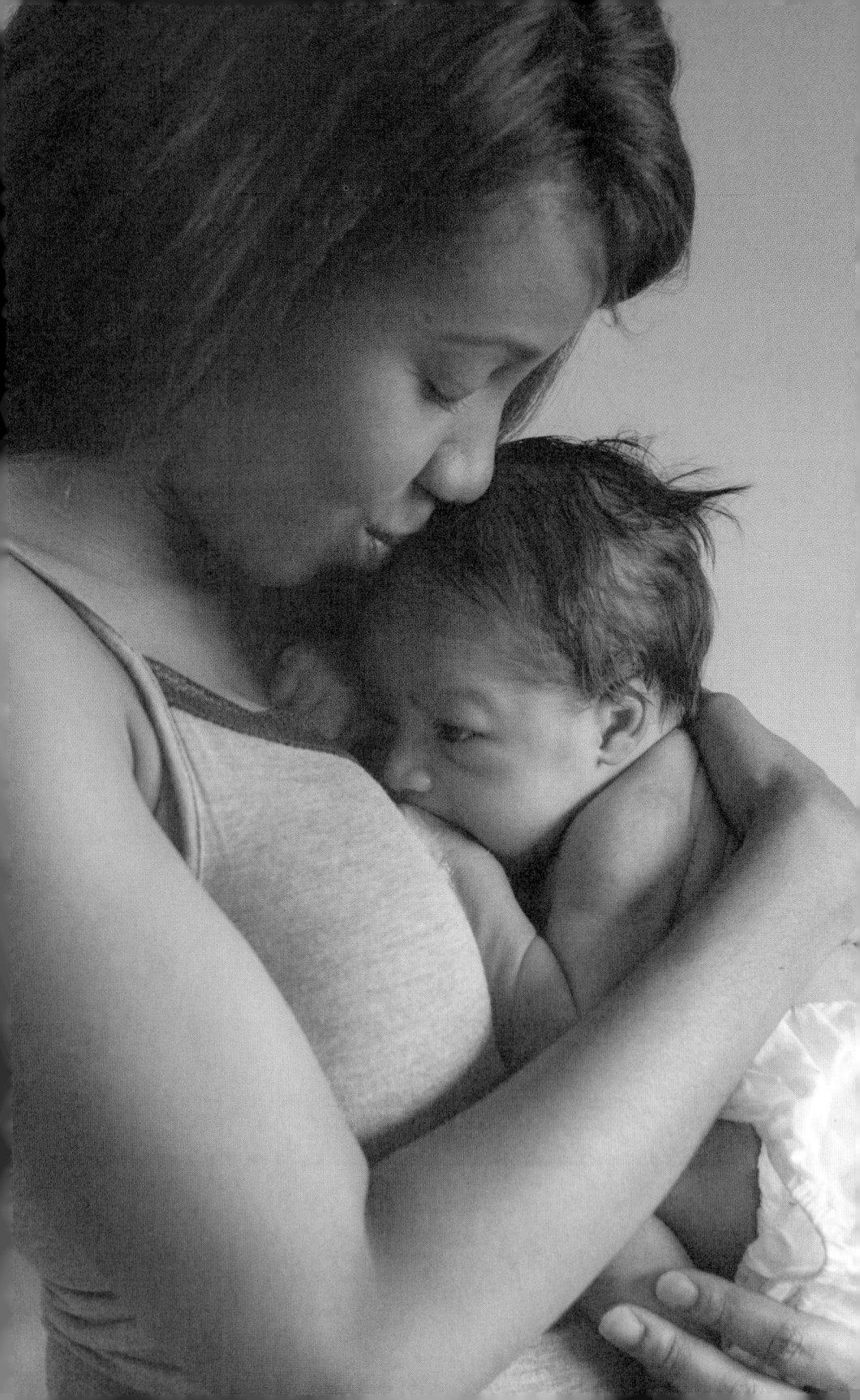

PART 4

Health During Pregnancy

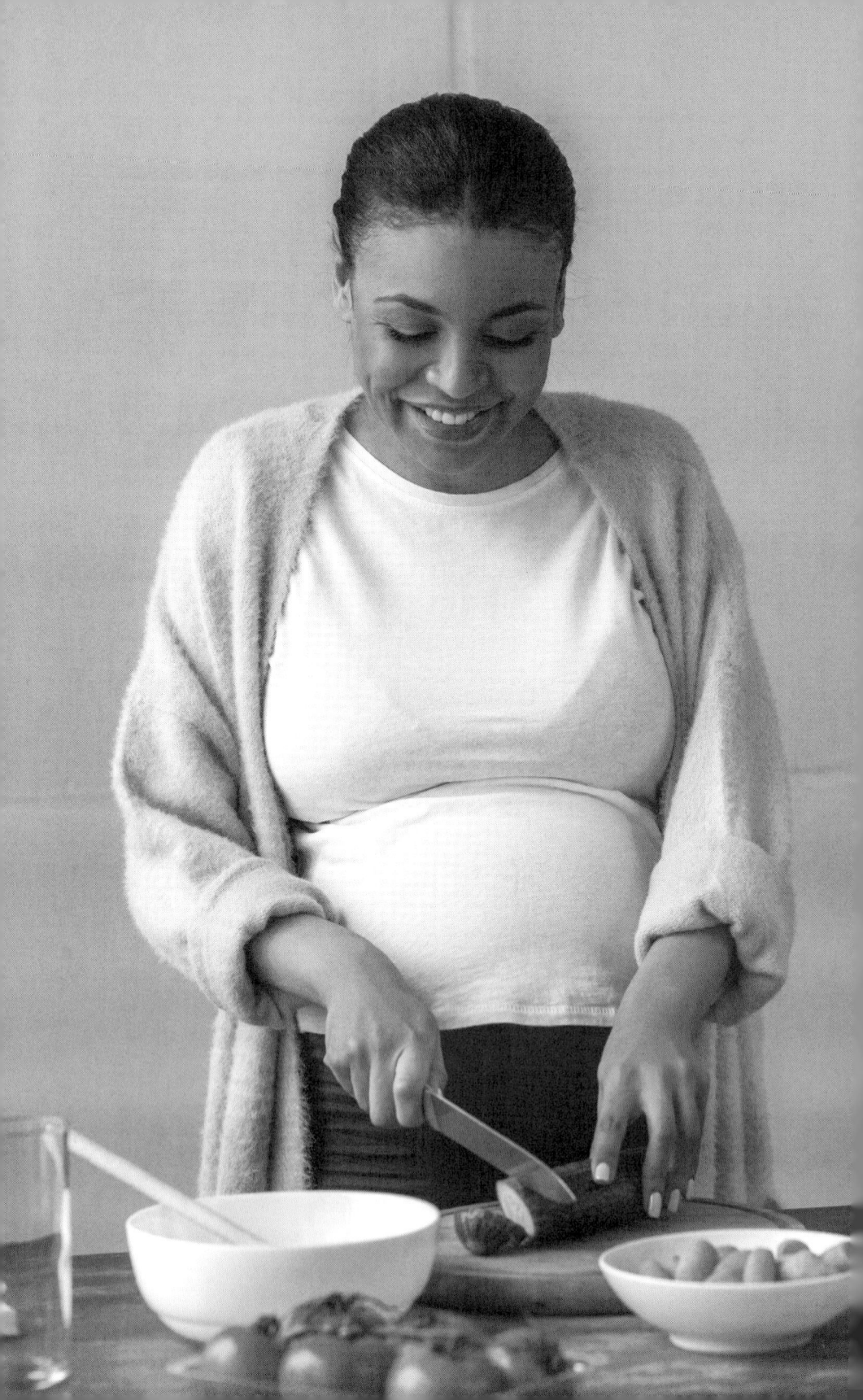

CHAPTER 22

Nutrition During Pregnancy

Eating well during your pregnancy is one of the best things you can do for yourself and your baby. Pregnant women used to be told to "eat for two." Now we know that it's not healthy to eat twice your usual amounts during pregnancy. You need to balance getting enough **nutrients** to fuel the baby's growth with maintaining a healthy pregnancy weight. The best approach: Don't eat for two, eat twice as healthy.

If you are carrying one baby, you need an average of 300 extra **calories** per day (and a bit more in the later stages of pregnancy). That's the number of calories in a glass of skim milk and half a sandwich. If you are pregnant with twins, you need to eat about 600 extra calories per day. For triplets, you need about 900 extra calories. These calories should come from healthy foods.

Balancing Your Diet

Nutrients are the building blocks of the body. When you're pregnant, you need to maintain your own body with nutrients and support the growth of your baby. A balanced diet includes

- protein, carbohydrates, and fat
- vitamins and minerals, including **folic acid**, vitamin D, calcium, and iron
- water and fiber

Major Nutrients

Proteins, carbohydrates, and fats are important nutrients that provide most of the energy in your food, in the form of calories.

Protein

Protein helps with muscle growth and repair. Protein is found in

- beef, pork, and fish
- poultry
- eggs
- milk, cheese, and other dairy foods
- beans and peas
- nuts and seeds

For vegetarians, protein can be found in nuts, seeds, nut butters, legumes such as beans and chickpeas, and soy products such as tempeh and tofu. Vegetarians who include dairy products in their diets also can get needed protein from milk and egg products.

Carbohydrates

All carbohydrates are broken down into *glucose* (blood sugar), the body's main fuel. There are two types of carbohydrates: simple carbohydrates and complex carbohydrates. Simple carbohydrates provide a quick energy boost because they are digested rapidly. They are found in naturally sweet foods like fruits, table sugar, honey, and maple syrup. Simple carbohydrates often are high in calories. It is best to limit your intake of simple carbohydrates to those found naturally in food. Avoid sugary drinks and foods with added sugar.

Complex carbohydrates include fiber and starches. It takes your body longer to process them, so complex carbohydrates provide longer-lasting energy than simple carbohydrates. Complex carbohydrates are found in

- whole grains
- rice
- pasta
- some fruits
- starchy vegetables, such as potatoes and corn

Fiber is found in plant foods. It is the part of the plant that your body cannot digest. Fiber passes relatively unchanged through your digestive system. It can help prevent constipation by adding bulk to the stool, making it easier to pass. You should eat about 25 grams of fiber per day. Good sources of fiber include

- fruits (especially dried fruits, berries, oranges, apples, and peaches with the skin)
- vegetables (such as dried beans, peas, lentils, and leafy vegetables like spinach and kale)
- whole-grain products (such as whole-wheat bread, whole-wheat pasta, and brown rice)

Check the labels on packaged foods to see how much fiber is in a serving.

Fiber also helps maintain a stable blood sugar level because it is digested slowly. Foods that do this are described as "low glycemic" because they do not cause blood sugar levels to spike. Eating low-glycemic foods can help you feel full and reduce the feeling of hunger. Low-glycemic foods also may help

- reduce **cholesterol** levels
- lower your risk of **diabetes mellitus** and heart disease

If you have not been getting your 25 grams a day, it's best to slowly and gradually increase the amount of fiber you eat. Too much, too soon can cause bloating and gas. Drink lots of water as you increase your fiber intake.

Fats

The body needs a certain amount of fat to function normally. Some types of fats, called omega-3 fatty acids, play an important role in brain development. Fats also help your body use vitamins A, D, E, and K.

The fat in the foods you eat is digested and sent to the liver. The liver then assembles the fat into lipoproteins. These lipoproteins carry fat through your bloodstream for use by or storage in other parts of the body. There are different types of fat in foods:

- Unsaturated fats tend to be liquid and come mostly from plants and vegetables. Olive, canola, peanut, sunflower, and fish oils are all unsaturated fats. So is the fat in avocados.
- Saturated fats come mainly from meat and dairy products. They tend to be solid when chilled. Examples include butter and lard. There also are two plant-based saturated fats: palm oil and coconut oil.
- Trans fats are unsaturated fats that have been processed to be solid at room temperature. This is done to make foods last longer and give them better flavor. Vegetable shortenings, margarines, crackers, cookies, and snack foods like potato chips often contain trans fats.

Oils and fats give you important nutrients. During pregnancy, the fats you eat provide energy and help build some of the baby's organs and the **placenta**. But too much saturated fat and trans fat can lead to health problems, including heart disease. Fats should make up about 20 to 35 percent of your total calorie intake—that's about 6 tablespoons per day. Most of the fats and oils in your diet should be unsaturated fats, such as olive oil and peanut oil. Limit saturated fats, such as butter and fatty red meats. Avoid trans fats, which have no nutritional value. Check the labels of processed and packaged foods to see how much fat and what kind of fat they contain.

Vitamins and Minerals

Eating healthy foods and taking a prenatal vitamin every day should supply all of the vitamins and minerals you need during pregnancy (see Table 22-1, "Key Vitamins and Minerals During Pregnancy"). If you have food restrictions or if you have trouble absorbing certain nutrients, your **obstetrician–gynecologist (ob-gyn)** may recommend that you take a supplement as well as your regular prenatal vitamin. See the "Special Diets and Food Restrictions" section in this chapter.

Take your prenatal vitamin only as directed on the bottle. Some prenatal vitamins are meant to be taken two or three times day to get the full doses of vitamins and minerals. Do not take more than recommended per day. If you need an extra amount of a vitamin or mineral, such as iron or folic acid, take it as a separate supplement. Some multivitamin ingredients, such as vitamin A, are needed at low doses but can cause **birth defects** at higher doses. If you take more than what is recommended for your brand of prenatal vitamin, you could get an overdose of some of the ingredients.

Calcium

Calcium is a mineral that helps build your baby's bones and teeth. Women who are age 18 or younger need 1,300 milligrams (mg) of calcium per day. Women who are 19 or older need 1,000 mg per day. Milk and other dairy products, such as cheese and yogurt, are the best sources of calcium. If you have trouble digesting milk or do not eat dairy foods, you can get calcium from other sources, including

- dark, leafy greens
- broccoli
- fortified cereals, breads, and juice
- almonds and sesame seeds
- sardines or anchovies with the bones
- calcium supplements

TABLE 22-1 Key Vitamins and Minerals During Pregnancy

Nutrient (Daily Recommended Amount)	Why You and Your Baby Need It	Best Sources
Calcium (1,300 milligrams [mg] for ages 14 to 18 years; 1,000 mg for ages 19 to 50 years)	Builds strong bones and teeth	Milk, cheese, yogurt, sardines, green leafy vegetables
Iron (27 mg)	Helps red blood cells deliver oxygen to your baby	Lean red meat, poultry, fish, dried beans and peas, iron-fortified cereals, prune juice
Iodine (220 micrograms [mcg])	Essential for healthy brain development	Iodized table salt, dairy products, seafood, meat, some breads, eggs
Choline (450 mg)	Important for development of your baby's brain and spinal cord	Milk, beef liver, eggs, peanuts, soybeans
Vitamin A (750 mcg for ages 14 to 18 years; 770 mcg for ages 19 to 50 years)	Forms healthy skin and eyesight. Helps with bone growth	Carrots, green leafy vegetables, sweet potatoes
Vitamin C (80 mg for ages 14 to 18 years; 85 mg for ages 19 to 50 years)	Promotes healthy gums, teeth, and bones	Citrus fruit, broccoli, tomatoes, strawberries
Vitamin D (600 international units [IU]; note that vitamin labels may show this as 15 mcg)	Builds your baby's bones and teeth. Helps promote healthy eyesight and skin	Sunlight, fortified milk, fatty fish such as salmon and sardines
Vitamin B_6 (1.9 mg)	Helps form red blood cells. Helps body use protein, fat, and carbohydrates	Beef, liver, pork, ham, whole-grain cereals, bananas
Vitamin B_{12} (2.6 mcg)	Maintains nervous system	Meat, fish, poultry, milk (vegetarians should take a supplement)
Folic acid (600 mcg)	Helps prevent birth defects of the brain and spine. Supports the general growth and development of the baby and placenta	Fortified cereal, enriched bread and pasta, peanuts, dark green leafy vegetables, orange juice, beans. It is difficult to get the recommended amount from diet alone, which is why taking a daily prenatal vitamin with 400 mcg of folic acid (667 mcg dietary folate equivalents [DFE]) is important.

Choline

Choline plays a role in your baby's brain development. It also may help prevent some common birth defects. Experts recommend that pregnant women get 450 mg of choline each day. It's important to get choline from your diet, because it is not found in most prenatal vitamins. Make sure your diet contains a healthy amount of foods rich in choline, including

- chicken
- beef
- eggs
- milk
- soy
- peanuts

Folic Acid

Folic acid, also known as folate or vitamin B_9, is a vitamin that helps prevent major birth defects of the baby's brain and spine called **neural tube defects (NTDs)**. Current guidelines recommend that pregnant women get at least 600 micrograms (mcg) of folic acid each day from all sources, including food and vitamin supplements.

To be sure you are getting enough, take a daily prenatal vitamin with at least 400 mcg of folic acid and eat foods rich in this vitamin, including

- fortified cereal
- enriched bread and pasta
- peanuts
- dark green leafy vegetables
- orange juice
- beans

Remember that it may be hard to get the folic acid you need from food alone. Pregnant women should take a prenatal vitamin with folic acid each day for at least 1 month before pregnancy and during pregnancy. Note that a vitamin containing 400 mcg of folic acid also may show 667 mcg DFE on the label.

NTDs, such as **spina bifida** and **anencephaly**, happen early in prenatal development when the coverings of the spinal cord do not close completely. You may have a higher risk of giving birth to a baby with this type of defect if:

- You have already had a baby with an NTD.
- You have certain health conditions, such as **sickle cell disease**.
- You are taking certain medications, such as drugs to treat epilepsy (especially valproate).

If any of these are true for you, your ob-gyn may recommend that you take 4 mg of folic acid each day—10 times the usual amount—as a separate vitamin supplement at least 3 months before pregnancy and for the first 3 months of pregnancy. You and your ob-gyn can discuss whether you need this amount of folic acid based on your health history.

Iron

Iron is used by your body to make the extra blood that you and your baby need during pregnancy. Women who are not pregnant need 18 mg of iron per day. Pregnant women need more, 27 mg per day. This increased amount is found in most prenatal vitamins. Vitamin supplements with higher iron levels may cause digestion problems, such as constipation.

You also can eat foods rich in a certain type of iron called heme iron. Heme iron is absorbed more easily by the body. It is found in animal foods, such as red meat, poultry, and fish. Non-heme iron is found in vegetables and legumes, such as soybeans, spinach, and lentils. Although it is not as easily absorbed as heme iron, non-heme iron is a good way to get extra iron if you are a vegetarian. Iron also can be absorbed more easily if iron-rich foods are eaten with vitamin C-rich foods, such as citrus fruits and tomatoes.

Your blood should be tested during pregnancy to check for **anemia**. If you have anemia, your ob-gyn may recommend extra iron supplements. The body can absorb supplemental iron only when it's part of a chemical compound. Look at the label to see how much elemental iron is in the supplement. There may be two numbers on the label: the weight of the compound, and the weight of the iron alone. For example, you may see these compounds and how much elemental iron they contain:

- Ferrous fumarate 200 mg contains 66 mg of elemental iron.
- Ferrous gluconate 325 mg contains 38 mg of elemental iron.
- Ferrous sulfate 325 mg contains 65 mg of elemental iron.

Knowing how much and what formulation of iron to take for anemia can be confusing. Check with your ob-gyn to see what he or she recommends.

Omega-3 Fatty Acids

Omega-3 fatty acids are a type of fat found naturally in many kinds of fish. Omega-3s may be important for your baby's brain development before and after birth. Women should eat at least two servings of fish or shellfish (about 8 to 12 ounces [oz]) per week before getting pregnant, while pregnant, and while breastfeeding.

Some types of fish have higher levels of a metal called mercury than others. Mercury has been linked to birth defects. To limit your exposure to mercury, follow a few simple guidelines. Choose fish and shellfish such as salmon, shrimp, pollock, and tilapia. Do not eat bigeye tuna, king mackerel, marlin, orange roughy, shark, swordfish, or tilefish. Limit white (albacore) tuna to only 6 oz a week. You also should check advisories about fish caught in local waters.

If you don't like fish or do not eat it, you can still get omega-3s from other foods. Flaxseed (either as whole seeds or oil) is a good source. Other sources of omega-3s include

- canola oil
- broccoli
- cantaloupe
- kidney beans
- spinach
- cauliflower
- walnuts

There also are supplements with omega-3s, but you should talk with your ob-gyn before taking one. High doses may have harmful effects.

B Vitamins

B vitamins, including B_1, B_2, B_6, B_9, and B_{12}, are key nutrients during pregnancy. These vitamins give you energy, supply energy for your baby's development, promote good vision, and help build the placenta.

Your prenatal vitamin should have the right amount of B vitamins that you need each day. Eating foods high in B vitamins is a good idea too. These foods include

- liver
- pork
- milk
- poultry
- bananas
- whole-grain cereals and breads
- beans

Vitamin C

Getting the right amount of vitamin C is important for a healthy *immune system*. Vitamin C also helps build strong bones and muscles. During your pregnancy, you should get at least 85 mg of vitamin C each day (80 mg if you are younger than 19). You can get the right amount in your daily prenatal vitamin, but you also can get vitamin C from

- citrus fruits and juices
- strawberries
- broccoli
- tomatoes

Vitamin D

Vitamin D works with calcium to help build your baby's bones and teeth. It also is key for healthy skin and eyes. All women, including those who are pregnant, need 600 IU of vitamin D a day. Good sources of vitamin D include

- fortified milk and breakfast cereal
- fatty fish, such as salmon and mackerel (avoid king mackerel)
- fish liver oils
- egg yolks

Vitamin D also can be made in the body through exposure to sunlight. But most people do not get enough vitamin D through sunlight alone. If your ob-gyn thinks that you may have low levels of vitamin D, a test can check the level in your blood. If it is below normal, you may need to take a vitamin D supplement. Some vitamin labels may show 600 IU as 15 mcg.

Water

Getting enough water and fiber in your diet are the keys to avoiding or relieving constipation. Water also

- allows nutrients and waste products to circulate within and out of the body
- aids digestion
- helps form *amniotic fluid* around the baby

It's important to drink water throughout the day, not just when you're thirsty. During pregnancy you should drink 8 to 12 cups (64 to 96 oz) of water every day.

Planning Healthy Meals

If you want help planning a healthy diet, start with the U.S. Department of Agriculture's MyPlate food-planning guide (see the "Resources" section at the end of this chapter). MyPlate can show you the foods and amounts that you need to eat each day during each *trimester* of pregnancy. The amounts are calculated according to

- height
- ***body mass index (BMI)*** before pregnancy
- due date
- how much you exercise during the week

The amounts of food are given in standard sizes that most people are familiar with, such as cups and ounces.

The Five Food Groups

Table 22-2, "Daily Food Choices," shows the foods and amounts that a pregnant woman with a normal BMI before pregnancy should eat for each trimester of pregnancy. (Use the "Body Mass Index Chart" at the back of this book to look up your prepregnancy BMI.) You'll notice that food is broken down into the following five food groups:

1. Grains—Bread, pasta, oatmeal, cereal, and tortillas are all grains. Half of the grains you eat should be whole grains. Whole grains are those that have not been processed and include the whole grain kernel. They include

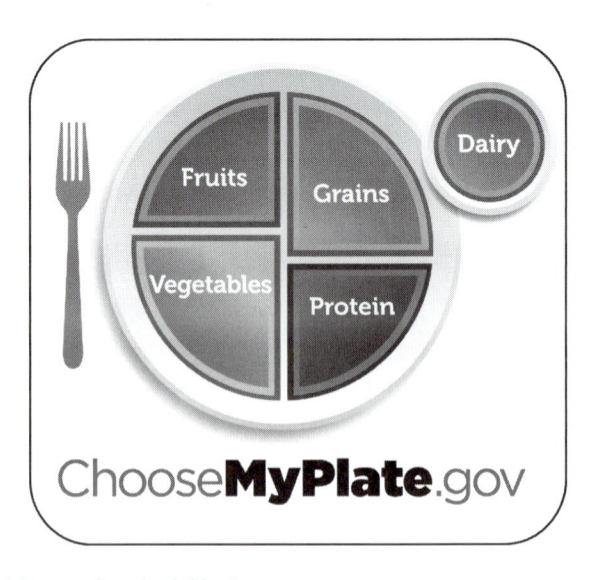

What should your plate look like? Half should be fruits and vegetables. The other half should be lean protein and whole grains. Each day you also should take a prenatal vitamin that has folic acid and iron. Courtesy of the U.S. Department of Agriculture.

oats, barley, quinoa, brown rice, and bulgur. Products made with these foods also count as whole grains. Look for the words "whole grain" on the product label.

2. Fruits—Fruits can be fresh, canned, frozen, or dried. Juice that is 100 percent fruit juice also counts. Make half of your plate fruits and vegetables.

3. Vegetables—Vegetables can be raw or cooked, frozen, canned, dried, or 100 percent vegetable juice. Use dark, leafy greens to make salads.

4. Protein foods—Protein foods include meat, poultry, seafood, beans and peas, eggs, processed soy products, nuts, and seeds. Include a variety of proteins and choose lean or low-fat meat and poultry.

TABLE 22-2 Daily Food Choices

Recommended daily food intake for a pregnant woman who is a normal weight and who gets less than 30 minutes of exercise each day.

Total Calories per Day	First Trimester 1,800	Second Trimester 2,200	Third Trimester 2,400	Comments
Grains	6 oz	7 oz	8 oz	1 oz is one slice of bread, ½ cup of cooked rice, ½ cup of cooked pasta, 3 cups of popped popcorn, or five whole-wheat crackers
Vegetables	2½ cups	3 cups	3 cups	2 cups of raw leafy vegetables count as 1 cup
Fruits	1½ cup	2 cups	2 cups	One large orange, one small apple, eight large strawberries, or ½ cup of dried fruit count as 1 cup
Dairy	3 cups	3 cups	3 cups	Two small slices of swiss cheese or ⅓ cup of shredded cheese count as 1 cup
Protein foods	5 oz	6 oz	6½ oz	1 oz of lean meat or poultry, one egg, 1 tablespoon of peanut butter, or ½ oz of nuts or seeds count as 1 oz
Fats and oils	5 teaspoons	7 teaspoons	8 teaspoons	Olives, some fish, avocados, and nuts

5. Dairy—Milk and milk products, such as cheese, yogurt, and ice cream, make up the dairy group. Choose fat-free or low-fat (1 percent) varieties. Make sure any dairy foods you eat are pasteurized. Pasteurization is a process that uses heat to kill **bacteria** that can cause disease. Foods that are pasteurized should say so on the label.

Tips for Healthy Eating

The following tips can help guide you when you are making food choices and ensure that you're eating in a healthy way:

- Choose a variety of foods and drinks to make sure you are getting a balanced diet with all the nutrients you need.
- Make half of your plate fruits and vegetables. Include dark green, red, and orange vegetables.
- Drink low-fat milk (skim or 1 percent).
- Make half of your grains whole grains.
- Vary your protein sources. Eat fish two to three times a week. See the "Fish and Shellfish" section later in this chapter for information about the types of fish to avoid. Choose lean meats and poultry. Vegetarians can get protein from plant-based foods such as nuts, seeds, and soy products.
- Limit foods with "empty" calories. These are foods that have a lot of calories but little nutritional value, such as candy, chips, and sugary drinks.
- Take a prenatal vitamin that contains 27 mg of iron and at least 400 mcg of folic acid. Note that some vitamin labels may say 667 mcg dietary folate equivalents (DFE) instead of 400 mcg of folid acid.
- Read the Nutrition Facts label on processed and packaged food. Limit foods that are higher in saturated fat, trans fat, added sugar, and sodium.

When planning your meals, remember to add snacks, which are a good way to get needed nutrition and extra calories. Choose snacks that have the right nutrients and are low in fat and sugar. Fruit and yogurt are healthy snack choices.

You may find it easier to eat six smaller meals during the day, especially later in pregnancy, when you may have indigestion after larger meals. To make these mini meals, just divide the daily recommended amount of foods from each of the food groups into small portions. Milk and half a sandwich made with meat, fish, peanut butter, or cheese make a good mini meal. Other ideas are low-fat milk and fresh fruits, cheese and crackers, and soups.

Healthy Eating on a Budget

MyPlate also has useful information on shopping to make the most of your food budget. Many people need help with buying healthy food. Depending on your income, you may qualify for help through the Supplemental Nutrition Assistance Program (SNAP) or the Special Supplemental Nutrition Program for Women, Infants, and Children (WIC). See the "Resources" section at the end of this chapter for more details.

Weight Gain During Pregnancy

Weight gain depends on your health, your BMI before pregnancy, and how many babies you are carrying (see Table 22-3, "Weight Gain During Pregnancy"). Weight gain should be gradual. During your first 12 weeks—the first trimester—you may gain only 1 to 5 pounds or no weight at all. In your second and third trimesters, if you were a healthy weight before pregnancy, you should gain between half a pound and 1 pound per week.

The key to healthy weight gain is to slowly increase your calories. In the first trimester, when weight gain is minimal, usually no extra calories are needed. In the second trimester, you need an extra 340 calories a day, and in the third trimester, about 450 extra calories a day.

TABLE 22-3 Weight Gain During Pregnancy

Body Mass Index (BMI) Before Pregnancy	Rate of Weight Gain in the Second and Third Trimesters* (Pounds Per Week)	Recommended Total Weight Gain With a Single Baby (in Pounds)	Recommended Weight Gain With Twins (in Pounds)
Less than 18.5 (underweight)	1.0 to 1.3	28 to 40	Not known
18.5 to 24.9 (normal weight)	0.8 to 1.0	25 to 35	37 to 54
25.0 to 29.9 (overweight)	0.5 to 0.7	15 to 25	31 to 50
30.0 and above (obese)	0.4 to 0.6	11 to 20	25 to 42

*Assumes a first-trimester weight gain between 1.1 and 4.4 pounds
Source: Institute of Medicine and National Research Council. 2009. *Weight Gain During Pregnancy: Reexamining the Guidelines*. Washington, DC: The National Academies Press.

Your weight should be checked at each **prenatal care** visit, and your ob-gyn should keep track of how much weight you have gained. A woman who gains too few pounds is more likely to have a small baby (less than 5½ pounds). These babies often have health problems after birth. Women who gain too much weight also are at risk of health problems. These problems include **gestational diabetes**, **high blood pressure**, and a baby that's too large (**macrosomia**).

If you are overweight or gaining weight too quickly, you may need to adjust your nutrition and exercise plan. Talk with your ob-gyn before making any major changes. Usually, you can start by cutting down on the "extra" calories that you get from extra fats and sugars. Watch your portion size and avoid second helpings. Focus on eating foods that have lots of nutrients, such as beans, leafy greens, and nuts.

Foods to Avoid or Limit During Pregnancy

Eating a variety of healthy foods is the best way to get all the nutrients you need. But there are some foods that you should eat only in moderation, and some that you should not eat at all during your pregnancy.

Alcohol. Alcohol can harm your baby's health. It's best to stop drinking before you get pregnant. If you did have some alcohol before you knew you were pregnant, it most likely will not harm your baby. The important thing is to stop drinking alcohol once you know you're pregnant. See the "Healthy Decisions" section of Chapter 3, "Months 1 and 2 (Weeks 1 to 8)."

Also, no types of alcoholic drinks are safe. One beer, one shot of liquor, one mixed drink, or one glass of wine all contain about the same amount of alcohol.

Watch out for foods that are cooked with alcohol as well. Depending on the cooking method, alcohol may or may not "cook out" of food. Simmering for a long time in a wide pan appears to remove the most alcohol. Baking removes the least alcohol.

Caffeine. There have been many studies on whether caffeine increases the risk of **miscarriage**, but the results are unclear. Most experts believe that consuming less than 200 mg of caffeine a day during pregnancy is safe. That's the amount in one 12-ounce cup of coffee. Remember that caffeine also is found in teas, colas, and chocolate. Make sure you count these sources in your total caffeine for the day.

Fish and Shellfish. Fish and shellfish are excellent sources of omega-3 fatty acids. Three of these fatty acids—DHA, EPA, and ALA—are considered "essential," meaning you can get them only through your diet. But there are some types of fish you should never eat while you are trying to get pregnant, when you are pregnant, and when you are breastfeeding. These fish have too much mercury, which has been linked to birth defects. These fish include

- bigeye tuna
- king mackerel
- marlin
- orange roughy
- shark
- swordfish
- tilefish

These fish also should not be fed to young children.

Sushi. Eat only cooked sushi or vegetable sushi during your pregnancy. Avoid all raw or seared fish when you're pregnant. Raw fish, including sushi and sashimi, is more likely to contain parasites or bacteria than cooked fish (see the "Food Safety" section in this chapter).

Sodium, Salt, and Monosodium Glutamate. Current guidelines recommend getting no more than 2,300 mg of sodium per day. That's the equivalent of about 1 teaspoon of table salt. Foods that are very high in sodium include

- frozen processed foods
- canned soups and broths
- other processed products

Check the label on packaged foods to see how much sodium is in them.

Another seasoning used in many foods is monosodium glutamate (MSG). It is used to enhance the flavor of many foods, especially Asian food. The U.S. Food and Drug Administration (FDA) requires that all foods that contain MSG list this ingredient on the label because some people develop a bad reaction to it, pregnant or not. But the FDA hasn't found any evidence that MSG is harmful during pregnancy.

Sugar and Sugar Substitutes. Limit the amount of simple sugars you eat each day. Simple sugars are found in foods such as table sugar, honey, syrup, fruit juices, soft drinks, and many processed foods. Although they may give you a quick energy boost, the energy they give is used up quickly.

The following artificial sweeteners are 200 to 600 times sweeter than sugar. They are safe to use while you are pregnant. Just use them in moderation:

- Saccharin (Sweet'N Low)
- Aspartame (Equal and NutraSweet)
- Sucralose (Splenda)
- Acesulfame-K (Sunett)
- Stevia (Truvia and SweetLeaf)

Special Diets and Food Restrictions

Many people do not eat certain foods. Their reasons may include

- a medical condition such as celiac disease, **lactose intolerance**, or a food allergy
- religious, cultural, or ethical concerns
- personal preference

If there are foods you do not or cannot eat, you still can get all the nutrients you need for a healthy pregnancy.

Before you get pregnant or early in your pregnancy, let your ob-gyn know if you have any food restrictions. They may suggest that you see a nutritionist or a dietitian to review what you normally eat. This will help make sure you are getting enough of all the nutrients you need. In some cases, you may need to take extra vitamins or minerals in addition to your prenatal vitamin.

Celiac Disease

Women who have celiac disease are unable to eat foods containing gluten, which is found in wheat, barley, and rye. There are many foods that are gluten-free, so pregnant women with celiac disease can choose fruits, vegetables, meats, potatoes, poultry, rice, and beans. There also are many gluten-free products sold in grocery and natural food stores or online.

Review your gluten-free diet with your ob-gyn and a dietitian to make sure that it gives you and the baby enough nutrients to grow and stay healthy. You may need to make changes if you are not gaining enough weight or if you develop **complications**, such as anemia. You also may need to add more vitamin D or calcium to your diet. Your ob-gyn will let you know if this is the case. Some vitamin supplements contain gluten, so be sure to find a gluten-free brand.

Food Allergies

Allergies are caused by the body's immune system overreacting to something that is normally harmless. Some food allergies can cause a life-threatening condition called anaphylaxis. Nearly any food can cause an allergy, but some of the more common allergens are eggs, wheat, milk, soy, nuts, fish, and shellfish.

People with a food allergy need to avoid foods that might trigger the allergy. But this can make it more difficult to eat a balanced diet. Let your ob-gyn know if you have a food allergy. Your ob-gyn may suggest that you see a nutritionist or a dietitian to help you plan meals that are nutritious and safe for you.

Lactose Intolerance

Lactose intolerance means you cannot fully digest the milk sugar (lactose) in dairy products. Pregnant women with this condition still need to get the daily amount of calcium to nourish their baby's growth. Here are some tips:

- Try different kinds of dairy products. Not all dairy products have the same amount of lactose. For example, hard cheeses such as Swiss or cheddar have small amounts of lactose and generally cause no symptoms.
- Buy lactose-free milk, cheese, and other dairy products. They contain the nutrients found in regular milk and dairy products.
- Get calcium from other foods. Good sources are canned pink salmon, nuts and seeds, leafy greens, molasses, and calcium-fortified breads and juices.

Talk with your ob-gyn if you are having trouble getting 1,000 mg of calcium each day. You may be advised to take a calcium supplement.

Vegetarian Diets

There are different types of vegetarian diets. Some include dairy products. Others strictly avoid all products that come from animals. If you are a vegetarian, you may need a little extra planning to get the nutrients that you and your baby need during pregnancy. Tell your ob-gyn at your first prenatal care visit that you are a vegetarian and ask for a recommended diet you can follow.

The following tips can help you maximize the key nutrients you need while still eating a vegetarian diet:

- Get enough protein from foods such as soy milk, tofu, and beans. Eggs, milk, and cheese also are good protein sources if you eat some animal foods.

- Eat lots of iron-rich vegetables and legumes, such as spinach, white beans, kidney beans, and chickpeas. You can increase the amount of iron that your body absorbs if you also eat foods high in vitamin C, such as oranges or tomatoes, at the same time.
- If you don't eat dairy foods, eat dark leafy greens, calcium-enriched tofu, and other calcium-enriched products (soy milk, almond milk, and orange juice) to get the recommended amount of calcium every day.
- Eat fortified cereal to get vitamin B_{12}. Drink milk if you eat dairy foods.

Food Safety

Pregnant women can get foodborne illness (also known as food poisoning) just like anyone else. But foodborne illness in a pregnant woman can cause serious problems for her and her baby. Contact your ob-gyn right away if you think you may have a foodborne illness (see the box "Signs and Symptoms of Foodborne Illness").

Certain foods are more likely to carry bacteria that cause foodborne illness, and you should not eat them while you are pregnant. Preparing and storing food safely also can reduce your risk.

Common Types of Foodborne Illness

Several types of bacteria can cause foodborne illness. Some of the more common types are discussed in this section.

> ### Signs and Symptoms of Foodborne Illness
>
> The following can be signs of foodborne illness. See your ob-gyn as soon as possible if you have
> - vomiting
> - diarrhea
> - abdominal pain
> - abdominal cramps that can last for a couple of days
> - fever
> - flu-like symptoms, such as chills and aches

Listeriosis. *Listeriosis* is a serious infection caused by *Listeria* bacteria. *Listeria* can be found in

- unpasteurized (raw) milk
- soft cheeses made with unpasteurized milk, such as queso, feta, and Brie
- hot dogs
- luncheon meats
- smoked seafood

Pregnant women are 13 times more likely to get listeriosis than other people. Listeriosis can cause mild, flu-like symptoms such as fever, muscle aches, and diarrhea, but it also may not cause any symptoms at all. But if it's not treated right away, listeriosis can lead to serious complications for your baby, including miscarriage, **stillbirth**, and **preterm** birth. Babies can get infected during passage through the birth canal during delivery.

If you think you have eaten food contaminated with listeria or if you have symptoms of listeriosis, call your ob-gyn. **Antibiotics** can be given to treat the infection and protect your baby.

Salmonellosis. *Salmonella* bacteria often are found in raw poultry, fish, eggs, and milk. Salmonellosis (infection with *Salmonella* bacteria) causes vomiting, diarrhea, fever, and abdominal cramps that can last for a couple of days. People with salmonellosis can get dehydrated because of the loss of body fluids. In addition, one type of *Salmonella* bacteria, called *Salmonella typhi*, can be passed to the baby if you are infected during pregnancy.

If you have signs and symptoms of salmonellosis, see your ob-gyn as soon as possible. You may get fluids through an **intravenous (IV) line** to prevent dehydration. Medication also may be needed in some cases.

Campylobacteriosis. This infection is caused by bacteria known as *Campylobacter*. Most people who get ill with campylobacteriosis have diarrhea, cramping, abdominal pain, and fever within 2 to 5 days after being exposed to the bacteria. The illness usually lasts about 1 week. Most cases of the infection are from eating raw or undercooked poultry or from contamination of other foods by raw poultry. Animals also can be infected, and some people have gotten campylobacteriosis from contact with the stool of a sick dog or cat.

Escherichia coli. *Escherichia coli* (*E. coli*) are a large and diverse group of bacteria. Although most strains of *E. coli* are harmless, others can make you sick. Some kinds of *E. coli* can cause diarrhea. Others can cause urinary tract infections, respiratory illness, **pneumonia**, and other illnesses. Most often, people are exposed to *E. coli* by eating or drinking contaminated food, unpasteurized milk, or water that has not been disinfected.

Foods to Avoid

To help avoid foodborne illness, do not eat any of the following foods while you're pregnant:

- Sushi made with raw fish
- Unpasteurized milk and foods made with unpasteurized milk, including soft cheeses such as feta, queso blanco, queso fresco, Camembert, Brie, or blue-veined cheeses, unless the label says "made with pasteurized milk"
- Hot dogs, luncheon meats, cold cuts, or smoked or pickled fish, unless they are heated until steaming hot just before serving
- Refrigerated pâté and meat spreads
- Refrigerated smoked seafood
- Raw and undercooked seafood and meat
- Raw eggs, which can be found in homemade mayonnaise and caesar salad dressing. Also avoid undercooked eggs.

Safe Food Preparation

Bacteria can transfer easily from one surface to another, and they multiply fastest in the "Danger Zone" between 40°F and 140°F. To reduce the risk of foodborne illness, remember these four steps when preparing food: Clean, Separate, Cook, and Chill.

1. Clean.
    - Wash your hands with soap and water before and after handling raw food.
    - Wash fruits and vegetables under running tap water before eating, cutting, or cooking.
    - Keep your kitchen clean. Wash your utensils, countertops, and cutting boards with soap and hot water after handling and preparing uncooked foods. You can sanitize them by applying a solution of 1 teaspoon of liquid chlorine bleach per gallon of water. Allow the surface to air dry.

2. Separate.
    - Keep raw meat, poultry, eggs, and seafood and their juices away from ready-to-eat food.
    - Separate raw meat, poultry, and seafood from produce in your shopping cart by placing them into plastic bags.
    - Keep raw meat, poultry, and seafood on a plate, in a container, or in a sealed plastic bag in the refrigerator.
    - Do not wash raw poultry or meat before cooking. Bacteria in raw meat and poultry juices can be spread to other foods, utensils, and surfaces.
    - Use a separate cutting board for raw meat, poultry, and seafood.
    - Never put cooked food back on the same plate that previously held raw food unless the plate has been washed in hot, soapy water. Do not use sauce used to marinate raw food on cooked food unless it is boiled first.
3. Cook.
    - Use a food thermometer to check doneness of meat, poultry, seafood, and egg products. These items should be cooked to a safe minimum temperature (see www.foodsafety.gov/keep/charts/mintemp.html).
    - Place the food thermometer in the thickest part of the food, away from bone, fat, and gristle.
4. Chill.
    - Keep your refrigerator at 40°F or below and the freezer at 0°F or below.
    - Thaw food in the refrigerator, microwave, or in cold (not hot) water.
    - Do not leave food at room temperature for more than 2 hours (1 hour when the temperature is above 90°F).
    - Meat and poultry defrosted in the refrigerator may be refrozen before or after cooking. If thawed in the microwave or cold water, cook before refreezing.
    - Only buy eggs from a refrigerator or refrigerated case. Store eggs in the refrigerator in their original carton and use within 3 to 5 weeks.
    - When selecting precut produce, choose only those items that are refrigerated or surrounded by ice and keep them refrigerated at home to maintain quality and safety.

RESOURCES

Choose Fish and Shellfish Wisely
www.epa.gov/choose-fish-and-shellfish-wisely/
Information from the U.S. Environmental Protection Agency about safe fish consumption.

How to Understand and Use the Nutrition Facts Label
www.fda.gov/food/labelingnutrition/ucm274593.htm
Illustrated guide from the U.S. Food and Drug Administration. Helps with understanding the Nutrition Facts label on processed and packaged foods.

Lactose Intolerance
www.niddk.nih.gov/health-information/health-topics/digestive-diseases/lactose-intolerance/Pages/facts.aspx
Webpage from the National Institute of Diabetes and Digestive and Kidney Diseases. Offers detailed information about the causes, signs and symptoms, diagnosis, and management of lactose intolerance.

MyPlate
www.ChooseMyPlate.gov
Website from the U.S. Department of Agriculture. The customized MyPlate Plan lets you enter your information for tips on what and how much to eat.

National Foundation for Celiac Awareness
www.beyondceliac.org
Patient awareness and advocacy website that gives comprehensive information about living with celiac disease, including an extensive guide to gluten-free food.

People at Risk: Pregnant Women
www.foodsafety.gov/people-at-risk/pregnant-women
Guide from the U.S. Department of Health and Human Services that provides practical information for avoiding foodborne illness during pregnancy (and at any time).

Supplemental Nutrition Assistance Program (SNAP)
www.fns.usda.gov/snap
Webpage from the U.S. Department of Agriculture. Explains how to apply for food assistance. Your state health department also can tell you how to locate a SNAP office, or you can go to the website to link to your state's SNAP application process.

Women, Infants, and Children (WIC) Breastfeeding Support Program
https://wicbreastfeeding.fns.usda.gov
The WIC breastfeeding campaign from the U.S. Department of Agriculture offers moms information, resources, and support for breastfeeding.

Your Pregnancy and Childbirth
www.acog.org/MyPregnancy
Website from the American College of Obstetricians and Gynecologists (ACOG) with information on pregnancy, labor, delivery, and postpartum care. Includes the latest information from the experts in women's health care, questions answered by ACOG ob-gyns, pregnancy stories from real women, and an A–Z directory of health topics covering pregnancy and beyond.

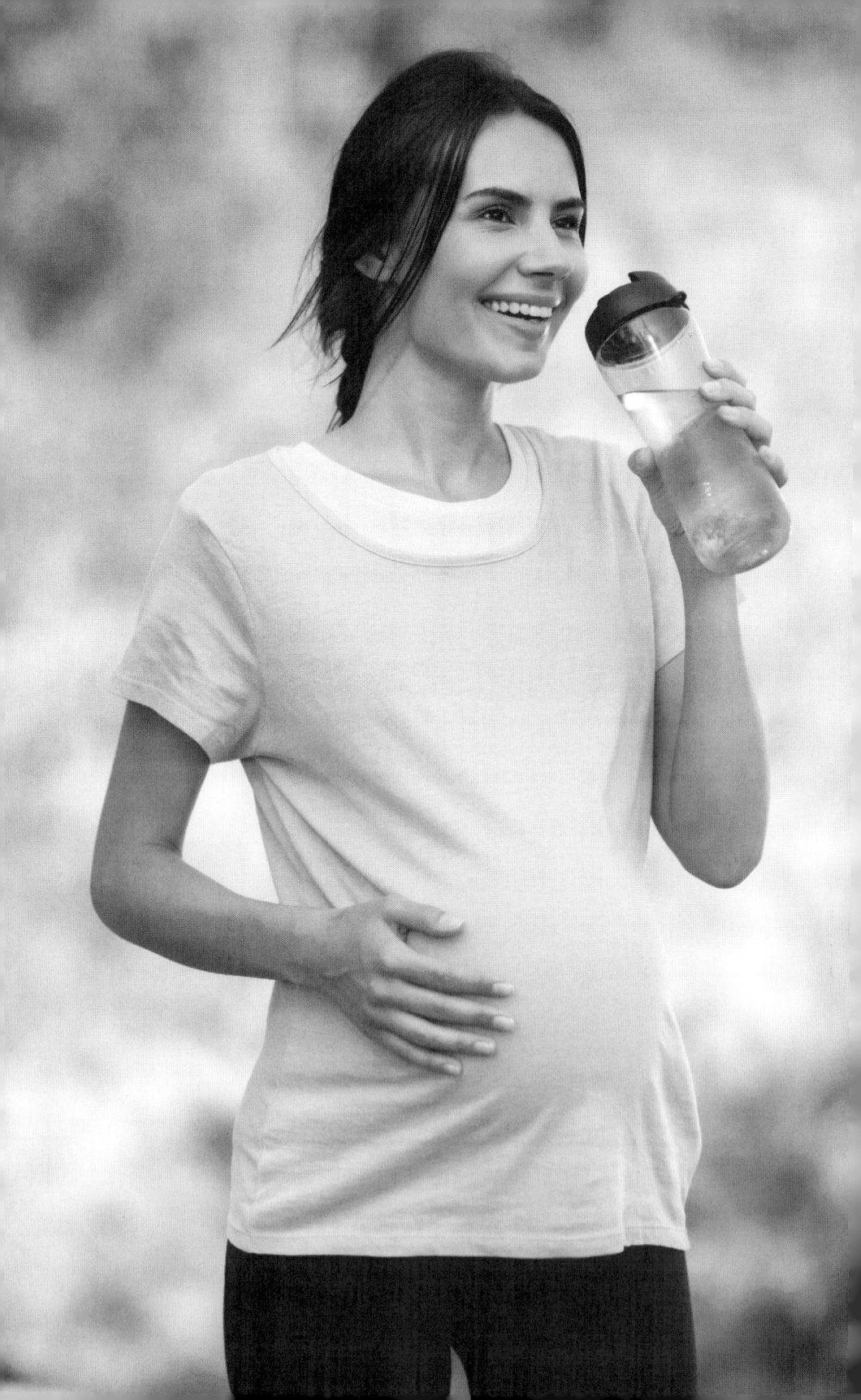

CHAPTER 23

Exercise During Pregnancy

Being active and exercising at least 30 minutes on most days of the week can help your pregnancy in many ways. Exercise can benefit you by

- reducing backaches, constipation, bloating, and swelling
- boosting your mood and energy levels
- building muscle tone, strength, and endurance
- helping you sleep better

Exercise also may reduce your risk of certain pregnancy **complications**, including

- *gestational diabetes*
- *preeclampsia*
- *cesarean birth*

The ideal exercise routine gets your heart pumping, keeps you limber, and controls your weight gain without causing too much physical stress for you or the baby. Exercising now also will make it easier for you to get back to your prepregnancy weight after the baby is born.

Some exercise routines can help you relieve pregnancy-related aches and pains. For instance, the extra weight you are carrying affects your posture and can be hard on your back. Exercise may help ease back pain by toning muscles and making them stronger.

This chapter discusses safe ways to exercise during pregnancy. Plus, at the end of the chapter there are a few core exercises you can do after pregnancy.

Who Should Not Exercise During Pregnancy?

Before you start exercising, talk with your **obstetrician–gynecologist (ob-gyn)**. Women with certain medical conditions may be advised not to exercise. These conditions may include

- some forms of heart and lung disease
- *cervical insufficiency* with or without a *cerclage*
- *multiple pregnancy* with risk factors for *preterm* labor
- *placenta previa* after 26 weeks of pregnancy
- vaginal bleeding
- risk of preterm labor
- *prelabor rupture of membranes (PROM)*
- preeclampsia or *high blood pressure* that happens for the first time during pregnancy
- severe *anemia*

You and your ob-gyn should discuss what activities you can do safely.

Guidelines for Physical Activity During Pregnancy

Ideally, pregnant women should get 150 minutes of moderate-intensity aerobic activity per week. An aerobic activity is exercise in which you move large muscles of the body (like those in the legs and arms) in a rhythmic way, which increases the heart rate. Moderate-intensity means you are moving enough to raise your heart rate and start sweating. At the desired intensity you should still be able to speak in full sentences.

Examples of moderate-intensity aerobic activity include brisk walking and gardening (raking, weeding, or digging). You can divide the 150 minutes into 30-minute workouts on 5 days of the week or into smaller 10-minute workouts throughout each day.

If you have not been active lately, start with a few minutes each day. Add 5 minutes each week until you can stay active for 30 minutes a day.

If you were very active before pregnancy, you can keep doing the same workouts with the approval of your ob-gyn. But be realistic. Your exercise endurance will decrease as your pregnancy progresses. Listen to your body and don't "push through" or overdo it. You might hurt yourself. And keep in mind that high-intensity exercise can lead to weight loss. If you are losing weight, you may need to take in more calories.

Pay attention to your body while you exercise. If you have any of the signs or symptoms listed in the box "Warning Signs to Stop Exercise," stop exercising and call your ob-gyn right away.

Tips for Safe and Healthy Exercise

It's important to protect yourself from injury while exercising. For starters, make sure you have all the equipment you need for a safe workout. Wear shoes that have plenty of padding and support. Wear a sports bra that fits well. Later in pregnancy, a belly support belt may reduce discomfort while walking or running. Here are a few more tips for keeping exercise safe:

- Drink enough fluids. Take a bottle of water with you for a drink before, during, and after your workouts. If you're getting hot or feeling thirsty, take a break and drink more water or a low-sugar sports drink.
- Avoid getting overheated, especially in the first trimester. To be on the safe side while working out, drink plenty of water, wear loose-fitting clothing, and exercise in a temperature-controlled room. Do not exercise outside when it is very hot or humid.

Warning Signs to Stop Exercise

Whether you're a seasoned athlete or a beginner, watch for the following warning signs when you exercise. Stop and call your ob-gyn if you have

- bleeding from the vagina
- feeling dizzy or faint
- shortness of breath before starting exercise
- chest pain
- headache
- muscle weakness
- calf pain or swelling
- regular, painful contractions of the uterus
- fluid gushing or leaking from your vagina

- Begin your workout with stretching and warming up for 5 minutes to prevent muscle strain. Slow walking or riding a stationary bike are good warm-ups.
- Work out on a wooden floor or a firmly carpeted surface. This gives you better footing. Also watch where you walk in general, especially in a gym. Gyms have a lot of equipment that is easy to trip over.
- Don't do jerky, bouncy, or high-impact motions. Jumping, jarring motions, or quick direction changes can strain your joints and cause pain.
- Get up slowly after lying or sitting on the floor. This will help keep you from feeling dizzy or faint. Once you're standing, walk in place briefly.
- Don't do deep knee bends, full sit-ups, double leg lifts (raising and lowering both legs at once), or straight-leg toe touches.
- Follow intense exercise with cooling down for 5 to 10 minutes. Slow your pace little by little and end your workout by gently stretching. Don't stretch too far, though. Intense stretching can injure the tissue that connects your joints.
- Avoid standing still or lying flat on your back as much as possible. When you lie on your back, your **uterus** presses on a large vein that returns blood to the heart. Standing motionless can cause blood to pool in your legs and feet. These positions may cause your blood pressure to drop for a short time.

Activities to Avoid

Although there are many sports that you can do while you're pregnant, such as walking and swimming, there are some activities that you should avoid because they can be too risky for you and the baby. Some types of exercise involve positions and movements that may be uncomfortable or harmful. While pregnant, do not do any activity that puts you at higher risk of injury, such as:

- Contact sports and sports that put you at risk of getting hit in the belly, including soccer, basketball, boxing, and hockey
- Activities that may result in a fall, such as downhill snow skiing, water skiing, surfing, off-road cycling, gymnastics, and horseback riding
- "Hot yoga" or "hot Pilates," which may cause you to get overheated
- Scuba diving, which puts your baby at risk of decompression sickness

Some sports should be avoided if you haven't done them before. In racquet sports, such as badminton, tennis, and racquetball, your changing body may affect your balance and put you at risk of falls. If you're an experienced player, though, you may be able to adjust to your body's changes. But no matter how skilled you are at a sport, you can't predict what another player or (if outdoors) the weather will do. It's best to always play it safe. Minimize any risk of hurting yourself and the baby.

Pregnancy Changes That Can Affect Your Exercise Routine

Some of the changes in your body during pregnancy affect the kinds of activities you can do safely. Consider the following things when choosing how to exercise:

- Joints—Some pregnancy hormones cause the ligaments that support your joints to stretch. This makes them more prone to injury.

- Balance—The weight you gain in the front of your body shifts your center of gravity, especially during the second and third trimesters. This puts stress on your joints and muscles, mostly those in the lower back and pelvis. It also can make you less stable and more likely to fall.

- Heart rate—Extra weight also makes your body work harder than it did before you were pregnant. This is true even if you are working out at a slower pace. Intense exercise boosts *oxygen* and blood flow to the muscles and away from other parts of your body, such as your uterus. If you can't talk normally in full sentences during exercise, you are working too hard.

Starting an Exercise Program During Pregnancy

If you don't get regular exercise, pregnancy is a great time to start. Discuss your plan to start exercising with your ob-gyn. Also, start slowly. Begin with as little as 5 minutes of exercise a day and add 5 minutes each week until you can stay active for 30 minutes per day.

If you're not used to exercising regularly, it may be tough to get started. There are simple ways of adding movement to your daily life. While you're at the grocery store, do a couple of laps inside the store. Or, if you have a shopping mall nearby, try walking to the farthest end and back. Take the stairs instead of the elevator. The important thing is to get moving a little more each day to get the best benefits.

Staying Motivated

If you need motivation, ask a friend to join you on your walks or workouts. If you have other small children, try walking them in their stroller. Make it a family activity.

Another way to stay motivated is to keep track of your progress. If you're a beginner, gradually increasing the time and distance that you walk can be a great incentive to keep at it. Some smartphone apps and websites are available that track your distance, speed, calories burned, and other factors (see the box "Which Fitness App Should You Use?"). Some use a tracking device or bracelet that you can wear all day to monitor your daily activity.

The rest of this chapter has suggestions for activities that are generally safe for pregnant women, plus some exercises you can try after your baby is born. Find out what's offered at your local gym or community center. Think about trying something new. The best physical activity is one that you enjoy and want to keep doing.

Aerobic Activities

Aerobic activities ("cardio") are ones in which you move large muscles of the body (like those in the legs and arms) in a rhythmic way. This type of activity increases your heart rate and strengthens your heart and blood vessels. You should aim to get about 30 minutes of moderate-intensity aerobic activity on most days of the week.

Many aerobic sports and activities are safe during pregnancy, even for beginners. The following are good aerobic activities:

- Walking is a great form of exercise, and one of the easiest. All you need is a good pair of shoes and comfortable clothing. Wear walking shoes or tennis shoes that fit well and give good support, flexibility, and cushioning. Brisk walking gives a total body workout and is easy on the joints and muscles. And remember you can swing your arms while you walk for an extra workout.

- Swimming is great for your body because it works so many muscles at the same time. The water supports your weight so you avoid injury and muscle strain. It also helps you stay cool and may prevent your legs from swelling. Many women swim right up to the end of their pregnancies.

- Water workouts (also known as "aqua aerobics") give many of the same benefits as swimming. If you have a local pool, find out if there are classes.

> ## Which Fitness App Should You Use?
>
> Various smartphone apps are available that track your steps, distance, speed, heart rate, calories eaten, calories burned, weight, and more. Here are some things to keep in mind when selecting a fitness app to track your progress during pregnancy:
>
> - Do you want to use the apps that come with your phone, or apps that you purchase and download?
> - Do you also use step counters, heart rate monitors, scales, or other devices? Do you want these to connect to the app?
> - Does the app have a "pregnancy mode"? For example, if your app tracks your weight and calorie intake, will it take into account the weight you need to gain during your pregnancy?
> - If social networking and sharing are important to you, does the app support that?
>
> It's a good idea to let your ob-gyn know you are using a fitness app during pregnancy. He or she may be able to recommend useful ones.

- Cycling provides a good aerobic workout. But your growing belly can affect your balance and make you more prone to falls. You may want to stick with stationary or recumbent biking later in pregnancy.
- Low-impact aerobics classes also can give a good workout. Find out what is available at your local gym or community center.
- If you are an experienced runner, jogger, or racket-sports player, you may be able to keep doing these activities during pregnancy. Discuss these activities with your ob-gyn. Try to avoid any racket sport in which you need to move and pivot quickly or risk getting hit by someone else's racket.

Activities for Balance, Strength, and Flexibility

Some activities don't necessarily get your heart pumping faster, but they have other benefits. They build muscle strength and help lower stress. You may wish to try one or more of the following activities:

- Yoga can stretch and strengthen muscles and develop good breathing techniques. Yoga also helps you learn to breathe deeply and relax, which may be helpful during labor and delivery. Yoga is safe for pregnant women, but you should not do "hot yoga." Also, some poses aren't recommended for pregnant women, such as those in which you lie flat on your back (after the first trimester) and those that require a lot of abdominal stretching.

  Tell your yoga instructor that you are pregnant. You may want to consider joining a yoga class that is designed especially for pregnancy. These classes often teach modified poses that accommodate a pregnant woman's shifting balance.

- Pilates focuses on healthy breathing and improving flexibility. A Pilates exercise program is a good way to improve posture and build muscle strength. As with yoga, some Pilates moves shouldn't be done during pregnancy. Tell your instructor that you are pregnant or join a special class for pregnant women.

- Tai chi involves performing a series of movements in a slow, graceful manner. Each posture flows into the next without pausing. Anyone can do tai chi. It's known to reduce stress, increase flexibility and energy, and improve muscle strength and balance.

- Exercises to improve upper body strength are important. Babies, car seats, strollers, and extra bags all can be heavy. You can lift light weights at home, just 5 to 10 pounds, to improve arm and shoulder strength. Talk with your ob-gyn about the correct movements.

- Weight training also may be safe if you did this regularly before your pregnancy. Talk with your ob-gyn.

Exercises You Can Do at Home

During pregnancy, the muscles in your abdomen and lower back—your core muscles—stretch. The following exercises are designed to gradually help tone and strengthen these muscles and help you stay flexible. Most of them can be done at home without any special equipment. A few use an exercise ball. As with any physical activity, make sure you are safe and protect yourself from injury while doing these exercises.

Kegel Exercises

Kegel exercises help tone the muscles of the pelvic floor. These muscles support your **urethra**, **bladder**, uterus, and **rectum**. Strengthening these muscles may help improve bladder control. After delivery, they may help tighten vaginal muscles that are stretched from childbirth. Here is how Kegel exercises are done:

- Squeeze the muscles that you use to stop the flow of urine. This pulls the **vagina** and rectum up and back.
- Hold for 3 seconds, then relax for 3 seconds.
- Do 10 contractions three times a day.
- Increase your hold by 1 second each week. Work your way up to 10-second holds.

Make sure you are not squeezing your stomach, thigh, or buttock muscles. You also should breathe normally. Do not hold your breath as you do these exercises.

You can do Kegel exercises anywhere—while working, driving in your car, or watching television. But you should not do these exercises when you are urinating.

4-Point Kneeling

This exercise strengthens and tones the abdominal muscles.

1. Kneel on all fours. Make sure that your hips are positioned directly over your knees and your shoulders are positioned directly over your hands. Your back should be straight, not curved upward or downward.

2. Inhale deeply. Then exhale. As you exhale, pull your abdominal muscles in. Imagine that you are pulling your belly button inward up to your spine. This is called engaging your abdominal muscles. Do not hold your breath. Make sure your back stays straight.

3. Repeat 5 times.

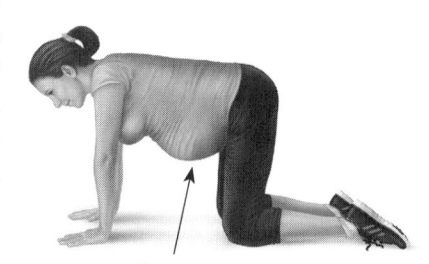

Engage abdominals

Seated Leg Raises

This exercise strengthens abdominal muscles and helps with balance and stability.

1. Sit on a chair, keeping your spine in neutral position. Your feet should be flat on the floor, about hip-width apart.

2. Engage your abdominal muscles by imagining that you are pulling your belly button inward to your spine. Your tailbone should relax. Do not hold your breath. Your arms should be relaxed.

3. Raise your left foot off the ground by extending your knee. At the same time, raise your right arm. Hold for a few seconds.

4. Return to the starting position. Repeat with your right leg and left arm. Do this 4 to 6 times per side, switching sides each time.

Seated Overhead Triceps Extension

This exercise stretches and strengthens the triceps (upper arm muscle) and chest muscles. Also works abdominal and hip muscles.

1. While seated, keep your spine straight and your feet flat on the floor.

2. Hold the resistance band in your right hand and raise your arm, then bend your arm at the elbow. Reach your left hand behind your back and hold the other end of the resistance band at the back of your waist.

3. With your elbow close to your head, raise and lower your right arm by bending the elbow. Keep the other end of the resistance band anchored behind your waist. Repeat 4 to 6 times.

4. Return to starting position. Then repeat with the opposite side.

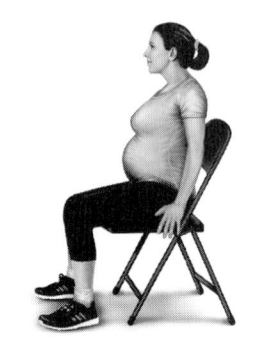

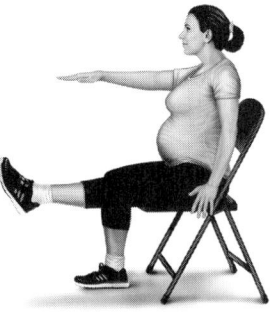

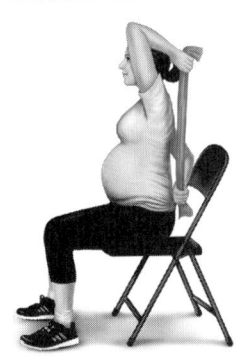

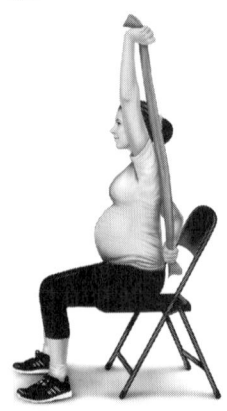

Ball Wall Squat

This exercise stretches the muscles of the legs and buttocks. Caution: If you have any knee pain, do not do this exercise.

1. Place exercise ball against wall. Stand and firmly press the ball into the wall using your lower back.

2. Distribute your weight between both feet. With a slow, controlled movement, squat down while firmly pressing against the ball. Do not let your knees collapse inward. Keep your feet flat and avoid lifting the heels. Maintain an open chest and avoid rounding your shoulders.

3. Start with squatting halfway if you cannot squat all the way down.

4. Repeat 4 to 6 times, working up to 10 to 12 times.

Ball Shoulder Stretch

This exercise stretches the upper back, arms, and shoulders.

1. Kneel on the floor with the exercise ball in front of you. Put your hands on either side of the ball.

2. Move your buttocks back toward your hips while rolling the ball in front of you. Keep your eyes on the floor. Do not arch your neck. Go only as far as is comfortable for you to feel a gentle stretch. Hold the stretch for a few seconds.

3. Return to starting position. Repeat 4 to 6 times.

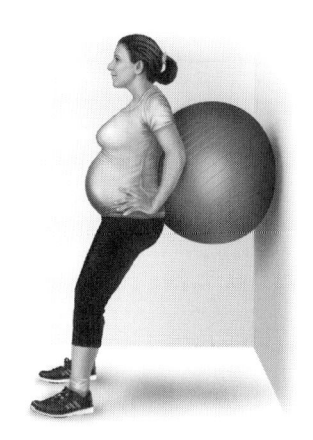

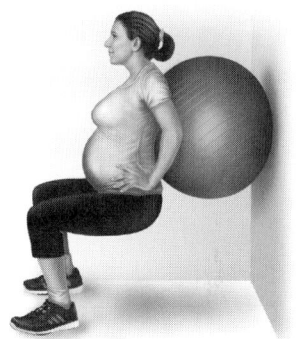

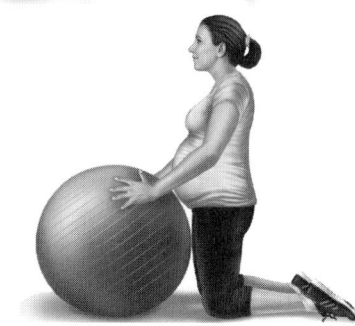

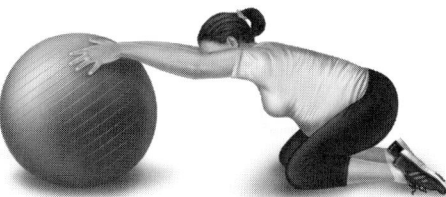

Seated Side Stretch

This exercise eases tension on the sides of your body and stretches your hip muscles.

1. Sit up tall on a chair, keeping your spine in a neutral position and your abdominals engaged. Your feet should be flat on the floor, about as wide as your hips. Put your left hand on your right knee.

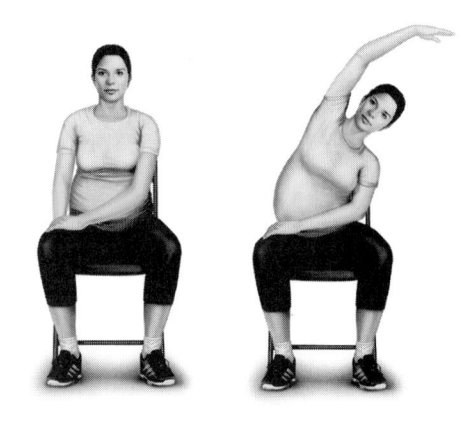

2. Raise your right arm and bend it toward your left side until you feel a gentle stretch. Breathe normally. Do not hunch down or round your shoulders. Hold the stretch for a few seconds.

3. Return to the starting position. Repeat with your left arm. Do this 4 to 6 times per side, switching sides each time.

Kneeling Heel Touch

This exercise tones muscles of the upper back, lower back, and abdomen.

1. Kneel on an exercise mat.

2. Using a slow, controlled movement, rotate your torso to the right. Bring your right hand back and touch your left heel. You can place a yoga block next to each ankle and aim to touch them instead of your heels. Extend your left arm above your head for balance.

3. Return to starting position. Repeat on the other side. Do this 4 to 6 times per side, switching sides each time.

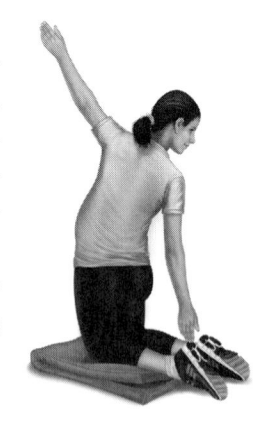

Standing Back Bend

This exercise helps counteract the increased forward bending that happens during pregnancy as your uterus grows.

1. Stand with your palms on the back of each hip.
2. Slowly bend backward about 15 to 20 degrees. Hold for 20 seconds. Repeat 5 times. Do not bend your neck back too far. If needed, you can hold on to a chair for support.

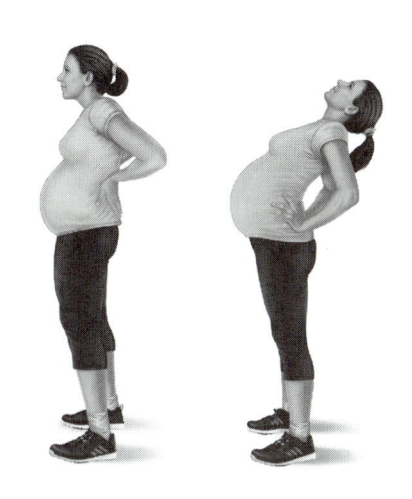

Exercising After Childbirth

When you are caring for a newborn, finding time for exercise can be a challenge. Hormonal changes and sleepless nights can affect your energy level. You may feel too tired to exercise but being active can give you more energy. Even exercising for a few minutes each day has benefits, including

- strengthening and toning your abdominal muscles
- helping you sleep better
- relieving stress
- helping prevent **postpartum depression**

Another benefit of exercise is that it can help you lose the extra pounds that you may have gained during pregnancy and help you to keep them off. Getting back to a healthy weight now will increase your chances of a healthy pregnancy the next time you decide to get pregnant. Staying at a healthy weight throughout your life also reduces your risk of health problems, including

- **diabetes mellitus**
- heart disease
- certain types of cancer

When to Start Exercising

If you had a healthy pregnancy and a normal vaginal delivery, you should be able to start exercising again soon after the baby is born. Usually, it is safe to begin exercising a few days after giving birth, or as soon as you feel ready. If you had a cesarean birth or other complications, ask your ob-gyn when it is safe to exercise.

Guidelines for Exercise After Childbirth

Aim to stay active for 20 to 30 minutes a day. When you first start exercising after childbirth, try simple ***postpartum*** exercises that help strengthen major muscle groups, including abdominal and back muscles. Gradually add moderate-intensity exercise. Even 10 minutes of exercise benefits your body. Stop exercising if you feel pain or dizziness.

Walking is a good way to ease back into fitness. So is swimming, once your postpartum bleeding has stopped. There also are exercise classes designed just for new mothers. To find one, check with local health and fitness clubs, community centers, and hospitals.

No matter what sort of exercise you do, design a program that meets your needs. You may want to strengthen your heart and lungs, tone your muscles, lose weight, or do all three.

Also, try to choose exercises that you'll keep doing. Staying fit over time is more important than getting into shape right after birth. Your ob-gyn may be able to suggest forms of exercise that will help you meet your fitness goals.

Postpartum Exercises

During pregnancy, the growing uterus stretches the muscles in your abdomen and your lower back—your "core" muscles. The following exercises are designed to gradually help tone and strengthen these muscles. When you master one exercise—you can do 20 repetitions without stopping—move on to the next one. Make sure you get your ob-gyn's approval before exercising after pregnancy.

4-Point Kneeling

This exercise strengthens and tones the abdominal muscles.

1. Kneel on all fours. Make sure that your hips are positioned directly over your knees and your shoulders are positioned directly over your hands. Your back should be straight, not curved upward or downward.

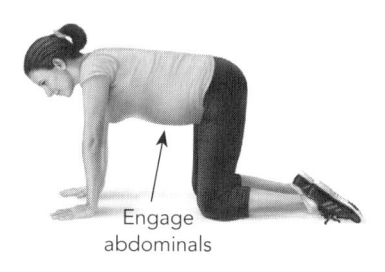

2. Inhale deeply. Then, exhale. As you exhale, pull your abdominal muscles in. Imagine that you are pulling your belly button inward up to your spine. This is called engaging your abdominal muscles. Do not hold your breath. Make sure your back stays straight.

3. Repeat 5 times.

Leg Slides

This exercise tones abdominal and leg muscles.

1. Lie flat on your back, bending your knees slightly, with your feet flat on the floor. Imagine that you are pulling your belly button inward up to your spine. This is called engaging your abdominal muscles.

2. Inhale, and slide one leg from a bent to a straight position.

3. Exhale, and bend it back again. Do not hold your breath.

4. Be sure to keep both feet on the floor and keep them relaxed.

5. Repeat with your other leg.

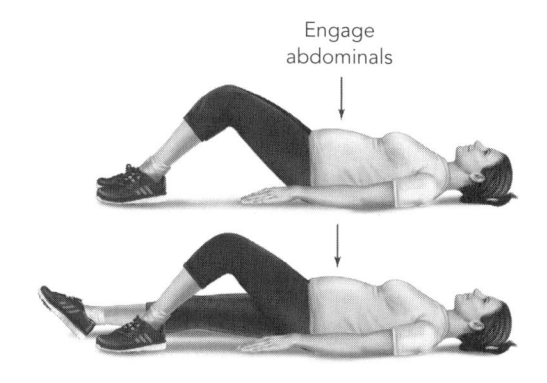

Knee Raises

This exercise strengthens core and lower back muscles.

1. Lie flat on your back, bending your knees slightly, with your feet flat on the floor.
2. Raise one leg with the knee bent so that your knee is above your hip. Slide the other leg from a bent position to a straight position.
3. Keep your abdominal muscles engaged. Focus on drawing your belly button inward. Do not move your back. Do not hold your breath.
4. Return to starting position. Repeat with opposite leg.

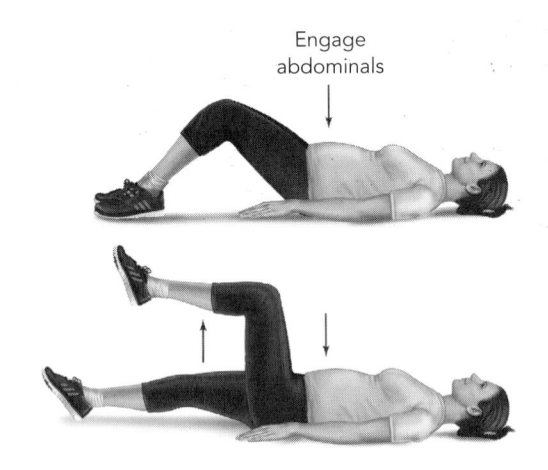

Heel Touches

This exercise strengthens core and lower back muscles.

1. Lie flat on your back, bending your knees slightly, with your feet flat on the floor.
2. Raise both legs with knees bent. Your knees should be at a 90-degree angle above your hips. The lower part of your legs should be parallel to the floor.
3. Lower one leg to the floor, keeping your knee bent, and touch your heel to the floor. Make sure that the knee stays bent at a 90-degree angle.
4. Keep your abdominal muscles engaged. Focus on drawing your belly button inward. Do not move your back. Do not hold your breath.
5. Bring the leg back up to the starting position.
6. Repeat with the opposite leg.

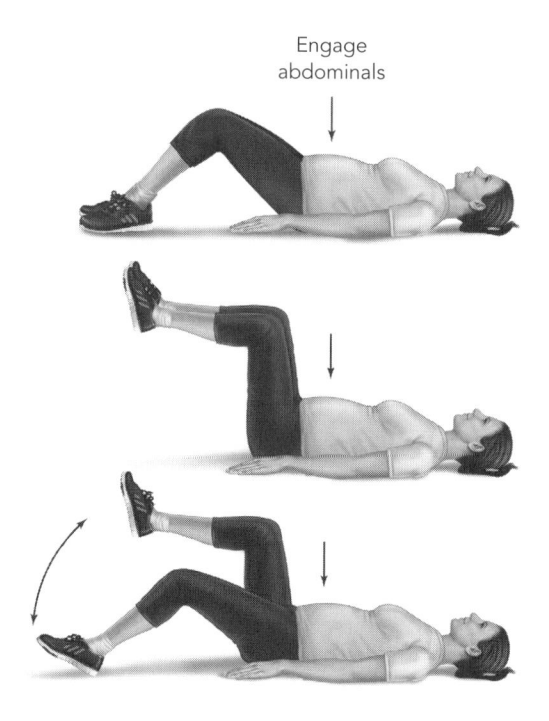

Leg Extensions

Leg extensions strengthen core, hip, and lower back muscles.

1. Lie flat on your back, bending your knees slightly, with your feet flat on the floor.
2. Raise both legs with knees bent at a 90-degree angle above the hips. The lower part of your legs should be parallel to the floor.
3. Extend one leg out with the foot 12 to 24 inches off the floor. Keep your abdominal muscles engaged. Do not hold your breath.
4. Return your extended leg to the starting position. Repeat with the opposite leg.

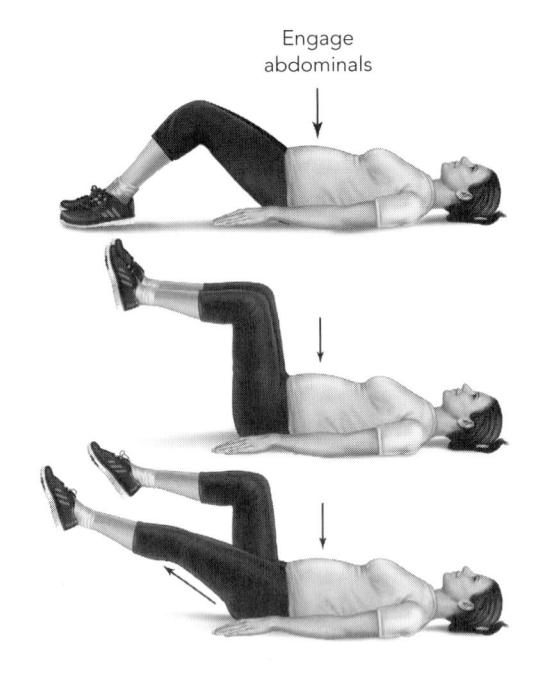

RESOURCES

Exercise and Physical Fitness
https://medlineplus.gov/exerciseandphysicalfitness.html
General exercise information from the U.S. National Library of Medicine, with links to other resources.

Your Pregnancy and Childbirth
www.acog.org/MyPregnancy
Website from the American College of Obstetricians and Gynecologists (ACOG) with information on pregnancy, labor, delivery, and postpartum care. Includes the latest information from the experts in women's health care, questions answered by ACOG ob-gyns, pregnancy stories from real women, and an A–Z directory of health topics covering pregnancy and beyond.

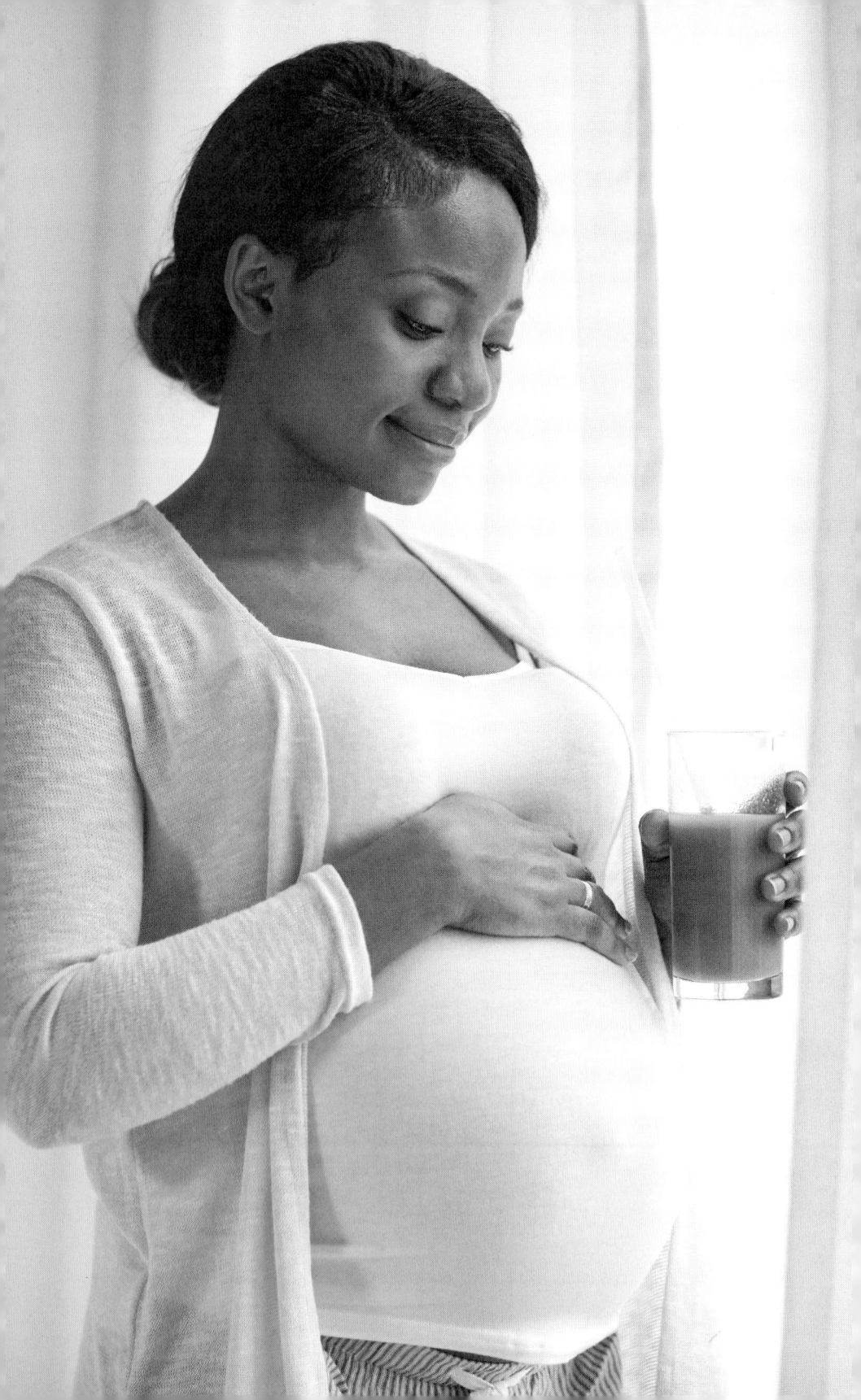

CHAPTER 24

Reducing Risks of Birth Defects

Each year about 1 in 33 babies in the United States is born with a **birth defect**. A birth defect is a condition that is present at birth. Most babies with birth defects are born to couples with no special risk factors. For some birth defects, steps can be taken before and during pregnancy to reduce the risk of having an affected child.

More than 4,000 birth defects, ranging from mild to severe, are known. Some birth defects can be seen right after the baby is born, such as **cleft lip**, **clubfoot**, or extra fingers or toes. Special tests may be needed to find others, such as heart defects or hearing loss. Some birth defects may not be noticed until later in life.

A small number of birth defects are caused by exposure during pregnancy to certain medications, infections, and chemicals. Only a few of these agents are known. How these agents cause birth defects is not completely understood. But for some birth defects, you may be able to decrease your risk by taking certain steps.

This chapter reviews birth defects caused by exposure during pregnancy. See Chapter 33, "Genetic Disorders, Screening, and Testing," for information on birth defects caused by **genetic disorders**.

Teratogens and Pregnancy

A *teratogen* is a drug, chemical, infection, or medical condition that can increase the risk of birth defects. Examples of teratogens include the following:

- Alcohol
- Chemicals and **toxins**, such as lead and mercury
- Some illegal drugs, such as methamphetamines
- Some prescription medications, such as warfarin
- Large amounts of some vitamins and minerals, such as vitamin A
- Some over-the-counter medications
- Infections, such as **chickenpox** (see Chapter 25, "Protecting Yourself From Infections")

Doctors use the word "exposure" when a person comes into contact with something harmful. You can be exposed to toxic agents

- in the air you breathe
- in things you eat or drink, like food, water, and medications
- through direct contact with your skin

Some medical conditions—such as **diabetes mellitus**, **high blood pressure**, and **seizure disorders**—also may be "teratogenic." This means they may increase the risk of certain birth defects. Some of the risk may be due to the condition itself or the medications used to treat it.

Exactly how teratogens may affect your health and the health of your baby depends on many factors, including

- the amount you are exposed to
- how long you were exposed
- how far along you are in your pregnancy
- how your body reacts to the exposures

Many, but not all, agents can be passed from you to the baby through the **placenta**. In some cases, such as with lead, chemicals can build up in the tissues of the baby. This can mean the baby has a much higher exposure than you.

Being exposed to toxic agents at certain times during pregnancy may do more harm than at other times. For example, the baby's major organs form during the first 8 weeks of pregnancy. During these early weeks the baby may be most at risk of harm from exposure. Exposures very early in pregnancy can happen even before you know that you are pregnant.

What Is an Exposure History?

Before you get pregnant, or as soon as you learn you are pregnant, talk with your **obstetrician–gynecologist (ob-gyn)** about agents that you may be exposed to at home or work. This is called an environmental exposure history. Use the "Environmental Exposure History Form" at the back of this book to think about places and situations in which you may be exposed to toxic substances. Think about things such as

- foods you eat
- pesticides for your home or garden
- flea control products for your pets
- personal care products
- household cleaners
- building materials
- supplies for arts, crafts, or other hobbies
- office supplies or other materials in your workplace

Your ob-gyn can help you think about your possible environmental exposure. Once you have a list of the agents you may have contact with, you can find ways to reduce your exposure or to avoid them altogether.

Many pregnant women have questions about potential hazards. Some of the concerns in this chapter include

- medications
- alcohol
- environmental toxins
- infections
- X-rays
- high body temperatures

You can find more information about these and other hazards from the "Resources" section at the end of this chapter. If you have questions about your specific situation, talk with your ob-gyn. He or she may recommend you see a specialist. Remember that not all birth defects can be prevented. Still, it makes sense to avoid known risks.

Medications

Taking a medication during pregnancy is common. Half of all pregnant women take at least one prescription or over-the-counter medication. But not all medications are safe to take when you are pregnant. It's important to know which medications are safe to use and which should be avoided.

Prescription Medications

The U.S. Food and Drug Administration (FDA) requires makers of prescription medications to give detailed information about risks. This information can help ob-gyns and patients make decisions about the known and potential risks of taking a drug during pregnancy. If new information becomes available about a drug, the drug label must be revised to include it.

Before pregnancy or early in your pregnancy, talk with your ob-gyn about the medications you take. Some women need to continue their medications during pregnancy to protect their own health and the health of their babies. How much of a medicine you take during pregnancy may need to be increased or decreased. Or you may need to take a different drug altogether. All decisions should be made with your ob-gyn.

Most medications are considered safe for use during pregnancy. Only a small number of medications are known to cause birth defects. These medications include (but are not limited to)

- *isotretinoin*, used to treat serious, cystic acne
- warfarin, used to manage certain blood conditions
- valproic acid (valproate) and carbamazepine, used to prevent seizures
- angiotensin-converting enzyme inhibitors (ACE inhibitors), used to treat some heart conditions and high blood pressure

For many other prescription medications, the evidence about their effects during pregnancy is not clear or not strong enough to draw a conclusion. The MotherToBaby website and other organizations have information about the safety of many common prescription medications (see the "Resources" section at the end of this chapter).

Remember to tell any health care practitioners who prescribe drugs for you that you are pregnant or thinking about getting pregnant. This includes doctors you see for health conditions, mental health care, and dental problems. Some medications may increase the risk of birth defects slightly, but the benefits of continuing to take the medication during pregnancy may outweigh any risk to your baby.

For example, asthma is a chronic condition that can decrease the level of *oxygen* in your body and the amount of oxygen that reaches your baby. Uncontrolled asthma can lead to growth problems and a smaller-than-normal baby. Problems with a baby's growth also increase the risk of *preterm* birth. It's very important to control asthma, which often involves taking medications.

These considerations also apply to mental illnesses, such as **depression.** If you are taking an **antidepressant** and you get pregnant, you and your ob-gyn should talk about whether you should continue your medication. Sometimes, not taking an antidepressant can cause more problems during pregnancy than taking the medication. If your depression returns, you may have trouble eating, sleeping, and exercising, all of which could affect your pregnancy.

As you can see in these examples, the decision to continue or stop taking a medication is a complex one and depends on several factors, including

- how severe your illness is
- if you currently are having symptoms
- what is known about your medication's risk of causing birth defects

You and your ob-gyn should discuss these factors and weigh the risks and benefits. Do not make decisions about medications on your own. The benefits of continuing to take medication during pregnancy may outweigh any risk to your baby.

Over-the-Counter Medications

You can buy many medications for minor problems at the store without a prescription. These are called over-the-counter medications. Examples include

- pain relievers
- *laxatives*
- antacids
- cold and allergy remedies
- skin treatments
- patches (including heat wraps for pain relief)
- nasal sprays
- smoking cessation aids
- herbal medications
- vitamin supplements

Remember that just because a medication is sold over-the-counter, that doesn't mean it is safe during pregnancy. Also, some over-the-counter medications can affect how your prescription medications work. You and your ob-gyn can talk about over-the-counter medications to avoid.

Cold and indigestion medicines. What should you do if you have a cold or indigestion and want to take an over-the-counter medication? Always talk with your ob-gyn first. You also can try relieving your symptoms without taking medicine. For nasal congestion, drink a lot of water, put a warm washcloth on your face, and use a humidifier to put moisture in the air. For heartburn, do not lie down right after eating. Your ob-gyn may suggest other ideas for you to try, depending on your specific symptoms.

Herbal medications. The FDA considers herbal remedies to be dietary supplements, not drugs. Manufacturers are required to conduct their own safety studies. But the FDA does not oversee this process. There also are no standards for purity or regulation of the ingredients in herbal supplements. For these reasons, it is best to avoid taking herbal supplements during pregnancy.

Prenatal vitamins. You should take one dose of prenatal vitamin every day, as recommended by your ob-gyn. A dose may mean just one vitamin pill or several pills, depending on the brand. If you need an extra amount of a specific vitamin or mineral (such as iron or *folic acid*), take it separately from your prenatal vitamin as a single supplement. Do not take more than one dose of your daily prenatal vitamin. Some ingredients, such as vitamin A, are safe at low doses but can cause birth defects at higher doses.

Alcohol

Drinking alcohol during pregnancy is a leading cause of birth defects. There is no safe level of alcohol use during pregnancy. Alcohol can affect a baby throughout pregnancy, including before many women even know they are pregnant.

Fetal alcohol spectrum disorders (FASD) is a group of physical, mental, behavioral, and learning disabilities that can happen to a baby whose mother drank alcohol during pregnancy. The most severe form of FASD is *fetal alcohol syndrome (FAS)*. FAS causes

- growth problems
- intellectual and behavioral problems
- abnormal facial features

Drinking heavily means having three or more drinks per occasion or more than seven drinks per week. Moderate drinking means having one drink per day. Women who drink heavily throughout pregnancy have the highest risk of having a baby with FAS. But even moderate drinking during pregnancy can affect a child's growth and lead to behavioral and learning problems.

Alcohol-related birth defects are 100 percent preventable by not drinking during pregnancy or when trying to get pregnant. No types of drinks are safe. One beer, one shot of liquor, one mixed drink, or one glass of wine all contain about the same amount of alcohol.

If you drank a small amount of alcohol before you knew you were pregnant, talk with your ob-gyn. There is no need to panic. It is unlikely that drinking a small amount of alcohol very early in pregnancy will cause serious birth defects. The important thing is that you stop drinking alcohol as soon as you find out you are pregnant.

For some women, it may be hard to stop drinking alcohol. If you have trouble stopping, some questions to ask yourself are listed in the box "Do You Have a Drinking Problem?" in Chapter 3, "Months 1 and 2 (Weeks 1 to 8)." Talk with your ob-gyn about your alcohol habits. If you are dependent on alcohol, you may need counseling and medical care. Your ob-gyn can help you connect with these resources.

Environmental Toxins

Exposure to some toxic agents in the environment may have lasting effects on reproductive health. Unfortunately, there is limited information about what things to avoid and how to minimize your risk. Still, there are steps that you can take to reduce your exposure to some of the known chemical teratogens during pregnancy.

Lead

Although lead has not been used in paint and gasoline for a long time, 1 percent of women who are of childbearing age still have unsafe levels of lead in their blood. Lead can be found in

- older homes
- old paint
- water pipes
- soil
- imported pottery, toys, jewelry, candy, medicine, and cosmetics

Also, lead still is used in some manufacturing jobs.

Lead exposure during pregnancy has been linked to high blood pressure and preterm birth. Lead exposure also can affect a baby's brain development. It is not known how much lead is necessary to cause these effects.

If you are at risk of lead exposure, the Centers for Disease Control and Prevention (CDC) recommends that you have a blood test to measure the level of lead in your body. If you have high levels of lead, the source should be found so that you can avoid further contact. Often, avoiding the lead source is enough to decrease the lead levels in your blood to a safe level. If you have a very high level of lead in your body, treatment with medication may be recommended. Lead testing is not recommended for women who are not at risk of lead exposure.

Most women are not exposed to high levels of lead. Follow these tips to reduce your risk:

- Never eat nonfood items such as clay, paint, or soil, because they could be contaminated with lead. A craving for nonfood items is known as **pica**. This craving may be a sign of **anemia** or a nutrient deficiency. If you think you may have pica, talk with your ob-gyn.
- If your home was built before 1978, stay away from repair or remodeling work, including sanding or scraping paint.
- If anyone who lives with you works with lead, they should change into clean clothing before coming home, leave work shoes outside, and wash their work clothes separately.
- Avoid hobbies that use lead glaze.
- Some containers may have lead in them, including imported glazed pottery, pewter, brass, and lead crystal. Do not use them to store, cook, or serve food.

Mercury

Mercury can affect the development of a baby's nervous system. Mercury exposure during pregnancy can lead to

- learning difficulties
- problems with thinking and reasoning
- problems with language and motor skills

A baby can be exposed to mercury if a pregnant woman

- eats certain fish
- uses alternative or traditional remedies containing mercury
- inhales mercury vapors at work

Some fish has higher levels of mercury than others. Fish is a healthy food, and you should eat 8 to 12 ounces (oz) per week to get the benefits of omega-3 fatty acids, which may help your baby's brain development. That's two to three servings per week. To decrease your exposure to mercury in fish, follow these guidelines:

- Eat a variety of fish that have lower levels of mercury, such as salmon, shrimp, pollock, and tilapia.
- Do not eat bigeye tuna, king mackerel, marlin, orange roughy, shark, swordfish, or tilefish.
- Limit albacore tuna to 6 oz a week. Canned light tuna has lower levels of mercury than albacore tuna.

- Check local advisories about the safety of fish caught in waters near where you live. If there is no information available, limit your intake of fish from these waters to no more than 6 oz a week (and do not eat any other fish during that week). See the "Resources" section at the end of this chapter for more information about mercury and fish.

Pesticides

Pesticides are chemicals used to kill bugs, weeds, rodents, and mold. You can be exposed to pesticides from eating fruits or vegetables and from using chemicals in your home or on your pets. Exposure during pregnancy can affect your baby's brain development and may cause childhood leukemia (cancer of the blood). Follow these tips to reduce exposure:

- Do not use pesticides in your home.
- Do not buy chemical tick and flea collars or dips for your pets. Ask your veterinarian about safe options, such as flea tablets for your dog or cat.
- Wash all fruits and vegetables before you eat them, even if you peel them or don't eat the skin.

Infections

Several infections can cause birth defects. These include

- chickenpox
- *cytomegalovirus (CMV)*
- *rubella*
- *syphilis*
- *toxoplasmosis*
- *Zika* virus

It is important to avoid infections and take steps to prevent them if you can. Some infections can be prevented with vaccines (shots), but others cannot.

If you have been exposed to an infection, or if you think you might be at risk, talk with your ob-gyn. See Chapter 25, "Protecting Yourself From Infections."

X-Rays and Other Radiation

Ionizing radiation is the type of *radiation* used in X-rays. There is a belief that exposure to any amount of ionizing radiation will cause birth defects. This is not true. The risk of birth defects is related to the dose. So the higher the dose of radiation, the higher the risk of birth defects.

If you are pregnant or think you might be pregnant, tell the radiology center. The amount of radiation used in a standard X-ray is well below the level needed to harm a baby during pregnancy. In fact, you are exposed to more radiation from a day at the beach or the pool than from a standard X-ray. If you need an X-ray or other type of imaging test while you are pregnant, it is safe to do so provided that certain guidelines are followed:

- The lowest dose of radiation is used (this guideline applies to everyone, not just pregnant women).
- If you need an X-ray that doesn't involve your pelvis, your uterus should be shielded from radiation with a special cover.
- If multiple X-rays or a **computed tomography (CT)** scan are needed, ask if **magnetic resonance imaging (MRI)** is an option for you. MRI does not use radiation.
- **Contrast agents** are substances that are injected into the body during some X-ray or MRI procedures. These agents make it easier to see organs and structures. Contrast agents are not likely to harm the baby. But because not much is known about this, these agents should be used only when the benefits of doing so outweigh the risks.
- There is some concern about contrast agents that contain iodine. In theory, these agents can damage the baby's **thyroid gland**. These agents should be used during pregnancy only if the potential benefit justifies the potential risk to the baby.

Radioisotopes are chemicals that give off radiation. They are used in certain tests and treatments. The amount of radiation given off by radioisotopes in these tests is low. Also, most of them leave the body quickly, so they usually are not dangerous to the baby. But iodine-131 should not be used. High doses of iodine-131 can cause defects in the baby's thyroid gland.

Talk with your ob-gyn about the risks and benefits of procedures that need radiation. Remember that if you do not get a test that you need, it may not be possible to make an important diagnosis. Missing a diagnosis can be harmful to you and your baby, especially if you need treatment.

Also, many pregnant women wonder about radiation during air travel. Radiation exposure increases at higher altitudes, but the level of exposure generally isn't a concern for pregnant women. If you are a frequent flier, talk with your ob-gyn about how much flying is safe for you.

Elevated Core Body Temperature

There is evidence that an elevated body temperature during pregnancy is associated with birth defects. Limit exposure to saunas (no more than 15 minutes) and hot tubs (no more than 10 minutes). Make sure that your head, arms, shoulders, and upper chest are not under the water while you are in a hot tub, so that less of your body area is exposed to heat. Also, talk with your ob-gyn about a safe temperature for bath water.

Hazards in the Workplace

Workplace exposure to toxins is a concern for many women. Some jobs have a higher risk of exposure to chemicals, infections, pesticides, and radiation (see the box "Jobs That Could Be Hazardous During Pregnancy"). If you are concerned about your exposure at work, talk with your ob-gyn.

Jobs That Could Be Hazardous During Pregnancy

Some jobs come with risks of exposure to radiation, toxic chemicals, and infections. Some of these jobs include

- airline staff (pilots, flight attendants, baggage handlers, mechanics)
- animal care worker (veterinarian, vet tech)
- artist (including fine arts and pottery)
- auto shop worker
- beauty salon specialist
- dry-cleaning worker
- electronics worker
- factory worker
- farmer or greenhouse worker
- firefighter
- health care worker
- home renovation worker
- laboratory technician
- printing press worker

If you think you have been exposed to a harmful agent at work, talk with your employer. The Occupational Safety and Health Act protects workers from unsafe and unhealthy conditions in the workplace. As part of this act, the Occupational Safety and Health Administration (OSHA) sets and enforces standards and provides training, outreach, and education. OSHA says the following:

- Employers are responsible for placing warning labels on all hazardous materials. They also must train workers who are at risk of occupational exposure to these materials. Employers must issue personal protective equipment (PPE) at no cost to employees whose job duties put them in contact with workplace hazards.
- Employees are responsible for learning about the hazards in their workplace and for following the established guidelines for protecting themselves.

The National Institute for Occupational Safety and Health (NIOSH) researches workplace hazards and makes recommendations for preventing worker injury and illness. The job of NIOSH is to

- find workplace hazards
- decide how to control them
- suggest ways to limit the dangers

You or your union can request that NIOSH conduct a Health Hazard Evaluation. At the NIOSH website, you can ask an occupational safety and health question or learn more about specific hazards and PPE (see the "Resources" section at the end of this chapter).

Certain state and city laws also give workers and unions the right to ask for the names of chemicals and other substances used in the workplace. If you have questions or concerns, ask your employer or review the websites for OSHA or NIOSH.

Also, when it comes to coronavirus (COVID-19), your employer should follow guidelines from local and state health departments and the CDC. These guidelines can help reduce the risk of infection for employees. If there is a chance you could be exposed to COVID-19 at work, ask your employer about PPE, such as masks, gloves, and other equipment, that can help protect you. See www.acog.org/COVID-Pregnancy for more information.

RESOURCES

Choose Fish and Shellfish Wisely
www.epa.gov/choose-fish-and-shellfish-wisely/
Information from the U.S. Environmental Protection Agency about safe fish consumption.

Lead
www.epa.gov/lead
Information from the U.S. Environmental Protection Agency about lead and how to protect yourself and your family.

MotherToBaby
www.mothertobaby.org
1-866-626-6847
1-855-999-3525 (text messages only)

Fact sheets on the safety of specific medications during pregnancy and breastfeeding, available in English and Spanish. The site, run by the Organization of Teratology Information Specialists (OTIS), also offers information by phone, email, or online chat.

Workplace Safety and Health
National Institute for Occupational Safety and Health: www.cdc.gov/niosh
Occupational Safety and Health Administration: www.osha.gov/workers
Government websites that provide information about workers' rights, workplace safety, and occupational health. Includes information about hazardous chemicals in the workplace.

Your Pregnancy and Childbirth
www.acog.org/MyPregnancy
Website from the American College of Obstetricians and Gynecologists (ACOG) with information on pregnancy, labor, delivery, and postpartum care. Includes the latest information from the experts in women's health care, questions answered by ACOG ob-gyns, pregnancy stories from real women, and an A–Z directory of health topics covering pregnancy and beyond.

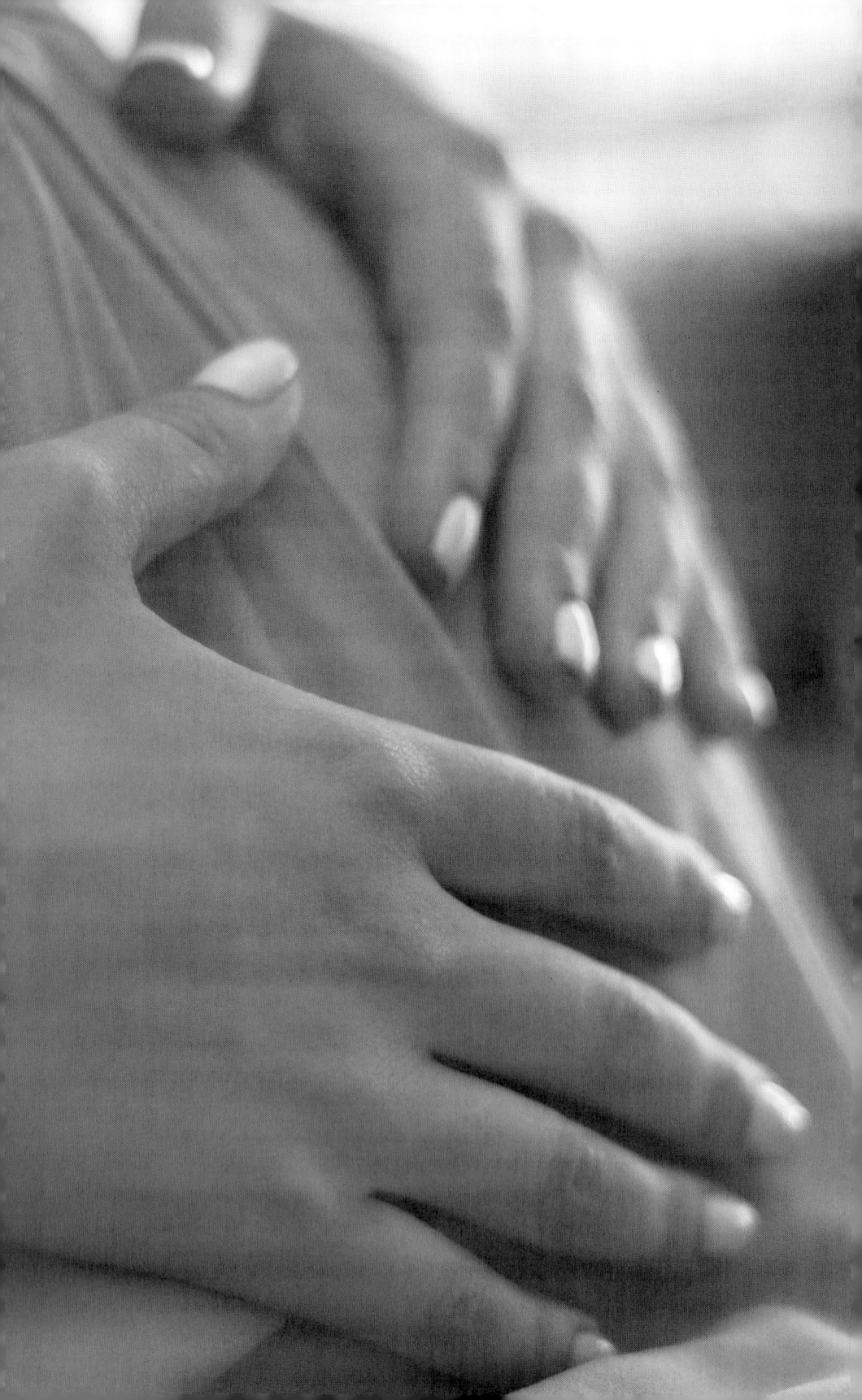

CHAPTER 25

Protecting Yourself From Infections

Certain infections pose risks to you and your baby. Some infections can be passed from you to the baby during pregnancy. Others can be passed to the baby during childbirth. Many of the tests and exams done during **prenatal care** visits are used to detect these infections.

Early diagnosis of infections may help reduce **complications** for you and your baby. But it's better to prevent infection if you can. You can take steps to reduce your risk of some infections by

- getting **vaccines** before and sometimes during pregnancy
- avoiding people who are sick
- practicing safe sex
- washing your hands often
- handling food safely

What Happens During an Infection

Infections are diseases caused by **pathogens**. Pathogens include **bacteria**, **viruses**, fungi, and parasites. When your body is invaded by a pathogen, the **immune system** swings into action. It identifies the pathogen and attacks the infection. Sometimes the immune system makes **antibodies**. These antibodies "tag" pathogens so the immune system can find and kill them.

Some blood tests can show whether antibodies have formed in your body. If they have, it means you have been exposed to that infection or you have had a vaccine to prevent it. In many cases, once the body makes antibodies to a disease, you become *immune* to the disease. This means you will not get that disease in the future.

An infection may not cause any signs or symptoms. For some infections, symptoms happen only as the infection gets worse. If you have any unusual symptoms during pregnancy, tell your **obstetrician–gynecologist (ob-gyn)** right away. Infections caused by bacteria or parasites often can be treated with medications. Some medications can make certain viral infections less severe. The sooner you start treatment, the better.

Vaccine Safety

Vaccines train the immune system to attack specific viruses and bacteria. This makes *vaccination* an important part of preventing infections during pregnancy. Pregnant women and women who are thinking about getting pregnant need certain vaccines. At different points during their lives, babies, children, teens, adults, and seniors all need certain vaccines, too.

Vaccines are subject to strict safety standards. They are approved by the U.S. Food and Drug Administration (FDA) and have been thoroughly researched. But as with any medication, vaccines may have some risks. People react differently. There is no way to predict how a person will react to a specific vaccine.

Most side effects of vaccines are mild, such as a sore arm or a low fever, and go away within a day or two. Severe side effects and reactions are rare. The Centers for Disease Control and Prevention (CDC) monitors reactions for all vaccines given in the United States.

When you get a vaccine, you should get an information sheet that lists the possible side effects associated with that vaccine. If you have ever had a reaction to a vaccine, or if you have concerns about side effects, talk with your ob-gyn. You also can report side effects to the CDC.

How Vaccines Are Made

Most vaccines are made with inactivated (killed) versions of a pathogen. Some vaccines are made with parts of the pathogen or with an inactivated *toxin* made by the pathogen. None of these things can cause the disease itself when given as a vaccine.

Most vaccines also contain some other ingredients. These ingredients may include

- water or other fluids
- preservatives and stabilizers

- chemicals added to inactivate the virus or bacteria
- substances called **adjuvants**, which help create a stronger immune response to the vaccine
- small amounts of the material that was used to grow the virus or bacteria

The amounts of these ingredients are very small. All of them are tested extensively to make sure they are safe. You can learn more about these ingredients at the CDC's website (www.cdc.gov/vaccinesafety).

Certain vaccines should not be given to pregnant women, because they contain live, attenuated viruses. "Attenuated" means that the virus has been weakened so that it cannot cause disease in a healthy person. The vaccines that women should not get during pregnancy include

- ***live, attenuated influenza vaccine*** given as a nasal spray (but the flu shot is safe)
- ***measles–mumps–rubella (MMR) vaccine***
- ***varicella (chickenpox) vaccine***

Coping With Fear of Needles

If you don't like getting shots, you're not alone. As many as 1 in 5 adults have at least some fear of needles. In severe cases, fear of needles can cause light-headedness, nausea, and fainting. Here are some ways to cope:

- Let your ob-gyn know ahead of time that you don't like needles. Also let him or her know if you have ever fainted during or after an injection. You may get a numbing cream or gel for the injection site.
- Remind yourself that getting the shot will take only a few seconds, and that it will help protect you and your baby against infection.
- Don't watch while you get the shot. Distract yourself with music or a game on your smartphone or talk about something else with the person giving you the shot.
- Relaxation techniques and deep breathing may be helpful. But if you have fainted in the past, these techniques may make things worse. Talk with your ob-gyn about other ways to cope.
- Your ob-gyn or a nurse may ask you to sit quietly for 15 minutes after getting the vaccine, in case you have any side effects. Speak up if you feel dizzy, or if you have vision changes or ringing in the ears.

If you need the MMR vaccine or the chickenpox vaccine, get these shots at least 1 month before getting pregnant. During this month, keep using **birth control**.

Vaccine-Preventable Diseases

If possible, you and your ob-gyn should make sure you have had all the vaccines recommended for your age group before you try to get pregnant. But it still is safe to get many of the needed vaccines during pregnancy. See Table 25–1, "Vaccinations and Pregnancy," for the vaccines that are recommended for pregnant women.

Two vaccines that are especially important for pregnant women are the flu vaccine and the **tetanus toxoid, reduced diphtheria toxoid, and acellular pertussis (Tdap) vaccine** (see the sections on "Influenza (Flu)" and "Pertussis (Whooping Cough), Tetanus, and Diphtheria" in this chapter). Other diseases for which there are vaccines include

- **hepatitis A** and **hepatitis B**
- **human papillomavirus (HPV)**
- measles, mumps, and **rubella**
- **meningococcal disease**
- **pneumococcal disease**
- chickenpox

Influenza (Flu)

The flu is a contagious infection of the **respiratory system**. It is caused by a virus. Signs and symptoms include

- fever
- headache
- fatigue
- muscle aches
- coughing
- congestion
- runny nose
- sore throat

The flu is much more serious than a cold. Because of changes to the immune system during pregnancy, pregnant women who get the flu can get much sicker than nonpregnant women who get the flu. It can cause serious complications,

TABLE 25–1 Vaccinations and Pregnancy

Vaccine	When You Should Get It	Can You Get It During Pregnancy?	Notes
Influenza (flu)	Every year, especially if you are pregnant or have risk factors for serious infection	*Injection:* Yes *Nasal spray:* No, because it is a live vaccine	The flu virus changes often, so the vaccine is different every year.
Tetanus, diphtheria, whooping cough (pertussis) (Tdap, Td)	One dose of Tdap vaccine with every pregnancy, preferably during the third trimester. Td booster dose every 10 years	Yes	Talk with your ob-gyn if you haven't had at least three tetanus- and diphtheria-containing shots sometime in your life or if you have a deep or dirty wound. Family members who will be in contact with your baby also should get a dose of Tdap, if they have not been vaccinated.
Hepatitis A*	If you have a specific risk factor for hepatitis A virus infection or simply want to be protected from this disease	Yes	
Hepatitis B*†	If you have a specific risk factor for hepatitis B virus infection or simply want to be protected from this disease	Yes	It's also important that your newborn baby gets started on his or her hepatitis B vaccination series before leaving the hospital.
Human papilloma-virus (HPV)	Before you get pregnant or after you give birth.	No, because it has not yet been studied enough. But if you got it before you realized you are pregnant, this is not a cause for concern.	If you are older than 26, have not been vaccinated, and are at risk of a new HPV infection, you and your ob-gyn can talk about whether you need the HPV vaccine. The vaccine is approved for people through age 45.

continued

TABLE 25–1 **Vaccinations and Pregnancy,** *continued*

Vaccine	When You Should Get It	Can You Get It During Pregnancy?	Notes
Measles–Mumps–Rubella (MMR)	At least 1 month before you get pregnant or after you give birth, if you have never had the vaccine or you have only ever had 1 dose	No, because it is a live vaccine. But if you got it before you realized you are pregnant, this is not a cause for concern.	If you get rubella or are exposed to rubella during your pregnancy, talk with your ob-gyn right away.
Meningo-coccal*	If you have a specific risk factor for meningo-coccal infection: for example, if you are a first-year college student living in a residence hall, you are a military recruit, or you have certain health conditions	Yes	
Pneumo-coccal*	If you have a specific risk factor for pneumo-coccal disease, such as **diabetes mellitus** or lung disease	Yes	
Varicella* (chickenpox)	At least 1 month before you get pregnant or after you give birth, if you have never had chickenpox or the vaccine	No, because it is a live vaccine. But if you got it before you realized you are pregnant, this is not a cause for concern.	If you get varicella or are exposed to varicella during your pregnancy, talk with your ob-gyn right away.

*Talk with your ob-gyn to determine if you need this vaccine.
† Note there is no vaccine for hepatitis C.

such as **pneumonia**. Pregnant women, postpartum women, and babies are at high risk of serious illness from the flu.

The flu vaccine does "double duty" by protecting you and your baby. Babies can't be vaccinated against the flu until they are 6 months old. When you get a flu shot during pregnancy, your body makes antibodies that transfer to your baby. These antibodies will protect your newborn from the flu until he or she is old enough to get the vaccine. And remember, a newborn's immune system is not developed at birth. Any infection that a newborn gets can be very serious and even life-threatening.

How the flu vaccine protects you and your baby

1. Flu vaccine is injected.
2. Antibodies are made.
3. Antibodies are transferred to the baby.

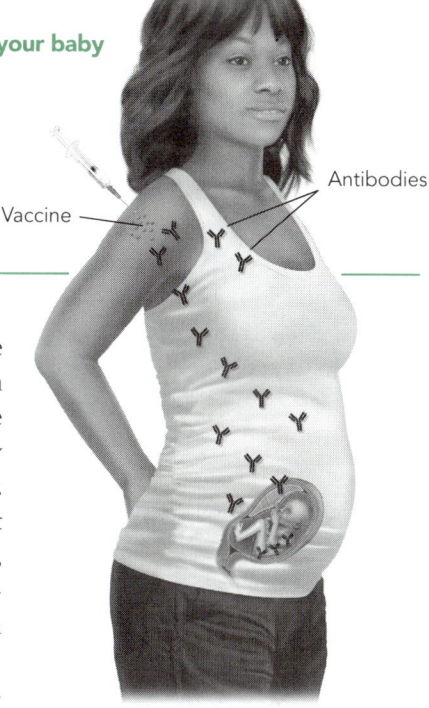

All pregnant women should be vaccinated early in the flu season (October through May) as soon as the vaccine is available, regardless of how far along they are in their pregnancy. Women with medical conditions that increase the risk of flu complications, such as asthma, should consider getting the vaccine before the flu season starts.

Getting the flu shot during pregnancy will not make you sick or harm your baby. Current research shows that approved vaccines do not cause pregnancy problems, **birth defects**, or autism in children. The flu vaccine has been used safely for many years in millions of pregnant women. But pregnant women should not get the flu vaccine that comes as a nasal spray. The nasal spray flu vaccine is not approved for use during pregnancy.

If you do get the flu, or if you have close contact with someone who has the flu, call your ob-gyn right away. He or she may prescribe antiviral medication to reduce your risk of complications. This medication is most effective if you start taking it within 48 hours of having symptoms. But it still may be helpful even if you miss this window.

Pertussis (Whooping Cough), Tetanus, and Diphtheria

Pertussis (whooping cough), tetanus, and diphtheria are caused by bacteria:

- Whooping cough is a highly contagious disease that causes severe coughing. Newborns and babies are at high risk of severe whooping cough, which can be life-threatening.

- Tetanus bacteria can enter the body through a break in the skin. Tetanus can paralyze the breathing muscles. In some cases, tetanus can cause death.
- Diphtheria can restrict breathing and cause death.

The Tdap vaccine is safe and effective against all three diseases.

Because whooping cough is so dangerous for newborns, all pregnant women should get the Tdap vaccine during each pregnancy. The vaccine helps your body make antibodies to protect you from the disease. Just like the flu vaccine, the Tdap vaccine allows antibodies to transfer to your baby. These antibodies can protect your baby until he or she can get the Tdap vaccine at 2 months old.

It is best to get the Tdap vaccine between 27 and 36 weeks of each pregnancy. If you do not get Tdap during pregnancy, you should get it right after you have your baby. If you have family members who will be in close contact with your baby, and they have not been vaccinated with Tdap, they also should get a single dose of Tdap. This dose should be given at least 2 weeks before they have any close contact with the baby.

Hepatitis

Hepatitis is a viral infection that affects the liver. The four common kinds of virus that can cause infection include

- hepatitis A
- hepatitis B
- hepatitis C
- hepatitis D

Hepatitis A virus cannot be passed to a baby during pregnancy, and hepatitis D virus is rare. Hepatitis B virus and hepatitis C virus are of the greatest concern during pregnancy because they are most likely to be passed to the baby.

Hepatitis A and hepatitis B infections can be prevented with vaccines. There currently is no vaccine for hepatitis C. Hepatitis C is discussed in the section "Other Infections" later in this chapter.

Hepatitis A. Hepatitis A is spread by eating food or drinking water that has the virus or through direct contact with an infected person. Signs of hepatitis A infection include

- sudden fever
- loss of appetite
- nausea

- stomach ache
- dark urine
- *jaundice*
- a general feeling of being unwell

The hepatitis A vaccine is recommended for people at increased risk of infection. People at higher risk include those who

- travel to areas where hepatitis A is common
- have a liver disease

The vaccine is safe for women who are pregnant or breastfeeding. A combination vaccine for hepatitis A virus and hepatitis B virus also is available for people 18 and older.

Hepatitis B. Hepatitis B is passed through contact with body fluids. This can happen during unprotected sex or while sharing needles used to inject ("shoot") drugs. Women who work in the health care field also may be exposed to body fluids. A baby can be infected during birth if the pregnant woman has hepatitis B.

Hepatitis B often causes no symptoms. Some people have signs and symptoms, including

- fever
- nausea
- tiredness
- loss of appetite

In most people, the virus goes away by itself. But in some people, the virus does not go away. These people become carriers of the virus who can infect others. Carriers also may develop chronic hepatitis, which can lead to cirrhosis (liver damage), liver cancer, and early death.

If no preventive steps are taken, as many as 9 in 10 women infected with hepatitis B virus will pass the infection to their babies during pregnancy. Hepatitis may be severe in babies and can be life-threatening. Even babies who appear well may be at risk of serious health problems. Infected newborns have a high risk of becoming carriers of the virus.

The hepatitis B vaccine is a series of three shots. The vaccine is safe for pregnant women, postpartum women, and women who are breastfeeding. All babies should get their first dose of hepatitis B vaccine before leaving the hospital after birth. The second dose is given when the baby is 1 to 2 months old. The third dose is given when the baby is 6 to 18 months old.

All pregnant women are tested for hepatitis B infection as part of early *prenatal care*. If you test negative for hepatitis B virus but you have risk factors for getting infected, you should be offered the hepatitis B vaccine. If you test positive, you should be tested again during your third *trimester* to determine how much virus is in your system. Depending on the results of this test, you may be offered antiviral therapy to lower the risk that your baby will be infected.

Babies born to infected mothers will get the first dose of hepatitis B vaccine within 12 hours of birth. They also will get a medication called **hepatitis B immune globulin** (HBIG) soon after birth. HBIG contains antibodies to the virus and may give extra protection against infection. The rest of the shots then will be given over the next 6 months. With this treatment, the chance of the baby getting the infection is much lower. A woman who has hepatitis B infection can breastfeed her baby as long as the baby gets the hepatitis B vaccine and HBIG at birth.

Human Papillomavirus

Human papillomavirus (HPV) is a very common virus that can be passed from person to person. There are more than 150 types of HPV. About 40 types infect the genital area of men and women and are spread by skin-to-skin contact during vaginal, anal, or oral sex. Genital HPV infection can occur even if you do not have *sexual intercourse.* HPV can cause the following diseases:

- Genital warts—Most cases of genital warts are caused by just two types of HPV: 1) type 6 and 2) type 11. Genital warts are growths that can appear on the outside or inside of the **vagina** or on the **penis** and can spread to nearby skin. Genital warts also can grow around the **anus**, on the **vulva**, or on the **cervix**. Genital warts are not cancer and do not turn into cancer. Warts can be removed with medication or surgery.

- Cancer—At least 13 types of HPV are linked to cancer of the cervix, anus, vagina, penis, mouth, and throat. Types of HPV that cause cancer are known as "high-risk types." Most cases of HPV-related cancer are caused by just two high-risk types of HPV: 1) type 16 and 2) type 18.

There is no cure for HPV, so it is best to try to prevent it. There is a vaccine that protects against the HPV types that are the most common cause of cancer and genital warts.

Girls and boys should get the HPV vaccine as a series of shots. Vaccination works best when it is done before a person is sexually active and exposed to HPV. But it still can reduce the risk of getting HPV if given after a person has become sexually active.

The CDC recommends routine HPV vaccination between age 9 and 26. If you are older than 26, have not been vaccinated, and are at risk of a new HPV infection, you and your ob-gyn can talk about whether you need the HPV vaccine. The vaccine is approved for people through age 45.

HPV vaccination during pregnancy is not recommended. It's best to get all HPV shots before getting pregnant. If you get pregnant in between doses of the HPV vaccine, you can complete the shots after having your baby. The vaccine is safe for women who are breastfeeding.

Measles, Mumps, and Rubella

These three diseases are discussed together because they are prevented with a combination vaccine known as the MMR vaccine:

- Measles infection causes fever, runny nose, cough, and a rash all over the body. In more serious cases, ear infection, seizures, pneumonia, or brain damage can result. Some people who get measles can die. Measles spreads easily from person to person.

- Mumps infection starts out with flu-like symptoms including fever, headache, muscle aches, fatigue, and loss of appetite. The salivary glands become swollen and painful. Serious cases of mumps can result in deafness or fertility problems.

- Rubella infection causes a high fever and a rash that last a few days. Pregnant women who get rubella are at risk of *miscarriage*, *stillbirth*, or *preterm* birth. In newborns, rubella can cause a very serious disease called **congenital rubella syndrome (CRS)**. CRS can cause deafness, growth problems, and serious defects of the eyes, heart, and brain. Babies with CRS also are highly contagious and can spread the disease to others.

The MMR vaccine is a live, attenuated vaccine. This means it should not be given during pregnancy. You should use birth control for 1 month after getting the MMR vaccine.

All pregnant women are tested early in their prenatal care to see if they are immune to rubella. If you are not immune (if you do not have antibodies showing a past infection or vaccination against rubella), it is recommended that you get the MMR vaccine right after you give birth. If you get rubella or are exposed to rubella while you are pregnant, contact your ob-gyn right away.

Meningococcal Meningitis

Meningitis is an infection of the coverings of the brain and spinal cord. Meningitis is caused by a type of bacteria called meningococcus and is very serious. The bacteria multiply quickly and can cause severe illness in just 1 or 2 days. Signs and symptoms of meningococcal meningitis include

- high fever
- headache
- stiff neck
- small, dark spots on the arms and legs
- confusion
- nausea
- vomiting
- trouble looking into bright lights

This disease can cause death or serious complications. Some people are more at risk of catching meningococcal meningitis than others. Groups at higher risk include

- babies, teens, and young adults
- people who live in a group setting, such as college students and military personnel
- people who have **human immunodeficiency virus (HIV)**
- people who do not have a working spleen

Getting a vaccine is the best way to prevent meningococcal meningitis infection. You may need this vaccination if

- you have been exposed to someone with meningococcal meningitis
- you're traveling to an area where the illness is common
- you are at higher risk for any reason

Pneumococcal Pneumonia

A type of bacteria called *Streptococcus pneumoniae* spreads easily among people. It can cause lower respiratory tract infections, ear infections, and sinus infections. These infections can be more serious or life-threatening in some people, especially older adults and people with long-term illnesses. In serious cases, the infection can cause bacteremia (bacteria in the bloodstream), meningitis, or pneumonia. The infection also can cause brain damage or hearing loss.

A vaccine is available that prevents pneumococcal pneumonia. The vaccine is recommended for people age 65 and older or for younger adults who have risk factors for pneumonia, such as smoking or **diabetes mellitus.** If you are in a high-risk group and could get pregnant, you should get the vaccine before getting pregnant. If you are already pregnant, talk with your ob-gyn about whether you should get this vaccine. There have been no reports of any harmful effects when the vaccine has been given during pregnancy.

Varicella (Chickenpox) and Herpes Zoster (Shingles)

Varicella, also known as chickenpox, is caused by the **varicella zoster virus**. It causes fever and an itchy rash with fluid-filled blisters, and it can spread easily from person to person. In children, chickenpox usually does not cause serious illness, but there is a risk that the blisters can get infected with bacteria. In adults, chickenpox may cause severe complications, such as pneumonia. Pregnant women are at higher risk of severe chickenpox.

A pregnant woman infected with chickenpox also can pass the virus to her baby. When this happens in the first 28 weeks of pregnancy, it can lead to a rare condition called **congenital varicella syndrome**. This syndrome may cause

- **low birth weight**
- scarring of the baby's skin
- small limbs
- brain and eye defects

When transmission happens later in pregnancy, the baby may develop a painful skin rash known as **herpes zoster (shingles)** early in life.

The chickenpox vaccine is given in two doses 4 to 8 weeks apart. Because the vaccine contains a live, attenuated virus, it is not recommended for pregnant women. If you have never had chickenpox and you have not had the vaccine, it's best to get vaccinated before you try to get pregnant. You also should avoid pregnancy for 1 month after each dose. But if you get the vaccine before you realize that you are pregnant, do not worry. There have been no reports of the baby getting infected when a pregnant woman is vaccinated.

If you are already pregnant and have not had the vaccine, you should have the first dose of vaccine right after you have your baby, before you leave the hospital. It is safe to get the vaccine right away, even if you are breastfeeding. If you have had chickenpox in the past, you do not need to get the vaccine.

If you get chickenpox during pregnancy, symptoms can be treated with an antiviral medication. If you are pregnant and have been near someone with chickenpox, talk with your ob-gyn right away.

Once you've had chickenpox, the virus never leaves your body. It stays in an inactivated state in certain nerves. The virus can be activated later in life and cause shingles. Shingles causes a skin rash and can lead to other complications. People with shingles should stay away from pregnant women who have not been vaccinated and from preterm or low-birth-weight babies until the rash has formed crusts. There is a shingles vaccine, but it is not given to pregnant women.

Sexually Transmitted Infections

Sexually transmitted infections (STIs) are infections that are spread by sexual contact. They can be caused by bacteria, viruses, or parasites. STIs can cause severe damage to the body if they are not diagnosed and treated. Some STIs can be harmful during pregnancy. Pregnant women are screened for some STIs as part of their routine prenatal care. It is important to protect yourself against STIs by following these guidelines:

- Know your sexual partners—The more partners you or your partners have, the higher your risk of getting an STI.
- Use a latex or polyurethane condom—Using a latex or polyurethane condom every time you have vaginal, oral, or anal sex reduces the risk of infection.
- Know that some sex practices increase the risk—Sexual acts that tear or break the skin carry a higher risk of STIs. Anal sex poses a high risk because tissues in the rectum break easily. Body fluids also can carry STIs. Having any unprotected sexual contact with an infected person poses a high risk of getting an STI.

It's a good idea to get tested for STIs before trying to get pregnant. See Chapter 1, "Getting Ready for Pregnancy."

Genital Herpes

Genital herpes is a viral infection that is spread through sexual contact. Symptoms include painful sores and blisters on or around the ***genitals***, anus, and mouth. Other symptoms may include

- swollen glands
- fever
- chills
- muscle aches
- fatigue
- nausea

PROTECTING YOURSELF FROM INFECTIONS • 423

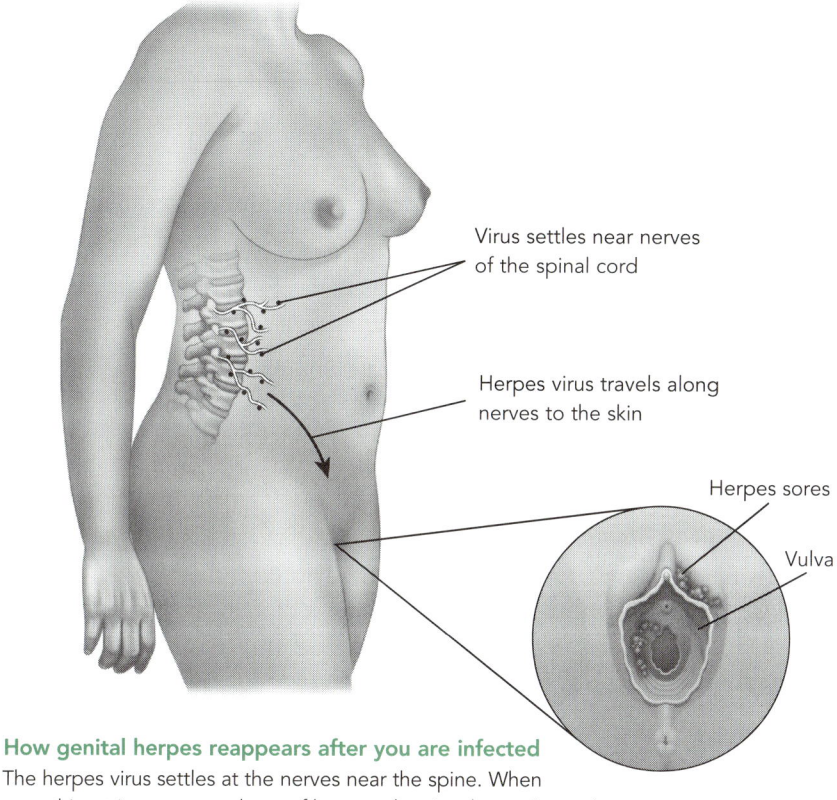

How genital herpes reappears after you are infected
The herpes virus settles at the nerves near the spine. When something triggers a new bout of herpes, the virus leaves its resting place and travels along nerves to the skin. This leads to an outbreak of herpes sores around the vulva.

Sometimes, though, there are no symptoms. There is no cure for genital herpes, but it can be managed.

Herpes infection can cause serious illness in newborns. Herpes can damage a baby's brain and eyes. If a pregnant woman is infected with herpes, it can be passed to the baby during birth when he or she passes through the woman's infected birth canal. The risk is highest when a woman gets herpes for the first time late in pregnancy. The risk is lower in women with a repeated outbreak at the time of delivery.

If you are infected with herpes for the first time during pregnancy, you may be prescribed antiviral medication. This medication may reduce the severity of symptoms and the length of the outbreak. If you have had outbreaks before, you may take antiviral medication during the last several weeks of pregnancy to help reduce the risk of an outbreak at the time of delivery.

If you have sores or warning signs of an outbreak (tingling or burning sensations) at the time of delivery, you may need to have a **cesarean delivery**. A cesarean delivery can reduce the chance of the baby getting infected. The decision depends on many factors, including

- where the sores are on your body
- whether the baby would come into contact with them during delivery

In most cases, you can still breastfeed if you have genital herpes. The herpes virus cannot be passed to a baby through breast milk. But the baby could get infected by touching a sore somewhere else on your body. Make sure any sores that the baby could have contact with are covered when you hold your baby or while breastfeeding. Wash your hands with soap and water before and after feeding your baby. If you have sores on your breast, feed from the other breast.

Gonorrhea and Chlamydia

Both *gonorrhea* and *chlamydia* are caused by bacteria. Women 25 and younger are at greater risk of both infections, although they can happen at any age. Women with these infections often have only mild symptoms or no symptoms at all. Symptoms may include

- discharge from the vagina
- painful or frequent urination
- pain in the pelvis or abdomen
- burning or itching in the vaginal area
- redness or swelling of the vulva
- bleeding between periods
- sore throat with or without fever
- swollen or enlarged lymph nodes

Chlamydia and gonorrhea can cause infections in the mouth, reproductive organs, and *rectum*. In women, the most common place these infections happen is the cervix. From the cervix, the bacteria can spread into the *uterus* and *fallopian tubes* and cause **pelvic inflammatory disease (PID)**. PID is a serious infection that can lead to scarring in the fallopian tubes. This scarring increases the risk of *infertility* and *ectopic pregnancy*. A pregnant woman with untreated chlamydia or gonorrhea has an increased risk of

- *prelabor rupture of membranes (PROM)*
- preterm birth
- fetal growth problems (having a small baby)

Gonorrhea also has been linked to miscarriage and infection of the ***amniotic fluid.***

Gonorrhea and chlamydia can be passed from mother to baby during childbirth. Babies born to infected women may have ***conjunctivitis*** (an infection of the eyes). To prevent conjunctivitis, the eyes of all newborns are treated with eyedrops at birth, regardless of whether the mother is infected. Chlamydia also may cause pneumonia in an infected baby, and gonorrhea may cause infection of the baby's heart, brain, joints, and skin.

If a newborn has signs and symptoms of gonorrhea or chlamydia infection, he or she will be treated with ***antibiotics.*** The mother and her sex partner or partners also need to be treated.

All pregnant women are tested for chlamydia early in pregnancy. Women with certain risk factors also are screened later in pregnancy. Women who are at increased risk of gonorrhea, or who have symptoms, are tested for this infection early in pregnancy and may be tested again in the third trimester. Both infections can be treated with antibiotics during pregnancy. Sex partners also need to be treated.

Human Immunodeficiency Virus

Human immunodeficiency virus (HIV) is the virus that causes ***acquired immunodeficiency syndrome (AIDS).*** HIV is passed through contact with an infected person's body fluids, such as ***semen***, vaginal fluid, or blood. This can happen during sex or by sharing needles used to inject ("shoot") illegal drugs. An infected woman who is pregnant can pass the virus to her baby during labor. Women with HIV also can pass the virus to their babies through breast milk.

Once HIV is in your body, it attacks the immune system. As the immune system weakens, it is less able to resist disease and infections. AIDS is diagnosed when a person infected with HIV develops diseases that the immune system normally would fight off. These diseases include

- pneumonia
- certain types of cancer
- harmful infections

There is no cure for HIV infection, but it can be managed. Drugs are available that can help people with HIV stay healthy for a long time. The earlier treatment is started, the better for your long-term health. Early treatment also reduces your risk of giving the virus to uninfected sex partners. HIV testing is recommended for women who are pregnant or who are thinking about getting pregnant.

If you are pregnant and have HIV, you and your ob-gyn should talk about things you can do to reduce the risk of passing HIV to your baby. They include the following:

- Taking a combination of anti-HIV drugs during your pregnancy as prescribed.
- Having your baby by cesarean delivery if lab tests show that your level of HIV is high.
- Taking anti-HIV drugs during labor and delivery as needed.
- Giving anti-HIV drugs to your baby after birth.
- Not breastfeeding.

By following these guidelines, 99 percent of HIV-infected women will not pass HIV to their babies.

Babies who are born to HIV-positive mothers are tested for HIV several times in the first few months. The test looks for the virus in the baby's blood. The baby has HIV infection if two of these test results are positive. The baby does not have HIV if two of these test results are negative. Another type of HIV test is done when the baby is 12 to 18 months old.

If you are HIV-negative, you have a male partner who is HIV-positive, and you want to get pregnant, talk with your ob-gyn about how to prevent HIV infection. One option may be a medication called **pre-exposure prophylaxis (PrEP)**. PrEP is a pill that you take once a day. If you are exposed to HIV, PrEP may prevent HIV from causing infection. You also can consider taking PrEP while pregnant.

Most experts agree that PrEP is safe to take during pregnancy and while breastfeeding. The drugs in PrEP are used to safely treat women with HIV during pregnancy. There are no reports of birth defects caused by PrEP.

Syphilis

Syphilis is caused by bacteria. The disease happens in stages and is spread more easily in some stages than in others. If it is not treated, syphilis can cause heart and brain damage, blindness, paralysis, and death. If it is found early and treated, syphilis may cause less damage.

Syphilis can be passed from a woman to her baby through the *placenta*. If this happens, there is an increased risk of preterm birth, stillbirth, and death. Babies who are born infected and who survive may have serious health problems involving the brain, eyes, teeth, skin, and bones.

Syphilis causes very few signs or symptoms in the early stage of the disease. A small sore may develop at the site of infection. This sore—called a *chancre*—is painless. It may be in the vagina where it cannot be seen. The chancre heals by itself, but the infection remains. Later symptoms include a rash, sluggishness, or slight fever.

In the very early stages of syphilis, a blood test may or may not find the disease. If you have a chancre, a sample of it can be tested to diagnose syphilis. The chancre will go away even without treatment. After the chancre goes away, the only sure way to diagnose syphilis is with a blood test.

All women are tested for syphilis early in pregnancy. The test may be repeated later in pregnancy if a woman lives in an area where syphilis is common. Syphilis infection during pregnancy is treated with antibiotics. Blood tests are needed to ensure that the treatment is working. Babies born to women who have syphilis or have been treated for syphilis during pregnancy are tested for the infection. If a baby has the infection, he or she is treated.

Trichomoniasis

Trichomoniasis is caused by the microscopic parasite *Trichomonas vaginalis*. Women who have trichomoniasis are at an increased risk of infection with other STIs. There is some research that suggests a link between trichomoniasis and certain pregnancy problems, including

- prelabor rupture of members (PROM)
- preterm birth
- low birth weight

Signs of trichomoniasis may include

- yellow-gray or green vaginal discharge with a fishy odor
- burning, irritation, redness, and swelling of the vulva
- pain during urination

Often, there are no symptoms. To diagnose trichomoniasis, your ob-gyn should take a sample of vaginal discharge and look at it under a microscope. Trichomoniasis can be treated during pregnancy with medication.

Other Infections

Other infections that can affect pregnancy are discussed in this section. These infections cannot be prevented by vaccines. But other steps often can be taken to help prevent them.

Yeast Infection

Yeast infection is caused by the overgrowth of yeast in the vagina. Symptoms may include

- vaginal discharge that is thick and white (like cottage cheese)
- itching around the vagina
- painful urination

To diagnose a yeast infection, your ob-gyn should take a sample of vaginal discharge and look at it under a microscope. Yeast infections can be treated with oral or vaginal antifungal medications.

If you have had a yeast infection before and recognize the symptoms, talk with your ob-gyn before using an over-the-counter medication. If this is the first time you've had vaginal symptoms, it's best to see your ob-gyn.

Bacterial Vaginosis

An imbalance of the bacteria growing in the vagina can cause **bacterial vaginosis (BV)**. It is the most common cause of a vaginal discharge that has a fishy odor. Symptoms may include

- thin grayish or white discharge
- worse odor after having sex
- itching of the vulva and vagina

Half of women with BV do not have any symptoms. BV is not an STI.

To diagnose BV, your ob-gyn should take a sample of vaginal discharge and look at it under a microscope. The acidity of your vagina also may be tested using a pH test strip. If BV is diagnosed in a pregnant woman who has symptoms, treatment is recommended. Treatment involves oral medication or medication inserted into the vagina.

Some studies suggest that women who have BV during pregnancy are at higher risk of prelabor rupture of membranes (PROM) or preterm birth. At this time, routine screening of pregnant women without symptoms is not recommended. But in women with high-risk pregnancies, some research shows that screening for and treating BV with oral antibiotics may reduce the risk of preterm PROM and preterm birth.

Urinary Tract Infection

Urinary tract infections (UTIs) are common. These are infections of the **bladder**, **kidney**, or **urethra**. Severe infections can cause problems for both you and the baby, so it is important to treat these infections early. Because some UTIs may not cause symptoms, you will be tested at your first prenatal visit. If an infection is found, it can be treated with antibiotics.

When an infection of the bladder does cause symptoms, they may include

- burning pain when you urinate
- an increased urge to urinate
- blood in the urine
- abdominal pain

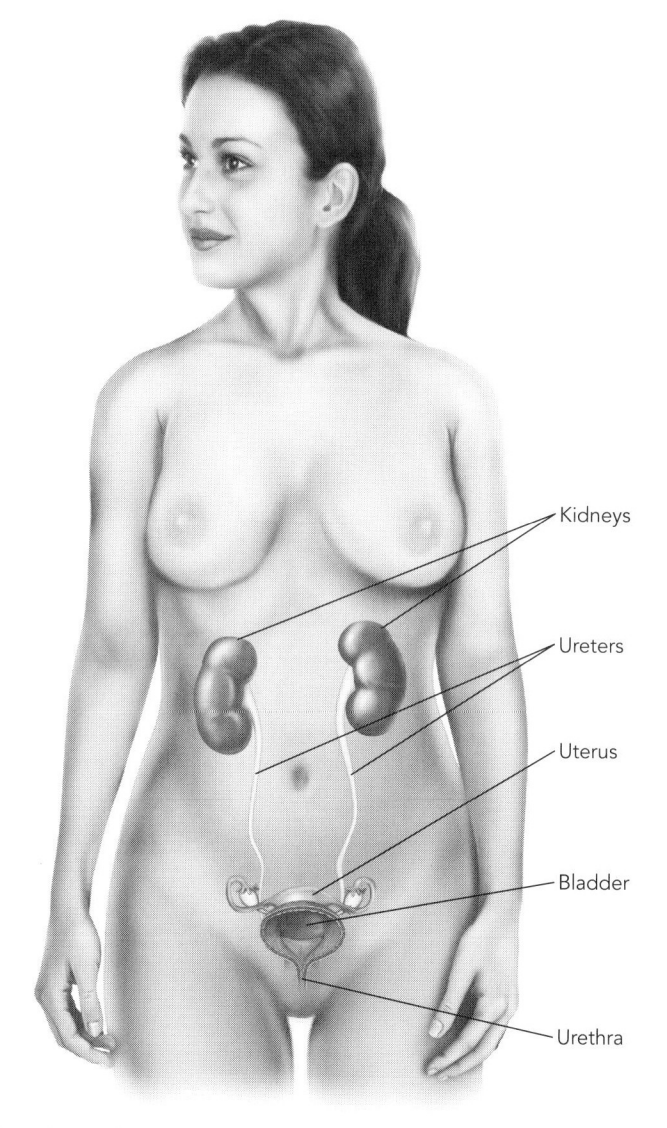

Female urinary tract. If not treated, an infection of the bladder can spread to the kidneys.

It is very important to finish medications prescribed for a bladder infection, even after your symptoms go away.

If a bladder infection is not treated or is not cured by treatment, it may result in a kidney infection called *pyelonephritis*. This infection can cause

- chills
- fever
- back pain
- rapid heart rate
- nausea
- vomiting

Contact your ob-gyn right away if you have any of these symptoms so that you can be treated with antibiotics. If left untreated, pyelonephritis can lead to preterm labor or severe infection.

Cytomegalovirus

Cytomegalovirus (CMV) is a common virus. As many as 8 in 10 women in the United States get infected with CMV by age 40. Some women are infected for the first time during pregnancy. CMV is hard to detect because it rarely causes symptoms. When it does, the symptoms include

- fever
- sore throat
- fatigue

Healthy people generally do not need treatment for CMV infection. But those who have other illnesses may need treatment with antiviral medications.

Women usually get infected through contact with an infected person's body fluids, such as urine, saliva, blood, and semen. Health care workers and people who work with children are most at risk of getting the infection. The virus can pass to the baby through the placenta or after birth through contact with the mother's infected body fluids. This is more likely to happen if the infection happens for the first time during pregnancy or if a past infection has been reactivated, especially in the last trimester of pregnancy.

CMV infection can cause serious problems in babies who are infected before birth. These problems include

- jaundice
- neurologic problems
- hearing loss

Cytomegalovirus is the leading cause of hearing loss in children in the United States. Developmental delays are common. There is no treatment for CMV. Some people who are sick with other diseases may be given antiviral medication if they get CMV. Babies who are infected with CMV at birth may be treated with an antiviral, but this treatment carries significant risks.

If you are concerned about CMV infection, talk with your ob-gyn about being tested. You can take some simple steps to avoid CMV infection:

- Wash your hands with soap and water after changing diapers, feeding a child, or handling a child's toys.
- Be careful when kissing a child to avoid contact with the child's saliva.
- Do not share eating utensils or toothbrushes with children.

Preterm babies and low-birth-weight babies are at risk of being infected through breast milk. Breastfeeding is not recommended if you are infected with CMV and your baby is preterm.

Group B Streptococcus

Group B streptococcus (GBS) is one of the many bacteria that live in the body. In women, GBS most often is found in the **vagina** and **rectum**. GBS usually does not cause problems in adults. But if GBS is passed from a woman to her baby during birth, the baby may get sick. This is rare and happens to 1 or 2 babies out of 100 when the mother does not receive treatment with antibiotics during labor. The chance of a newborn getting sick is much lower when the mother receives treatment.

Pregnant women should have a screening test for GBS between 36 and 38 weeks of pregnancy as part of routine prenatal care. A swab is used to take a sample from the vagina and rectum. The sample is sent to a lab for testing.

If the results show that GBS is present, most women will receive antibiotics through an *intravenous (IV) line* once labor has started. The best time for treatment is during labor. This is done to help protect the baby from being infected.

You likely will have a GBS test during each pregnancy no matter what your test results were in a past pregnancy. In some cases, you automatically will be given antibiotics during labor without testing for GBS. Antibiotics may be given without testing if

- you had another child who had GBS disease
- you have GBS bacteria in your urine at any point during your pregnancy
- your GBS status is not known when you go into labor and you have a fever

- your GBS status is not known and you go into labor before 37 weeks
- your GBS status is not known and it has been 18 hours or more since your water broke
- your GBS status for this pregnancy is not known but you tested positive for GBS in a past pregnancy

Penicillin is the antibiotic that is most often given to prevent GBS disease in newborns. If you are allergic to penicillin, tell your ob-gyn before you are tested for GBS. You may have a skin test to determine the severity of your allergies. If needed, other antibiotics can be used.

If you are having a planned cesarean delivery, you do not need antibiotics for GBS during delivery as long as your labor has not started and your water has not broken. But you should still be tested for GBS because labor may happen before the planned delivery. If your test result is positive, your baby may need to be monitored for GBS disease after birth.

It's important for you to know your GBS test result. If you go into labor away from home, you can tell your caregivers if you need antibiotics during labor.

Hepatitis C Infection

Hepatitis is a viral infection that affects the liver. Hepatitis A and hepatitis B infections are discussed earlier in this chapter under "Vaccine-Preventable Diseases." To date, there is no vaccine for hepatitis C virus. Hepatitis B and hepatitis C are of the greatest concern during pregnancy because they are the most likely to be passed to the baby.

The hepatitis C virus is spread by direct contact with infected blood. This can happen by

- sharing needles used to inject ("shoot") drugs
- sharing household items that come into contact with blood
- accidentally being stuck with a needle (for health care workers)

A baby can be infected during birth if the pregnant woman has a hepatitis C infection. It also can be spread during unprotected sex, but it is harder to spread the virus this way. It is not spread by casual contact or breastfeeding.

Hepatitis C virus infection can cause signs and symptoms similar to those of hepatitis B virus infection, or it can cause no symptoms. Unlike hepatitis B virus infection, most adults infected with the hepatitis C virus become carriers. Most carriers develop long-term liver disease. A smaller number will develop cirrhosis (liver damage) and other serious, life-threatening liver problems. About 4 in 100 pregnant women who are infected with the hepatitis C virus will pass it to their babies. The risk is related to how much of the virus a woman has and whether she also is infected with HIV.

The CDC recommends testing for hepatitis C virus for all adults. If you are infected with the hepatitis C virus, your baby will be tested, usually when he or she is at least 18 months old. There is no newborn vaccine as there is with hepatitis B. Babies who get infected with the hepatitis C virus will need ongoing medical care. You also will need long-term health care. Various antiviral drugs are used to treat people infected with the hepatitis C virus, but they are not currently approved for use during pregnancy.

Cesarean birth does not lower the risk of transmission to the baby. You can still breastfeed your baby if you are infected with hepatitis C.

Listeriosis

Listeriosis is a serious infection caused by eating food contaminated with the bacterium *Listeria monocytogenes*. Pregnant women are about 20 times more likely than other healthy adults to get listeriosis. About 1 in 3 listeriosis cases happen during pregnancy.

If you get infected during pregnancy, you may have symptoms similar to the flu. The infection is very serious and can lead to miscarriage, stillbirth, preterm birth, or infection of the baby. Prompt diagnosis and treatment may prevent the baby from getting infected. Listeriosis is diagnosed with a blood test and is treated with antibiotics. See Chapter 22, "Nutrition During Pregnancy," for tips on reducing your risk of listeriosis.

Parvovirus

Parvovirus is a contagious infection also known as "fifth disease." It's common among school children. If you had it during your childhood, you aren't likely to get it again. Symptoms of parvovirus include

- cold-like symptoms
- rash on the cheeks, arms, and legs
- pain and swelling in the joints that can last from days to weeks

Parvovirus may cause miscarriage or anemia of the baby that can lead to heart failure and stillbirth.

If you think you have been exposed to parvovirus or have any of the symptoms, see your ob-gyn. A test can be done to see if you have the infection. If you do, you may need to have **ultrasound exams** for a few weeks to check the health of the baby.

Toxoplasmosis

Toxoplasmosis is a disease caused by a parasite that lives in soil. People can be infected by

- eating raw or undercooked meat
- eating unwashed vegetables
- having contact with animal feces, especially from cats that spend time outdoors

Toxoplasmosis may cause no symptoms. When symptoms do appear, they are like flu symptoms, such as fatigue and muscle aches.

If you are infected for the first time while you are pregnant, you can pass the disease to your baby. Toxoplasmosis can cause birth defects, including hearing loss, vision problems, and intellectual disability.

To protect against toxoplasmosis, make sure that you eat well-cooked meat and wear gloves while gardening or handling unwashed vegetables. Wash cutting boards, counters, utensils, and hands with hot soapy water after contact with raw meat, poultry, seafood, or unwashed fruits or vegetables (see the "Food Safety" section in Chapter 22, "Nutrition During Pregnancy.")

If you have an outdoor cat that uses a litter box, have someone else empty it. If you must empty the litter box, use gloves and wash your hands well after doing so. Do not adopt or handle stray cats, especially kittens. Do not get a new cat while you're pregnant.

If you are infected during pregnancy, medication may be available. You and your baby should be monitored closely during your pregnancy and after your baby is born.

Tuberculosis

Tuberculosis (TB) is a disease caused by bacteria. These bacteria are carried through the air when infected people cough or sneeze. TB infection usually happens in the lungs.

If your ob-gyn determines that you have risk factors for TB, such as moving from a country that has a high rate of TB infection, you should be tested with a skin test or a blood test during pregnancy. If the test results are positive, you will need a chest X-ray or sputum culture test to confirm the result.

TB can be either active or latent. Active TB symptoms include

- fever
- weight loss
- night sweats
- cough

- chest pain
- fatigue

Active TB usually shows up on a chest X-ray.

Latent TB usually does not cause any symptoms and will not show up on a chest X-ray. Most people who are infected with TB have latent TB. Their bodies stop the bacteria from growing. The bacteria become inactive but remain in the body and can become active later.

In pregnant women with latent TB who have a normal chest X-ray, treatment of latent TB may be delayed until 2 to 3 months after delivery. Women with latent TB that threatens to become active should get treatment during pregnancy. Most experts recommend waiting until the second trimester of pregnancy to begin treatment. Medication needs to be taken for 2 to 9 months. It is safe to breastfeed while getting treatment for latent TB.

For women with active TB, treatment with several different drugs (called multidrug therapy) is given. Therapy lasts at least 6 months. There is no published information about the safety of the drugs used to treat active TB in pregnancy. But they have been used in pregnant women with no clear problems for either the woman or the baby.

TB can be passed to the baby before birth through the placenta or after birth if the baby inhales infected body fluids. In these rare cases, the baby will be treated after birth. Women with TB can breastfeed, but they need to be careful not to expose their babies to coughing or sneezing. Talk with your ob-gyn or your baby's doctor if you have questions.

Zika Virus

Zika virus has been found in South America, Central America, and North America. Infection with the virus during pregnancy can cause serious birth defects, including ***microcephaly*** (a birth defect in which a baby's head and brain are smaller than normal) and other brain abnormalities. These birth defects can lead to lifelong problems, including seizures, feeding problems, hearing loss, vision problems, and learning difficulties. There still are many things that researchers do not know about Zika virus.

Zika virus can be transmitted through the bite of an infected mosquito or through sex with an infected partner. Many people infected with Zika virus will not have symptoms or will have only mild symptoms, including

- fever
- rash
- joint pain
- red, itchy eyes

Infection during pregnancy, even infection without symptoms, can be passed from a woman to her baby. There is no vaccine against Zika virus, and as of 2020, there is no treatment for it.

To avoid Zika virus, take strict steps to avoid mosquito bites. If your male partner lives in or travels to an area where Zika virus is spreading, use a condom each time you have sex. Do not travel to areas where Zika virus is known to be active.

If you or your partner must travel to an area where Zika virus is active, strictly follow these four steps to prevent mosquito bites:

1. Use EPA-registered bug spray with DEET, picaridin, IR3535, oil of lemon eucalyptus, para-menthane-diol, or 2-undecanone. Used as directed, these sprays are safe for pregnant and breastfeeding women.

2. Wear long-sleeved shirts and long pants.

3. Treat clothing and gear with permethrin or buy permethrin-treated items.

4. Stay in air-conditioned or screened-in areas during the day and at night.

Follow these steps at all times. Mosquitoes are active during the day and night. (These steps also can be taken to protect yourself if you are traveling in an area with *malaria*, another disease that is spread by mosquitoes.)

If you or your sexual partner have traveled or live in an area where Zika is present, or if one of you has symptoms of Zika virus infection, see your ob-gyn. You may need to be tested for Zika virus infection, although this test cannot always confirm or rule out infection. If you have had Zika virus in the past, this may make it harder to interpret the results.

If you do test positive for Zika virus infection, you and your ob-gyn should discuss what it means for your pregnancy and talk about your options. Your ob-gyn may need to follow your baby's growth more closely. You may be referred to a ***maternal–fetal medicine (MFM) specialist*** or an infectious disease specialist. After your baby is born, tell your baby's doctor that you had Zika virus during pregnancy.

The CDC and the World Health Organization recommend that women breastfeed, even if they have Zika virus or live in an area where the virus is common. If you have questions about Zika virus and breastfeeding, talk with your ob-gyn and your baby's doctor.

There are many things you can do to stay healthy and avoid infections when you travel. See Chapter 26, "Work and Travel During Pregnancy."

RESOURCES

Coronavirus (COVID-19)
www.cdc.gov/coronavirus/2019-ncov/index.html
Website from the Centers for Disease Control and Prevention (CDC) with the most up-to-date information on the coronavirus.

Coronavirus (COVID-19), Pregnancy, and Breastfeeding: A Message for Patients
www.acog.org/COVID-Pregnancy
Webpage from the American College of Obstetricians and Gynecologists (ACOG) with frequently asked questions about coronavirus, pregnancy, and breasfeeding.

People at Risk: Pregnant Women
www.foodsafety.gov/people-at-risk/pregnant-women
Guide from the U.S. Department of Health and Human Services that provides practical information for avoiding foodborne illness during pregnancy (and at any time).

Pregnancy and Vaccination
www.cdc.gov/vaccines/pregnancy/pregnant-women
Information from the CDC on vaccination before, during, and after pregnancy. Includes a quiz to help you figure out which vaccines you need.

Pregnant Travelers
wwwnc.cdc.gov/travel/page/pregnant-travelers
Advice from the CDC on staying healthy during international travel.

Sexually Transmitted Diseases (STDs)
www.cdc.gov/std
Provides current information from the CDC about sexually transmitted infections, including signs and symptoms, treatment, and prevention.

Vessel Sanitation Program
www.cdc.gov/nceh/vsp/
CDC website that lists sanitation inspection scores for national and international cruise ship lines.

Zika Virus: Pregnancy
www.cdc.gov/zika/pregnancy/
Frequently updated CDC site with the latest news about Zika virus and pregnancy, how to protect yourself, and travel information.

Your Pregnancy and Childbirth
www.acog.org/MyPregnancy
Website from ACOG with information on pregnancy, labor, delivery, and postpartum care. Includes the latest information from the experts in women's health care, questions answered by ACOG ob-gyns, pregnancy stories from real women, and an A–Z directory of health topics covering pregnancy and beyond.

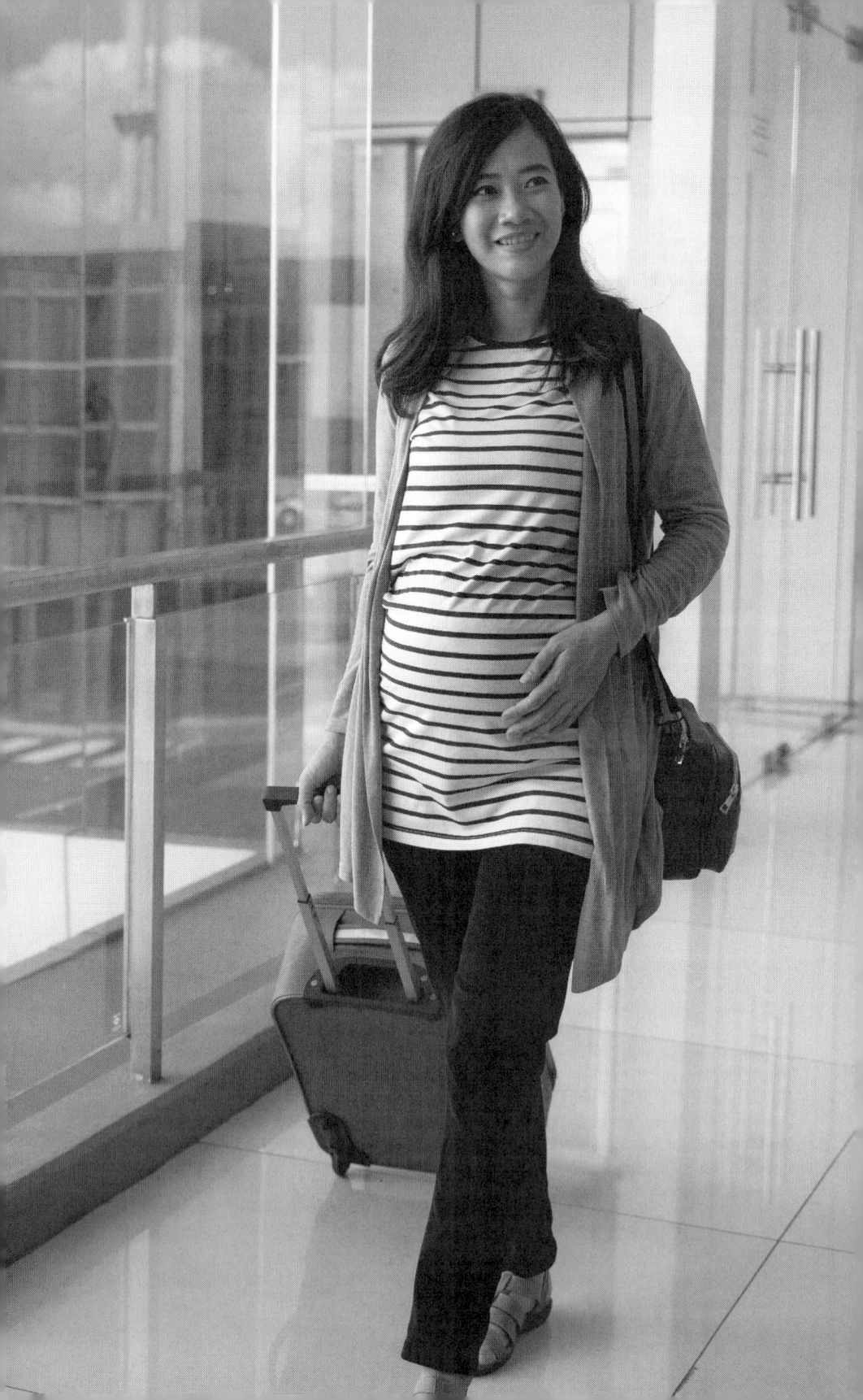

CHAPTER 26

Work and Travel During Pregnancy

When you're pregnant, you need to think about things that may not have occurred to you before. This includes safety in your workplace and safety when you travel. Along with work concerns, you also may be thinking about health insurance for your newborn or yourself. This chapter looks at workplace concerns and health insurance coverage. The chapter also discusses tips for safe domestic and international travel during pregnancy.

As this book went to press, many women had questions about travel during the coronavirus (COVID-19) health crisis. Before making any plans to travel while COVID-19 is spreading, talk with your ***obstetrician–gynecologist (ob-gyn)***. Together you can talk about whether your travel is essential or could be avoided. If it is essential that you travel, together you can make a plan to help you minimize risk.

For more information, visit the COVID-19 travel website of the Centers for Disease Control and Prevention (CDC): www.cdc.gov/coronavirus/2019-ncov/travelers/index.html. You also can read about COVID and pregnancy at the website of the American College of Obstetricians and Gynecologists (ACOG): www.acog.org/COVID-Pregnancy.

Your Workplace Rights

Several federal laws protect the health, safety, and employment rights of many pregnant working women. Many states also have laws that protect pregnant workers.

Requesting Workplace Accommodations

Working during pregnancy generally is safe. But you may need to ask your employer to modify the work you do if

Lifting, Bending, and Standing

For most women, normal amounts of physical activity aren't a problem during pregnancy. But some studies have found that some activity may increase the risk of miscarriage or preterm birth, including

- heavy lifting
- bending a lot
- standing or walking for 3 hours or more a day

Some demanding activities can cause low back pain or injury, including

- heavy lifting
- repetitive motions
- awkward postures
- long periods of sitting or standing

If your job requires any of these things, discuss it with your ob-gyn.

The National Institute for Occupational Safety and Health (NIOSH) has lifting recommendations for pregnant workers. Here are some guidelines for lifting safely:

- Always try to lift with both hands.
- Do not twist your body while you lift.
- Do not lift anything lower than about the middle of your shins.
- Do not lift anything higher than your head. Ideally, whatever you are lifting should be 28 to 52 inches above the ground before, during, and after the lift.
- It is safest to lift close to your body.
- Objects you lift should weigh no more than 36 pounds before 20 weeks of pregnancy and no more than 26 pounds after 20 weeks. The weight limits are lower for women who lift more often, higher, lower, or farther from the body. Your ob-gyn can help you figure out your limits.

- your job exposes you to hazards such as heavy metals, solvents, pesticides, infections, or **radiation** (see Chapter 24, "Reducing Risks of Birth Defects")
- you need to do heavy lifting, stand, or walk for 3 hours or more a day, or bend a lot (see the box "Lifting, Bending, and Standing")
- you have a higher risk of falls or injuries, especially later in your pregnancy when your balance and center of gravity have changed
- you have any pregnancy **complications** that are affected by your work conditions

In these situations, workplace accommodations can help you continue to work safely. A workplace accommodation is a change in your work environment or the way you do your job. Examples of reasonable accommodations include

- sitting if you normally stand
- more frequent bathroom breaks
- time off for medical appointments
- help with lifting

You and your ob-gyn should discuss your work and figure out whether you need any accommodations. In some cases, your ob-gyn may need to write a note to your employer. It's important to be as specific as possible about your situation and your needs. The Pregnant@Work website has state-by-state guidance to help ob-gyns write work accommodation notes. See the "Resources" section at the end of this chapter.

Some tasks are considered "essential functions" of a job, which means that your employer may not be able to accommodate a change. For example, if you have a desk job, lifting may not be considered an essential function. But if you work in a warehouse, lifting may be required. In some cases, your employer may be able to find a different, less strenuous job that you can do while you are pregnant. But if not, you may need to take medical leave (if it is available) or risk losing your job. There are hotlines that can help you understand your rights and your options (see the "Resources" section at the end of this chapter). Discuss any concerns with your ob-gyn.

Pregnancy Discrimination Act

The Pregnancy Discrimination Act prohibits discrimination against women who are affected by pregnancy, childbirth, or related medical conditions. The act applies to employers with 15 or more employees. If you have questions, contact the U.S. Equal Employment Opportunity Commission (see the "Resources" section at the end of this chapter).

Occupational Safety and Health Act

The Occupational Safety and Health Act (OSH Act) requires employers to provide a safe workplace. This means a workplace free from things that can or may be likely to cause serious physical harm or death, such as chemicals and radiation. The OSH Act also requires employers to give workers facts about harmful agents (see Chapter 24, "Reducing Risks of Birth Defects"). If you have concerns about safety in your workplace, visit the OSHA website (see the "Resources" section at the end of this chapter).

The National Institute for Occupational Safety and Health (NIOSH) researches workplace hazards and makes recommendations for preventing injury and illness. Established by OSHA, NIOSH finds workplace hazards, decides how to control them, and suggests ways to limit the dangers. You or your union can request that NIOSH conduct a Health Hazard Evaluation. If you have questions, go to the NIOSH website (see the "Resources" section at the end of this chapter).

Family and Medical Leave Act

The Family and Medical Leave Act (FMLA) provides eligible employees with up to 12 work weeks of leave without pay in any 12-month period. Under FMLA, you have a right to return to your same job or to an equivalent job at the end of your leave. To qualify for FMLA, you must meet the following conditions:

- Work for a company where there are at least 50 employees of the same employer within a 75-mile area (branch offices included)
- Have worked there for at least 12 months (these months do not need to be consecutive but need to have been within the last 7 years)
- Have worked at least 1,250 hours during the past 12 months

During pregnancy and after your baby is born, FMLA can be taken for

- *prenatal care* visits
- incapacity due to pregnancy (such as severe morning sickness)
- recovery from childbirth
- caring for a newborn (until the baby is 12 months)

Partners can use FMLA during pregnancy to care for spouses who have an illness or other condition related to pregnancy or childbirth. Partners also can use FMLA to care for their newborns.

The 12 weeks do not have to be taken all at once. They can be taken in segments, but your FMLA leave cannot exceed a total of 12 weeks per 12-month period. This means that if you use some of the 12 weeks for a difficult pregnancy, you will have fewer than 12 weeks to take after the baby is born.

You may have to use vacation time or personal or sick leave for some or all of your FMLA leave. If your employer provides health care benefits, this coverage must be kept at the same level during the leave period. Many states have laws that are like FMLA. In some cases, a state's FMLA gives more weeks of job-protected leave than the federal FMLA. See the "Resources" section at the end of this chapter for more on FMLA.

Break Time for Nursing Mothers Law

The Break Time for Nursing Mothers Law is part of the Affordable Care Act. Most hourly workers and some salaried workers are covered. Under this law, most employers must provide reasonable break time and a private space (not a bathroom) to express or pump breast milk for up to a year after birth (see Chapter 20, "Feeding Your Baby").

Health Insurance

There are many options for health insurance. If you are employed, you may have health insurance through your employer. Most employers with 50 or more full-time employees must provide insurance to their full-time employees or pay a tax penalty.

If you are not employed, or if your employer does not offer health insurance, you can purchase a health insurance plan through the health insurance Marketplace. Marketplace plans are offered through State Health Insurance Exchanges. You usually must sign up for this coverage during an open enrollment period. But you may be able to sign up outside this period if you recently moved, lost qualifying health coverage, or had a baby. Insurance plans cannot deny you coverage because you are pregnant or have a preexisting medical condition. See the "Resources" section at the end of this chapter for information on the website Healthcare.gov.

With some exceptions, all health insurance plans must provide certain benefits, including

- maternity care
- preventive care
- pediatric care services

All health insurance plans must provide breastfeeding support, counseling, and equipment (such as breast pumps) for as long as you breastfeed your baby. Talk with your ob-gyn about how to access benefits and services. See Chapter 20, "Feeding Your Baby," for information on how to get a breast pump through your insurance plan.

Tax credits are available to help qualified people and families purchase insurance through the Marketplace. People at certain income levels may qualify for government-funded health care, such as Medicaid. When you sign up for health insurance coverage at Healthcare.gov, you will answer questions about your annual income to see if you qualify. The government-funded health care offered in the United States includes the following programs:

- Medicaid—Medicaid is a state-run program that is funded by the federal government. Medicaid provides medical assistance for low-income families and single people.

- State Children's Health Insurance Program—The State Children's Health Insurance Program (SCHIP) provides health coverage to children, up to age 19 years, whose families have incomes too high to qualify for Medicaid but can't afford private coverage. SCHIP gives federal matching funds to states to provide this coverage. See the Insure Kids Now information in the "Resources" section to find out more about SCHIP in your state.

Travel During Pregnancy

As this book went to press, many women had questions about travel during the coronavirus (COVID-19) health crisis. Before making any plans to travel while COVID-19 is spreading, talk with your ob-gyn. Together you can talk about whether your travel is essential or could be avoided. If it is essential that you travel, together you can make a plan to help you minimize risk.

In terms of pregnancy, most women can travel safely until close to their due dates. But travel may not be recommended for women who have pregnancy complications.

The best time to travel is mid-pregnancy (14 to 28 weeks). During these weeks, your energy has returned, morning sickness is over or improved, and you are still easily mobile. After 28 weeks, it may be harder to move around or sit for a long time.

When choosing how you will travel, think about how long it will take to get where you are going. The fastest way often is the best. Whether you go by train, plane, car, or boat, think ahead about your comfort and safety. Here are some tips for healthy travel:

- Have a *prenatal care* checkup before you leave.
- If you'll be far from home, take a copy of your health record with you.
- Wear comfortable shoes and clothing that doesn't bind. Wear a few layers of light clothing that can easily be added or removed.

- Eat regular meals to boost your energy. Be sure to get plenty of fiber to ease constipation, a common travel problem.
- Drink extra fluids. Take some water with you. The air on airplanes is very dry. If you are offered a drink, choose water instead of a soft drink.
- Know how to locate a health care practitioner in case you need one. If you need a doctor while traveling in the United States, visit the American Medical Association's website and use the DoctorFinder tool. You also can find an ob-gyn at the website of the American College of Obstetricians and Gynecologists (ACOG). See the "Resources" section at the end of this chapter.
- Buy travel insurance to cover tickets and deposits that can't be refunded. Pregnancy problems can come up at any time and prevent you from leaving.

A concern for all travelers—not just pregnant women—is ***deep vein thrombosis (DVT)***. Learn about preventing this condition before you start your trip (see the box "Deep Vein Thrombosis and Travel").

Deep Vein Thrombosis and Travel

Deep vein thrombosis (DVT) is a condition in which a blood clot forms in the veins, usually in the leg. DVT can lead to a dangerous condition called pulmonary embolism, in which a blood clot travels to the lungs. Research shows that any type of travel lasting 4 hours or more—whether by car, train, bus, or plane—doubles the risk of DVT. Being pregnant is an extra risk factor for DVT.

If you are planning a long trip, take the following steps to reduce your risk of DVT:

- Drink lots of fluids without caffeine.
- Wear loose-fitting clothing.
- Walk and stretch at regular intervals. For example, when traveling by car, make frequent stops so you can get out and stretch your legs.

Special stockings that compress the legs, either below the knee or full length, also can be worn to help prevent blood clots from forming. Talk with your ob-gyn before you try these stockings. Some people should not wear them (for example, those with diabetes and other circulation problems). Also, compression stockings can increase the risk of DVT if they are too tight or worn incorrectly.

International Travel

If you are planning a trip out of the country, visit your ob-gyn at least 4 to 6 weeks before your trip. During this visit, you can

- go over your travel plans
- get advice about specific health issues (such as food and water precautions)
- get any vaccines that are recommended for the area you are traveling to (see Chapter 25, "Protecting Yourself From Infections")

The CDC Travelers' Health website offers safety tips, vaccination facts, and information for pregnant travelers (see the "Resources" section at the end of this chapter).

Even if you are in perfect health before going on a trip, you never know when an emergency will come up. Carry a copy of your health record with you. Also, before leaving home, locate the nearest hospital or medical clinic in the place you are visiting. The International Association for Medical Assistance to Travelers has a worldwide directory of doctors who provide health care for travelers. See the "Resources" section at the end of this chapter for more information. You must be a member to view their directory of doctors, but membership is free.

After you arrive at your destination, register with an American embassy or consulate. This will help if you need to leave the country because of an emergency.

By Plane

For healthy pregnant women, occasional air travel is almost always safe. Most airlines allow pregnant women to fly domestically until about 36 weeks of pregnancy. If you are planning an international flight, the cut-off for traveling may be earlier. Check with your airline.

Avoid flying if you have a medical or pregnancy condition that may be made worse by flying or could require emergency medical care. Keep in mind that most common pregnancy emergencies usually happen in the first and third trimesters.

Lower air pressure during a flight may slightly reduce the amount of *oxygen* in your blood, but your body will adjust. Radiation exposure increases at higher altitudes, but the level of exposure isn't a concern for pregnant women. If you are a frequent flier, talk with your ob-gyn about how much flying is safe for you.

When traveling by air, follow these tips:

- If you can, book an aisle seat. This will make it easier to get up and stretch your legs during a long flight.

- Avoid gas-producing foods and carbonated drinks before your flight. Gas expands at high altitude and can cause discomfort.

- Wear your seat belt at all times (see the box "Buckling Up During Pregnancy"). Turbulence can happen without warning during air travel.

- Move your feet, toes, and legs often. If you can, get up and walk around a few times during your flight.

Buckling Up During Pregnancy

Wear a lap–shoulder belt every time you travel. The safety belt will not hurt your baby. You and your baby are far more likely to survive a car crash if you are buckled in correctly. Follow these rules when wearing a safety belt:

- Always wear both the lap and shoulder belts.
- Buckle the lap belt low on your hip bones, below your belly.
- Never put the lap belt across your belly.
- Place the shoulder belt off to the side of your belly and across the center of your chest (between your breasts).
- The upper part of the belt should cross your shoulder without chafing your neck. Never slip the upper part of the belt off your shoulder.
- Make sure the belts fit snugly.
- If you're driving, keep as much distance as possible between your belly and the steering wheel. Make sure you can still comfortably reach the pedals.
- Don't recline your seat more than necessary. This will help reduce the gap between the belt and your shoulder.

Safety belts worn too loose or too high on the belly can cause broken ribs or injuries to your belly if you are in an accident. If your car's seat belts don't fit you properly, ask the dealer or manufacturer about seat belt adjusters. If you are in a car accident, get medical attention even if you are not injured.

By Ship

If you are thinking about a cruise, check with the cruise line about their policy on pregnancy. Most cruise ships won't allow pregnant passengers after 28 weeks of pregnancy. Some won't accept them past 24 weeks. Before you book your trip, make sure a doctor or nurse will be on board the ship. Also, check that your scheduled stops are places with modern medical facilities in case there is an emergency.

Many travelers on cruise ships have symptoms of seasickness (motion sickness). Seasickness causes nausea and dizziness, and sometimes weakness, headache, and vomiting. If seasickness usually is not a problem for you, traveling by sea during pregnancy may not upset your stomach. To be on the safe side, ask your ob-gyn about which medications are safe for you to carry along to calm seasickness.

Another concern for cruise ship passengers is norovirus infection, which can cause severe nausea and vomiting for 1 or 2 days. This infection can spread rapidly. People can be infected by eating food, drinking liquids, or touching surfaces that are contaminated with the norovirus.

There is no vaccine or drug that prevents norovirus. You can help protect yourself by washing your hands often and washing any fruits and vegetables before you eat them. If you are pregnant and get this infection (or any other illness that causes diarrhea and vomiting), see a health care practitioner. **Dehydration** can lead to certain pregnancy problems. You may need to have fluids through an **intravenous (IV) line**.

By Car

During a car trip, try to limit car time to less than 6 hours each day. Stop every few hours to stretch, get a drink, and empty your bladder. Be sure to wear your seat belt every time you ride in a car or truck (see the box "Buckling Up During Pregnancy"). If you are in an accident, get medical attention right away, even if you are not injured.

RESOURCES

DoctorFinder
https://doctorfinder.ama-assn.org/doctorfinder
Directory from the American Medical Association that can help you find a doctor in the United States.

Family and Medical Leave Act
www.dol.gov/whd/fmla
Website from the U.S. Department of Labor offers detailed information about FMLA for workers and employers.

Find an Ob-Gyn
www.acog.org/FindAnObGyn
This directory from the American College of Obstetricians and Gynecologists (ACOG) can help you find an ob-gyn near you.

Healthcare.gov
www.healthcare.gov
Portal for the Health Insurance Marketplace that provides information about coverage under the Affordable Care Act. Includes information about how to sign up.

Insure Kids Now
www.insurekidsnow.gov
Provides information about finding free or low-cost health insurance coverage for your child.

International Association for Medical Assistance to Travelers
www.iamat.org
Nonprofit organization that provides medical information for international travelers. Membership is free and allows you to access detailed information for your destination, such as doctors and hospitals.

Pregnancy Discrimination
www.eeoc.gov/laws/types/pregnancy.cfm
Webpage from the U.S. Equal Employment Opportunity Commission (EEOC). The EEOC enforces federal laws that make it illegal to discriminate against applicants or employees because of race, color, religion, sex, national origin, age, or disability. The EEOC investigates charges of workplace discrimination.

Pregnant@Work
www.pregnantatwork.org
A website with state-by-state information for pregnant women and ob-gyns about pregnant workers' rights and how to access workplace accommodations.

Travelers' Health
www.cdc.gov/travel
Webpage from the CDC that offers medical advice for travelers going to national and international destinations. Includes food and water precautions, disease outbreak information, and vaccine recommendations.

Workplace Safety and Health
National Institute for Occupational Safety and Health: www.cdc.gov/niosh
Occupational Safety and Health Administration: www.osha.gov/workers
These government sites provide information about workers' rights, workplace safety, and occupational health. Includes information about hazardous chemicals in the workplace.

Your Pregnancy and Childbirth
www.acog.org/MyPregnancy
Website from ACOG with information on pregnancy, labor, delivery, and postpartum care. Includes the latest information from the experts in women's health care, questions answered by ACOG ob-gyns, pregnancy stories from real women, and an A–Z directory of health topics covering pregnancy and beyond.

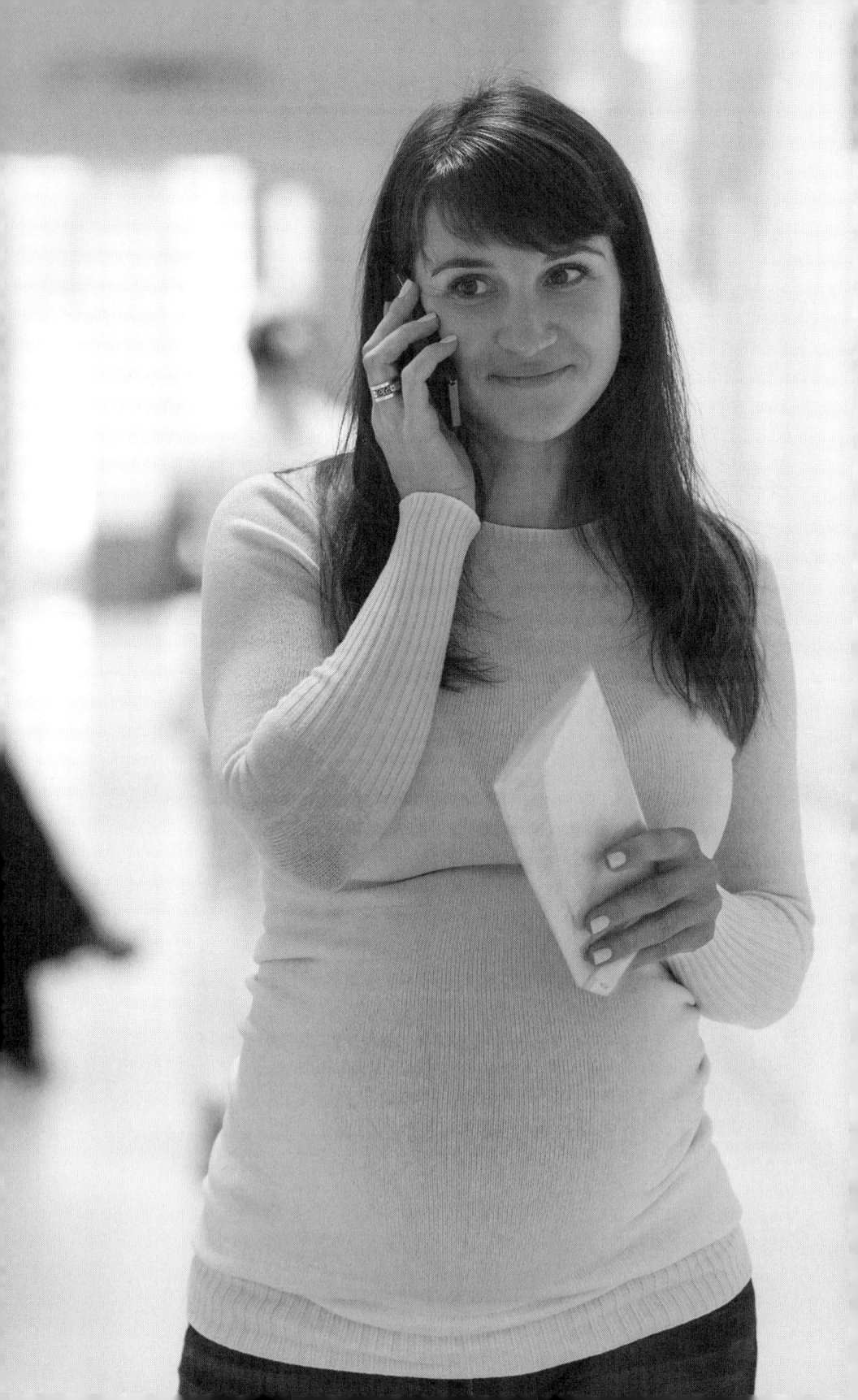

CHAPTER 27

Frequently Asked Questions

This chapter answers common questions that many women have about pregnancy. If you have a question that isn't covered here, check the index at the back of the book. Your question may be answered in another chapter.

If you have specific questions about your situation, your **obstetrician–gynecologist (ob-gyn)** is your best resource. Write down any questions you have so you can ask them during your regular appointments.

Personal Care

Is it safe to dye my hair during pregnancy?

Most experts think that using hair dye during pregnancy is not toxic for your baby. There are different types of hair coloring, including

- permanent color
- semipermanent color
- temporary color

These all contain chemicals. Studies on animals show that high doses of these chemicals do not cause serious **birth defects**. Also, only a small amount of chemicals from hair dye is absorbed through the scalp.

Can I get a massage?

Yes. Massage is a good way to relax and improve circulation. The best position for a massage while you're pregnant is lying on your side, rather than face-down. Some massage tables have a cut-out for the belly, allowing you to lie face-down comfortably. Tell your massage therapist that you're pregnant if you're not showing yet. Many health spas now offer special prenatal massages done by therapists who are trained to work on pregnant women.

Can I get infections from pedicures?
It's smart to avoid things that can cause infection when you're pregnant. Although it is true that you can get fungal infections if the instruments used for your pedicure are not sanitized, this happens very rarely. To reduce the small risk of a fungal infection, bring along your own pedicure tools. Also, ask if the soaking tub has been disinfected before you put your feet in it.

Is there anything I can do about my varicose veins?
Not really. **Varicose veins** tend to run in families. Also, they are more likely to come back with each pregnancy. For some women, varicose veins shrink or go away after giving birth. In the meantime, prop up your legs when you can. If you must sit or stand for long periods, move around often. This may help reduce swelling.

Varicose veins

Is it safe to douche during pregnancy?
No. Do not douche, whether you're pregnant or not.
Women do not need to douche to wash away blood, **semen**, or vaginal discharge. It's better to let your **vagina** clean itself naturally. Keep in mind that healthy vaginas may have a mild odor. If you feel a need to clean the **vulva** while you are in the shower or bath, plain water is all you need. To avoid irritation, do not use soaps or body washes on the vulva.

Can I use a sauna or hot tub early in pregnancy?
It's best not to. Some studies suggest that using saunas and hot tubs early in pregnancy, especially for long periods of time, is associated with birth defects. Your core body temperature rises when you use saunas and hot tubs. This rise in temperature can be harmful for your baby.

What causes stretch marks?
Stretch marks are caused by changes in the elastic supportive tissue that lies just under the skin. The skin on your belly and breasts may become streaked with reddish brown, purple, or dark brown marks, depending on your skin

FREQUENTLY ASKED QUESTIONS • 453

Stretch marks

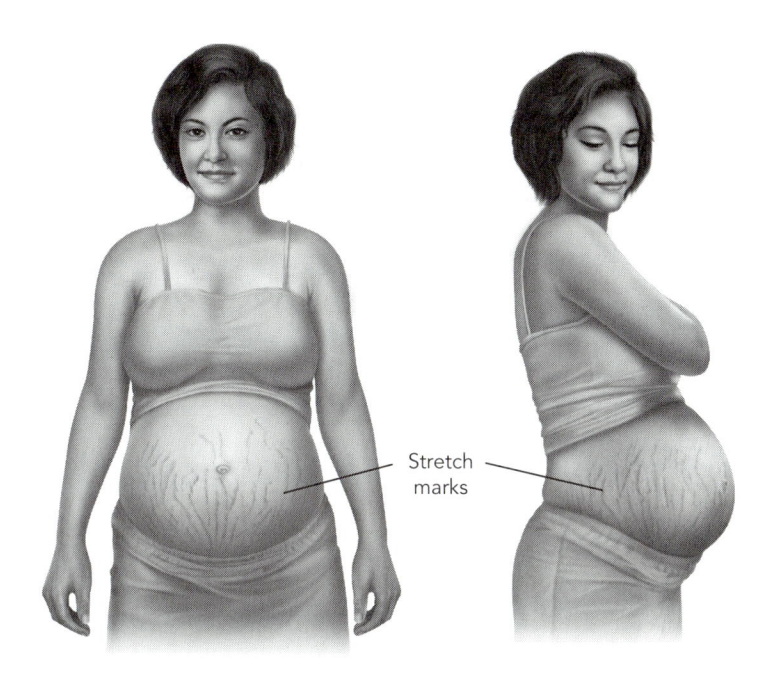

color. Some women also get them on their buttocks, thighs, and hips. There are no proven remedies that keep them from appearing or that make them go away. Keeping your belly well moisturized as it grows may reduce itching. After your baby is born, some of theses streaks may slowly fade in color.

Health and Health Care

Where can I find information on coronavirus (COVID-19) and pregnancy?

You can find information on COVID-19 and pregnancy at the website of the American College of Obstetricians and Gynecologists (ACOG): www.acog.org/COVID-Pregnancy. The Centers for Disease Control and Prevention (CDC) also has up-to-date information: www.cdc.gov/coronavirus/2019-ncov/need-extra-precautions/pregnancy-breastfeeding.html.

Should I tell my ob-gyn that I have an eating disorder?

Yes, you should talk with your ob-gyn if you have an eating disorder. Pregnancy raises body image issues for many women. You and your ob-gyn can be alert to any signs that the disorder has returned. It may be helpful to continue with counseling or start counseling when you get pregnant. See Chapter 29, "Weight During Pregnancy: Obesity and Eating Disorders."

What if I need surgery while I'm pregnant?

If you need urgent surgery during pregnancy, your ob-gyn should explain how you and your baby will be monitored. If your surgery is not urgent, having it in the second *trimester* is best. If you are thinking about elective surgery, it's best to wait until after you have your baby. Elective surgery is a planned procedure that will benefit your health but is not absolutely necessary.

Is it safe to see my dentist during pregnancy?

Yes, seeing your dentist is safe and important when you are pregnant. Pregnancy can cause mouth and gum changes that your dentist can treat. Regular teeth cleaning can reduce the *bacteria* in your mouth. This can improve your overall health. *Local anesthesia*, which is often used before filling cavities, is safe during pregnancy.

Can I have dental X-rays?

Yes. The amount of *radiation* in a dental X-ray is very low. Let your dentist know that you are pregnant. Even though the amount of radiation is small, your dentist should give you lead aprons or covers to put over your abdomen, pelvis, and neck area (where the *thyroid gland* is located). These covers help shield you and the baby from radiation.

What medicine can I take for allergies?

Many people with allergies take antihistamines for relief. Studies show that several over-the-counter allergy medications are safe to use during pregnancy, including

- chlorpheniramine
- dexchlorpheniramine
- hydroxyzine

Newer antihistamines, such as cetirizine and loratadine, also may be safe. There also is a *corticosteroid* nasal spray that is safe to use during pregnancy. But one of the most common decongestants, pseudoephedrine, has been linked to a small risk of abdominal wall birth defects. Do not use pseudoephedrine during the first 3 months of pregnancy. Check with your ob-gyn before taking any over-the-counter allergy medication.

Is it normal for my partner to be controlling and jealous?

Disagreements and arguments, even heated ones, are part of a normal relationship. Abusive behavior is not. Extreme jealousy, constant criticism, and not allowing you to make your own decisions are all signs of an unhealthy or abusive relationship.

Abuse puts both the pregnant woman and her baby at risk. If you are in a violent relationship—whether that violence is physical, emotional, verbal, or sexual—it's vital to take steps to protect yourself and your baby.

If you are concerned about your partner's behavior, talk with a friend, a family member, your ob-gyn, or someone else you trust. You can seek out resources in your area, such as crisis hotlines, **intimate partner violence** programs, legal aid services, and shelters for abused women. Many counselors and health care practitioners are specially trained to deal with intimate partner violence. Call the 24-hour, toll-free National Domestic Violence Hotline: 1-800-799-SAFE (7233) or 1-800-787-3224 (TTY). You also can find help online at www.thehotline.org.

Intimate partner violence is more common than most people think. It is a serious threat to the lives of many women. No woman has to live with abuse. There is help. Your life can be better.

Pregnancy and Technology

What should I know about pregnancy apps?

Some smartphone apps are useful for tracking your fertility, fitness, nutrition, and of course your pregnancy. Here are a few things to keep in mind when using apps:

- Do you also use step counters, heart rate monitors, scales, or other devices? Do you want these to connect to the app?
- Does the app have a "pregnancy mode"? For example, if your app tracks your weight and calorie intake, will it take into account the weight you need to gain during your pregnancy?
- If social networking and sharing are important to you, does the app support that?
- How does the app use and store your personal data?

Using apps during pregnancy can be fun and informative. But apps should not replace the advice of your ob-gyn. If you have questions about anything mentioned in your app, ask your ob-gyn at your next visit.

Can I trust the information I read in pregnancy chat rooms?

Online chat rooms can help you feel part of a community. You can find support from women going through similar experiences. But you cannot know the health situation of anyone who visits a chat room. Remember that every woman and every pregnancy is unique. For this reason, chat room advice should never replace the advice of your ob-gyn.

Your Pregnancy

How long does pregnancy last?

Pregnancy is counted from the first day of your **last menstrual period (LMP)**. This means an extra 2 weeks are counted at the beginning of your pregnancy when you aren't actually pregnant. So pregnancy lasts 10 months (40 weeks)—not 9 months—because of these extra weeks.

How much weight should I gain during pregnancy?

Weight gain depends in part on your **body mass index (BMI)** before pregnancy. During your first 12 weeks—the first trimester—you may gain only 1 to 5 pounds or no weight at all. In your second and third trimesters, if you were a healthy weight before pregnancy, you should gain between half a pound and 1 pound per week.

For women who were a healthy weight when they got pregnant, the key to healthy weight gain is to slowly increase your calories. In the first trimester, when weight gain is minimal, usually no extra calories are needed. In the second trimester, you need an extra 340 calories a day, and in the third trimester, about 450 extra calories a day. See Chapter 22, "Nutrition During Pregnancy," for a chart showing healthy weight gain by BMI.

What causes nausea and vomiting during pregnancy?

No one knows for sure what causes the nausea and vomiting. Increasing levels of **hormones** may play a role. Hormonal changes also may heighten your sense of smell and make you much more sensitive to certain odors. These changes can cause your sense of taste to be "off"—you may have a sour or bitter taste in your mouth, or nothing may taste good to you.

How can I take care of my teeth after vomiting?

Vomiting can cause some of your tooth enamel to wear away. This happens because your stomach contains a lot of acid. Make a rinse with a teaspoon of baking soda dissolved in a cup of water. Rinsing your mouth with this mixture may help neutralize the acid and protect your teeth.

How can I tell if my sadness is normal or a sign of depression?

It's normal to feel blue sometimes. But if you are feeling a loss of interest in things that used to make you happy, talk with your ob-gyn. Other signs of *depression* include

- feeling hopeless or worthless
- sleeping more than normal
- having trouble paying attention or making decisions

Tell your ob-gyn how you are feeling. He or she can determine if your sadness is depression and get you the help you need.

Does a positive ultrasound exam guarantee that my baby will be healthy?

It's good when an ***ultrasound exam*** shows no sign of trouble for the baby. But this isn't a guarantee that a baby will be born healthy. Ultrasound cannot detect all problems that a baby may have. Ultrasound may not find a birth defect and is not designed to tell how well a baby's organs will work after birth.

Sometimes an ultrasound exam will show minor problems or uncertain results. If this happens, your ob-gyn should discuss the results with you. If a clear problem is found, your ob-gyn may order more tests to understand what the results may mean for your baby.

What is expanded carrier screening?

Expanded carrier screening is a blood test that screens for many ***genetic disorders*** at one time. If you are interested in this type of screening, talk with your ob-gyn. See Chapter 33, "Genetic Disorders, Screening, and Testing."

What should I know about "keepsake" ultrasound pictures?

There is a type of business that creates baby portraits using ultrasound technology. You may have seen a business like this in a shopping mall. These businesses are not medical facilities. Employees may not be trained to interpret the ultrasound images for you. You may be falsely reassured that your baby is doing well after one of these ultrasounds, when there may be a problem that was not detected. Or you may be worried that the image shows a problem, and you will not get an expert medical opinion. There also is concern about the safety of using ultrasound for a nonmedical reason. If you want an image of your baby, you can ask for one during a standard ultrasound exam arranged by your ob-gyn.

Will I need bed rest near the end of pregnancy?

For most women, bed rest is not recommended. There is no scientific evidence that bed rest reduces the risk of ***preterm*** labor or ***preeclampsia***. Being completely inactive can increase the risk of other problems, including blood clots. If your ob-gyn suggests bed rest because you have a specific medical condition, ask if you can do some activity.

Is it safe to have sex during pregnancy?

Most sexual activity is safe for women having healthy pregnancies. This includes **sexual intercourse** or **penetration** with fingers or sex toys. The **amniotic sac** and the strong muscles of the **uterus** protect the baby. If you have pregnancy **complications** or questions about what may be safe sexual activity for you, talk with your ob-gyn.

It is normal to have cramps or spotting after sex with penetration. Also, **orgasm** can cause cramps. If you have severe, persistent cramping, or if your bleeding is heavy (like normal menstrual bleeding), call your ob-gyn.

Nutrition and Exercise

How much exercise should I get early in my pregnancy?

Unless your ob-gyn tells you not to, you should do moderate exercise for 30 minutes or more on most days, if not every day. The 30 minutes do not have to be all at one time. For example, you could take two 10-minute walks and do 10 minutes of stretching, for a total of 30 minutes. If you have not been active, start with a few minutes each day and build up to 30 minutes or more. See Chapter 23, "Exercise During Pregnancy."

How much caffeine can I have per day?

Research suggests that moderate caffeine consumption (less than 200 milligrams per day) does not cause **miscarriage** or preterm birth. That's the amount in one 12-ounce cup of coffee. Remember that caffeine also is found in tea, chocolate, energy drinks, and soft drinks. Caffeine can interfere with sleep and contribute to nausea and light-headedness. Caffeine also can increase urination and lead to **dehydration**.

What can I do about the smell of my prenatal vitamins?

If the odor of your vitamins upsets your stomach, or if you find it difficult to keep them down, you can take two children's chewable vitamins. Be sure to tell your ob-gyn that you're taking children's vitamins.

Can I eat sushi while I'm pregnant?

Many fish are safe to eat when fully cooked, but you should avoid all raw or undercooked fish when you're pregnant. Raw fish, including sushi and sashimi, is more likely to contain parasites or **bacteria** than fully cooked fish. See Chapter 22, "Nutrition During Pregnancy," for more on safe fish to eat during pregnancy.

What is vitamin D deficiency?

Vitamin D deficiency happens when a person does not get enough of the vitamin in her daily diet. Although vitamin D can be made in the body through exposure to sunlight, most people do not get enough vitamin D through sunlight exposure alone. Food sources of vitamin D include

- fortified milk
- fish liver oils
- fatty fish, such as salmon and mackerel (but avoid king mackerel, which may have high levels of mercury)

Look for a prenatal vitamin with 600 international units (IU) of vitamin D. Note that the label may say 15 micrograms (mcg), which is the same as 600 IU. If your prenatal vitamin doesn't have this much vitamin D, talk with your ob-gyn about getting what you need from foods.

How can I get all the calcium I need if I can't eat dairy products?

Lactose intolerance means you cannot fully digest the milk sugar (lactose) in dairy products. Pregnant women with this condition still need to get the daily amount of *calcium* to nourish their baby's growth. Here are some tips:

- Try different kinds of dairy products. Not all dairy products have the same amount of lactose. For example, hard cheeses such as Swiss or cheddar have only small amounts of lactose and generally cause no symptoms.
- Buy lactose-free products, such as Lactaid. They contain all of the *nutrients* found in regular milk and dairy products.
- Get calcium from other foods. Good sources are canned pink salmon, nuts and seeds, leafy greens, molasses, and calcium-fortified breads and juices.

See the section "Special Diets and Food Restrictions" in Chapter 22, "Nutrition During Pregnancy."

How much water should I be drinking each day?

During pregnancy you should drink 8 to 12 cups (64 to 96 ounces) of water every day. Water has many benefits. It aids digestion and helps form the *amniotic fluid* around the baby. Water also helps nutrients circulate in the body and helps waste leave the body.

Why is fiber important in the third trimester?

Constipation is common near the end of pregnancy. Eating more foods with fiber can help fight constipation. Fiber is found mostly in fruits, vegetables, whole grains, beans, and nuts and seeds. You should aim for about 25 grams of fiber in your diet each day. Good sources of fiber include

- apples
- bananas
- lentils
- raspberries
- split peas
- whole-wheat pasta

Check the labels on packaged foods and choose higher-fiber options if possible. If you have not been getting your 25 grams a day, increase the amount of fiber you take in a little each day. Drink a lot of water as you increase your fiber intake. See Chapter 22, "Nutrition During Pregnancy."

Potentially Harmful Substances

Why should I tell my ob-gyn about my medications and supplements?

Some medications, including over-the-counter medications and herbal supplements, should not be taken while you are pregnant. For example, *isotretinoin* is a prescription medication used to treat severe acne. It can cause severe birth defects if used during pregnancy. Another example is vitamin A, which has been shown to cause severe birth defects if taken in large doses during pregnancy. Your ob-gyn can determine the safety of anything you are taking. See Chapter 24, "Reducing Risks of Birth Defects."

What can I do to avoid secondhand smoke?

Be direct about asking others to not smoke around you. If your partner or family members are not willing to quit smoking, ask them to smoke outside. Do not allow anyone to smoke in your car or your home.

What do I need to know about Zika virus?

You can get *Zika* virus from the bite of an infected mosquito or during sex with an infected partner. Many people infected with Zika virus have no symptoms or only mild symptoms. Infection during pregnancy can be passed from a woman to her baby. Zika virus can cause severe brain damage in a baby. If you or your partner live in an area with active Zika virus or will be traveling to an area with Zika, talk with your ob-gyn about ways to protect yourself. See Chapter 25, "Protecting Yourself From Infections."

Is it safe to keep a cat during pregnancy?

You may have heard that cat feces can carry the infection **toxoplasmosis**. This infection is only found in cats who go outdoors and hunt prey, such as mice and other rodents. If you have an indoor cat who eats only cat food and doesn't have contact with outside animals, your risk of toxoplasmosis is very low. If you do have a cat that goes outdoors or eats prey, have someone else take over daily cleaning the litter box. This will keep you away from any cat feces.

What should I do if I've been exposed to chickenpox?

Tell your ob-gyn right away if you've been around someone who has **chickenpox**, you've never had the illness, and you have never gotten the **varicella** vaccine. Sometimes steps can be taken to avoid problems and reduce any risk to your baby. See Chapter 25, "Protecting Yourself From Infections."

Labor and Delivery

Do I have to write a birth plan?

A birth plan is a way for you to share your wishes with those who will care for you during labor and delivery. Some women like to have a plan, even though unexpected things can happen and the plan may need to change. See Chapter 12, "Preparing for Birth," for tips on writing a plan. You also can use the "Sample Birth Plan" at the back of this book as a guide. But you don't need to have a birth plan before your baby is born. It's not a requirement. If the idea of writing a birth plan doesn't appeal to you, that's OK.

If coronavirus (COVID-19) is spreading as I get close to delivery, would it be safer to have a home birth?

ACOG believes that the safest place for you to give birth is a hospital, hospital-based birth center, or accredited freestanding birth center. Even the healthiest pregnancies can have problems arise with little or no warning during labor and delivery. If problems happen, a hospital setting can give you and your baby the best care in a hurry. Keep in mind that hospitals, hospital-based birth centers, and accredited freestanding birth centers follow strict infection control procedures.

How can I remember everything I need to do before I give birth?

You may feel overwhelmed as you get ready for childbirth. One way to take control is to write a checklist of everything you need to do before you give birth. Your checklist can include things like filling out work forms for your maternity leave and making sure you have a caregiver for your other children and pets until you come home. See Chapter 12, "Preparing for Birth."

Is there anything I can do to start labor?

You may have heard other women talk about ways you can make labor start on your own. Many women believe that taking long walks, having sex, taking herbal medications, or eating spicy foods can bring on labor. But there is no evidence that any of these methods work.

One nonmedical method of labor induction that is somewhat effective is nipple stimulation. Research on this method found that it did bring on labor in some women, but only when the *cervix* was ready for labor. Do not try to bring on labor with nipple stimulation without your ob-gyn's approval.

What is "back labor"?

Back labor refers to the intense lower back pain that many women have during labor and delivery. Some women even feel this pain between contractions. The pain is caused by the pressure of the baby's head on the lower back. Your childbirth classes should teach you ways to deal with back labor, including changing positions or partner massage. See Chapter 13, "Pain Relief During Childbirth."

What is assisted vaginal delivery?

When a vaginal delivery is assisted, it means the ob-gyn uses *forceps* or a *vacuum device* to help deliver the baby. *Assisted vaginal delivery* may be done if you have pushed for a long time without progress. It also may be done if there is a problem with the baby, such as a slow heartbeat. Talk with your ob-gyn about assisted vaginal delivery at one of your *prenatal care* visits. See Chapter 16, "Assisted Vaginal Delivery and Breech Presentation."

What is an episiotomy?

Episiotomy is a procedure in which a small cut is made to widen the opening of the vagina when a woman is giving birth. It may be done to avoid tearing of the skin at the opening of the vagina. It also may be done to help with delivery of the baby. The types include

- mediolateral, a cut that is made to the side of the vagina and **vulva**
- midline, a cut that is made in the vagina and vulva in the direction of (but not all the way down to) the **anus**

Talk with your ob-gyn about episiotomy at one of your prenatal care visits. ACOG recommends that episiotomy be done only when it is absolutely necessary. This might include situations when the baby is stressed and needs to be delivered more quickly, or to prevent larger tears that may happen during delivery. Ask your ob-gyn

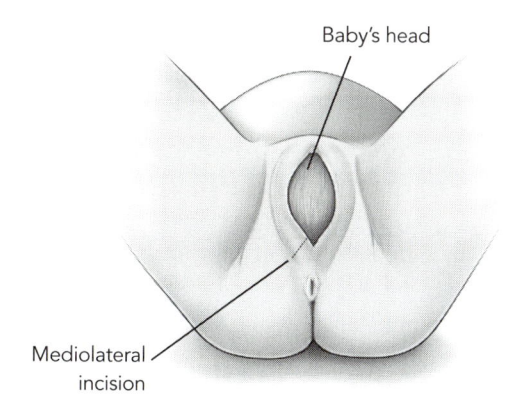

- how often he or she does episiotomies
- what type is most often done
- what type of situations call for this procedure

Together you can make a decision about your particular situation.

After the Baby Is Born

What is delayed cord clamping?

Delayed cord clamping is the practice of waiting a short time before cutting the **umbilical cord** after birth. This allows blood from the umbilical cord, along with extra iron, **stem cells**, and **antibodies**, to flow back into the baby. Delayed cord clamping appears to be helpful for both full-term and **preterm** babies. For this reason, ACOG recommends delayed cord clamping for at least 30 to 60 seconds after birth for most babies. See Chapter 12, "Preparing for Birth," for more on cord clamping and cord blood banking.

What are the benefits of breastfeeding?

Breastfeeding is good for your baby and good for you. Breast milk has the right amount of fat, sugar, water, and protein needed for your baby's growth. Breast milk contains antibodies that protect babies from infections. Breastfed babies have a lower risk of **sudden infant death syndrome (SIDS)**. For you, breastfeeding triggers the release of a hormone called **oxytocin**. This hormone makes the uterus contract and return to its original size. These mild contractions also reduce the amount of bleeding you may have after giving birth. See Chapter 20, "Feeding Your Baby," for more details on the many benefits of breastfeeding.

How soon after delivery can I breastfeed?

If you feel up to it, you can start breastfeeding as soon as the baby is born. A healthy baby is able to breastfeed in the first hour after birth. Keeping your baby on your chest (called skin-to-skin contact) is the best way to get breastfeeding started. Your labor nurses can help you and your baby get into the right position. See Chapter 18, "After the Baby Is Born."

What kind of birth control should I use after I have the baby?

You have many **birth control** options after pregnancy. Some, like the **intrauterine device (IUD)** and the **birth control implant**, can be inserted before you go home from the hospital.

In some cases, what you were using before pregnancy might not be a good choice now. For example, birth control pills that contain **estrogen** may affect your milk supply while you are starting to breastfeed. If you were using a diaphragm or cervical cap before pregnancy, you'll need to be refitted several weeks after delivery, when the uterus and cervix have gone back to their normal size. See Chapter 21, "Birth Control After Pregnancy and Beyond," for a discussion of birth control options.

RESOURCES

Birth Control
https://medlineplus.gov/birthcontrol.html
Overview of birth control and related information from the U.S. National Library of Medicine. Includes links to other resources.

Coronavirus (COVID-19)
www.cdc.gov/coronavirus/2019-ncov/index.html
CDC website with the most up-to-date information on the coronavirus.

Coronavirus (COVID-19), Pregnancy, and Breastfeeding: A Message for Patients
www.acog.org/COVID-Pregnancy
ACOG webpage with frequently asked questions about coronavirus, pregnancy, and breastfeeding.

Exercise and Physical Fitness
https://medlineplus.gov/exerciseandphysicalfitness.html
General exercise information from the U.S. National Library of Medicine, with links to other resources.

La Leche League International
www.llli.org

Provides information and support for breastfeeding women. Offers referrals to local support groups.

National Cord Blood Program
www.nationalcordbloodprogram.org

Website for the largest public cord blood bank in the United States. Provides information about cord blood collection, storage, banking, and retrieval.

National Domestic Violence Hotline
1-800-799-SAFE (7233)
(TTY 1-800-787-3224)
Text LOVEIS to 22522
www.thehotline.org

Website, phone lines, and online chat service that let you talk confidentially with a counselor about domestic violence and finding help. Phone lines and chat are available 24 hours a day.

National Eating Disorders Association
www.nationaleatingdisorders.org/pregnancy-and-eating-disorders

Gives an overview of the risks that eating disorders pose during pregnancy. Maintains an extensive list of resources to find help and support.

Postpartum Support International Helpline
www.postpartum.net
1-800-944-4773
Text 1-503-894-9453 (English) or 1-971-420-0294 (Spanish)

Non-emergency helpline for support, information, or referrals to postpartum mental health practitioners. The helpline is open 7 days per week. Leave a confidential message at any time, and a volunteer will return your call or text as soon as possible. PSI also offers online support group meetings to connect with other pregnant and postpartum women. You also can join PSI's weekly Chat with an Expert.

Zika Virus: Pregnancy
www.cdc.gov/zika/pregnancy/

Frequently updated CDC site with the latest news about Zika virus and pregnancy, how to protect yourself, and travel information.

Your Pregnancy and Childbirth
www.acog.org/MyPregnancy

Website from ACOG with information on pregnancy, labor, delivery, and postpartum care. Includes the latest information from the experts in women's health care, questions answered by ACOG ob-gyns, pregnancy stories from real women, and an A–Z directory of health topics covering pregnancy and beyond.

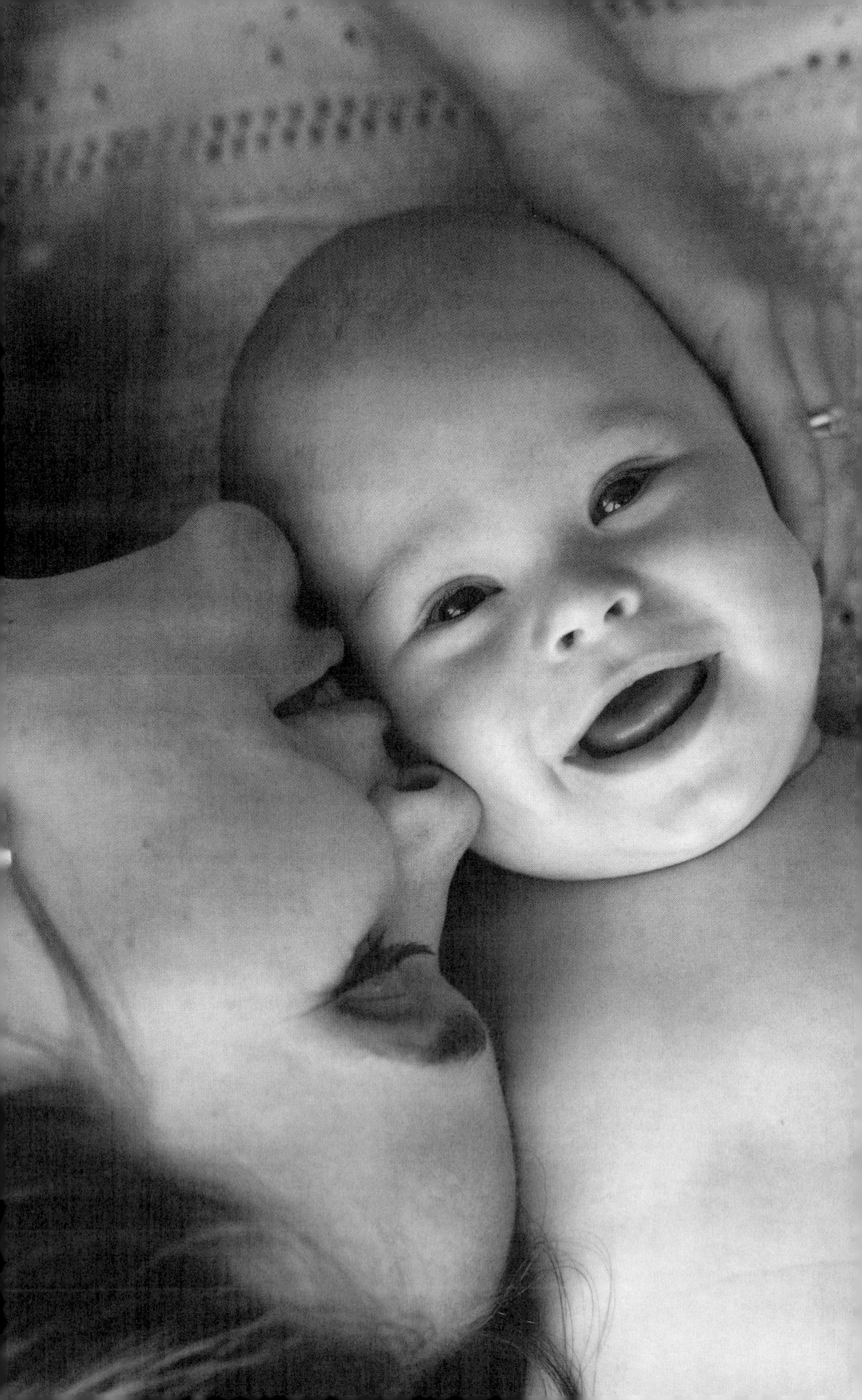

PART 5

Special Considerations

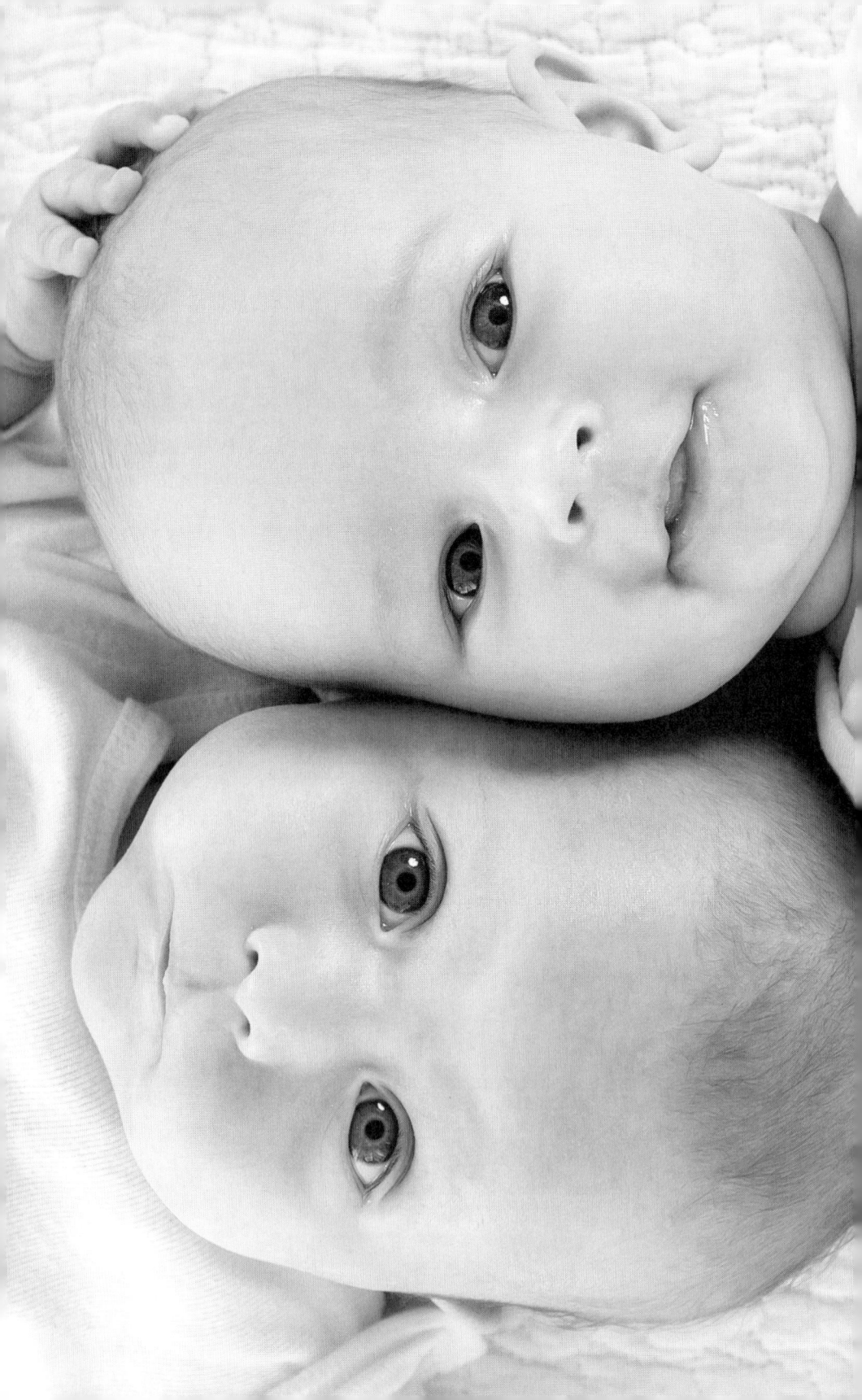

CHAPTER 28

Multiples
When It's Twins, Triplets, or More

When a woman is carrying more than one baby, it is called a ***multiple pregnancy***. In the past 40 years, multiple pregnancies have become more common. The twin birth rate in 2017 was 33 twins for every 1,000 births. That's nearly double the twin birth rate in 1980. Meanwhile, the birth rate for three, four, or more babies rose 400 percent from 1980 to 1998, but in recent years this rate has fallen.

Why the increase in multiple pregnancies? One reason is because more women are having babies later in life. Women over 35 have a higher chance of having twins. Another reason is that more women are having fertility treatments to get pregnant. These treatments can increase the risk of multiple pregnancy. If you are having fertility treatments, talk with your fertility specialist or ***obstetrician–gynecologist (ob-gyn)*** about the risks of multiple pregnancy.

Making Multiples

Multiple births happen when more than one ***embryo*** grows in the ***uterus***. This process can happen naturally, or it can happen artificially during fertility treatments.

Fraternal and Identical Twins

The most common kind of multiple pregnancy is twins, and twins come in two types:

Fertility Treatments and Multiple Pregnancy

Fertility treatments are a major factor in the increase in multiple pregnancy in the United States. **Assisted reproductive technology (ART)** includes all fertility treatments in which both eggs and sperm are handled. ART usually involves *in vitro fertilization (IVF)*. With IVF, sperm are combined with the egg in a laboratory, and later the **embryo** is transferred to the uterus.

In some cases, more than one embryo is transferred. The risk of multiple pregnancy increases as the number of transferred embryos increases. When two or more embryos are transferred, about 45 percent of pregnancies result in twins and about 7 percent result in triplets or more.

Because of the risks associated with multiple pregnancy, the American Society for Reproductive Medicine recommends trying to prevent multiples when fertility treatments are used. If you are considering fertility treatments, talk with a fertility specialist about the risks of a multiple pregnancy and how you may avoid having more than one baby.

A pregnancy is called "higher order" if the woman is carrying three or more fetuses. When this happens, a procedure called **multifetal pregnancy reduction** may be considered. This procedure reduces by one or more the total number of fetuses.

There are risks with this procedure, including the risk of losing all of the fetuses. But with higher-order pregnancies, experts generally feel that these risks are outweighed by the possible benefits. Reducing a pregnancy reduces the risks associated with **preterm** birth. It also reduces risks to the pregnant woman, which include **gestational diabetes**, **high blood pressure**, and **preeclampsia**.

- *Fraternal twins*—Most twins are fraternal. These babies grow from separate fertilized *eggs* and *sperm*. Because each twin grows from the union of a different egg and a different sperm, these twins are similar only in the way any siblings are similar. These twins can be boys, girls, or one of each.

- *Identical twins*—When one fertilized egg splits early in pregnancy and grows into two embryos, identical twins are formed. Identical twins are the same sex and have the same inherited traits including blood type, hair color, and eye color. They usually look very much alike.

How Twins Are Formed

Fraternal twins are formed from two eggs and each has a placenta. Identical twins are formed from one egg that splits into two. They may share the same placenta, but each usually has its own amniotic sac.

Types of twins. Fraternal twins are formed from two eggs and each has a placenta. Identical twins are formed from one egg that splits into two.

Three or More Babies

A pregnancy with three or more babies can be formed

- by more than one egg being fertilized
- a single fertilized egg splitting
- both processes happening in the same pregnancy

This is called a higher-order pregnancy and rarely happens naturally. It is most often the result of fertility treatments.

Signs That It's More Than One Baby

There are signs that can tell your ob-gyn that you are pregnant with more than one baby. These signs include the following:

- Rapid weight gain during the first *trimester*
- Severe morning sickness
- Hearing cardiac sounds for more than one baby during a prenatal exam
- Your uterus being larger than expected during a prenatal exam

Most women learn they're carrying multiples early in their pregnancies. An *ultrasound exam* can detect most multiples by 6 to 8 weeks of pregnancy.

Terms to Know

Early in a multiple pregnancy, an ultrasound exam will be done to see how the babies are situated in the uterus. In a pregnancy with one baby, there is one *amniotic sac*, one *chorion* (membrane) around the sac, and one *placenta*. When there are two babies, there can be two amniotic sacs, two chorions, and two placentas, or these may be shared. Doctors use the terms *chorionicity* and *amnionicity* to refer to this sharing. The types of twins are explained this way:

- *Diamniotic–dichorionic*—Twins who have their own amniotic sacs and chorions. They may or may not share a placenta.

- *Diamniotic–monochorionic*—Twins who have separate amniotic sacs but share a chorion and placenta.

- *Monoamniotic–monochorionic*—Twins who share a chorion, placenta, and amniotic sac.

Triplets can all have their own placentas and amniotic sacs. Or two of the triplets may share an amniotic sac, a placenta, or both. Rarely, triplets may share one placenta and one amniotic sac. The amount of risk to the babies mainly depends on what they share in the uterus, so it's important to know as soon as possible.

Risks With Multiples

The risk of problems during a multiple pregnancy increases with the number of babies. This means that there is a higher risk of problems with twins than with a single baby, and a higher risk of problems with triplets than with twins. This is why prenatal care is so important. It allows your ob-gyn to manage any *complications* that may arise.

Chorion
Amnion
Placenta

Diamniotic–dichorionic,
two placentas

Diamniotic–dichorionic,
one placenta

Diamniotic–monochorionic,
one placenta

Monoamniotic–monochorionic,
one placenta

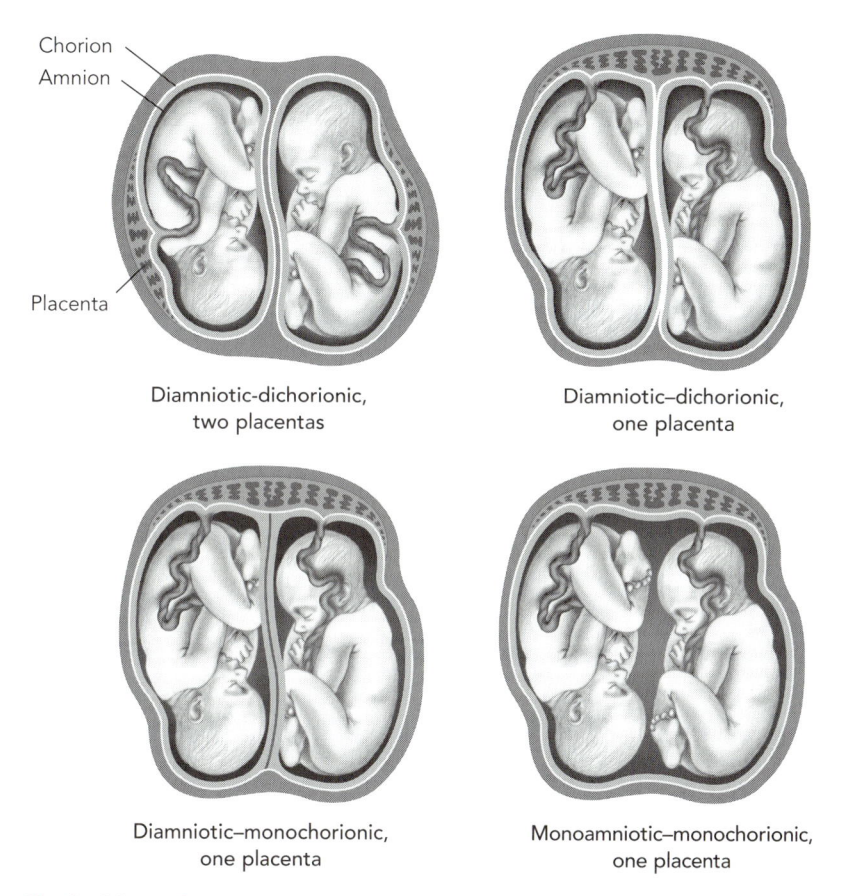

Chorionicity and amnionicity. When there are two babies, there can be two separate amniotic sacs, two chorions, and two placentas, or these may be shared. Ob-gyns use the terms chorionicity and amnionicity to refer to this sharing.

Preterm Birth

Preterm birth—birth before 37 weeks of pregnancy—is the most common problem of multiple pregnancies. More than half of twins and more than 90 percent of triplets are born preterm. With each extra baby, the average pregnancy is shorter and the average birth weight is lower (see Table 28-1, "Length of Multiple Pregnancies").

Preterm babies have not finished growing and developing. They are more likely to have health problems than babies born at *full term*. Some problems, such as learning disabilities, appear later in childhood or even in adulthood. Preterm multiples are at higher risk of brain damage and bleeding in the brain than preterm single babies. ***Cerebral palsy*** also is more common in preterm multiples than in preterm single babies.

> ## What Type of Ob-Gyn Should You See?
>
> Some women who are carrying more than one baby see a **maternal–fetal medicine (MFM) specialist** during pregnancy. These specialists, also called perinatologists, are doctors who specialize in caring for pregnant women who may be at high risk of health problems.
>
> Having a multiple pregnancy does not necessarily mean you need an MFM specialist. If you are healthy, you can choose to see an ob-gyn who has experience caring for women with multiple pregnancies. If you have conditions that put you at risk of complications, or if you have a history of pregnancy problems, your ob-gyn may refer you to an MFM. This specialist will help take care of you and your babies along with your ob-gyn.

TABLE 28-1 **Length of Multiple Pregnancies**

Type of Pregnancy	Average Gestational Age at Time of Delivery (in Weeks)	Average Birth Weight (in Pounds and Ounces)
Single	39	7 and 5
Twin	35	5 and 2
Triplet	32	3 and 11
Quadruplet	30	2 and 13

Twins need to be admitted to the **neonatal intensive care unit (NICU)** in about 1 in 4 deliveries, and triplets in about 3 in 4 deliveries. Very preterm babies (those who are born before 32 weeks of pregnancy) can die or have severe health problems, even with the best of care. But it's important to keep in mind that most twins and other multiple babies do survive.

There is no treatment that can be given to prevent preterm birth from happening in multiple pregnancies. The best thing is to be prepared for the possibility that your babies may be born early. If your labor does start early, some things can be done to help protect your babies' health:

- If you go into labor and are likely to give birth between 23 and 34 weeks of pregnancy, you may be given **corticosteroids**. These medications can help the babies' lungs, brain, and other organs mature.

- You also may be given a medication called a **_tocolytic_**. Tocolytics are drugs used to delay delivery for a short time (up to 48 hours). They are given to allow time for corticosteroids to do their job or to transport you to a hospital that offers higher-level care for babies who are born preterm or with other complications.

- If you are likely to give birth before 32 weeks of pregnancy, you may be given a medication called **_magnesium sulfate_**. It has been shown to reduce the risk and severity of cerebral palsy in preterm babies.

Tocolytics can have side effects for the pregnant woman, some of which can be serious and life-threatening. The risk of these side effects is higher in women with multiple pregnancies than in women with single pregnancies. For this reason, tocolytics are given to a woman with a multiple pregnancy only when preterm labor starts. Tocolytics are not recommended to prevent preterm labor.

If you are pregnant with more than one baby, make sure you know the signs of preterm labor (see the box "Signs of Preterm Labor" in this chapter). Call your ob-gyn right away if you have any of the signs or symptoms. See Chapter 35, "When Labor Starts Too Soon: Preterm Labor, Prelabor Rupture of Membranes, and Preterm Birth."

Signs of Preterm Labor

Call your ob-gyn right away if you have signs or symptoms of preterm labor, including

- change in vaginal discharge (gets watery, mucus-like, or bloody)
- increase in amount of vaginal discharge
- pelvic or lower-abdominal pressure
- constant low, dull backache
- mild abdominal cramps, with or without diarrhea
- regular or frequent contractions or uterine tightening, often painless (four times every 20 minutes or eight times an hour for more than 1 hour)
- ruptured membranes (your water breaks, with a gush or a trickle of fluid)

Problems With the Placenta and Umbilical Cords

Babies who share a placenta have a higher risk of complications than those with separate placentas. One problem that can happen is **twin–twin transfusion syndrome (TTTS)**. In TTTS, the blood flow between the twins becomes unbalanced because of a problem with the placenta. One twin donates blood to the other twin. The donor twin has too little blood, and the recipient twin has too much blood. This condition can lead to problems for both babies.

Treatment is available for TTTS. One treatment that can be done is to remove extra fluid from the recipient twin's amniotic sac. This procedure, done with **amniocentesis**, may need to be done every few days or weekly. Severe cases of TTTS that are diagnosed early may be treated with laser surgery on the placenta. This surgery should be performed in a hospital by an obstetrician who has experience with high-risk pregnancies.

It is rare for babies to share an amniotic sac, but when it happens, it is a very risky pregnancy. The most common problem is an **umbilical cord** complication. If the babies get tangled in their cords, they may not be able to move and grow and may die. Women with this type of pregnancy are monitored more often and need to have their babies by **cesarean birth.**

Gestational Diabetes

Women carrying multiple babies are more likely to have gestational diabetes. Gestational diabetes can increase the babies' weight, risk of breathing difficulties, and other problems during the newborn period. Managing gestational diabetes through diet, exercise, and sometimes medication can reduce the risk of these complications. See Chapter 31, "Diabetes During Pregnancy."

High Blood Pressure and Preeclampsia

Women carrying multiple babies have a higher risk of developing a high blood pressure condition during pregnancy called **preeclampsia**. This condition usually starts after 20 weeks of pregnancy, and it also can happen after childbirth. It can lead to damage to the woman's **kidneys** and liver. It also can increase the risk of heart disease later in life. Preeclampsia tends to happen earlier in multiple pregnancies.

If symptoms of preeclampsia become severe, the babies may need to be delivered right away, even if they are not fully grown. See Chapter 30, "Hypertension and Preeclampsia," for more information about preeclampsia.

Growth Problems

Multiples generally grow more slowly during pregnancy than single babies. About 25 percent of twins and 60 percent of triplets are born at a smaller-than-average size. Sometimes the placenta of one or more of the babies may not be in the best place. Sometimes the umbilical cord may not be formed normally. These problems can limit the amount of **nutrients** the babies receive.

Twins are called **discordant** if one is much smaller than the other. Discordant twins are more likely to have problems during pregnancy and after birth. Twins may be discordant because of problems with the placenta, genetic problems, or TTTS.

Beginning at about 24 weeks, ultrasound exams are used to check the growth of each baby. If a growth problem is suspected, ultrasound exams are done more often. If a problem is found, special tests also may be done to assess the babies' well-being. Ultrasound also may be used to check your **cervix** (whether it is opening) and assess your risk of preterm birth.

Everyday Health

If you are carrying more than one baby, you may need to adjust your diet and exercise routine. You also will be advised to gain more weight than a woman who is pregnant with a single baby.

Nutrition

When pregnant with multiple babies, you will need to eat a bit more than if you were carrying one baby. Eating well is important for your health and the health of your babies. A guideline to follow is that you need about 300 extra calories per baby per day. So, if you are pregnant with twins, you need to eat about 600 extra calories per day. For triplets, you need about 900 extra calories. These calories should come from healthy foods. See Chapter 22, "Nutrition During Pregnancy," for information on healthy eating.

Some women with twins may have more nausea and vomiting. It may be easier to eat smaller meals more often.

All pregnant women need to get extra amounts of iron (27 milligrams a day) and **folic acid** (600 micrograms [mcg] a day). The easiest way to make sure you are getting these recommended amounts is to take a prenatal vitamin every day. Note that the label may say 1,000 mcg dietary folate equivalents (DFE), which is the same as 600 mcg of folic acid.

Weight Gain

Along with eating well, gaining the right amount of weight is very important for the health of your babies. You will need to gain more weight when carrying twins than if you were carrying only one baby (see Table 28-2, "Weight Gain Recommendations for a Twin Pregnancy").

TABLE 28-2 **Weight Gain Recommendations for a Twin Pregnancy**

Body Mass Index (BMI) Before Pregnancy	Recommended Total Weight Gain With a Single Baby (in Pounds)	Recommended Weight Gain With Twins (in Pounds)
Less than 18.5 (underweight)	28 to 40	Not known
18.5 to 24.9 (normal weight)	25 to 35	37 to 54
25.0 to 29.9 (overweight)	15 to 25	31 to 50
30.0 and above (obese)	11 to 20	25 to 42

Source: Institute of Medicine and National Research Council. 2009. *Weight Gain During Pregnancy: Reexamining the Guidelines*. Washington, DC: The National Academies Press.

Gaining the necessary pounds during your pregnancy should be done gradually. With twins, you should gain about 1 pound per week in the first half of pregnancy. In the second half of pregnancy, you should aim to gain a little more than 1 pound each week.

Exercise

Getting regular exercise is important in every pregnancy. But when you're carrying multiple babies, most ob-gyns recommend some caution. Your ob-gyn may advise you to avoid strenuous activity and high-impact exercise, such as aerobics and running. Sports that are lower impact may be better for you. These include

- swimming
- prenatal yoga
- walking

Avoid getting out of breath when you exercise. See Chapter 23, "Exercise During Pregnancy," for information on exercising safely.

Health Care

If you are carrying more than one baby, you may see your ob-gyn more often than a woman carrying one baby. You also may need special care during pregnancy, labor, and delivery.

Prenatal Genetic Screening and Diagnosis

Having a multiple pregnancy means that there are special considerations for routine screening and diagnosis of **birth defects**. Each baby is at risk of having a birth defect. This means the risk that a birth defect will happen is higher in a multiple pregnancy.

Standard **screening tests** for chromosomal disorders, such as **Down syndrome (trisomy 21)**, involve taking a sample of your blood and measuring the level of certain substances. But if the results of a screening test indicate that there is a possibility of a disorder, it's not possible to tell from the test results if one or both babies are affected.

You may have heard about another type of screening called the **cell-free DNA** test. This blood test is based on the fact that a small amount of DNA from the placenta circulates in a pregnant woman's blood. The placenta DNA in a sample of the woman's blood can be screened for chromosome disorders. Cell-free DNA screening for Down syndrome can be done for women carrying twins, but its accuracy for **Patau syndrome (trisomy 13)** and **Edwards syndrome (trisomy 18)** is not known.

Because of the increased risk of birth defects and the limitations of screening tests in a multiple pregnancy, your ob-gyn may recommend **diagnostic testing** for fetal **aneuploidy**. Tests include **chorionic villus sampling (CVS)** or **amniocentesis**. These tests are invasive, meaning that a small amount of amniotic fluid or a very small piece of the placenta needs to be obtained. Before having one of these tests, you should know that

- a sample usually needs to be taken from each baby
- the risks of the procedures are increased with more than one baby
- results may show that one baby has a defect and another baby does not

These tests also are more difficult to do in multiple pregnancies. Only an experienced ob-gyn should do these tests for a multiple pregnancy.

Monitoring

You will need special prenatal care if you are pregnant with multiples. You should visit your ob-gyn more often. Your ob-gyn should monitor the health of your babies with exams and special tests. Some tests are routine. Others may be done only when a problem is suspected. Tests may include

- checking the cervix for signs of preterm labor
- more frequent ultrasound exams to check the babies' growth
- **nonstress test**, in which the babies' cardiac activity is measured
- **biophysical profile (BPP)**, with or without a nonstress test, which includes checking the babies' body movements, breathing movements, muscle tone, and amount of amniotic fluid

Bed Rest and Hospitalization

Recent studies suggest that routine hospitalization or bed rest for women with healthy twin pregnancies does not result in healthier babies or healthier moms. In fact, bed rest can increase the risk of a woman developing **deep vein thrombosis (DVT)**, a condition in which a blood clot forms in the deep veins in the body. For these reasons, routine bed rest and hospitalization are not recommended for women with multiple pregnancies.

Delivery

When and how your babies are born depends on certain factors, including

- the position of each baby
- the weight of each baby
- your health
- the health of the babies
- the location of your placenta

After about 38 weeks of pregnancy, the placenta does not function as efficiently in women carrying twins compared with women carrying one baby. There also is a slightly increased risk of **stillbirth**. But delivering the babies preterm may increase the risk of health problems for them. So, you and your ob-gyn should discuss the best timing for delivery of your babies.

The chance of needing a **cesarean delivery** is higher when you're pregnant with twins than when you're pregnant with one baby. But you have a good chance of having a normal vaginal delivery if

- the presenting twin (the one nearest to the cervix) is in a head-down position
- the placenta is in a normal position
- there are no other complications
- you are at least 32 weeks pregnant

If you're carrying three or more babies, a cesarean birth is recommended because it is safer for the babies (see Chapter 17, "Cesarean Delivery and Vaginal Birth After Cesarean Delivery"). If you are able to give birth vaginally, be prepared for a long labor. The pushing stage may take longer with twins.

Getting Ready

Having more than one baby can be exciting and overwhelming. It is important for you and your partner to be as prepared as possible to care for more than one baby. It may be helpful to talk with other parents who have multiple babies. Having help and support will make life with multiples go much smoother.

Although it's impossible to be prepared for everything, many families of multiple babies encounter the following challenges:

- High health care costs—Because multiple babies often are born with health problems, they may need short-term and long-term specialized health care. Contact your health insurance company to learn what types of care will be covered under your plan.

- Breastfeeding—Breastfeeding any baby takes practice, and the same goes for multiples. Nurses, **certified lactation consultants**, and your ob-gyn can help you get started and work out any problems you may have.

Breast milk has the right amount of all the nutrients the babies need and adapts as your babies' needs change. When you breastfeed, your milk supply will increase to the right amount. If your babies are preterm, you can pump and store your milk until they are strong enough to feed from the breast. See Chapter 20, "Feeding Your Baby," for information on breastfeeding multiples.

- Extra help—You will need some extra hands to help care for your babies. Line up your volunteers well before your due date. Also, make sure that at least some of your helpers are in for the long haul. You most likely will need helpers for several weeks or months, depending on how many babies you have.

- Stress and fatigue—Caring for multiples is stressful. Preterm babies need smaller, more frequent feedings, and sleep can be in short supply for the parents. Plan regular, daily rest periods for yourself. One parent most likely will need to stay at home to care for multiple babies.

- **Postpartum depression**—The "baby blues" are very common after pregnancy. About 2 to 3 days after childbirth, some women begin to feel depressed, anxious, and upset. These feelings usually go away after a week or two. If they do not, or if they get worse, it may be a sign of a more serious condition called postpartum depression. Having multiples may increase your risk of this condition. If you have intense feelings of sadness, anxiety, or hopelessness that keep you from being able to do your daily tasks or enjoy your babies, tell your ob-gyn right away. See Chapter 19, "Your Postpartum Care," for information on postpartum depression.

It may help to take a childbirth class for parents that are expecting more than one baby. Plan to take the class between your fourth and sixth months of pregnancy, when you are likely to be most comfortable. Ask your ob-gyn to help you find a class.

RESOURCES

Challenges of Parenting Multiples
www.reproductivefacts.org/news-and-publications/patient-fact-sheets-and-booklets/documents/fact-sheets-and-info-booklets/challenges-of-parenting-multiples/
Information from the American Society for Reproductive Medicine that addresses the social, economic, and psychological issues of multiple pregnancy.

Raising Multiples
www.raisingmultiples.org
Nonprofit national organization that provides information and support for parents of multiples. The website that covers all aspects of having multiples—not just twins.

What Do Maternal–Fetal Medicine Subspecialists Do?
www.smfm.org/whatwedo
Webpage that explains the role of an MFM specialist in pregnancy care.

Your Pregnancy and Childbirth
www.acog.org/MyPregnancy
Website from the American College of Obstetricians and Gynecologists (ACOG) with information on pregnancy, labor, delivery, and postpartum care. Includes the latest information from the experts in women's health care, questions answered by ACOG ob-gyns, pregnancy stories from real women, and an A–Z directory of health topics covering pregnancy and beyond.

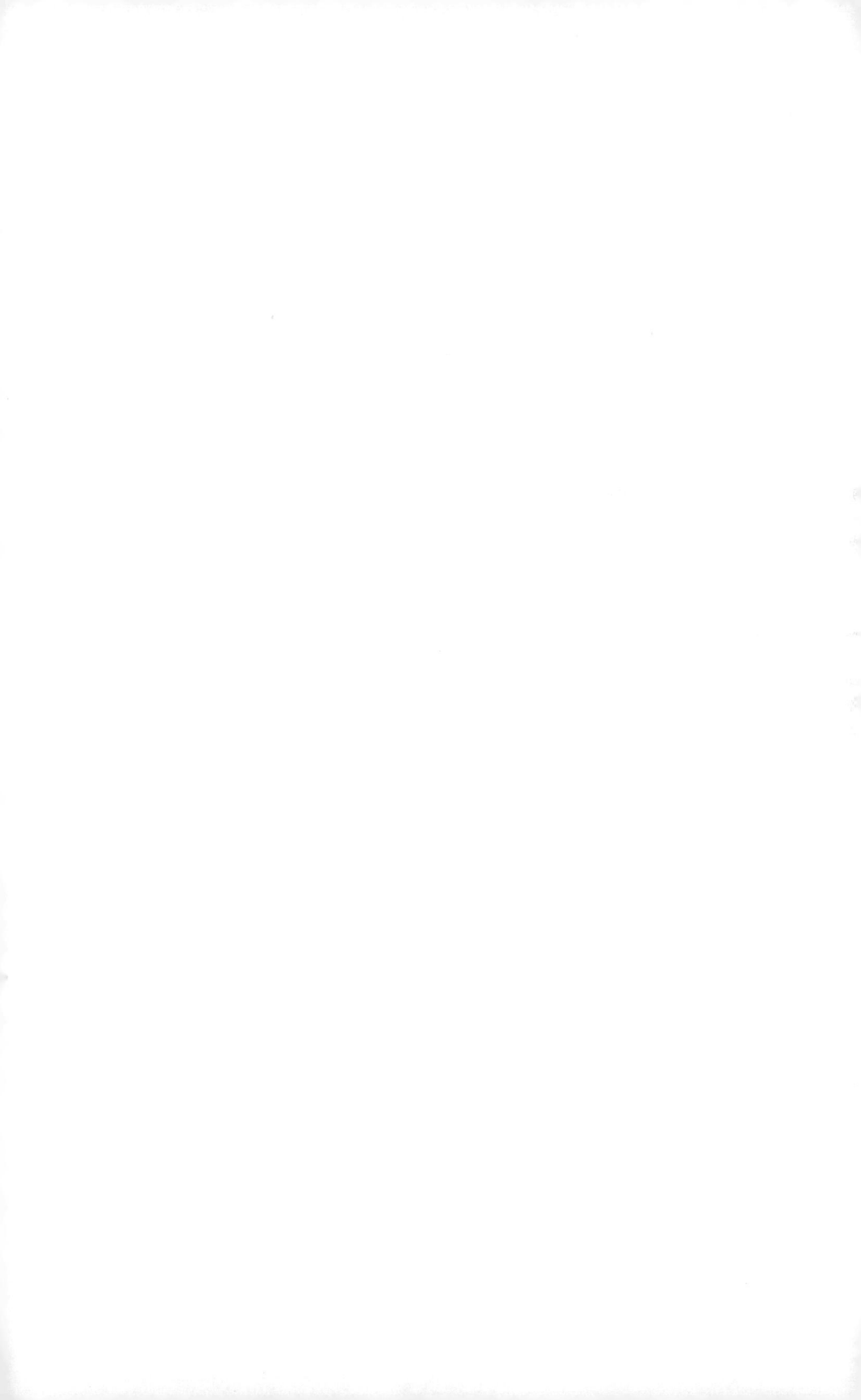

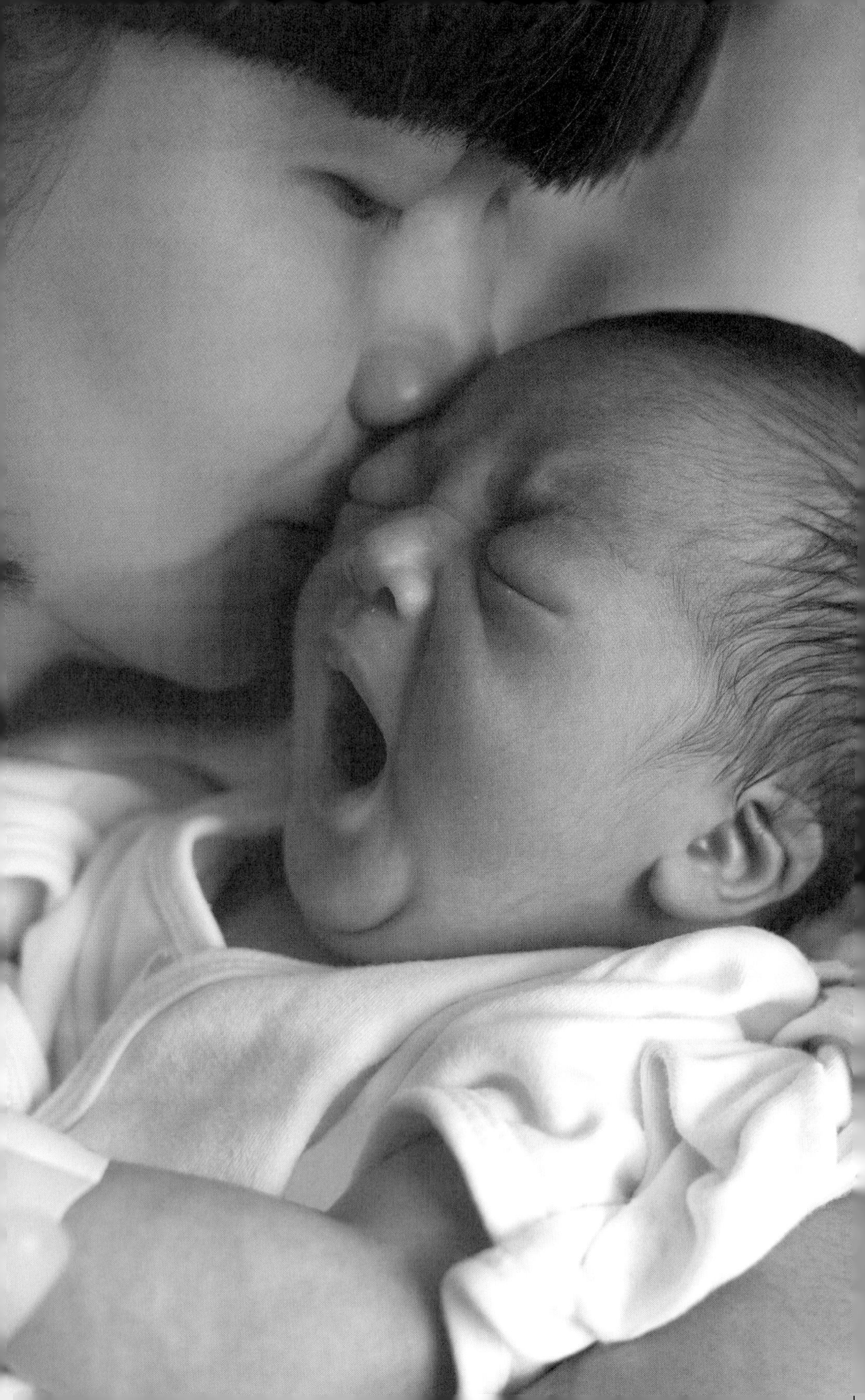

PART 6

Medical Problems During Pregnancy

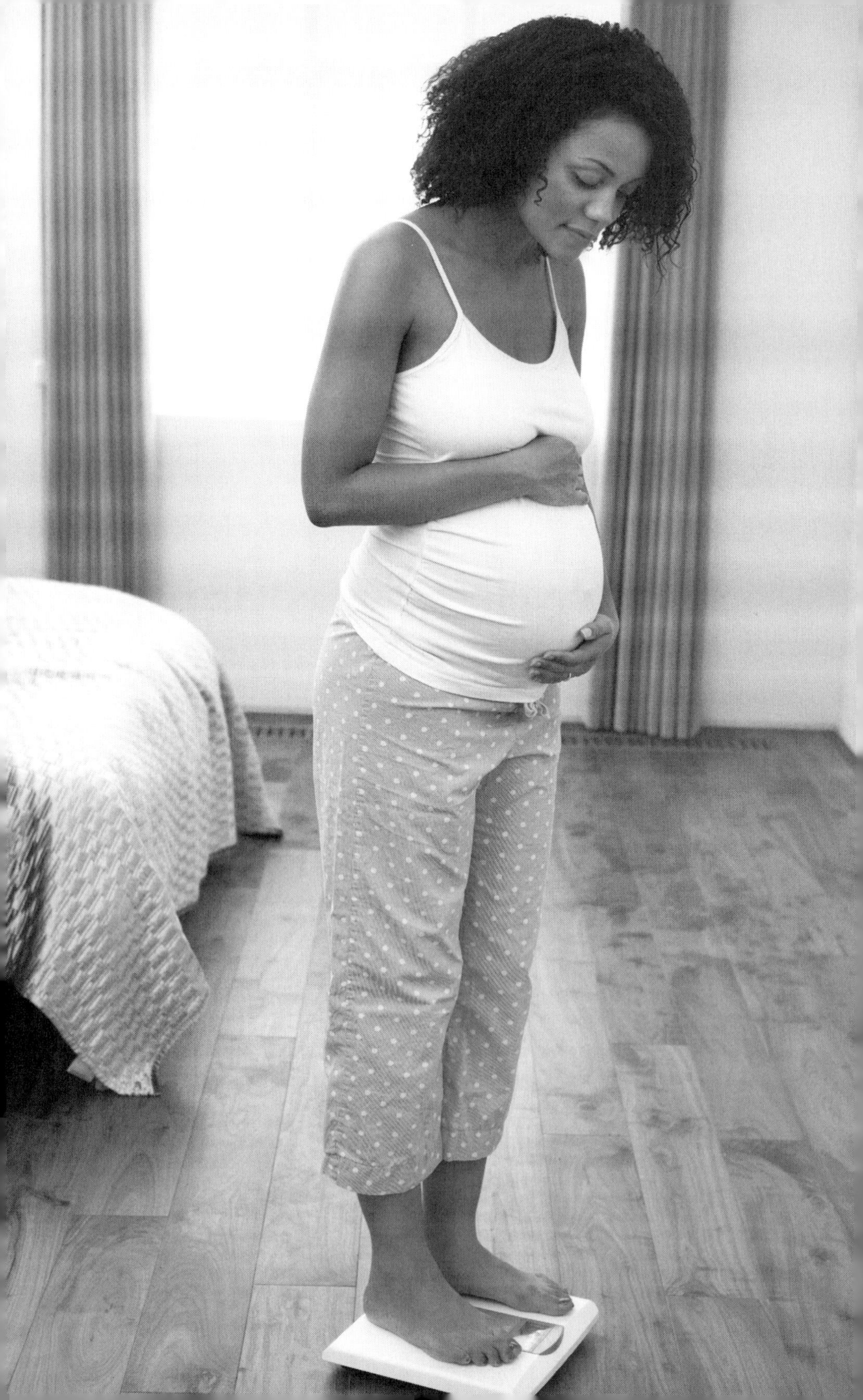

CHAPTER 29

Weight During Pregnancy
Obesity and Eating Disorders

Women are often judged by their weight. Society projects an image of a woman's "ideal" weight that does not match reality. For women whose bodies don't fit the ideal, this stigma can be harmful to their health. Regardless of your weight, you have a right to respectful, nonjudgmental, high-quality care from all your health care practitioners. But being underweight or obese can pose risks for you and your pregnancy. So you and your **obstetrician–gynecologist (ob-gyn)** should talk about these risks and how they can be minimized.

Most of what you need to know about pregnancy, labor, and delivery is discussed in the "Pregnancy Month by Month," "Labor and Delivery," and "Postpartum Care" sections of this book. This chapter focuses on the things that may be different about your pregnancy if you are obese or have an eating disorder.

Why Your Weight Is Important

When you eat more **nutrient**-rich foods during pregnancy, you increase your intake of **calories**. You also are providing what your baby needs to develop. Early in pregnancy, you may have some weight loss if you are unable to eat or drink due to nausea and vomiting. Later in pregnancy, too much weight gain can have negative effects.

Remember that when you are weighed during pregnancy, it includes the weight of

- the baby
- the **placenta**

> ### Dealing With Comments About Your Weight
>
> Sometimes people, including family members, comment on a pregnant woman's weight. They may mean well, but these comments can make you feel bad or unsure about whether you have or haven't gained the right amount of weight for your baby.
>
> To cope with comments, remember that your pregnancy and your weight are your private concerns. Also, remember that other people do not know how big or small you should be, how much weight you have gained or lost, or what your weight should be for your current stage of pregnancy. A well-timed reply, such as "Thank you for your concern" or "My doctor thinks I'm doing fine," can let your questioner know that his or her comments are off-limits.
>
> For women who begin pregnancy overweight or obese, and for women with an eating disorder, these comments can be especially challenging. You may want to work on scripts to deal with unwanted comments so that you'll have them when you need them. Your ob-gyn or a trusted family member or friend can help you with this.

- *amniotic fluid*
- fluid that is retained, usually as swelling in the legs

So looking at your stomach and measuring your actual weight are only general assessments. What is most important is whether you are able to eat enough healthy foods to support you and your baby, and whether that nutrition is helping the baby grow over time.

At your first **prenatal care** visit, you and your ob-gyn should discuss your current weight and recent changes. The National Academy of Medicine has published guidelines for weight gain during pregnancy. These weight gain ranges are based on extensive research and are associated with the best possible outcomes for pregnant women and their babies (see Table 29-1, "Weight Gain Recommendations for Pregnancy").

Experts recommend an initial weight gain of 2 to 4 pounds in the first *trimester*. In the second and third trimesters, women who are overweight should gain a little over half a pound each week, on average. Women who are obese should gain a little under half a pound each week. Women who are underweight should aim to gain about a pound a week, on average, in the second and third trimesters.

TABLE 29-1 **Weight Gain Recommendations for Pregnancy**

Body Mass Index (BMI) Before Pregnancy	Rate of Weight Gain in the Second and Third Trimesters* (Pounds Per Week)	Recommended Total Weight Gain With a Single Baby (in Pounds)	Recommended Weight Gain With Twins (in Pounds)
Less than 18.5 (underweight)	1.0 to 1.3	28 to 40	Not known
18.5 to 24.9 (normal weight)	0.8 to 1.0	25 to 35	37 to 54
25.0 to 29.9 (overweight)	0.5 to 0.7	15 to 25	31 to 50
30.0 and above (obese)	0.4 to 0.6	11 to 20	25 to 42

*Assumes a first-trimester weight gain between 1.1 and 4.4 pounds
Source: Institute of Medicine and National Research Council. 2009. *Weight Gain During Pregnancy: Reexamining the Guidelines*. Washington, DC: The National Academies Press.

You and your ob-gyn should talk about your weight gain at each prenatal visit. You also may talk about poor appetite, nausea and vomiting, or other digestive concerns. The growth of your baby also should be checked. If your baby is not growing well, your ob-gyn may recommend changes in your diet or exercise plan that may be helpful.

Good nutrition is key to a healthy pregnancy. A healthy diet relies on the foods you eat and portion size. If you need help planning a healthy diet, or if your weight gain is not enough or too much, your ob-gyn may recommend nutrition counseling. See Chapter 22, "Nutrition During Pregnancy," for a guide to healthy eating during pregnancy.

Obesity and eating disorders both can affect pregnancy. If you have either of these conditions, learn about the risks that they pose. You and your ob-gyn can work together to manage your pregnancy and avoid some of these risks.

Obesity and Pregnancy

Obesity is one of the country's fastest-growing health problems. The number of people with obesity in the United States has increased steadily over the past 25 years. Today, about 1 in 4 pregnant women in the United States is considered obese. Obesity can have serious effects on a pregnant woman's health and the health of her baby.

If you are obese and already pregnant, certain things can help reduce the risk of problems for you and your baby. These include

- prenatal care visits with an ob-gyn
- healthy eating (see Chapter 22, "Nutrition During Pregnancy")
- regular exercise

If you are planning a pregnancy, the best way to prevent problems is to lose weight before you get pregnant. Of course, this is not always easy. It's important to work with your ob-gyn on a plan of care that is right for you.

Defining Obesity

Body mass index (BMI) is a number calculated from height and weight. BMI is used to determine whether a person is underweight, normal weight, overweight, or obese. You are considered obese if your BMI before pregnancy is 30 or higher. Use the "Body Mass Index Chart" at the back of this book to look up your prepregnancy BMI. You also can find an online BMI calculator at www.nhlbi.nih.gov/health/educational/lose_wt/BMI/bmicalc.htm.

There are four categories of weight that are based on BMI:

1. Underweight—BMI of less than 18.5
2. Normal weight—BMI of 18.5 to 24.9
3. Overweight—BMI of 25 to 29.9
4. Obese—BMI of 30 or greater

Within the general category of obesity, there are three subcategories that also are based on BMI:

- Obesity category I—BMI of 30 to 34.9
- Obesity category II—BMI of 35 to 39.9
- Obesity category III—BMI of 40 or greater

Risks for You

Pregnancy carries some risk for all women, whatever their weight. But women who are obese are more likely to have certain health problems during pregnancy. The more severe her obesity, the more likely that a woman will have one or more of these problems during pregnancy, delivery, or the ***postpartum*** period.

- ***Gestational hypertension***—High blood pressure that starts during the second half of pregnancy is called gestational hypertension. It can lead to serious ***complications*** (see Chapter 30, "Hypertension and Preeclampsia").

- ***Preeclampsia***—Preeclampsia is a serious form of gestational hypertension that usually happens in the second half of pregnancy, or soon after childbirth (see Chapter 30, "Hypertension and Preeclampsia"). This condition can cause the woman's **kidneys** and liver to fail. In rare cases, seizures, heart attack, and **stroke** can happen. Other risks include problems with the **placenta** and growth problems for the baby. In extremely severe cases, preeclampsia can cause death for the woman, her baby, or both.

- *Gestational diabetes*—High levels of **glucose** (blood sugar) during pregnancy increase the risk of having a very large baby. This also increases the chance of a **cesarean birth**. Women who have had gestational diabetes have a higher risk of **diabetes mellitus** in the future. So do their children (see Chapter 31, "Diabetes During Pregnancy").
- *Obstructive Sleep Apnea*—Sleep apnea is a condition in which a person stops breathing for short periods during sleep. During pregnancy, sleep apnea can cause fatigue and increase the risk of high blood pressure, preeclampsia, **eclampsia**, and heart and lung problems.

Obesity also can interfere with certain tests. For example, higher amounts of body fat can make it harder for an ob-gyn to measure the ***fundal height*** of the **uterus**. This measurement can help determine the size of the baby. ***Ultrasound exams*** may be used to follow the baby's growth if measuring the uterus is difficult.

Risks for the Baby

Women who are obese are at greater risk of having a large baby (***macrosomia***). This can increase the risk of the baby being injured during delivery. For example, the baby's shoulder can get stuck after the head is delivered (***shoulder dystocia***). Macrosomia also increases the chance that a ***cesarean delivery*** will be needed (see the "Risks for Childbirth" section on the next page).

Babies born to women who are obese also have a slightly higher risk of several problems, including

- heart defects
- **neural tube defects (NTDs)**
- **stillbirth**, though the risk overall is low

Preterm birth is another risk with obesity, particularly when the woman also has medical conditions such as diabetes or high blood pressure. Babies born preterm are at increased risk of

- breathing problems
- eating problems
- developmental and learning difficulties later in life

Risks for Childbirth

Obesity increases the risks of complications during labor and delivery. Being obese can lower the chance of a successful vaginal delivery. It can be harder to monitor the baby during labor. For these reasons, obesity increases the chance that a cesarean delivery will be needed.

If a cesarean delivery is needed, it can be riskier for an obese woman than for a thinner woman, and the time it takes to perform the surgery may be longer. Complications may include

- problems with the *anesthesia* used for the procedure
- excessive bleeding during surgery
- poor wound healing
- infection

Surgery and obesity also increase the risk of blood clots developing in the veins of the legs (*deep vein thrombosis [DVT]*).

Exercise

Exercise is important for all pregnant women. Women who are obese should start with low-intensity, short periods of exercise and gradually increase as they can. Walking is an excellent form of exercise. A good plan is to work up to 20 to 30 minutes per day on most days or every day of the week. You also should do some strengthening exercises. Talk with your ob-gyn about what's best for you. See Chapter 23, "Exercise During Pregnancy."

Testing for Gestational Diabetes

Your ob-gyn may test you for gestational diabetes during the first 3 months of your pregnancy. Women who are overweight or obese have a higher risk of this complication. You also may be given the test again in the later months of your pregnancy.

Labor and Delivery

Depending on your health and the health and size of your baby, your ob-gyn may suggest a planned cesarean birth (see Chapter 17, "Cesarean Delivery and Vaginal Birth After Cesarean Delivery"). You and your ob-gyn should discuss the risks and benefits of this procedure well before your due date so that you can make an informed decision.

Women who are obese may need extra attention before, during, and after cesarean birth to decrease the risk of certain problems, such as blood clots. For example, you may be given a medication to prevent blood clots or special stockings or boots to wear before, during, and after surgery. All pregnant women receive **antibiotics** to prevent infection during a cesarean birth, but women who are obese may receive a higher dose. Even with antibiotics, women who are obese are at higher risk of infection, including wound infection.

If you are suspected of having sleep apnea, your ob-gyn may have you see an **anesthesiologist** before delivery. He or she may monitor you closely for breathing problems after delivery, particularly if cesarean delivery is needed.

Losing Weight After Pregnancy

Many women find it hard to lose the weight they gain during pregnancy. If you are overweight or obese and planning another pregnancy in the future, talk with your ob-gyn about weight loss. It's important to reach a healthier weight between pregnancies. Losing excess weight before getting pregnant again is especially important if you had complications in your last pregnancy.

Losing weight is not easy. In general, it involves using up more calories than you take in. You can do this by getting regular exercise and eating smaller portions. Even if you do not lose much weight, making these changes may reduce your risk of serious medical problems, such as diabetes and high blood pressure. Your ob-gyn may refer you to a dietitian or a nutritionist who can help you plan healthy meals and snacks.

Exercise should be an important part of your weight loss plan. Most people who have lost weight and kept it off get 60 to 90 minutes of moderate-intensity activity on most days of the week. Moderate-intensity activities include biking, brisk walking, and yard work.

You do not have to do this amount all at once. For example, you can exercise for 20 to 30 minutes three times a day. If you do not have access to healthy food or a safe place to exercise, talk with your ob-gyn about options that might work for you.

Your ob-gyn may suggest medications to help with weight loss if you have tried to lose weight through diet changes and exercise and you still have

- a BMI above 30, or
- a BMI of at least 27 with certain medical conditions, such as diabetes or heart disease

Weight loss medications should not be taken during pregnancy.

If diet and exercise or medications do not work, **bariatric surgery** may be an option for people who either are very obese (a BMI of 40 or greater) or are moderately obese (a BMI between 35 and 39) and have major health problems caused by obesity, such as diabetes or heart disease.

Future Health Risks

If you had gestational diabetes, you should be tested 4 to 12 weeks after you give birth. If your blood sugar is normal, you will need to be tested for diabetes every 1 to 3 years. Maintaining a healthy weight, eating a balanced diet, and staying active after pregnancy may reduce your risk of getting diabetes in the future.

Pregnancy After Weight-Loss Surgery

Bariatric surgery may help some people with weight loss when diet and exercise alone aren't enough. After bariatric surgery, many people lose a lot of weight. Losing weight can restore normal *ovulation* in women and increase the chance of becoming pregnant. Bariatric surgery can be divided into two types:

- Restrictive surgery reduces the amount of food the stomach can hold. Weight loss with restrictive surgery tends to be slow and steady.
- Malabsorptive surgery changes the way food is absorbed through the intestines. Weight loss with malabsorptive surgery may be faster. People who have had malabsorptive surgery may lose more weight overall.

Like any surgery, each type of weight-loss surgery has different risks, benefits, and success rates, which you should discuss with your surgeon. If you had or plan to have weight-loss surgery, keep the following in mind and discuss with your ob-gyn:

- You should wait 12 to 24 months after surgery before you try to get pregnant. This is the time when you will have the fastest weight loss.
- If you have had fertility problems, they may resolve on their own as you lose weight. It is important to know about this possibility. The increase in fertility can lead to an unplanned pregnancy if you have a male partner and are not using birth control.
- Some types of weight-loss surgery may affect how the body absorbs medications taken by mouth, including birth control pills. You may need to switch to another form of birth control until you are ready for pregnancy.

Most women who have had weight-loss surgery in the past do well during pregnancy. Still, you may need to pay attention to a few special issues:

- You may need to be monitored for vitamin deficiencies, especially if you have had malabsorptive surgery. If deficiencies are found, you may need to take extra amounts of iron, vitamin B_{12}, folic acid, vitamin D, and calcium.

There may not be enough of these vitamins and minerals in your prenatal vitamin. It is best to get these vitamins as separate supplements. Do not take extra prenatal vitamins. Extra doses of the other vitamins in supplements, such as vitamin A, can be harmful (see Chapter 22, "Nutrition During Pregnancy.")

- Nutritional counseling may be recommended to be sure that you are getting enough **nutrients** and to help you cope with the nutritional demands of pregnancy.
- Your ob-gyn may recommend that you visit your bariatric surgeon for an evaluation after you get pregnant. If you've had gastric band surgery (a type of restrictive surgery), adjustments may need to be made to the band during pregnancy. The surgeon who did your bariatric surgery can help monitor you for any problems.
- If you've had malabsorptive surgery, you may not be able to tolerate the test commonly used to screen for gestational diabetes, which involves drinking a sugary mixture. You may need to have a different type of test to screen for gestational diabetes.

Eating Disorders and Pregnancy

Each year in the United States, 10 million women struggle with eating disorders. Some women with eating disorders may have a temporary improvement in their symptoms when they get pregnant. For other women, eating disorders that were under control before pregnancy may start again during pregnancy. And sometimes an eating disorder may begin during pregnancy.

Like any health problem, an eating disorder can cause problems for you and your baby. It's important to be open with your ob-gyn and let him or her know if you are worried about your eating or exercise habits, weight, or body image for any reason. Don't be afraid to ask for help. With proper support, many women with eating disorders can have healthy babies.

How Eating Disorders Can Affect You

- Calorie restriction can affect memory, concentration, and mental skills.
- Vomiting or using laxatives excessively can cause dehydration and interfere with the body's electrolyte balance, including levels of sodium, calcium, and potassium. This can cause seizures, heart rhythm problems, or kidney failure.
- Over time, eating disorders can damage all parts of the body, including the heart, bones, muscles, digestive system, and brain.

- Women with eating disorders who are underweight often have problems getting pregnant. With treatment and weight gain, fertility often returns as well.

How Eating Disorders Can Affect Your Baby

Having an eating disorder can affect your pregnancy in many ways. Gaining a healthy amount of weight and getting enough nutrients are important for a healthy pregnancy. If you do not take in enough nutrients or gain enough weight while you're pregnant, it can lead to problems for both you and your baby, including

- slow growth of the baby
- *low birth weight*
- preterm birth
- *miscarriage*
- gestational diabetes
- preeclampsia
- problems during labor
- difficulty with breastfeeding
- *depression*

If you take *laxatives*, diuretics, or medications to purge your meals, they also can harm your baby. These substances take away nutrients and fluids before your body is able to absorb them and pass them to your baby.

Types of Eating Disorders

There are many different types of eating disorders. They often have different warning signs and result in different health problems.

Anorexia Nervosa. A person with *anorexia nervosa* diets to an extreme because she feels overweight even when she is not. Most women with anorexia nervosa have an intense fear of being overweight. They want to be thin so badly that they may starve themselves—sometimes to death. They may diet nonstop, refuse to eat except in small portions, or want to eat alone. They also may exercise excessively.

People with anorexia nervosa go through many physical changes:

- They may lose a lot of weight and still think they are overweight.
- They may have fine hair growing on their face and arms.
- They may lose hair from their head.
- Their skin may be dry, pale, and yellowed.

Women with anorexia nervosa may stop having **menstrual periods**. They also may have fertility problems.

Bulimia Nervosa. People with ***bulimia nervosa*** binge eat. This means they eat large amounts of food in a short time. They may feel like they cannot control what they eat or how much they eat during a binge. Then they purge the excess food by forcing themselves to vomit. Or they do things to compensate for overeating, including taking laxatives, fasting, or exercising too much.

People with bulimia also go through physical changes:

- They may have a constant sore throat.
- They may have swollen salivary glands in the neck and jaw.
- They may have worn tooth enamel and decaying teeth from stomach acid.
- They may have acid reflux and intestinal problems.
- They may have dehydration and an imbalance of the minerals needed to be healthy.

Binge Eating Disorder. Binge eating disorder is the most common eating disorder in the United States. People with this disorder eat a lot of food in a short time. They may eat when they are not hungry and to the point where they feel uncomfortable. They may feel like they cannot control what they eat or how much they eat. Then they may feel disgusted, depressed, or guilty after overeating. People with binge eating disorder usually do not purge the way people with bulimia do.

Other Eating Disorders. Other eating disorders include the following:

- Avoidant Restrictive Food Intake Disorder (ARFID) is extreme restriction of food that is not related to problems with body image or fears of weight gain. People with this disorder may eat only a small number of foods, or only foods with certain textures. They may be afraid of choking or vomiting. If you have this problem, let your ob-gyn know so you can be evaluated, ideally before pregnancy.
- ***Pica*** (pronounced "pike-uh") is a strong urge to eat nonfood items, such as clay, chalk, paint chips, or laundry starch. Eating nonfood items can be harmful. It also can prevent you from getting the nutrients you need. Pica often starts during pregnancy. It can be a sign that you lack one or more nutrients, such as iron or zinc. You may need to be tested for **anemia** or other health problems. Pica often goes away if the underlying problem is

treated. Your ob-gyn may not be aware of this problem if you do not share your urge to eat nonfood items.

- Rumination disorder involves regularly regurgitating food (bringing it back up from the stomach). The person may then re-chew or re-swallow the food, or they may spit it out. This is not caused by another medical condition, such as a stomach problem. It does not happen as part of another eating disorder.

Risk Factors and Warning Signs

People who tend to be perfectionist or obsessive may be more likely to develop an eating disorder. Having a close relative with an eating disorder or another mental health condition also may be a risk factor.

Different eating disorders have different warning signs, but any of the following can mean there is a problem:

- Feeling preoccupied with weight, food, calories, or dieting
- Feeling shame or guilt about your eating habits
- Body image distortion—an unrealistic view of how your body looks
- Dieting nonstop (even when you are a normal weight or are underweight)
- Skipping meals to lose weight
- Refusing to eat except in small portions
- Wanting to eat alone
- Eating until you feel uncomfortable or sick
- Making yourself vomit
- Using diet pills, laxatives, or diuretics to control your weight
- Exercising compulsively or excessively

If you have any of these warning signs, talk with your ob-gyn. You also should let them know if you are worried about your eating or exercise habits, weight, or body image.

Getting Help

If you have an eating disorder or think you might have one, tell your ob-gyn right away. The sooner you can address and resolve the problem, the better. The good news is that many women with eating disorders can have healthy babies.

If you need it, your ob-gyn may refer you to a special health care practitioner that can help treat your disorder. Individual and group therapy also may help. You may need medication as well.

Remember that gaining the right amount of weight is crucial to having a healthy baby. Ask your ob-gyn to refer you to a nutritionist with experience in eating disorders. They can help you plan for healthy eating and weight gain during your pregnancy. You also may want to continue seeing a nutritionist after you give birth.

Some of the activities associated with pregnancy—like getting weighed or enrolling in a prenatal exercise class—may be difficult for you if you have an eating disorder. Discuss these issues with your ob-gyn so that you can find ways to address them. For example, you may prefer not to know your weight unless there is a problem.

If You Have a History of Eating Disorders

Pregnancy raises body image issues for just about every woman. For a woman with a past eating disorder, these issues can trigger the return of the disorder.

If you have a history of an eating disorder, tell your ob-gyn early in pregnancy. Together, you can monitor your feelings and be alert to any signs that the disorder has returned. It may be a good idea to continue counseling or seek out a counselor when you get pregnant.

Recovering from an eating disorder is not always easy, especially in a body-conscious world. If you need more support, don't be afraid to ask for it.

RESOURCES

Being Overweight During Pregnancy
www.marchofdimes.com/pregnancy/overweight-and-obesity-during-pregnancy.aspx
March of Dimes webpage that provides information and advice about managing obesity before, during, and after pregnancy.

National Eating Disorders Association
www.nationaleatingdisorders.org/pregnancy-and-eating-disorders
Gives an overview of the risks that eating disorders pose during pregnancy. Maintains an extensive list of resources to find help and support.

Your Pregnancy and Childbirth
www.acog.org/MyPregnancy
Website from the American College of Obstetricians and Gynecologists (ACOG) with information on pregnancy, labor, delivery, and postpartum care. Includes the latest information from the experts in women's health care, questions answered by ACOG ob-gyns, pregnancy stories from real women, and an A–Z directory of health topics covering pregnancy and beyond.

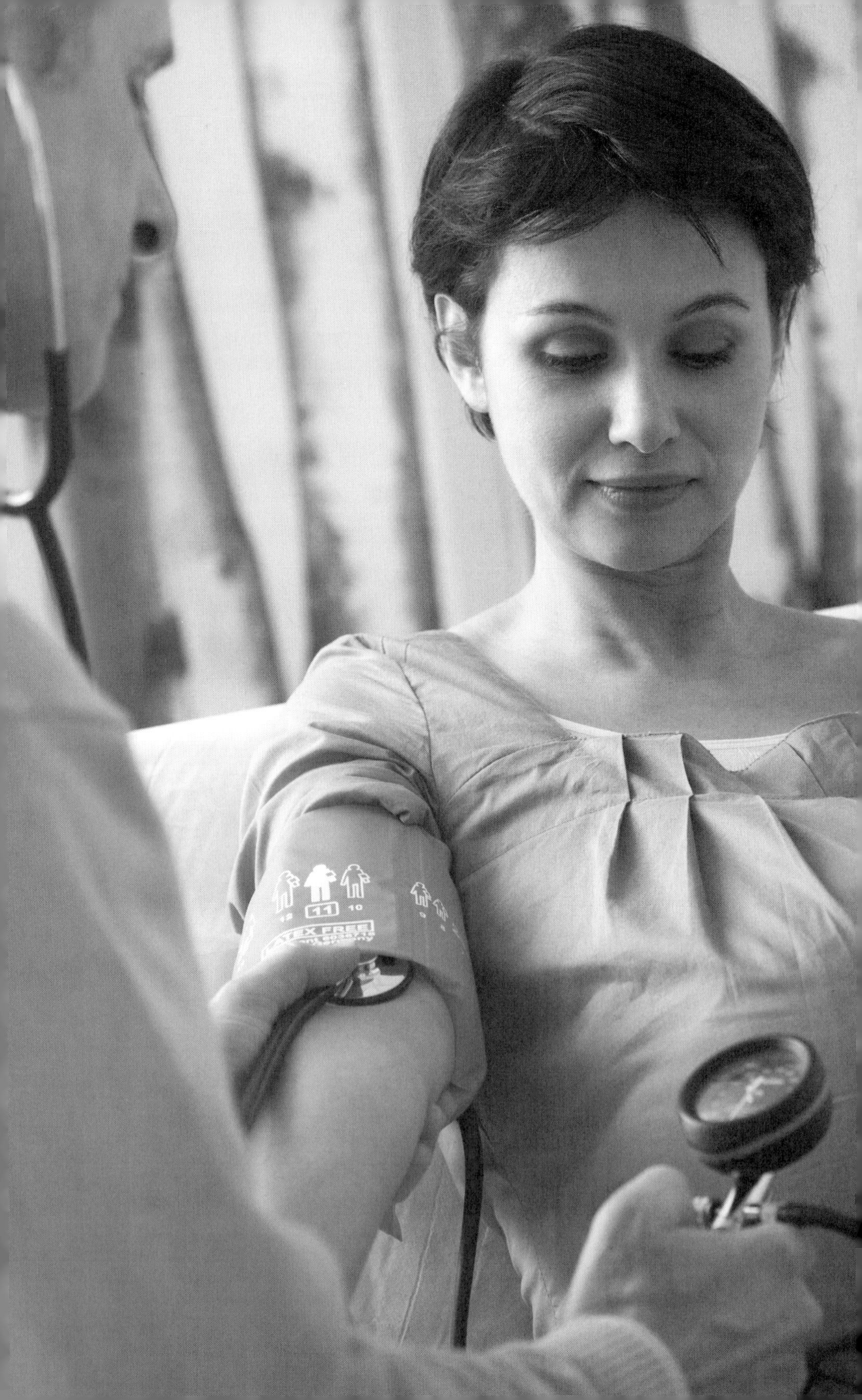
11
10

CHAPTER 30

Hypertension and Preeclampsia

Hypertension can lead to health problems at any time in life. Hypertension (also called **high blood pressure**) is a "silent disease" because it usually does not cause symptoms. During pregnancy, severe or uncontrolled hypertension can cause problems for you and your baby.

Some women have hypertension before they get pregnant. Others develop it for the first time during pregnancy. A serious high blood pressure disorder called **preeclampsia** also can happen during pregnancy or soon after childbirth.

No matter when high blood pressure starts, it usually happens without any signs or symptoms. This is one reason why it is so important to see your **obstetrician–gynecologist (ob-gyn)** when planning a pregnancy and during pregnancy. Your blood pressure should be checked at every office visit.

Blood pressure often goes up in the weeks after childbirth as your body adjusts. This means you also will need to watch for the signs of preeclampsia for 7 to 10 days after you give birth. See the box "Signs and Symptoms of Preeclampsia."

Blood Pressure

Blood pressure is the force of blood pushing against the walls of blood vessels called **arteries**. The arteries bring blood from the heart to your lungs, where it picks up **oxygen** and then moves to your organs and tissues. The organs and tissues use the oxygen to power their activities. Blood vessels called **veins** return the blood to the heart.

> **Signs and Symptoms of Preeclampsia**
>
> If you have any of the following symptoms, especially if they happen in the second half of pregnancy, contact your ob-gyn right away:
>
> - Swelling of face or hands
> - A headache that will not go away
> - Seeing spots or changes in eyesight
> - Pain in the upper abdomen or shoulder
> - Nausea and vomiting (in the second half of pregnancy)
> - Sudden weight gain
> - Difficulty breathing

To measure your blood pressure, a cuff with a balloon inside is wrapped around your upper arm. Air is pumped into the balloon. Your pressure reading is taken while the air is slowly released from the cuff.

A blood pressure reading has two numbers separated by a slash: 110/80 mm Hg. You may hear this referred to as "110 over 80." The first number is the pressure against the artery walls when the heart contracts (squeezes). This is called the ***systolic blood pressure***. The second number is the pressure against the artery walls when the heart relaxes between contractions. This is called the ***diastolic blood pressure*** (see the box "Your Blood Pressure Reading"). Blood pressure is expressed in "millimeters of mercury" (mm Hg) because the original blood pressure meters used a column of mercury to measure pressure.

Your ob-gyn should check your blood pressure at each ***prenatal care*** visit. Blood pressure changes often during the day. It can go down when you are resting. It can go up

- if you are excited
- when you exercise
- after you drink caffeine
- after you use tobacco
- with certain over-the-counter medications

> **Your Blood Pressure Reading**
>
> $\dfrac{110}{80}$ = $\dfrac{\text{systolic}}{\text{diastolic}}$ = $\dfrac{\text{force of blood in the arteries when heart contracts}}{\text{force of blood in the arteries when heart relaxes}}$

Some people have what is known as "white coat hypertension." This means that their blood pressure is higher when they are in a health care practitioner's office than when they are at home. It is called "white coat" because seeing the white coat of a doctor triggers an increase in blood pressure.

Short-term changes in blood pressure are normal. Because of the normal ups and downs in blood pressure, if you have one high reading, another reading may be taken a little later to confirm the result. In some cases, you may be asked to monitor your blood pressure at home.

Hypertension

Hypertension means one of the following:

- The systolic blood pressure (top number) is high.
- The diastolic blood pressure (bottom number) is high.
- Both are high.

The box "Measuring Blood Pressure" shows blood pressure categories as defined by the American College of Cardiology and the American Heart Association. A blood pressure reading of less than 120/80 mm Hg is considered normal.

Measuring Blood Pressure

The chart below shows different blood pressure readings and how they are classified for adults age 18 and older. Find your systolic and diastolic pressure readings to see whether your blood pressure is normal.

Normal: Less than 120/80 mm Hg

Elevated: Systolic between 120 and 129 and diastolic less than 80 mm Hg

Stage 1 hypertension: Systolic between 130 and 139 or diastolic between 80 and 89 mm Hg

Stage 2 hypertension: Systolic 140 or higher or diastolic 90 or higher mm Hg

Hypertensive crisis: Systolic over 180 and/or diastolic over 120 mm Hg

Abbreviation: mm Hg, millimeters of mercury.
Source: New ACC/AHA High Blood Pressure Guidelines Lower Definition of Hypertension. American College of Cardiology. November 2017.

Hypertension during pregnancy is classified as either chronic hypertension or **gestational hypertension**. These conditions are defined this way:

- Chronic hypertension is present before pregnancy or diagnosed in early pregnancy.

- Gestational hypertension comes on during pregnancy, typically in the second half of pregnancy and most often near the end of pregnancy.

Chronic Hypertension

Chronic hypertension is high blood pressure that was present before a woman got pregnant or that happens before 20 weeks of pregnancy. If you were taking blood pressure medication before you got pregnant—even if your blood pressure is currently normal—you have been diagnosed with chronic hypertension.

Risks

When a woman is pregnant, her body makes more blood to support the baby's growth. If blood pressure goes up during pregnancy, it can place extra stress on her heart and **kidneys**. This can lead to heart disease, kidney disease, and **stroke**.

High blood pressure also may reduce blood flow to the **placenta**. As a result, the baby may get fewer **nutrients** and less oxygen than he or she needs to grow. This can lead to a condition called **fetal growth restriction**, where the baby does not grow normally.

Other risks of chronic hypertension during pregnancy include the following:

- Gestational hypertension, including preeclampsia—This condition is more likely to happen in women with chronic hypertension than in women with normal blood pressure.

- **Preterm** birth—If the placenta is not getting enough nutrients and oxygen to the baby, early delivery may be better for the baby than allowing the pregnancy to continue. Early delivery also may be needed to prevent more health problems for the woman.

- **Placental abruption**—In this condition, the placenta comes away from the wall of the uterus too soon. This is a medical emergency that requires treatment right away (see Chapter 37, "Placenta Problems").

- **Cesarean birth**—Women with high blood pressure are more likely to have a cesarean birth than women with normal blood pressure. A cesarean

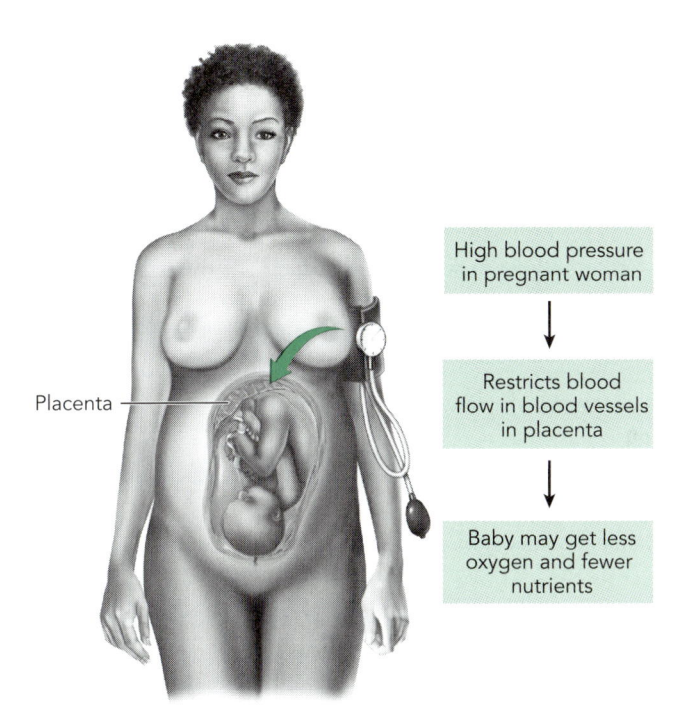

Hypertension. Hypertension during pregnancy can decrease the amount of oxygen and nutrients the baby receives.

birth may be needed if the baby is very small or if there are other problems that require avoiding labor. Cesarean birth carries risks for the woman, including infection, injury to internal organs, and bleeding. It also can affect the way that a woman gives birth later if she decides to have more children (see Chapter 17, "Cesarean Delivery and Vaginal Birth After Cesarean Delivery").

Treatment

Treatment depends on whether your chronic hypertension is mild or more severe. In the first half of pregnancy, blood pressure normally goes down as your blood circulation adapts to supply the baby with oxygen and nutrients. If your hypertension is mild, your blood pressure may stay that way or even return to normal during pregnancy. If this happens, your ob-gyn may lower your medication dose or advise you to stop taking your medication during pregnancy. If you have more severe hypertension or have health problems related to your hypertension, you may need to start or continue blood pressure medication during pregnancy.

Whether your hypertension is mild or more severe, your blood pressure should be monitored throughout pregnancy. You may need to monitor your blood pressure at home. **Ultrasound exams** may be done throughout pregnancy to track the growth of the baby. If growth problems are suspected, you may have extra tests that monitor the health of the baby. This testing usually begins in the third **trimester** of pregnancy. It also is important to watch for signs of preeclampsia (see the box "Signs and Symptoms of Preeclampsia" in this chapter).

If your condition remains stable, delivery of the baby 1 to 3 weeks before your due date (about 37 to 39 weeks of pregnancy) generally is recommended. If you or the baby develop **complications**, the baby may need to be delivered even earlier.

After delivery, you will need to keep monitoring your blood pressure at home for 1 to 2 weeks. Blood pressure often goes up in the weeks after childbirth. You may need to go back to taking medication, or your medication dosage may need to be adjusted. Talk with your ob-gyn about blood pressure medications that are safe to take when you're breastfeeding. Do not stop any medications without talking with your ob-gyn.

Gestational Hypertension

A woman has gestational hypertension when:

- She has a systolic blood pressure of 140 mm Hg or higher and/or a diastolic blood pressure of 90 mm Hg or higher.
- The high blood pressure first happens after 20 weeks.
- She had normal blood pressure before pregnancy.

Most women with gestational hypertension have only a small increase in blood pressure. But some women develop severe hypertension (defined as systolic blood pressure of 160 mm Hg or higher and/or diastolic blood pressure of 110 mm Hg or higher). These women are at risk of very serious complications. All women with gestational hypertension are monitored for signs of preeclampsia and to make sure that their blood pressure does not go too high.

Although gestational hypertension usually goes away after childbirth, it may increase the risk of developing hypertension in the future. If you had gestational hypertension, keep this risk in mind as you make decisions about your health. Healthy eating, weight loss, and exercise may help prevent high blood pressure in the future.

Preeclampsia

Preeclampsia is a serious blood pressure disorder that can affect all organs in a woman's body. Like gestational hypertension, it usually happens after 20 weeks of pregnancy, typically in the third trimester. When it happens before 34 weeks of pregnancy, it is called early-onset preeclampsia. It also can happen after delivery.

It is not clear why some women develop preeclampsia. Doctors refer to high risk and moderate risk of preeclampsia. Risk factors for women at high risk include

- preeclampsia in a past pregnancy
- carrying more than one baby
- chronic hypertension
- kidney disease
- ***diabetes mellitus***
- autoimmune conditions, such as ***lupus*** (systemic lupus erythematosus or SLE)

Risk factors for women at moderate risk include

- pregnant for the first time
- ***body mass index (BMI)*** over 30
- family history of preeclampsia (mother or sister)
- being older than 35

Risks

Preeclampsia is a leading cause of death worldwide for women and babies. ***Eclampsia*** is a complication of preeclampsia that causes seizures and ***stroke***. Another complication of preeclampsia is ***HELLP syndrome***. HELLP stands for **h**emolysis, **e**levated **l**iver enzymes, and **l**ow **p**latelet count. In this condition

- red blood cells are damaged or destroyed
- the blood does not clot well
- the liver can bleed internally, causing chest or abdominal pain

HELLP syndrome is a medical emergency. Women can die from HELLP or have lifelong health problems from the condition.

When preeclampsia happens during pregnancy, the baby may need to be delivered right away, even if he or she is not fully grown. Preterm babies have an increased risk of serious complications, including:

- breathing problems
- problems with eating or staying warm
- vision or hearing problems

Some preterm complications last a lifetime and require ongoing medical care. Babies born very early also may die.

Hypertension and preeclampsia also can happen after the baby is born, even in women who did not have these conditions during pregnancy. Be aware of the signs and symptoms of preeclampsia in the ***postpartum*** period (see the box "Signs and Symptoms of Preeclampsia").

Having preeclampsia once increases the risk of having it again in a future pregnancy. Also, women who have had preeclampsia have an increased risk of health problems later in life. These problems may include

- high blood pressure
- heart attack
- heart failure
- stroke
- artery disease

Signs and Symptoms

Preeclampsia can develop quietly without you being aware of it. When symptoms do happen, they can be confused with normal symptoms of pregnancy (see the box "Signs and Symptoms of Preeclampsia"). A woman has preeclampsia when she has high blood pressure and other signs that her organs are not working normally. One of these signs is ***proteinuria*** (an abnormal amount of protein in the urine). A woman with preeclampsia whose condition is worsening will develop other signs and symptoms known as "severe features." Severe features include

- low number of ***platelets*** in the blood
- abnormal kidney or liver function
- pain over the upper abdomen
- changes in vision
- fluid in the lungs
- severe headache
- blood pressure of 160/110 mm Hg or higher

Diagnosis

A high blood pressure reading may be the first sign of preeclampsia. If your blood pressure reading is high, a repeat blood pressure check may be done in a few minutes to confirm the results. You should have a urine test to check for protein. If you are diagnosed with preeclampsia, you may have tests to check how your liver and kidneys are working and to measure the number of platelets in your blood. You also will be asked whether you have any of the symptoms of preeclampsia.

Treatment of Gestational Hypertension and Preeclampsia

Based on your test results, you and your ob-gyn should talk about treatment. The goal of treatment is to

- limit complications for you
- deliver the healthiest baby possible

Gestational Hypertension or Preeclampsia Without Severe Features

If you have gestational hypertension or preeclampsia without severe features, you may be treated either in a hospital or as an outpatient. This means you can stay at home with close monitoring by your ob-gyn. If you are treated at home, strict bed rest usually is not necessary. But you may be advised to limit heavy physical activity.

You may be asked to keep track of your baby's movement by doing a daily **kick count.** You also may need to measure your blood pressure at home. You will need to see your ob-gyn at least once a week and sometimes two times per week. At these visits, you may have tests that include

- blood pressure check
- blood tests to check your liver and kidney function and platelet counts
- **nonstress test** or **biophysical profile** to check the baby's general well-being
- ultrasound exam to check the baby's growth and measure the amount of **amniotic fluid**

Once you reach 37 weeks of pregnancy, delivery may be recommended. Labor may need to be induced (see Chapter 14, "Labor Induction"). If test results show that the baby is not doing well, you may need to have the baby earlier.

Preeclampsia does not mean that you cannot have a vaginal delivery. But if you have problems during labor or if there are problems with the baby, you may need a **cesarean delivery** (see Chapter 17, "Cesarean Delivery and Vaginal Birth After Cesarean Delivery").

Preeclampsia With Severe Features

If you have preeclampsia with severe features, you may be treated in the hospital. If you are at least 34 weeks pregnant, it may be recommended that you have your baby as soon as your condition is stable. If you are less than 34 weeks and your condition is stable, it may be possible to wait to deliver your baby.

Delaying delivery for just a few days can be helpful in some cases. It allows time for you and your ob-gyn to get ready for delivery:

- You may be transferred to a hospital with a special high-risk maternity unit and a high-level **neonatal intensive care unit (NICU)**. These units have doctors and nurses with advanced training in caring for complicated pregnancies and preterm babies.
- You may be given **corticosteroids** to help the baby's lungs mature.
- You may be given medications to help reduce your blood pressure and help prevent seizures.

If your condition or the baby's condition gets worse, you will need to deliver as soon as possible.

Prevention

Currently, there is no medical screening test that can accurately predict whether a woman will develop preeclampsia during pregnancy. For now, prevention involves identifying whether you have risk factors for preeclampsia, such as diabetes or preeclampsia in a past pregnancy, and taking steps to address these factors.

Prepregnancy Care

Ideally, you should see your ob-gyn for a **prepregnancy care** visit (see Chapter 1, "Getting Ready for Pregnancy"). At this visit, your ob-gyn can assess

- whether you have hypertension
- if your chronic hypertension is under control
- whether it has affected your health

Because hypertension may affect the heart and kidneys, you may be given tests to check the function of these organs. The information from these tests is used to assess the risks of pregnancy on your future health.

At this visit, you and your ob-gyn also can discuss steps that you can take to make your pregnancy safer. The goal is to lower your blood pressure and be as healthy as possible before pregnancy:

- If you are overweight, try to lose weight through diet and exercise. Avoid taking weight loss medications.
- Take your blood pressure medication as prescribed.

- Stop smoking.
- If you have diabetes, try to make sure it is well controlled before you get pregnant.

You also should learn about the signs and symptoms of preeclampsia so that you can watch out for them when you are pregnant. If you have had preeclampsia before, you and your ob-gyn should discuss factors that may increase the risk of having it again and work on a plan to reduce the risks, if possible.

Aspirin

Low-dose aspirin may reduce the risk of preeclampsia in some women. Talk with your ob-gyn about what a low dose of aspirin means for you. Your ob-gyn may recommend that you take low-dose aspirin if

- you are at high risk of developing preeclampsia
- you have two or more risk factors (see the "Preeclampsia" section in this chapter)

If your ob-gyn recommends taking low-dose aspirin, the best time to start is between 12 and 16 weeks of pregnancy. It should be taken every day until the baby is born. Do not start taking aspirin on your own without talking with your ob-gyn.

RESOURCES

High Blood Pressure in Pregnancy
https://medlineplus.gov/highbloodpressureinpregnancy.html
Information from the U.S. National Library of Medicine about the diagnosis and management of high blood pressure during pregnancy.

Preeclampsia Foundation
www.preeclampsia.org
National organization dedicated to preeclampsia education, advocacy, and research.

Your Pregnancy and Childbirth
www.acog.org/MyPregnancy
Website from the American College of Obstetricians and Gynecologists (ACOG) with information on pregnancy, labor, delivery, and postpartum care. Includes the latest information from the experts in women's health care, questions answered by ACOG ob-gyns, pregnancy stories from real women, and an A–Z directory of health topics covering pregnancy and beyond.

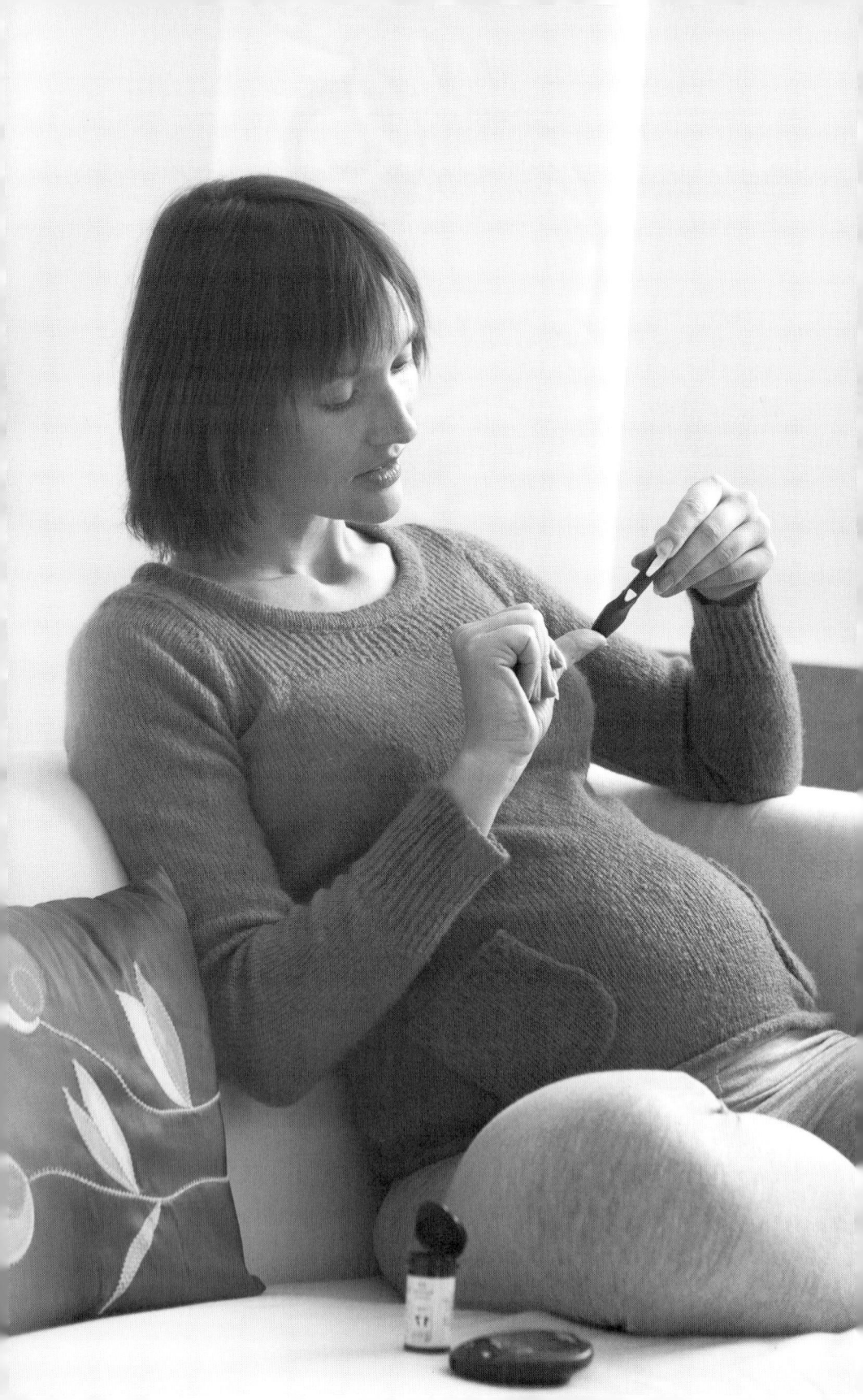

CHAPTER 31

Diabetes During Pregnancy

Glucose (blood sugar) is the body's fuel. *Insulin* is a *hormone* that helps cells absorb blood sugar. Blood sugar is needed to power the body's activities.

When a person has *diabetes mellitus*, the body does not make enough insulin, or the body's cells do not respond to insulin as they should. This means blood sugar cannot enter the body's cells. Instead, blood sugar stays in the blood. As a result, the amount of sugar in the blood can become too high. Over time, high blood sugar levels can damage the heart, eyes, *kidneys*, and other organs.

There are three types of diabetes:

- In type 1 diabetes, the body makes little or no insulin on its own.
- In type 2 diabetes, the body makes enough insulin, but the body's cells are insulin resistant. This means it takes more than the normal amount of insulin to manage the blood sugar level.
- *Gestational diabetes* is diabetes that is diagnosed during pregnancy.

Diabetes is common during pregnancy. In 2009, about 7 in 100 pregnant women had some form of diabetes, usually gestational diabetes. All three types of diabetes need to be carefully managed, especially during pregnancy. This includes

- keeping blood sugar in the normal range, neither too high nor too low
- getting tested regularly to check the well-being of the woman and the baby

Gestational Diabetes Mellitus

Some women develop diabetes for the first time during pregnancy. This is called gestational diabetes. Women with gestational diabetes need special care both during and after pregnancy.

During pregnancy, higher levels of pregnancy hormones can interfere with insulin. Usually the body can make more insulin during pregnancy to keep blood sugar levels normal. But in some women, the body cannot make enough insulin during pregnancy, and blood sugar levels go up. This leads to gestational diabetes.

Gestational diabetes goes away after childbirth, but women who have had this condition are at higher risk of developing diabetes later in life. Some women who develop gestational diabetes may have had mild diabetes before pregnancy and not known it. For these women, diabetes does not go away after pregnancy and may be a lifelong condition (see "Pregestational Diabetes Mellitus" in this chapter). These women will need to continue with diabetes treatment after giving birth.

Risk Factors

Several risk factors are linked to gestational diabetes. It also can happen in women who have no risk factors. But it is more likely in women who

- are overweight or obese
- are physically inactive
- had gestational diabetes in a past pregnancy
- had a very large baby in a past pregnancy
- have **high blood pressure**
- have a history of heart disease
- have **polycystic ovary syndrome (PCOS)**

How Gestational Diabetes Can Affect You

When a woman has gestational diabetes, her body passes more sugar to her baby than the baby needs. With too much sugar, the baby can gain a lot of weight. This condition is called **macrosomia**. A large baby may lead to **complications** for the woman, including

- labor difficulties
- **cesarean birth**
- **postpartum hemorrhage** (see the "Postpartum Hemorrhage" section in Chapter 39, "Problems During Labor and Delivery")

- severe tears in the *vagina* or the *perineum* with a vaginal birth
- *shoulder dystocia* (see the "Shoulder Dystocia" section in Chapter 39, "Problems During Labor and Delivery")

High blood pressure and *preeclampsia* also are more common in women with gestational diabetes.

How Gestational Diabetes Can Affect Your Baby

Babies born to women with gestational diabetes may have the following:

- Problems breathing
- *Jaundice*
- Low blood sugar at birth. This requires a stay in the *neonatal intensive care unit (NICU)* for a glucose drip that is gradually weaned.

Large babies are more likely to experience birth trauma, including damage to their shoulders, during vaginal delivery. Large babies may need special care in the NICU. There also is an increased risk of *stillbirth* with gestational diabetes.

Women who have had gestational diabetes are at higher risk of having diabetes in the future, and so are their children. Regular testing for diabetes after pregnancy is recommended for these women. Their children also will need

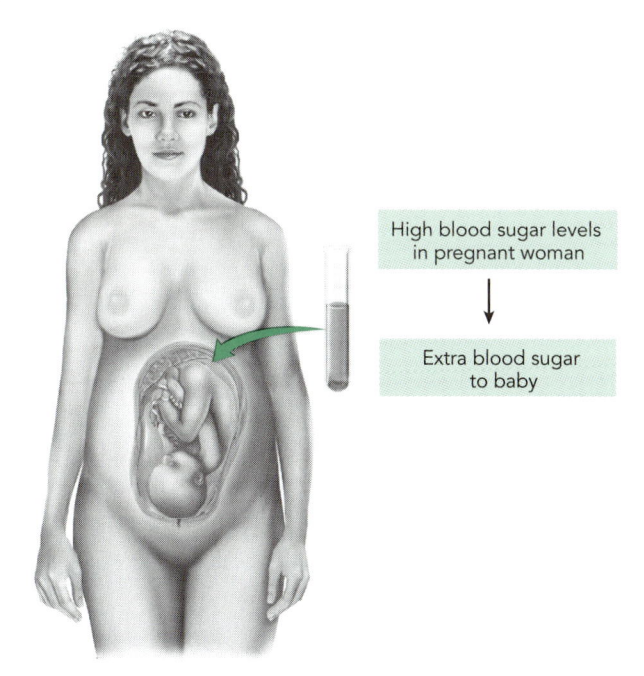

Diabetes during pregnancy. During pregnancy, high blood sugar levels can cause the baby to receive too much blood sugar. As a result, the baby can grow too large.

to be monitored for diabetes risks (see "Care After Pregnancy" later in this chapter).

Testing for Gestational Diabetes

All pregnant women should be screened for gestational diabetes. Your *obstetrician–gynecologist (ob-gyn)* should ask about your medical history, determine whether you have risk factors, and test your blood sugar levels.

- If you have certain risk factors, your blood sugar level may be measured early in pregnancy.
- If this early testing is negative, you will be tested again between 24 and 28 weeks of pregnancy.
- If you do not have risk factors, your blood sugar level may be measured between 24 and 28 weeks of pregnancy.

The most commonly used screening test is the 1-hour glucose challenge. To do this test, you first drink a sugary drink. A blood sample is taken 1 hour later. If the level of blood sugar is high, you will return on another day for a diagnostic glucose test. Once again, you will drink a sugary drink, but afterward your blood sugar will be tested hourly for a few hours.

Your ob-gyn also may order a blood test for hemoglobin A_{1C}. This test gives an estimate of how well your blood sugar level has been controlled during the past 4 to 6 weeks. Your A_{1C} should not be higher than 6 percent.

Controlling Gestational Diabetes

Treating gestational diabetes can greatly reduce the risk of complications for you and your baby. Treatment can reduce the risk of

- macrosomia
- birth injuries
- cesarean birth

The risk of preeclampsia and other high blood pressure disorders also is lower if your blood sugar levels are under control.

Treatment involves several things. If you are diagnosed with gestational diabetes, you will need more frequent **prenatal care** visits to monitor your health and your baby's health. You will need to keep your blood sugar under control. This will require

- eating healthy foods
- exercising regularly

- daily testing of blood sugar levels
- taking medications, if needed

Your ob-gyn may recommend that you see a diabetes educator or a dietitian. A diabetes educator is a health care practitioner who teaches people how to live with diabetes. A dietitian is an expert in nutrition and meal planning.

Later in pregnancy, special tests of the baby's growth and well-being may be done. You are more likely to have these tests if

- your gestational diabetes is not well controlled
- you need to take medications
- you develop problems

Tracking Blood Sugar Levels

You may be asked to use a glucose meter to test your blood sugar levels. This device measures blood sugar from a small drop of blood. Write down blood sugar levels and bring your log with you to each prenatal visit. Blood sugar logs also can be kept online, stored in phone apps, and emailed to your ob-gyn. Your blood sugar log will help your ob-gyn take the best care of you during your pregnancy.

Healthy Eating

A healthy diet is a key part of any pregnancy (see Chapter 22, "Nutrition During Pregnancy"). Your baby depends on the food you eat for its growth and **nutrients**. When women have gestational diabetes, making healthy food choices is even more important to keep blood sugar from getting too high. A dietitian can help you plan healthy meals that control your blood sugar.

Eat regular meals throughout the day. You may need to eat small snacks as well, especially at night. Eating regularly helps avoid dips and spikes in blood sugar levels. Often, three meals and two to three snacks per day are recommended.

Carbohydrates are an important part of a healthy diet. There are two types: 1) simple carbohydrates and 2) complex carbohydrates. Simple carbohydrates provide a quick energy boost because they are digested rapidly. Simple carbohydrates are found in

- fruits
- honey
- maple syrup
- sugary drinks
- foods with added sugar

Complex carbohydrates have dietary fiber and starches. It takes your body longer to process them, so complex carbohydrates provide longer-lasting energy than simple carbohydrates. Complex carbohydrates are found in

- whole wheat bread and pasta
- brown rice
- some fruits
- starchy vegetables, such as potatoes and corn

If you have gestational diabetes, complex carbohydrates are a better choice than simple carbohydrates. Carbohydrates should make up 40 to 50 percent of your total calories. Protein (15 to 30 percent) and fats (20 to 35 percent) should make up the rest.

It is important to gain a healthy amount of weight during pregnancy. Talk with your ob-gyn about how much weight gain is best for your pregnancy. For a woman with gestational diabetes, it can be harder to keep blood sugar levels under control if you

- gain too much weight
- gain weight too quickly

Exercise

Exercise helps keep blood sugar levels in the normal range. You and your ob-gyn can decide how much and what type of exercise is best for you. In general, 30 minutes of moderate-intensity aerobic exercise at least 5 days a week is recommended (or a minimum of 150 minutes per week). Brisk walking is a great exercise for all pregnant women. In addition to weekly aerobic exercise, taking a short walk after each meal may help control blood sugar.

Medications

Gestational diabetes often can be controlled with diet and exercise. But if diet and exercise are not enough, medication also may be needed to control blood sugar levels. Insulin is the recommended medication during pregnancy to help women control their blood sugar. Insulin does not cross the **placenta**, so it doesn't affect the baby. Your ob-gyn or diabetes educator will teach you how to give yourself insulin shots with a small needle. In some cases, your ob-gyn may prescribe a different medication to take by mouth.

If you take medication, keep monitoring your blood sugar levels. Your ob-gyn should review your blood sugar log to make sure that the medication is working, so remember to bring your blood sugar log to every appointment. Because your body gets more resistant to insulin as your pregnancy goes along, changes to your medications may be needed. This can help keep your blood sugar level in the normal range.

Special Tests

When a woman has gestational diabetes, she may need special tests to check the well-being of the baby. These tests may help your ob-gyn find possible problems and take steps to manage them. These tests may include the following:

- *Kick counts*—This is a record of how often you feel the baby move. A healthy baby tends to move the same amount each day. You may be asked to keep track of this movement late in pregnancy. You should contact your ob-gyn if you feel a difference in your baby's activity.

- *Nonstress test*—This test measures changes in the baby's heart rate when the baby moves. The term "nonstress" means that nothing is done to place stress on the baby. A belt with a sensor is placed around your abdomen. The sensor picks up the baby's heart rate and sends it to a machine that records it.

- *Biophysical profile (BPP)*—This test includes monitoring the baby's heart rate (the same way it is done in a nonstress test) and an **ultrasound exam**. The BPP checks the baby's heart rate and estimates the amount of **amniotic fluid**. The baby's breathing, movement, and muscle tone also are checked. A modified BPP checks only the heart rate and amniotic fluid level. See Chapter 34, "Ultrasound Exams and Other Testing to Monitor Fetal Well-Being," for details on these tests.

Labor and Delivery

Most women with controlled gestational diabetes can complete a full-term pregnancy. But if there are complications with your health or your baby's health, labor may be induced (started by drugs or other means) before the due date.

Although most women with gestational diabetes can have a vaginal birth, they are more likely to have a cesarean birth. If your ob-gyn thinks your baby is too big for a safe vaginal delivery, you may discuss a scheduled cesarean birth.

Care After Pregnancy

Gestational diabetes greatly increases your risk of developing diabetes in your next pregnancy and in the future when you are no longer pregnant. One third of women who had gestational diabetes will have diabetes or a milder form of elevated blood sugar soon after giving birth. Between 15 and 70 percent of women with gestational diabetes will develop diabetes later in life. If you had gestational diabetes, you should be tested 4 to 12 weeks after you give birth. If your blood sugar is normal, you will need to be tested for diabetes every 1 to 3 years.

Gestational diabetes also increases your risk of future heart disease. If you had gestational diabetes in a past pregnancy, let your health care practitioner know so your heart health can be monitored. There are several ways to maintain heart health, including

- eating a healthy diet
- limiting alcohol
- staying at a healthy weight
- not smoking
- getting daily exercise

A heart-healthy diet

- encourages vegetables, fruits, beans, and low-fat dairy products
- includes fish and poultry
- limits red meat, sodium, and sugary foods and drinks

Children of women who had gestational diabetes may be at risk of becoming overweight or obese during childhood. These children also have a higher risk of developing diabetes. Tell your baby's doctor that you had gestational diabetes, so your baby can be monitored. As your baby grows, his or her blood sugar levels should be checked throughout childhood.

Pregestational Diabetes Mellitus

Type 1 or type 2 diabetes before pregnancy is called **pregestational diabetes mellitus**. Some women who are first diagnosed with diabetes during pregnancy may have had mild diabetes already and not known it. This also is considered pregestational diabetes mellitus.

If you have diabetes and are planning to get pregnant, see your ob-gyn for a **prepregnancy care** visit. Your diabetes should be as well controlled as possible before you get pregnant. High blood sugar early in pregnancy increases the risk of problems for your baby.

Hormone changes during pregnancy make your body more resistant to insulin during the second and third trimesters. For women with diabetes, this often means that blood sugar is not as well controlled as it was before pregnancy. As a result, your diabetes treatment may change. Careful monitoring and regular visits with your ob-gyn are important.

Risks to Your Pregnancy

Women with poorly controlled diabetes before pregnancy are at risk of several complications during pregnancy, including the following:

- *Birth defects*—High blood sugar levels early in pregnancy increase the risk of birth defects, most often involving the baby's heart, brain, and skeleton.
- *Miscarriage* and *stillbirth*—Both miscarriage and stillbirth are more common in pregnant women with poorly controlled diabetes.
- *Hydramnios*—This is a condition in which there is too much *amniotic fluid* in the *amniotic sac* that surrounds the baby. The condition can lead to *preterm* labor and delivery.
- Preeclampsia—See Chapter 30, "Hypertension and Preeclampsia."
- Macrosomia—A condition in which the baby grows more than expected, often weighing more than 8 pounds and 13 ounces. Macrosomia can increase the risk of problems during labor and the need for a cesarean birth.
- *Respiratory distress syndrome (RDS)*—This syndrome can make it harder for the baby to breathe after birth. The risk of RDS is higher in babies whose mothers have diabetes.

Remember, the risk of developing these complications is lower if your blood sugar levels are well controlled before and during pregnancy.

Prepregnancy Care

If you have diabetes and want to get pregnant, see your ob-gyn for a prepregnancy visit. During this visit, you and your ob-gyn should discuss:

- Treating any medical problems that you may have because of your diabetes, such as high blood pressure, heart disease, **kidney disease**, and eye problems.
- Losing weight, if needed, through a healthy diet and exercise.
- Taking a prenatal vitamin with *folic acid* every day to help prevent *neural tube defects (NTDs).* Your prenatal vitamin should have at least 400 micrograms (mcg) of folic acid. The label may show this amount as 667 mcg dietary folate equivalents (DFE).

If you are seeing any health care practitioners with expertise in diabetes, they should continue to be involved while you are pregnant.

Controlling Your Diabetes During Pregnancy

Managing your diabetes while you are pregnant is a must. You can control your blood sugar with a combination of eating right, exercising, and taking medications as directed by your ob-gyn.

Women with diabetes need to see their ob-gyns more often than other pregnant women. Your ob-gyn should schedule frequent prenatal visits to check your blood sugar level and do other tests.

Tracking Blood Sugar Levels

Your ob-gyn may recommend that you check your blood sugar level several times a day to make sure it is in the normal range. Keep a log that lists your blood sugar levels with the time of day. Share this log with your ob-gyn at each prenatal visit. If you are not already doing so, your ob-gyn also may suggest keeping track of

- your carbohydrate counts
- how much you exercise
- when you take insulin or other medication

This information will help you and your ob-gyn adjust your treatment as your needs change during pregnancy.

Some people with diabetes use a "continuous glucose monitoring system" that constantly measures their blood sugar. Some use a closed loop system, which takes the information from a continuous glucose monitor and uses it to adjust an insulin pump. This technology is still fairly new, but some studies of pregnant women have shown promising results.

A hemoglobin A_{1C} test may be used to track your progress. Your A_{1C} should not be higher than 6 percent. During pregnancy you may need to have A_{1C} blood tests more often than you usually do.

Managing High and Low Blood Sugar

Even with careful monitoring, women with diabetes are more likely to have low blood sugar levels when they are pregnant. This is called hypoglycemia. Hypoglycemia can happen if you

- do not eat enough food
- skip a meal
- do not eat at the right time of day

- exercise too much
- feel sick or stressed

Late in the first trimester, your body may become more sensitive to insulin for a short time. This also can increase the risk of hypoglycemia, especially if you have morning sickness with nausea and vomiting. Signs and symptoms of hypoglycemia include

- dizziness
- feeling shaky
- sudden hunger
- sweating
- weakness

If you think you have symptoms of hypoglycemia, check your blood sugar level right away. If it is below 60 mg/dL, eat or drink something, such as a glass of milk, a few crackers, or special glucose tablets. Wait 15 minutes, then test your blood sugar again. Make sure your family members know what to do as well.

If you have repeated low blood sugar values, your ob-gyn may prescribe a glucagon pen. This device allows you to inject yourself with glucagon, a substance that causes blood sugar to be released into the bloodstream.

Your blood sugar level also can go too high despite treatment, which is called hyperglycemia. Hyperglycemia can happen if you

- don't take your medicine at the recommended times
- eat more food than usual or eat at irregular times
- are sick
- are less active than normal

It also can happen if there is a problem with your insulin pump. If you have repeatedly high blood sugar levels, talk with your ob-gyn. You may need to change your diet, exercise routine, or medications.

When the blood sugar level is very high, the body may make substances called ketones. Ketones can be harmful to you and your baby. They put you at risk of a life-threatening condition called diabetic ketoacidosis (DKA). If your blood sugar reading is above 200 mg/dL at any point, call your ob-gyn right away. You also should call if you have

- abdominal pain
- nausea
- vomiting
- trouble thinking clearly

It is a good idea to wear a medical bracelet or necklace that tells first responders and health care practitioners that you have diabetes.

Healthy Eating

Eating a well-balanced, healthy diet is a critical part of any pregnancy (see Chapter 22, "Nutrition During Pregnancy"). In women with diabetes, diet is even more important. Not eating properly can cause your blood sugar levels to go too high or too low.

Experts are still researching the best food balance for women with diabetes during pregnancy. Usually, it is recommended that you get

- 40 to 50 percent of your calories from complex, high-fiber carbohydrates
- 15 to 30 percent of your calories from protein
- 20 to 35 percent of your calories from fat (mainly unsaturated fats)

Carefully counting your carbohydrates at each meal also may be helpful. In most cases, your meal plan may include eating several small meals and snacks throughout the day and before bedtime. Your ob-gyn may recommend that you see a dietitian or diabetes educator to help with planning your meals.

Exercise

Another key part of a healthy pregnancy is exercise (see Chapter 23, "Exercise During Pregnancy"). Exercise helps keep your blood sugar level in the normal range and has many other benefits, including

- boosting your energy
- helping you sleep
- reducing backaches, constipation, and bloating

Exercise helps keep blood sugar levels in the normal range. You and your ob-gyn can decide how much and what type of exercise is best for you. In general, 30 minutes of moderate-intensity aerobic exercise at least 5 days a week is recommended (or a minimum of 150 minutes per week). Brisk walking is a great exercise for all pregnant women. In addition to weekly aerobic exercise, taking a short walk after each meal may help control blood sugar.

Medications

If you took insulin before pregnancy to control your diabetes, your insulin dosage may increase while you are pregnant. If you used an insulin pump before you became pregnant, you may be able to continue using the pump. Some women need to switch to insulin shots during pregnancy. Insulin is safe to use during pregnancy because it does not cross the ***placenta***.

Your ob-gyn should review your blood sugar log at each visit to make sure that your medication is working. Because your body gets more resistant to insulin as your pregnancy goes along, changes to your medications may be needed to help keep your blood sugar level in the normal range.

Your ob-gyn also may recommend that you take low-dose aspirin to help prevent preeclampsia. Talk with your ob-gyn about what a low dose of aspirin means for you. Ideally, this should start between 12 to 16 weeks of pregnancy and continue until the baby is born. Do not start taking aspirin on your own without talking with your ob-gyn.

Special Tests

As your pregnancy goes on, your ob-gyn may order special tests to check the well-being of the baby. These tests can help your ob-gyn find possible problems. Tests may include

- kick counts
- nonstress test
- biophysical profile (BPP)
- contraction stress test

These tests are discussed in detail in Chapter 34, "Ultrasound Exams and Other Testing to Monitor Fetal Well-Being." Your baby's growth and the amniotic fluid level around the baby also may be tracked throughout your pregnancy with ultrasound exams.

Labor and Delivery

You and your ob-gyn should discuss the timing of your delivery. You may go into labor naturally. If problems with the pregnancy arise, labor may be induced (started by drugs or other means) earlier than the due date (see Chapter 14, "Labor Induction"). If the baby is very large (more than 9 pounds, 15 ounces), you and your ob-gyn should discuss the risks and benefits of a cesarean birth.

If there is a risk of preterm birth, ***corticosteroids*** sometimes are given to help the baby's lungs mature. Corticosteroids can increase the need for insulin, so if you are given this medication, your blood sugar will be monitored closely.

While you are in labor, your blood sugar level will be monitored, typically every hour at first. If needed, you may receive insulin through an ***intravenous (IV) line***. If you use an insulin pump, you might use it during labor. Women who use insulin pumps will need to work with their medical team throughout labor to monitor blood sugar levels and adjust the pump settings.

Care After Pregnancy

Experts highly recommend breastfeeding for women with diabetes. Breastfeeding gives the baby the best nutrition to stay healthy, and it is good for the woman as well. It helps new mothers shed the extra weight that they gained during pregnancy (see Chapter 20, "Feeding Your Baby"). Taking insulin does not affect breast milk.

If you breastfeed, you will need to eat extra calories every day. Talk with your ob-gyn about the amount and types of foods that can give you these extra calories. Eating small snacks before breastfeeding may reduce the risk of hypoglycemia. Your ob-gyn also may suggest that you see a *lactation specialist*.

You should monitor your blood sugar levels after delivery. This will help determine what medication you should use and how much you will need. Most women who took insulin before pregnancy are able to go back to their prepregnancy insulin dosage soon after birth.

RESOURCES

Gestational Diabetes
www.diabetes.org/diabetes/gestational-diabetes
Webpage from the American Diabetes Association that focuses on gestational diabetes. Information also is available by phone at 800-DIABETES (800-342-2383).

Pregnancy If You Have Diabetes
www.niddk.nih.gov/health-information/diabetes/diabetes-pregnancy
Prepregnancy information for women with preexisting diabetes from the National Institute of Diabetes and Digestive and Kidney Diseases.

Your Pregnancy and Childbirth
www.acog.org/MyPregnancy
Website from the American College of Obstetricians and Gynecologists (ACOG) with information on pregnancy, labor, delivery, and postpartum care. Includes the latest information from the experts in women's health care, questions answered by ACOG ob-gyns, pregnancy stories from real women, and an A–Z directory of health topics covering pregnancy and beyond.

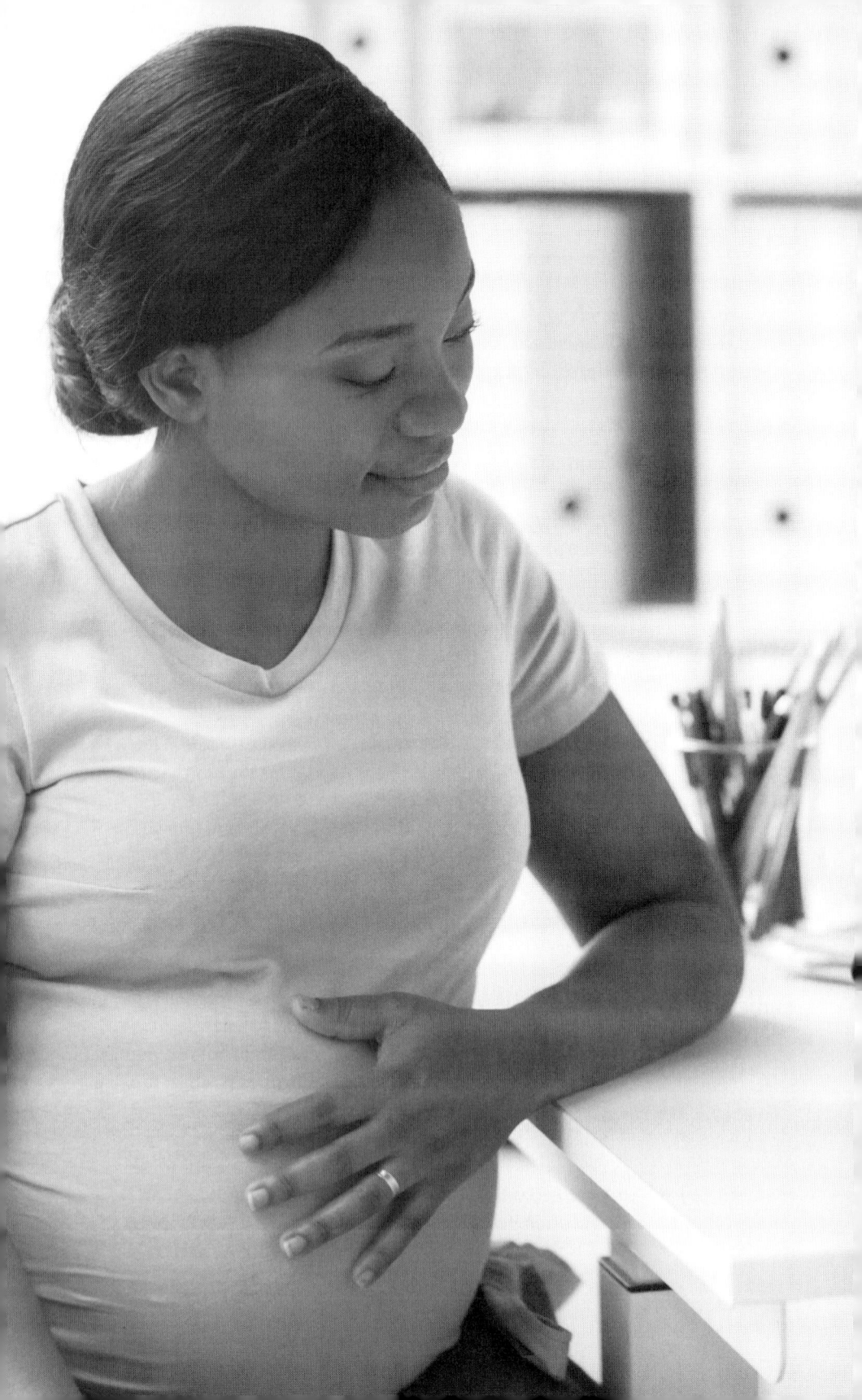

CHAPTER 32

Other Chronic Conditions

Pregnancy puts many demands on a woman's body. For women with medical conditions (often called chronic conditions), pregnancy may change the way their condition is managed. Women with certain medical conditions may need closer monitoring during pregnancy. This monitoring may help prevent problems for both a woman and her baby.

This chapter discusses the following conditions:

- Asthma
- **Autoimmune disorders**, including **multiple sclerosis (MS)**, **rheumatoid arthritis (RA)**, and **lupus** (systemic lupus erythematosus or SLE)
- Bleeding disorders and blood clotting disorders
- Digestive disorders, including celiac disease, **inflammatory bowel disease (IBD)**, and **irritable bowel syndrome (IBS)**
- **Epilepsy** and other **seizure disorders**
- Heart disease
- **Kidney disease**
- Mental illness
- Physical disabilities
- Thyroid disease

Other common health problems that may affect pregnancy are **high blood pressure** (discussed in Chapter 30, "Hypertension and Preeclampsia") and **diabetes mellitus** (discussed in Chapter 31, "Diabetes During Pregnancy").

If you have a medical problem, you may need to have extra tests. You may see your **obstetrician–gynecologist (ob-gyn)** more often. You may be able to monitor your condition from home. In some cases, you may need to stay in a hospital for part of your pregnancy.

Often, a team of health care practitioners will work together to care for you and your baby. If you are already seeing a specialist to manage your health condition, he or she should continue to care for you. Your ob-gyn may recommend that you see a ***maternal–fetal medicine (MFM) specialist***, a doctor who has specialized training in caring for pregnant women with medical problems.

Treatment for a chronic condition often includes taking medication. You and your health care practitioners should talk about the risks and benefits of your medication. You may need to change to a different medication or a different dosage.

Asthma

Asthma is a common condition. For many women, asthma symptoms stay the same or even improve during pregnancy. But for about 1 in 3 women with asthma, their symptoms get worse during pregnancy.

During an asthma episode, there is less ***oxygen*** in the blood. In a pregnant woman, this also means the baby gets less oxygen through the ***placenta***. Asthma symptoms that are severe and uncontrolled can increase the risk of certain pregnancy problems, including

- ***preeclampsia***
- growth problems for the baby
- ***cesarean birth***
- ***preterm*** birth

Controlling asthma symptoms during pregnancy is important. It's safer to use asthma medications than to have asthma symptoms while you are pregnant.

If you have a history of asthma, your health care practitioner should assess your condition. He or she may order tests of your lung function (see Table 32–1, "Asthma Severity and Control"). If you have been pregnant before, your health care practitioner should ask about how your asthma affected your past pregnancies. This may give some clues about how your asthma will affect your current pregnancy. With this information, you and your health care practitioner should discuss a treatment plan for you to follow throughout pregnancy. Treatment plans for asthma include

- seeing your health care practitioner for tests to monitor your lung function
- monitoring your lung function and breathing at home
- avoiding or controlling asthma triggers

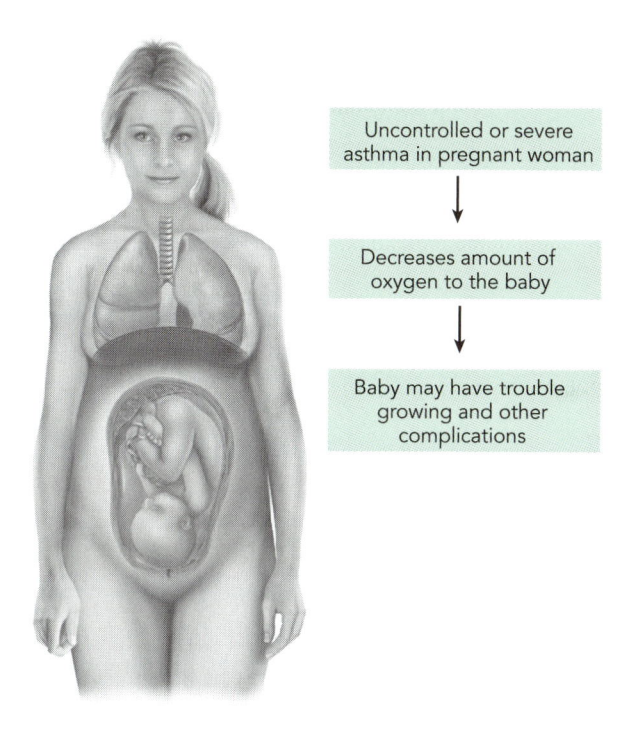

Uncontrolled or severe asthma in pregnant woman

↓

Decreases amount of oxygen to the baby

↓

Baby may have trouble growing and other complications

Asthma during pregnancy. If you have severe asthma episodes during pregnancy, the baby may get less oxygen.

- taking medications prescribed by your health care practitioner, including a rescue medication in case of emergency

If your asthma is mild and you have only occasional episodes, you may not need medication during pregnancy. But if you start having episodes more often and your symptoms are more severe, medications may be needed. Everyone is different, so you and your health care practitioner may need to try different medications to find what works best for you. If you have an inhaler, it is important to know how and when to use it. Check with your health care practitioner or your pharmacist if you are not sure. Also, never leave home without your inhaler.

Working closely with your ob-gyn to monitor your lung function can give a better picture of how well your medications are working. Your baby's growth and well-being may be tracked more closely if

- you have moderate or severe asthma
- your symptoms are not well controlled
- you have just had a severe asthma episode

TABLE 32-1 **Asthma Severity And Control**

Asthma Control	How Often You Have Symptoms	How Often You Wake Up At Night	How Much It Affects Normal Activity	FEV$_1$ or Peak Flow
Intermittent (well controlled)	2 days per week or less	2 times per month or less	None	More than 80 percent
Mild persistent (not well controlled)	More than 2 days per week, but not every day	More than 2 times per month	Minor limitation	More than 80 percent
Moderate persistent (not well controlled)	Every day	More than once per week	Some limitation	60 to 80 percent
Severe persistent (very poorly controlled)	Throughout the day	4 times per week or more	Extremely limited	Less than 60 percent

FEV$_1$: Forced expiratory volume in one second, a measure of breathing function

Most asthma medications are safe to use during pregnancy. Inhaled medications, such as albuterol and **corticosteroids**, are safe during pregnancy.

Autoimmune Disorders

Autoimmune disorders are triggered when the *immune system* attacks the body's own tissues. It's not clear what causes the immune system to go on the attack. Some common autoimmune disorders include

- certain types of thyroid disease
- inflammatory bowel disease (IBD)
- lupus
- celiac disease
- multiple sclerosis (MS)
- rheumatoid arthritis (RA)
- *antiphospholipid syndrome (APS)*

For some autoimmune disorders, pregnancy can increase symptoms and lead to certain **complications**. For others, pregnancy causes symptoms to be less severe. If you have an autoimmune disorder, you and your health care practitioners should work as a team to control your condition. This may increase your chance of having a healthy pregnancy.

Multiple Sclerosis

Multiple sclerosis (MS) is a disease that affects the central nervous system (the brain and spinal cord). The symptoms of the disease are different for every person, but they mostly include

- extreme fatigue
- vision problems
- loss of balance and muscle control
- stiffness

A person can have flare-ups when symptoms get worse. This is called relapse. Or a person can have periods with no symptoms. This is called remission.

Many women with MS have healthy pregnancies. Pregnancy does not make the disease worse. In fact, some women report that their symptoms get better when they are pregnant. If you have MS, the best treatment is to eat healthy food, exercise, rest, and follow a program of **prenatal care**.

Most medications for MS should not be used during pregnancy, either because they are harmful or because their safety is not known. Talk with your ob-gyn about whether and when to stop taking your medication.

The risk of having a flare-up increases in the weeks after pregnancy. Relapse in the **postpartum** period does not seem to change the course of the disease or make your prognosis worse. Breastfeeding does not seem to affect the risk of relapse.

Rheumatoid Arthritis

Rheumatoid arthritis (RA) causes pain and swelling in the joints. It also can cause stiffness in the morning and a general feeling of fatigue and discomfort. RA can flare up and then lessen for a time, or it can get worse and damage the joints. Some women with RA have fewer symptoms during pregnancy.

RA often is treated with anti-inflammatory medications, which can cause complications in pregnant women. Talk with your ob-gyn about which pain-relief medications you can use. There are some drugs that you should not take during pregnancy and breastfeeding. These drugs include methotrexate and cyclophosphamide.

Later in pregnancy, your joints may loosen. Let your ob-gyn know if you experience any new pain in your neck or the back of your head.

Lupus

Lupus (also called systemic lupus erythematosus or SLE) is an autoimmune disorder that affects various parts of the body, including

- skin
- joints
- blood vessels
- organs such as the **kidneys** or brain

Having lupus increases the risk of pregnancy complications, including

- ***miscarriage***
- ***stillbirth***
- preeclampsia
- preterm birth
- growth problems for the baby

Some women with lupus are more likely to develop blood clots (**deep vein thrombosis [DVT]**) than women who do not have the disease. Babies born to women with lupus may have symptoms of the disease. These babies also may have a higher risk of certain heart problems.

Today, more than half of women with lupus have uncomplicated pregnancies. One way to increase the chance of a healthy pregnancy is to make sure your lupus is under control for at least 6 months before trying to get pregnant. Still, pregnancy for a woman with lupus is considered high-risk. If you have lupus, you should be cared for by a maternal–fetal medicine (MFM) specialist or an ob-gyn who is experienced in treating lupus during pregnancy. You and your specialist may talk about the following:

- You may need to see your specialist often. Many problems that may happen during pregnancy can be treated more easily if found early.

- You may need tests later in pregnancy to see how the baby is growing and to monitor your condition.

- You may need to continue taking medications to control your condition throughout pregnancy.

- Your specialist should review your medications to see if they are safe enough to use during pregnancy. In some cases, you may need to take a different medication or adjust the dosage.

Blood Clotting and Bleeding Disorders

People with a blood clotting disorder (***thrombophilia***) tend to form blood clots too easily. People with bleeding disorders do not form blood clots easily enough. Both types of conditions can be dangerous in pregnancy. Blood clots can be life-threatening. Bleeding disorders can lead to miscarriage and ***postpartum hemorrhage***.

During pregnancy and for 4 to 6 weeks after delivery, the risk of forming blood clots is much higher for all women. A common location where blood clots develop is in the deep veins of the lower leg. If a piece of a clot breaks free and moves through the blood vessels to the lungs, it can be very serious. This condition, called pulmonary embolism, can be fatal. Blood clots also can form in organs such as

- the kidneys, leading to kidney disease
- the eyes, leading to vision problems
- the brain, leading to **stroke**

The risk of heart attack also may be increased with blood clots.

Symptoms of a Blood Clot

A deep vein thrombosis (DVT) or pulmonary embolism (PE) can be life-threatening. Signs and symptoms of DVT in an arm or leg include

- warmth or tenderness
- pain or sudden swelling
- redness of the skin
- constant pain in one leg while standing or walking

If you have symptoms of a DVT, call your ob-gyn right away or go to the emergency room (ER).

Signs and symptoms of a PE include

- sudden cough, which may produce blood
- sudden shortness of breath
- pain in the ribs when breathing
- sharp chest pain under the breast or on one side
- burning, aching, or dull heavy feeling in the chest
- rapid breathing
- rapid heart rate

If you have symptoms of a PE, go to the emergency room right away.

Inherited Thrombophilias

Clotting is a normal process that helps stop bleeding, such as from a cut in the skin. But people with a thrombophilia tend to form blood clots too easily.

Blood clotting is surprisingly complex. To work properly, blood needs the right amounts of certain proteins (called blood clotting factors, or simply factors). Having too much or too little of a factor can cause thrombophilias. Many of these diseases are caused by **mutations** in genes. This means they can be inherited (passed from parents to children). Inherited conditions that can cause thrombophilia include

- *factor V Leiden*
- prothrombin G20210A mutation
- antithrombin deficiency
- protein C deficiency
- protein S deficiency

Doctors also refer to whether a person has one or two faulty copies of a gene:

- **Heterozygous** means that a person has one defective copy and one normal copy of a gene.
- **Homozygous** means that a person has two defective copies of a gene.

The severity of a disease or the rate of complications is related to whether you are heterozygous or homozygous. Existing guidelines vary on the risk level of thrombophilias:

- Low-risk thrombophilias carry a small chance of causing a blood clot. They include factor V Leiden heterozygous and prothrombin G20210A mutation heterozygous.
- High-risk thrombophilias carry a higher risk of causing a blood clot. They include antithrombin deficiency, factor V Leiden homozygous, prothrombin G20210A mutation homozygous, and the combined double heterozygous factor V Leiden and prothrombin G20210A mutation.

Some other thrombophilias may be considered high-risk or low-risk depending on your personal or family history.

Most women who have a thrombophilia have healthy pregnancies. But there may be an association between thrombophilias and some pregnancy complications, including

- miscarriage
- *placental abruption*
- stillbirth

The risk of these complications during pregnancy or in the postpartum period may depend on

- the type of thrombophilia that you have
- whether you have ever had a blood clot
- if you have a close relative who has had a blood clot
- whether you are heterozygous or homozygous
- whether you are taking medication that prevents blood clots

Your ob-gyn should review your history and risk. This review will help him or her decide whether you should have treatment during pregnancy and, if so, the type of medication and dosage. A specialist who treats blood disorders may be involved in your care.

Women with low-risk thrombophilias may just need careful monitoring during pregnancy. Women with high-risk thrombophilias, a personal or family history of blood clots, or both, may need to take medication during pregnancy.

There also is a risk of blood clots in the postpartum period. Treatment with medication may be needed for at least 6 weeks after you have your baby. The drugs warfarin and heparin can be used by women who are breastfeeding.

You should talk with your ob-gyn if you have a

- history of blood clots, even if you have never been diagnosed with a thrombophilia
- parent or sibling with a history of blood clots or thrombophilia
- history of multiple miscarriages

It's best to have this conversation with your ob-gyn before you get pregnant. If you have symptoms of a DVT, call your ob-gyn right away or go to the emergency room (ER). If you have symptoms of a pulmonary embolism, go to the emergency room right away (see the box "Symptoms of a Blood Clot").

Antiphospholipid Syndrome

Antiphospholipid syndrome (APS) is an autoimmune disorder. APS develops when your immune system mistakenly creates ***antibodies*** that make your blood more likely to clot. During pregnancy, APS can have serious effects on you and your baby, including

- miscarriage
- preeclampsia
- problems with the baby's growth
- preterm birth

If you have APS and are pregnant, you should have special care throughout your pregnancy:

- Beginning in the third trimester, you may have tests to check the baby's health. You also may have a series of **ultrasound exams** to track the baby's growth.

- Depending on your history of blood clots, you may take a medication called heparin. Sometimes low-dose aspirin also is recommended. Heparin and low-dose aspirin help stop blood from clotting.

- You also may need to continue taking medication for at least 6 weeks after delivery, because there also is a risk of blood clots in the postpartum period.

Von Willebrand Disease

Von Willebrand disease is the most common inherited bleeding disorder that affects about 1 in 100 women. It is caused by a deficiency in von Willebrand factor (vWF), a protein that helps the blood to clot. Von Willebrand disease is passed from parent to a child. The most common symptom in women is heavy menstrual bleeding. Other symptoms may include bleeding

- from the nose
- of the gums
- after having a tooth removed
- from minor cuts
- after surgery
- in the digestive system
- in the joints

Von Willebrand disease can affect pregnancy, labor, and delivery. The disease increases the risk of miscarriage and postpartum hemorrhage. During labor and delivery, **anesthesiologists** take special care when giving an **epidural block** or **spinal block**. The needle used for these types of **anesthesia** may cause bleeding, bruising, and swelling. This can lead to compression of the spinal cord and nerve damage. For these reasons, the anesthesiologist may recommend another type of pain control.

Because von Willebrand disease is an inherited disorder, there is a chance the baby also could have the disease. For this reason, **assisted vaginal deliveries** should be avoided because of the potential risk of bleeding in the baby's brain. Also, during labor the heart rate of your baby may be monitored. In most cases, this is done with sensors placed on the woman's skin. Sometimes monitoring is done with a small device that is placed on the baby's scalp. But if you have von Willebrand disease, a sensor should not be placed on the scalp of the baby.

Levels of vWF and other blood clotting proteins should be measured throughout your pregnancy, especially as delivery gets closer. Your ob-gyn may talk with a *hematologist* (blood specialist) to plan the safest delivery for you.

Digestive Disorders

If you have a disorder that affects how your body digests food, work closely with your ob-gyn throughout your pregnancy. You will need to make sure you and your baby are getting enough of the vitamins and *nutrients* you both need.

Celiac Disease

Gluten is a protein found in wheat, rye, and barley. People with celiac disease cannot tolerate gluten. When gluten is eaten, the immune system reacts by damaging the lining of the small intestine. With this damage, nutrients cannot be absorbed properly.

Symptoms of celiac disease vary. Some people have no symptoms. Others may have

- diarrhea
- constipation
- fatigue
- abdominal pain
- bloating

If celiac disease is not managed, it can cause serious health problems. It may even affect your ability to get pregnant. Some studies have found links between celiac disease that is not managed and increased risk of repeated miscarriage.

Women with celiac disease can have healthy pregnancies. The key is to maintain a gluten-free diet before, during, and after pregnancy. Review your gluten-free diet with your ob-gyn and a dietitian to make sure that it gives you and the baby enough nutrients during pregnancy.

You may need to adjust your diet if you are not gaining enough weight or if you develop complications, such as *anemia*. You also may need to add more vitamin D or calcium to your diet, after consultation with your care team. Some vitamin supplements contain gluten, so look for a gluten-free brand. See Chapter 22, "Nutrition During Pregnancy," for more on healthy eating during pregnancy.

Inflammatory Bowel Disease

Inflammatory bowel disease (IBD) is a group of diseases that cause inflammation of the intestines. Researchers believe that IBD is an autoimmune disorder caused by the immune system attacking the normal **bacteria** in the digestive system. There are two kinds of IBD: 1) Crohn's disease and 2) ulcerative colitis. They cause similar symptoms, including

- diarrhea
- bloody stools
- abdominal pain
- fever
- bleeding from the **rectum**

If you have IBD, it may be hard to get the nutrients you need from the foods you eat. Your body may not be able to absorb enough protein, vitamins, or **calories**. You also may have intestinal damage.

Before you get pregnant, see your ob-gyn to talk about your condition and how you will manage it during your pregnancy. Discuss the medications that you are taking and whether you should continue to use the same drugs while you are pregnant. Talking with a nutritionist or dietitian also may be helpful.

Irritable Bowel Syndrome

Irritable bowel syndrome (IBS) is a disorder that causes digestive symptoms. For some people, the symptoms are mild. For others, they can be serious. It is not clear what causes IBS. Symptoms may include

- cramps
- gas
- bloating
- alternating diarrhea and constipation

Several things can trigger symptoms, including

- stress
- eating large meals
- travel
- certain medicines or foods

When you're pregnant, be aware of what triggers your IBS symptoms and try to avoid them.

There is no cure for IBS, but it can be managed to reduce symptoms. Your ob-gyn or a dietitian may suggest changes in your diet, such as eating more fiber or eating smaller meals more often, to help manage your symptoms. Some medications also may help.

Epilepsy and Other Seizure Disorders

Seizure disorders (including epilepsy) can cause several problems during pregnancy:

- Higher risk of birth defects, most commonly **cleft lip, cleft palate, neural tube defects (NTDs)**, and heart defects. The increased risk of birth defects may be related to the disorder itself or to the effects of medications to control the disorder.

- Injury and complications resulting from seizures. Seizure complications include injuries from falls, decreased oxygen to the baby during a seizure, and preterm birth.

- Increase in seizure frequency during pregnancy, which happens in about 1 in 3 pregnant women with epilepsy.

With medical care before and during pregnancy, many of these effects can be avoided.

Preparing for pregnancy is vital if you have a seizure disorder. Use of seizure medications can lower the levels of *folic acid* in the body. Low levels of folic acid before pregnancy and during early pregnancy may increase the risk of having a baby with an NTD.

Taking extra folic acid before and during the first weeks of pregnancy may lower this risk. Talk with your ob-gyn about taking extra folic acid, typically 4 milligrams every day and continuing through the first trimester of pregnancy. This amount is 10 times higher than the amount recommended for women who do not take seizure medications. To get the extra amount, you should take a separate folic acid supplement in addition to a prenatal vitamin.

Another important way to prepare for pregnancy is to review your medications with your health care practitioner. During pregnancy, the type, amount, or number of medications that you take may need to change. Ideally, any changes in medication should be made before pregnancy. This allows you and your health care practitioner to see how the medication changes affect you without putting the baby at risk. The changes that are made depend on your situation:

- If you have not had a seizure in at least 2 years, it may be possible for you to taper (gradually stop) the medication.

- The type of medication may be changed. Some medications are considered safer for the baby than others.

- It may be recommended that you take only one medication to control seizures. Taking only one medication may reduce the risk of birth defects. There also may be fewer side effects than if you take more than one medication.

During pregnancy, you will need more frequent visits with the health care practitioner who manages your seizure disorder. Blood tests may be done regularly to be sure that medication levels are constant. Levels that are too high can lead to side effects. Levels that are too low can lead to seizures. Keep in mind that after delivery, your medications may need to be adjusted again.

Having a seizure disorder may not affect how you will have your baby. Women with a seizure disorder may be able to give birth vaginally unless a problem happens during labor or delivery. If a labor problem happens, a cesarean birth may be needed.

Heart Disease

If you have a history of heart disease, heart murmur, or rheumatic fever, talk with your health care practitioner before you try to get pregnant. The risk of problems during pregnancy depends on

- the type of heart disease you have
- how serious your heart disease is

A woman who has **congenital** heart disease (meaning that it was present at birth) has a higher risk of having a baby with some type of heart defect. Testing may be needed after birth to determine whether your baby has a heart defect.

Pregnancy causes major changes in the circulatory system. Your blood volume (the amount of blood in your body) increases by 40 to 50 percent as early as 10 to 12 weeks into your pregnancy. This increased amount of blood makes the heart work harder during pregnancy. Your heart may continue to work harder for weeks or months after delivery.

Before you get pregnant, see your **cardiologist** or a maternal–fetal medicine (MFM) specialist to talk about how your condition may affect your heart during pregnancy. It's very important to have this conversation before you try to get pregnant. In some cases, pregnancy may not be recommended. In other cases, pregnancy can be attempted if you see your health care practitioners often and follow their instructions. You may need to see a cardiologist (heart doctor).

If you have heart disease and need to take medications during your pregnancy, you may be switched to medications that are considered safer. You may need tests during pregnancy to determine how well your heart is functioning. You also may be monitored for preeclampsia. If you are at risk of preeclampsia, your ob-gyn may recommend daily low-dose aspirin starting between 12 and 28 weeks and continuing until delivery.

You and your pregnancy care team should discuss how and where you should give birth. You should deliver your baby in a hospital that can manage complications. Also, it's important to see your health care practitioners regularly after you give birth, because the effects of pregnancy on your body can last for weeks or months. Talk with your ob-gyn and cardiologist about when to have heart check-ups after giving birth. Discuss any risks to your future health, especially if you had preeclampsia or gestational diabetes during pregnancy.

Kidney Disease

Your kidneys work almost 50 percent harder during pregnancy. The kidneys must filter wastes from your body and from the baby's body. This increased work means the kidneys need to work efficiently during pregnancy. If the kidneys are not working well, there is a greater risk of serious problems, including

- miscarriage
- hypertension (high blood pressure)
- preeclampsia
- preterm birth
- kidney failure

Pregnancy also can worsen any existing damage to your kidneys. This can greatly affect the length and quality of your life.

Kidney disease can be mild, intermediate, or severe. If you have mild kidney disease, you may be able to have a healthy pregnancy. See a maternal–fetal medicine (MFM) specialist or a kidney specialist for ***prepregnancy care***. These specialists can evaluate your condition and explain any health risks of pregnancy. They also can review your medications and suggest different medications, if needed. Throughout pregnancy, your health care practitioners should monitor your kidney function. You also may have tests to check the baby's health later in pregnancy.

If you have intermediate or severe kidney disease, you may have difficulty getting pregnant or staying pregnant. If pregnancy does happen, you may be at increased risk of

- serious pregnancy complications for you and the baby
- needing to be hospitalized
- preterm birth
- long-term kidney damage

Mental Illness

Millions of women in the United States are affected by mental illness. Some common mental illnesses include

- addiction and substance use disorders
- anxiety disorders (including panic disorder, obsessive–compulsive disorder, and phobias)
- bipolar disorder
- depression
- eating disorders (including **anorexia nervosa**, binge eating disorder, and **bulimia nervosa**)
- personality disorders
- schizophrenia

Most women with a mental illness can have successful pregnancies, but these conditions can affect pregnancy. If you have a mental illness or had one in the past, tell your ob-gyn. Being pregnant can cause some mental illnesses to get worse. In some cases, pregnancy can cause a mental illness to come back (called a recurrence). This may be a result of hormonal changes or stress.

If a mental illness is not treated, you may not be able to take care of yourself properly. For example, you could have trouble eating well or getting enough rest. You may be less likely to get regular prenatal care. You also may be at greater risk of **postpartum depression**.

Your ob-gyn needs to know about any medications you are taking to control your mental illness. Some medications are safe during pregnancy, but others can harm a baby during pregnancy (see the "Medications" section in Chapter 24, "Reducing Risks of Birth Defects"). If you are taking medication now, talk with your ob-gyn and mental health care professional about whether you should stop or continue the medication while you are pregnant. This decision should be based on several factors, such as

- whether you currently have symptoms
- whether the illness has come back
- the severity of your illness

You and your health care practitioners will need to decide if the benefit of using a medication to control your mental health condition outweighs any possible risks. If your medication is stopped, alternative therapies, such as psychotherapy, may be an option.

Women with mental health conditions before pregnancy are at risk of hospitalization for a psychiatric illness in the months after giving birth. These women also are more likely to have postpartum depression.

The first weeks after a newborn arrives are stressful for any new mother. During the early weeks, help and support are important to help you adjust to parenting (see Chapter 19, "Your Postpartum Care").

Physical Disabilities

If you have a physical disability, see your ob-gyn before trying to get pregnant. Prepregnancy care may reduce the chance that you will have medical complications during pregnancy. If your disability is an inherited condition, you may want to have genetic counseling (see Chapter 33, "Genetic Disorders, Screening, and Testing").

Special care also may be needed after pregnancy begins. Your health care practitioners may suggest occupational or physical therapy to help you cope with the stress that pregnancy puts on the body. Before the baby arrives, you may need to have special equipment installed at home to help you care for the baby. After you get home, you may need extra help as you care for yourself and your baby.

Thyroid Disease

Certain disorders cause the body's **thyroid gland** to release too much or too little **thyroid hormone**. **Hyperthyroidism** means the thyroid is too active. **Hypothyroidism** means the thyroid isn't as active as it should be. Either condition can harm you or your baby during pregnancy.

With treatment, most pregnant women with thyroid disease can have healthy babies. The chance of problems during pregnancy is greatest when thyroid disease is not under control.

Untreated hyperthyroidism has been associated with the following complications:

For the baby
- preterm birth
- **low birth weight**
- possible death

For the woman
- preterm labor
- stillbirth
- heart failure
- preeclampsia

These complications may mean you need to deliver the baby early. Preterm birth can increase the risk of serious health problems for the baby.

When women have hyperthyroidism, medications keep the level of thyroid hormone in the normal range during pregnancy. Propylthiouracil may be used in the first trimester. Methimazole may be used for the rest of the pregnancy. The lowest possible dosage of medication is used to minimize the baby's exposure to the medication.

Untreated hypothyroidism has been associated with the following complications:

For the baby
- preterm birth
- low birth weight
- possible death

For the woman
- miscarriage
- **gestational hypertension**

If you have hypothyroidism, you most likely will be prescribed levothyroxine. This medication helps increase the level of thyroid hormone in your body. For both hyperthyroidism and hypothyroidism, you should have regular blood tests to check your thyroid function during your pregnancy.

Some women who do not have thyroid problems during pregnancy may develop a thyroid condition after childbirth. This is called postpartum thyroiditis. It often is a short-term problem, and hormone levels quickly return to normal. But sometimes this condition can lead to long-term hypothyroidism, which requires treatment.

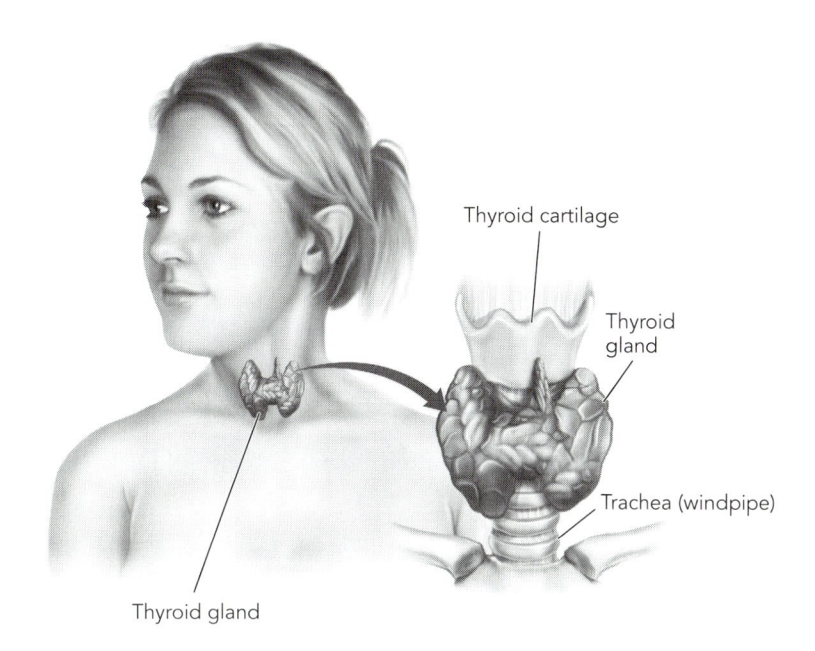

Thyroid gland. The thyroid gland is located in the neck. This gland releases thyroid hormone. Thyroid hormone plays many roles in the body, including maintaining heart rate and regulating body temperature.

Testing the function of the thyroid gland is not a routine part of prenatal care. But if you have a history or symptoms of thyroid disease, talk with your ob-gyn. He or she will decide how best to evaluate and manage your pregnancy.

RESOURCES

American College of Allergy, Asthma, and Immunology
https://acaai.org/allergies/who-has-allergies-and-why/pregnancy-and-allergies

American Heart Association
www.heart.org

American Psychiatric Association
www.psychiatry.org

Arthritis Foundation
www.arthritis.org

Crohn's and Colitis Foundation
www.ccfa.org

Epilepsy Foundation
www.epilepsy.com/living-epilepsy/women/epilepsy-and-pregnancy

Lupus Foundation of America
www.lupus.org/resources/planning-a-pregnancy-when-you-have-lupus

National Alliance on Mental Illness
www.nami.org

National Blood Clot Alliance
www.stoptheclot.org

National Institute of Diabetes and Digestive and Kidney Diseases (irritable bowel syndrome information)
www.niddk.nih.gov/health-information/digestive-diseases/irritable-bowel-syndrome

National Institute of Diabetes and Digestive and Kidney Diseases (thyroid disease information)
www.niddk.nih.gov/health-information/endocrine-diseases/pregnancy-thyroid-disease

National Foundation for Celiac Awareness
www.beyondceliac.org

National Kidney Foundation
www.kidney.org/atoz/content/pregnancy.cfm

National Multiple Sclerosis Society
www.nationalmssociety.org/Living-well-with-MS/Family-and-Relationships/pregnancy

Your Pregnancy and Childbirth
www.acog.org/MyPregnancy
Website from the American College of Obstetricians and Gynecologists (ACOG) with information on pregnancy, labor, delivery, and postpartum care. Includes the latest information from the experts in women's health care, questions answered by ACOG ob-gyns, pregnancy stories from real women, and an A–Z directory of health topics covering pregnancy and beyond.

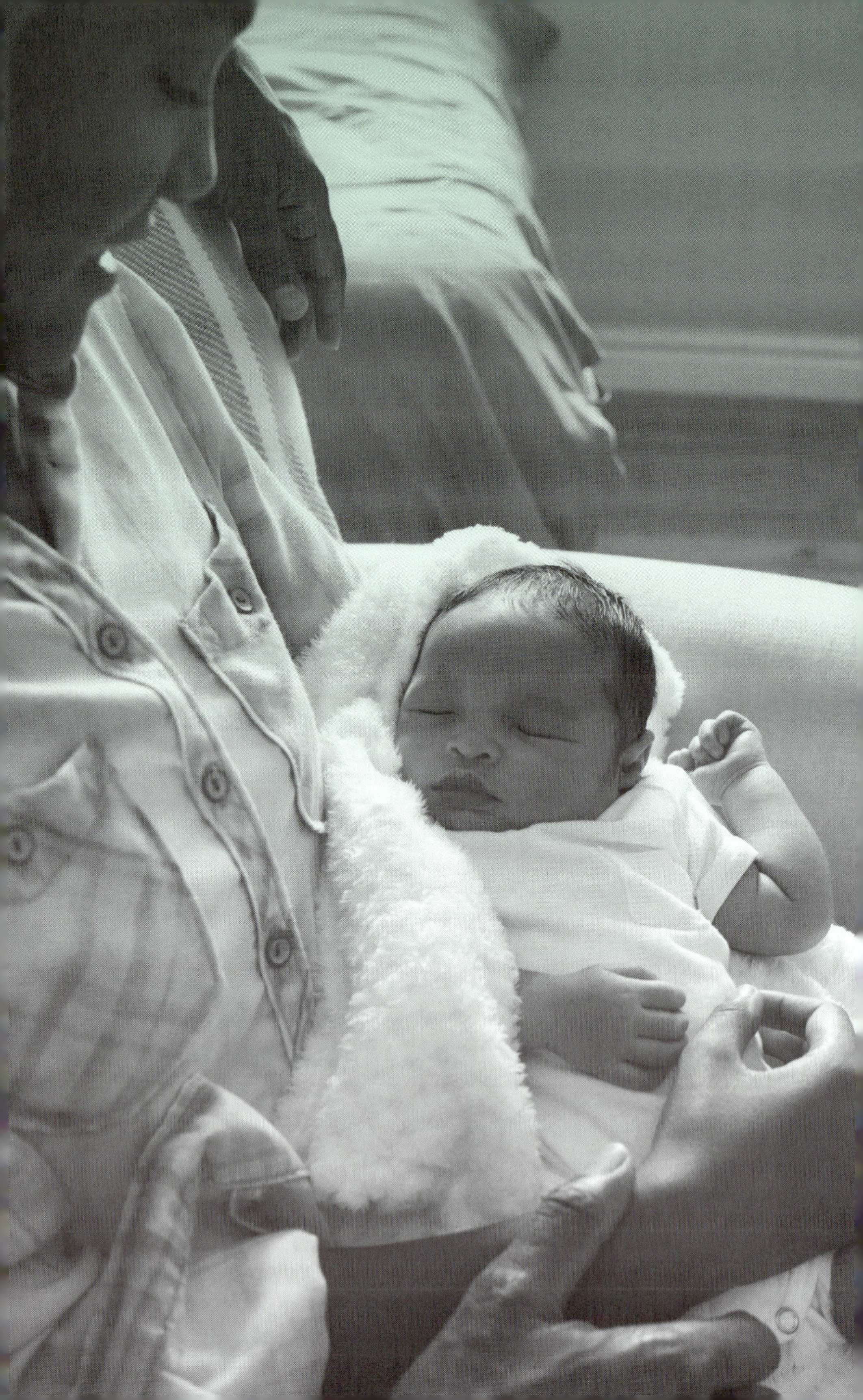

PART 7

Testing

CHAPTER 33

Genetic Disorders, Screening, and Testing

About 3 in 100 babies in the United States are born with a major **birth defect**. A birth defect is a physical or functional problem that is present at birth. Some birth defects are identified soon after birth. Others may not be noticed until the child is older.

Many birth defects are caused by problems with a person's **chromosomes** or **genes**. These types of disorders are called **genetic disorders**. Genetic disorders can range from mild to severe. An example of a mild genetic disorder is color blindness. Examples of more severe genetic disorders are some forms of **hemophilia** and **Tay–Sachs disease.**

Some genetic disorders are not harmful, and no special treatment is needed. For many genetic disorders, medical treatment and specialized care can greatly improve a child's quality of life. But for some genetic disorders, there is no effective treatment. See Table 33-1, "Common Genetic Disorders," for a list of common disorders.

Screening and Diagnostic Tests

There are tests to assess the risk of having a child with certain disorders. These **screening tests** can be done before you get pregnant or during pregnancy. Other tests can find out for sure if there are specific problems with the baby. These tests are called **diagnostic tests**. Both screening and diagnostic testing are offered to all pregnant women. You don't have to be a certain age or have a family history of a disorder to have these tests.

TABLE 33-1 **Common Genetic Disorders**

Disorder	What It Means	Most Often Affected
Dominant Disorders		
Neurofibromatosis	Disorder that causes growth of tumors in the nervous system	People with a family history of the disorder
Isolated polydactyly	Having extra fingers or toes	People with a family history of the disorder and people of African descent. Often happens without risk factors.
Recessive Disorders		
Thalassemia	Causes anemia. There are different types of the disorder, and some are more severe than others.	People of Mediterranean (especially Greek or Italian), Middle Eastern, African, and Asian descent
Sickle cell disease	A blood disorder in which the red blood cells can become crescent ("sickle") shaped rather than the normal doughnut shape. Because of their odd shape, these cells get caught in the blood vessels. This prevents oxygen from reaching organs and tissues, which causes episodes of severe pain and organ damage.	People of African, Mediterranean (especially Greek and Italian), Turkish, Arabian, Southern Iranian, and Asian Indian descent
Tay–Sachs disease	A disease in which harmful amounts of a fatty substance called ganglioside GM2 collect in the nerve cells in the brain. It causes severe intellectual disability, blindness, and seizures. Symptoms first show at about 6 months of age.	People of Eastern or Central European Jewish, French Canadian, and Cajun descent
Cystic fibrosis	Causes problems with digestion and breathing. Symptoms appear in childhood—sometimes right after birth. Some people have milder symptoms than others. Over time, the problems tend to get worse and harder to treat.	People of Northern European descent

continued

Screening and testing are a personal choice. Some people would rather not know if they are at risk or whether their child will have a disorder. Others want to know in advance. Knowing beforehand gives you time to learn about the particular disorder. It also gives you time to organize any special care that your child may need if you decide to get pregnant or continue a pregnancy.

TABLE 33-1 Common Genetic Disorders, *continued*

Disorder	What It Means	Most Often Affected
X-Linked Disorders		
Duchenne muscular dystrophy	Causes progressive muscle weakness, loss of muscle tissue, and abnormal bone development. The muscle problems cause problems with movement, especially walking, and breathing problems. Heart defects usually are present. Most affected people do not live beyond age 30.	Males
Color blindness	A condition in which a person cannot see certain colors	Males
Hemophilia	A disorder caused by the lack of a substance in the blood that helps it clot. Affected people are at risk of severe bleeding if they are injured.	Males

For a very small number of disorders, it may be possible to treat the condition during pregnancy (with fetal surgery, for example). You also may have the option of ending the pregnancy. Your *obstetrician–gynecologist (ob-gyn)* or a *genetic counselor* can discuss testing options and what the results may mean for you.

With any type of testing, *false-positive* and *false-negative* results are a possibility. Your ob-gyn can give you information about the rates of false-positive and false-negative results.

Genes and Chromosomes

Genes are the coded instructions that direct every process in your body. Genes also provide the "blueprints" for your physical traits. A gene is a short segment of *DNA*. DNA consists of two strands of different kinds of building blocks. The order in which these building blocks appear along the strands of DNA is the genetic code. The genetic code tells cells how to develop and function.

Genes are located on chromosomes, which come in pairs (normally one from each parent). Most cells have 23 pairs of chromosomes, making a total of 46 chromosomes. Chromosome pairs 1 to 22 are called *autosomes*. The 23rd pair of chromosomes are the *sex chromosomes*, which are called X and Y.

Genes are inherited, meaning that they are passed from parents to children. *Sperm* and *egg* cells each have a single set of 23 chromosomes—half as

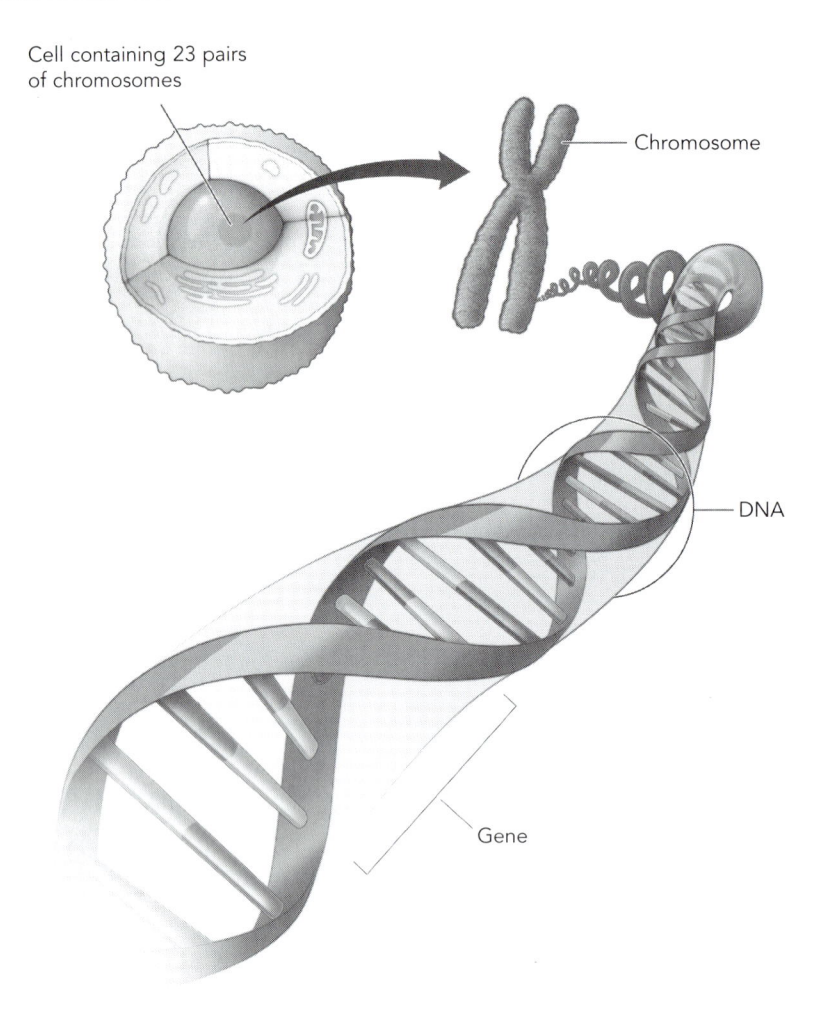

Chromosomes and genes. Chromosomes are the structures inside cells that carry a person's genes. Each person has 22 pairs of autosomes and one pair of sex chromosomes. A single gene is a segment of a large molecule called DNA.

many as other cells. During *fertilization*, when the egg and sperm join, the two sets of chromosomes come together. The cell that is formed contains the full set of 23 pairs of chromosomes. In this way, half of a baby's genes come from the mother and half come from the father.

A baby's sex is determined by the sex chromosomes. The egg always has an **X chromosome**, but the sperm can have either an X or a **Y chromosome**. A combination of XX results in a female and XY results in a male.

Inherited Disorders

Some genetic disorders are caused by a change in a gene. This change is called a ***mutation***. Most mutations are harmless. But some mutations can cause disease or can affect a child's appearance or physical function.

Mutations can be passed from parents to their children, or they can appear for the first time in a child. If a parent has a mutation, there is a 50 percent chance (1 in 2) that his or her child will have the mutation. When a child has a mutation, the chance of developing a disease or disability depends on whether the mutation is dominant or recessive.

Autosomal Dominant Disorders

With an ***autosomal dominant disorder***, just one mutated gene inherited from either parent can cause the disorder. A disorder is called autosomal dominant when the mutation is located on any of the 44 autosomes (the chromosomes that are not the sex chromosomes). If one parent has one copy of the mutated gene that causes an autosomal dominant condition, each child of the couple has a 50 percent chance (1 in 2) of inheriting the disorder.

Autosomal Recessive Disorders

With an ***autosomal recessive disorder***, two mutated genes (one inherited from each parent) are needed to cause the disorder. A person who has only one copy of a mutated gene for a recessive disorder is known as a ***carrier*** of the disorder. Carriers often do not know

Chromosomes

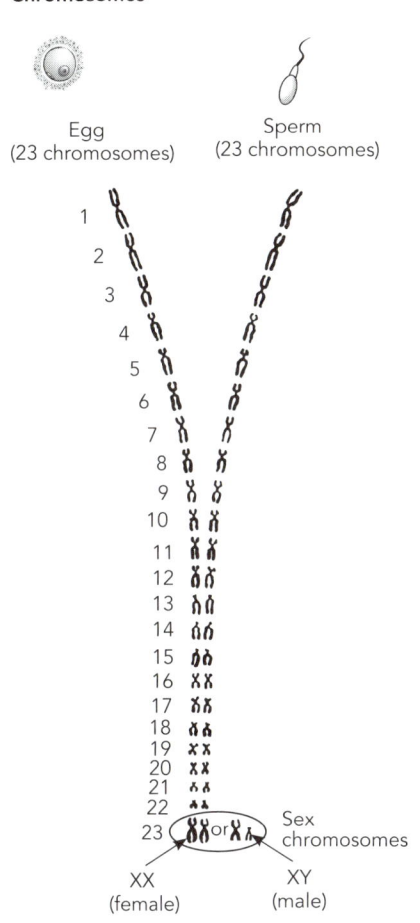

Egg (23 chromosomes)   Sperm (23 chromosomes)

1, 2, 3, 4, 5, 6, 7, 8, 9, 10, 11, 12, 13, 14, 15, 16, 17, 18, 19, 20, 21, 22, 23

XX (female)   XY (male)

Sex chromosomes

How genes are inherited. The chromosomes carry all of a person's genes. Egg and sperm cells have 23 chromosomes each—half as many as other cells. After fertilization, when an egg and sperm join, a baby gets half of its genes from the mother and half from the father. A baby's sex is determined by the sex chromosomes it has. The egg always has an X chromosome, but the sperm can have either an X or a Y chromosome. A combination of XX results in a female baby and XY results in a male baby.

that they have a recessive gene, because they usually do not have any symptoms of the disorder. But they are able to pass the mutated gene to their children.

- If only one parent is a carrier, there is a 50 percent chance (1 in 2) that the child also will be a carrier of the disorder.
- If both parents are carriers, there is a 25 percent chance (1 in 4) that the child will get the mutated gene from each parent and will have the disorder. There is a 50 percent chance (1 in 2) that the child will be a carrier of the disorder—just like the carrier parents. There is a 25 percent chance (1 in 4) that the child will not have the disorder and will not be a carrier.

The following are examples of autosomal recessive disorders:

- Cystic fibrosis—This disorder causes severe problems with breathing and digestion and can lead to early death.
- Sickle cell disease—A blood disorder in which the red blood cells can become crescent ("sickle") shaped rather than the normal doughnut shape. Because of their odd shape, these cells get caught in the blood vessels. This prevents *oxygen* from reaching organs and tissues, which causes episodes of severe pain and organ damage.
- *Spinal muscular atrophy (SMA)*—This disorder causes muscle wasting and severe weakness. It is the leading genetic cause of death in babies.
- Tay–Sachs disease—This disorder causes blindness, seizures, and death, often by age 5.

Sex-Linked Disorders

Disorders that are caused by genes on the sex chromosomes (the X or Y chromosome) are called *sex-linked disorders*. Often (but not always), these disorders are caused by a gene on the X chromosome, in which case they are called *X-linked disorders*.

Many X-linked disorders are recessive. Girls usually are not affected if they inherit a mutated copy of the gene, because their other X chromosome has a normal gene. This normal gene "cancels out" the mutated gene. But because boys have only one X chromosome, they will be affected by the disorder if they inherit a mutated copy of the gene.

- If a man has an X-linked disorder, his X chromosome has the mutated copy of the gene. This means he will pass the mutated gene to all his daughters, who will be carriers (if the gene is recessive) or will develop the disease (if the gene is dominant). He will pass the Y chromosome to his sons, so they will not have the disorder.

- If a woman is a carrier of an X-linked disorder, she has one normal copy and one mutated copy of the gene. This means that all her children have a 50 percent chance (1 in 2) of inheriting the mutated gene. In turn, this means that her sons have a 50 percent chance of developing the disorder. Her daughters have a 50 percent chance of being carriers (if the gene is recessive) or of developing the disease (if the gene is dominant). Some examples of X-linked recessive disorders include color blindness, Duchenne muscular dystrophy, and hemophilia.

Fragile X syndrome is an example of an X-linked dominant disorder, meaning that girls who inherit a copy of the mutated gene also can develop the condition. Girls with Fragile X syndrome usually are less seriously affected than boys.

Multifactorial Disorders

Multifactorial disorders are caused by different factors working together. Some factors are genetic and others are environmental. These disorders can run in families, but the way they are inherited is not completely understood. For example, many people are born with genes that give them a higher chance of developing cancer or *diabetes mellitus* but never develop these diseases. This may be because an environmental factor is needed to trigger the disease. These factors may include exposure to a cancer-causing chemical, smoking, a high-fat diet, or being overweight. Other disorder examples include

- *neural tube defects (NTDs)*
- heart defects
- cleft palate

Researchers have been able to identify environmental factors that trigger some of these disorders. For example, NTDs are a group of disorders that can happen when the baby's spine does not form correctly. NTDs have been linked to women not getting enough *folic acid* in the weeks before pregnancy and during early pregnancy.

For this reason, all women of childbearing age should take a vitamin supplement with 400 micrograms (mcg) of folic acid daily to help prevent NTDs if a pregnancy should happen (see the section "Taking Folic Acid" in Chapter 1, "Getting Ready for Pregnancy"). If the vitamin label lists dietary folate equivalents (DFE) instead, it should have 667 mcg DFE. But for most multifactorial disorders, the causes are not known.

Types of Genetic Disorders

Autosomal Dominant Disorder
If one parent has a dominant gene disorder, each child has a 50 percent chance (1 in 2) of inheriting the disorder.

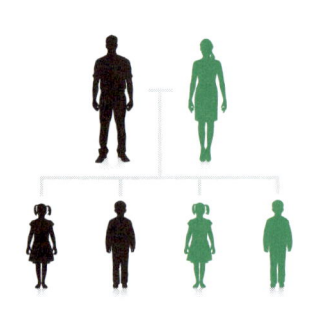

Autosomal Recessive Disorder
If both parents carry the recessive gene for a disorder, then for each child there is a 25 percent chance (1 in 4) that the child will have the disorder, a 50 percent chance (1 in 2) that the child will be a carrier, and a 25 percent chance (1 in 4) that the child will not get the gene at all.

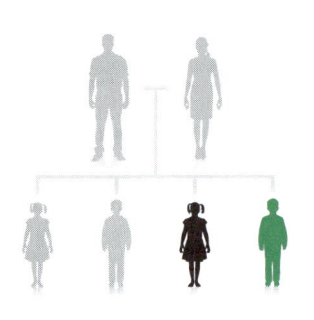

X-linked Disorder
If a woman is a carrier of an X-linked disorder and she has a son, there is a 50 percent chance (1 in 2) that he will have the disorder. If she has a daughter, there is a 50 percent chance (1 in 2) that the daughter will be a carrier. If the father has an X-linked disorder, all the daughters will be carriers and none of the sons will be affected.

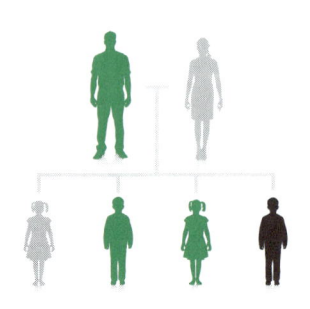

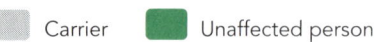

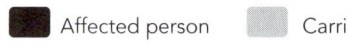

■ Affected person   ▨ Carrier   ■ Unaffected person

Chromosomal Disorders

Some genetic disorders are caused by having too many or too few chromosomes. Having an abnormal number of chromosomes is called ***aneuploidy***. As many as 1 in 5 fertilized eggs may have aneuploidy. In most cases, fertilized eggs with aneuploidy do not implant in the ***uterus***, or they cause ***miscarriage*** early in pregnancy.

Another type of genetic disorder is caused by problems with the structure of chromosomes. These sometimes are called "structural chromosomal disorders."

Aneuploidy

Most children with aneuploidy have physical defects and intellectual disabilities.

- The most common aneuploidy is a *trisomy*, in which there is an extra chromosome. Examples of trisomies include **Patau syndrome (trisomy 13)**, **Edwards syndrome (trisomy 18)**, and **Down syndrome (trisomy 21)**.
- Aneuploidy also can involve extra copies of the X or Y chromosomes. This means that instead of having an XX or XY combination, a baby may have an XXX, XXY, or XYY combination. People with these combinations may have fertility problems, but otherwise they may not be seriously affected.
- A *monosomy* is a condition in which there is a missing chromosome. Monosomies are much rarer than trisomies. An example of a monosomy is **Turner syndrome**, in which a baby has a single X chromosome rather than XX or XY. Babies with Turner syndrome develop female *genitals*, but they usually are infertile. The syndrome also may cause a webbed neck, short height, and heart problems.

Aneuploidy usually happens because the egg or sperm has an abnormal number of chromosomes. These errors usually happen by chance when the egg or sperm come together. But the chance of these errors occurring increases with age. The chance of aneuploidy therefore increases with age. For example, the risk of having a baby with Down syndrome is calculated according to the woman's age when the baby is born:

- 1 in 1,480 at age 20
- 1 in 940 at age 30
- 1 in 353 at age 35
- 1 in 85 at age 40
- 1 in 35 at age 45

Down syndrome is the most common trisomy in the United States. It happens in about 1 in 700 births. There are about 6,000 new cases each year. About 4 in 5 babies with Down syndrome are born to women who are younger than 35, simply because younger women have far more babies than older women.

Structural Chromosomal Disorders

Some structural chromosomal disorders are caused by abnormal chromosomes in eggs or sperm. Others happen during prenatal development or even later in life. There are several types of structural chromosomal disorders:

- Duplication means a part of a chromosome is repeated.
- Deletion means a part of a chromosome is missing. Deletions usually cause more serious problems than duplications.
- Translocation means a piece of a chromosome breaks off and relocates to another chromosome. This does not always cause a disease or physical disability. In some cases, genetic material is not lost, so there are no medical effects. In other cases, genetic material is lost. This can lead to repeated miscarriages.

Assessing Your Risk

Screening and diagnostic testing for genetic disorders are available to all women in pregnancy, regardless of whether they have risk factors. In the past, if a woman was 35 or older at the time of delivery, she was automatically considered at high risk of having a child with Down syndrome and offered diagnostic testing. But a woman of any age can give birth to a child with Down syndrome or another trisomy. For this reason, a woman's age is no longer used to determine whether she should be offered screening or diagnostic testing. Remember that it is your choice whether you want to have genetic testing.

To help guide the decision about testing, your ob-gyn may ask you certain questions about your health and your family history (see the box "Risk Factors for Genetic Disorders"). These questions are designed to find out whether you have risk factors that may increase your chance of having a baby with a genetic disorder. Risk factors that may increase the chance of having a child with a genetic disorder include

- older age in either the father or mother
- a genetic disorder in one or both parents
- a previous child with a genetic disorder
- family history of a genetic disorder
- one or both parents belonging to an ethnic group with a high rate of carriers of certain genetic disorders

Even if you have risk factors, it does not mean that your baby will have a disorder. In fact, most babies with a birth defect are born to couples with no known risk factors. An ob-gyn or a genetic counselor can study your family health history and make recommendations about which tests are most appropriate for you. An ob-gyn or counselor also can:

GENETIC DISORDERS, SCREENING, AND TESTING • 563

Risk Factors for Genetic Disorders

Before you talk with your ob-gyn about prenatal screening and diagnostic testing, review your risk factors for genetic disorders. You also may want to talk with family members about diseases or conditions that run in your families.

- What is your age?
- What is the baby's father's age?
- If you or the baby's father is of Mediterranean or Asian descent, do either of you or anyone in your families have thalassemia?
- Is there a family history of neural tube defects (NTDs)?
- Have you or the baby's father ever had a child with an NTD?
- Is there a family history of congenital heart defects?
- Is there a family history of Down syndrome?
- Have you or the baby's father ever had a child with Down syndrome?
- If you or the baby's father is of Eastern or Central European Jewish, French Canadian, or Cajun descent, is there a family history of Tay–Sachs disease?
- If you or your partner is of Eastern or Central European Jewish descent, is there a family history of Canavan disease or any other genetic disorders?
- Is there a family history of sickle cell disease or sickle cell trait?
- Is there a family history of hemophilia?
- Is there a family history of muscular dystrophy?
- Is there a family history of Huntington disease?
- Does anyone in your family or the family of the baby's father have cystic fibrosis?
- Does anyone in your family or the baby's father's family have an intellectual disability? Or have they had early menopause or tremors at an early age?
- If so, was that person tested for fragile X syndrome?
- Do you, the baby's father, anyone in your families, or any of your children have any other genetic diseases, chromosomal disorders, or birth defects?
- Do you have a metabolic disorder such as diabetes mellitus or phenylketonuria?
- Do you have a history of pregnancy issues (miscarriage or **stillbirth**)?

- interpret test results
- provide counseling about your options
- talk about any concerns you may have

Types of Tests for Genetic Disorders

Many types of tests are available to help address concerns about genetic disorders:

- *Carrier screening*—Carrier screening can show if you or your partner carries a gene for a disorder that could be passed to your children. It involves a simple blood test or a swab from the inside of the cheek, and it can be done before or during pregnancy. Sometimes people are screened based on their risk of being a carrier of a certain genetic condition. This screening often is based on race, ethnicity, or family history. But there also are screening panels that can test for 100 or more genetic disorders regardless of ethnic background (see the section "Carrier Screening" to learn more about *expanded carrier screening*).

- Prenatal screening tests—Tests of the pregnant woman's blood and findings from **ultrasound exams** can screen the baby for Down syndrome and other trisomies. These tests also can screen for NTDs and some defects of the abdomen, heart, and facial features. The tests do not tell whether the baby actually has these disorders. They only assess the risk that the baby has the disorders. Screening tests for birth defects are offered to all pregnant women. It is your choice whether you want to have them done.

- Diagnostic tests—Prenatal diagnostic tests can tell you, with as much certainty as possible, whether the baby has an aneuploidy or a specific genetic condition. These tests usually are done on cells from the baby or **placenta**. The cells are collected with **amniocentesis** or **chorionic villus sampling (CVS)**. Rarely, **fetal blood sampling** or fetal tissue sampling may be done. The cells can be analyzed in different ways. Diagnostic tests are available for all pregnant women, even for those who do not have risk factors.

Deciding Whether to Be Tested

It is your choice whether to have prenatal screening and diagnostic testing. A first step in making your decision is to learn the medical facts about the different kinds of testing (see Table 33–2, "Comparison of Screening Tests

GENETIC DISORDERS, SCREENING, AND TESTING • 565

and Diagnostic Tests"). Your ob-gyn or a genetic counselor can discuss testing options and recommend which tests may be best for your situation. You should understand the

- advantages, disadvantages, and limitations of each test
- risks of each test
- meaning and rates of false-positive or false-negative results
- timing of each test
- cost and whether it is covered by your health insurance plan

TABLE 33-2 **Comparison of Screening Tests and Diagnostic Tests**

	Screening Tests	Diagnostic Tests
Types of results	Screening tests give you the probability of your baby being born with or without a disorder. Results of prenatal screening tests often are given as a number such as 1 in 800, meaning that there is a 1 in 800 chance that your baby will have a defect. These results can be further described as being "high-risk" ("screen-positive") or "low-risk" ("screen-negative").	Diagnostic testing tells you whether or not the baby has a chromosome disorder or a specific **inherited disorder.**
Accuracy	If you decide to have screening tests, there is a possibility of false-positive and false-negative results.	With diagnostic testing, false-positive and false-negative results are rare.
Timing	Screening tests for birth defects can be done in the first or in the second trimester, but the accuracy of results is higher when first-trimester results and second-trimester results are combined.	Diagnostic tests also are done in the first trimester (between 10 and 13 weeks of pregnancy for CVS) and in the second trimester (between 15 and 20 weeks of pregnancy and beyond for amniocentesis).
Risks	The risks of having a screening test, which involves taking a blood sample from the woman and doing an ultrasound exam, are the possible anxiety after a false-positive test result and the possible false reassurance when a false-negative test result occurs.	Diagnostic tests are invasive. A sample needs to be taken from the amniotic fluid or part of the placenta using a needle. This can pose some risks to the pregnancy, although complications are rare.
Cost	Check with your health insurance plan to make sure that the tests that you and your ob-gyn or genetic counselor choose are covered. Some insurance plans cover diagnostic testing only if you have risk factors for having a baby with a genetic disorder or if you have a positive screening test result.	

A test result that shows there is a problem when one does not exist is called a false-positive result. A false-positive result can cause anxiety and may lead to unnecessary testing or treatment. A test result that shows there is not a problem when one does exist is called a false-negative result. A false-negative result can mean that you do not get the recommended counseling or preparation for having a child who has a medical condition or disability. Both of these errors, although rare, are more common with screening tests than with diagnostic tests.

Once you know the medical facts, you also need to consider how you will use the information from these tests. Your response to test results may depend on your personal beliefs, health history, and the specific disorders you are testing for. Your decision about test results may not be clear right away, or it may change as you go through the testing process.

Counselors, social workers, and faith leaders may be able to provide support. There also are parent support networks, such as the National Down Syndrome Society, March of Dimes, and the Cystic Fibrosis Foundation (see the "Resources" section at the end of this chapter).

Some people want to know beforehand if their pregnancy is affected by a genetic disorder. Knowing gives them time to learn about the disorder and plan for the medical care that the child may need.

Some people may decide to end the pregnancy in certain situations. The timing of tests is important for this reason. Having earlier results from diagnostic testing allows time to get more information from an ob-gyn or genetic counselor. Also, if you want to end the pregnancy, it may be safer and easier during the first trimester rather than later in the pregnancy.

But it's important that a decision to end a pregnancy not be made based on a screening test alone, because many at-risk pregnancies will not be affected. If you have a positive screening test and are considering ending your pregnancy, it is recommended that you have a diagnostic test first.

Other people do not want to know this information before the child is born. In this case, you may decide not to have any screening or diagnostic testing. There is no right or wrong choice. All of the decisions are yours.

If you choose to have one or more tests, you should meet with your ob-gyn or genetic counselor after testing. He or she can explain the results to you and help you make the best decisions for you and your family if you have a positive result.

Carrier Screening

Carrier screening detects if a person carries a gene for many, but not all, recessive disorders. If you are a carrier, it means that you can pass the gene to your children. For this test, a sample of blood, saliva, or cells from your inside cheek is sent to a lab for study. All women who are pregnant or thinking about getting pregnant are offered carrier screening for

- cystic fibrosis
- *hemoglobinopathies*
- spinal muscular atrophy (SMA)

Extra screening may be recommended based on certain factors. There are two general approaches to carrier screening: 1) targeted carrier screening and 2) expanded carrier screening.

Targeted carrier screening involves screening for certain disorders based on your ethnicity or family history. Traditionally, carrier screening has been recommended for people who belong to an ethnic group or race that has a high rate of carriers of a specific genetic disorder (see Table 33-3, "Recommended Carrier Screening Tests for People of Different Backgrounds"). Carrier screening for a specific disorder also may be recommended if you have a family history of that disorder. Targeted screening is highly accurate.

Expanded carrier screening is now possible to screen for a wide variety of disorders. It has a high degree of accuracy and usually is not expensive. Companies that offer expanded carrier screening create their own lists of

TABLE 33-3 **Recommended Carrier Screening Tests for People of Different Backgrounds***

Background and Ethnicity	Recommended Screening
All backgrounds	Cystic fibrosis Spinal muscular atrophy (SMA)
African descent	Alpha-thalassemia Sickle cell disease
Eastern or Central European Jewish descent	Tay–Sachs disease
French Canadian or Cajun descent	Tay–Sachs disease
Hispanic descent	Beta-thalassemia
Mediterranean descent (including Arab, Greek, southern Iranian, Italian, or Turkish)	Alpha-thalassemia Beta-thalassemia Sickle cell disease
Southeast Asian descent	Alpha-thalassemia Sickle cell disease
West Indian descent	Beta-thalassemia

*The tests that are available and who they should be offered to frequently change as a result of new research.

disorders that they test for. This list is called a screening panel. Some panels test for more than 100 different disorders. Screening panels usually focus on severe disorders that affect a person's quality of life from an early age. If you are interested in this type of screening, talk with your ob-gyn or genetic counselor.

Once you know your carrier status for a disorder, you do not need to be tested again in a future pregnancy for that disorder. If new carrier screening tests become available for a disorder that you have not been tested for and for which you may be at risk, you may want to discuss carrier screening for the disorder with your ob-gyn.

Results and What to Do Next

Let's say you have chosen carrier screening for a specific disorder:

- If your test result is negative, meaning that you do not have the gene for the disorder, no further testing is needed.

- If your test result is positive, meaning that you have the gene, the likely next step is to test your partner.

- If the result of your partner's test is positive too, a genetic counselor or your ob-gyn will help you understand your risk of having a child with the disorder.

Your ob-gyn or genetic counselor can explain the limitations of the screening tests that you decide to have. A negative screening test result does not necessarily mean that you do not have any gene for the disorder being tested. For example, with cystic fibrosis, the standard test looks only for a limited number of genetic changes. There are other, less common genetic changes that also can cause cystic fibrosis. So a negative carrier test result does not completely rule out the risk that a person is a carrier.

Timing

Carrier screening can be done either before pregnancy or during the early weeks of your pregnancy. If the screening is done before you are pregnant, you can use the results to decide if you want to get pregnant. If it's done after you get pregnant and you screen positive for being a carrier of a disorder, diagnostic testing may be possible to see if the baby has the disorder or is a carrier of the disorder.

If You or Your Partner Is a Carrier

Being a carrier of a disorder usually doesn't affect your own health. It also does not mean that all of your children will be affected. Your ob-gyn or genetic counselor can calculate the chances that a child will have the disorder or that a child will be a carrier. When you have this information, you can think about several options:

- If you have carrier screening before pregnancy, you may try to get pregnant with the option of considering prenatal diagnostic testing. You may choose to use *in vitro fertilization (IVF)* with donor eggs or sperm to achieve pregnancy. **Preimplantation genetic testing** can be used with this option. You also may choose not to get pregnant.

- If you are already pregnant, you may want to have diagnostic testing, if it is available, to see if the pregnancy is affected by the disorder.

You also may want to consider telling other family members if you or your partner is a carrier. They may be at risk of being carriers themselves. But you are not obligated to share this information. Your ob-gyn or genetic counselor can give you advice about the best way to do this. Telling others cannot be done without your consent.

Prenatal Screening Tests

A variety of tests that screen your pregnancy for aneuploidy and neural tube defects (NTDs) are available. Screening tests can be done in the first or second trimester (see Table 33-4, "Types of Screening Tests"). Results of these tests also can be combined in various ways. Combining results may give a better picture than just looking at individual results. The types of screening tests that you may be offered depend on

- which tests are available in your area
- how far along you are in your pregnancy
- your ob-gyn's assessment of which tests best fit your needs

First-Trimester Screening

First-trimester screening consists of a blood test combined with an ultrasound exam. This screening is done between 10 and 13 weeks of pregnancy to assess the risk of Down syndrome and other aneuploidies. The blood test measures the levels of at least two different proteins in the pregnant woman's blood. An ultrasound exam, called **nuchal translucency screening**, is used to measure the thickness at the back of the neck of the baby. An increase in the thickness of this space may be a sign of Down syndrome or other problems.

TABLE 33–4 **Types of Screening Tests**

Screening Test	Test Type	What Does It Screen For?	Down Syndrome Detection Rate
First-trimester screening (10 to 13 weeks of pregnancy)			
Combined screening	Blood test for two proteins in the pregnant woman's blood plus an ultrasound exam	• Down syndrome (trisomy 21) • Edwards syndrome (trisomy 18)	82 to 87 percent
First-trimester screening (10 weeks of pregnancy or later)			
Cell-free DNA test	Blood test that analyzes fetal DNA. This DNA circulates in the pregnant woman's blood.	• Down syndrome • Edwards syndrome • Patau syndrome (trisomy 13) • Sex chromosome abnormalities	99 percent
Second-trimester screening (15 to 22 weeks of pregnancy)			
Quad screen	Blood test for four proteins in the pregnant woman's blood	• Down syndrome • Edwards syndrome • Neural tube defects (NTDs)	81 percent
Maternal serum alpha-fetoprotein (MSAFP)	Blood test for a protein in the pregnant woman's blood	• NTDs	
Combined first- and second-trimester screening (10 to 13 weeks, then 15 to 22 weeks)			
Integrated screening	Blood test and an ultrasound exam in the first trimester, followed by quad screen in the second trimester	• Down syndrome • Edwards syndrome • NTDs • Patau syndrome	96 percent
Contingent sequential	First-trimester combined screening result: • Positive: diagnostic test offered • Negative: no further testing • Intermediate: second-trimester screening test offered	• Down syndrome • Edwards syndrome • NTDs • Patau syndrome	88 to 94 percent

Cell-Free DNA Testing

Another screening test, called the cell-free DNA test, is available. This blood test is based on the fact that a small amount of DNA from the placenta circulates in a pregnant woman's blood. The placenta DNA in a sample of the woman's blood can be screened for

- Down syndrome
- Edwards Syndrome
- Patau syndrome
- sex chromosome abnormalities

The cell-free DNA test can be done starting at 10 weeks of pregnancy. It takes about 1 week to get the results. A positive cell-free DNA test result should be followed by a diagnostic test with amniocentesis or CVS.

Cell-free DNA testing usually is not recommended for women carrying more than two babies. Also, cell-free DNA testing does not screen for NTDs.

Second-Trimester Screening

In the second trimester, a test called a "quadruple" or "quad" screen can be done to detect the presence of four different proteins in the pregnant woman's blood. This test screens for

- Down syndrome
- Edwards syndrome
- NTDs

The quad screen may be done between 15 and 22 weeks of pregnancy, but experts believe the ideal time for this screening is between 16 and 18 weeks. The stage of pregnancy at the time of the test is important because the levels of the substances measured change throughout pregnancy.

A standard ultrasound exam is recommended for all women between 18 and 22 weeks. This exam can provide information about whether certain structures are developing normally, including the baby's heart, abdomen, face, head, and spine. It can identify major physical defects, including NTDs.

Another blood test also screens for NTDs. It measures the levels of a substance called ***alpha-fetoprotein (AFP)*** in your blood. This test normally is done between 15 and 18 weeks, sometimes in combination with other tests. The screening also has several limitations and is less accurate for detecting NTDs than ultrasound exams.

Integrated and Sequential Screening

The results from first-trimester and second-trimester tests can be used together to screen for Down syndrome, Edwards syndrome, and NTDs. The tests can be done in the following ways:

- Integrated screening—Results of the first-trimester and second-trimester tests are analyzed together. The results are given only after the first-trimester and second-trimester screening tests are completed. Integrated screening is highly accurate and has a low rate of false-positive results.

- Sequential screening—Results of the first-trimester screening tests are used to determine further testing. If results show that you are at high risk, you can choose to have a diagnostic test. If results show that you are at low or intermediate risk, you can choose to have second-trimester screening or not. Compared with integrated screening, the chance of a false-positive result with sequential screening is slightly higher and accuracy is about the same.

If Screening Test Results Show an Increased Risk

In most cases, screening test results are normal. If the results of a screening test raise concerns about your pregnancy, you will need to think about the information and decide how to proceed. Your ob-gyn or genetic counselor can help guide you through your options. More evaluation, such as diagnostic testing, may be available for the disorder in question and can be done to provide more information.

The chance that you will have a positive diagnostic test result after a positive screening test result is low. If you are thinking about having a diagnostic test, you will need to balance the small risk of pregnancy **complications** that are associated with a diagnostic test against the risk of having a child with the disorder. Your ob-gyn or genetic counselor can explain these risks to you in detail. The goal is to help you make an informed decision.

Diagnostic Tests

Different methods are used to gather cells from the baby for diagnostic testing. The most common test is amniocentesis, followed by chorionic villus sampling (CVS). Once the cells are gathered, they can be studied in different ways.

Amniocentesis

Amniocentesis usually is done between 15 and 20 weeks of pregnancy, but it can be done at any later time during pregnancy. To do amniocentesis, a thin

GENETIC DISORDERS, SCREENING, AND TESTING • 573

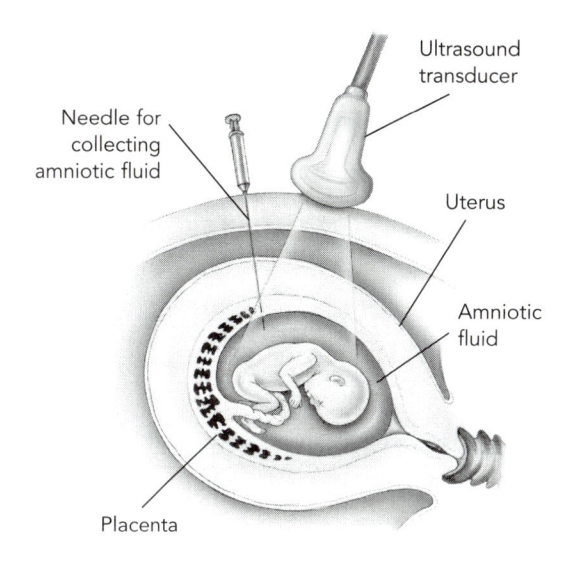

Amniocentesis. In this procedure, a small sample of amniotic fluid is removed with a needle to be studied.

needle is guided through the woman's abdomen and uterus. A small sample of amniotic fluid is withdrawn. Amniotic fluid contains cells from the baby. These cells are sent to a lab, where they are grown in a special culture. This takes about 10 to 12 days.

When the cells are ready, they are analyzed to find out whether the baby has certain disorders, such as Down syndrome or specific genetic disorders (see "How the Cells Are Analyzed" later in this chapter). The amniotic fluid also can be tested to detect NTDs. Complications of amniocentesis may include

- cramping
- vaginal bleeding
- infection
- leaking amniotic fluid

There is a very small chance of miscarriage (1 in 900 procedures).

Chorionic Villus Sampling

Chorionic villus sampling (CVS) is performed earlier than amniocentesis, generally between 10 and 13 weeks of pregnancy. This earlier time frame gives you more time to think about your options and to make decisions. But CVS is not as commonly done as amniocentesis and may not be available at all hospitals or centers.

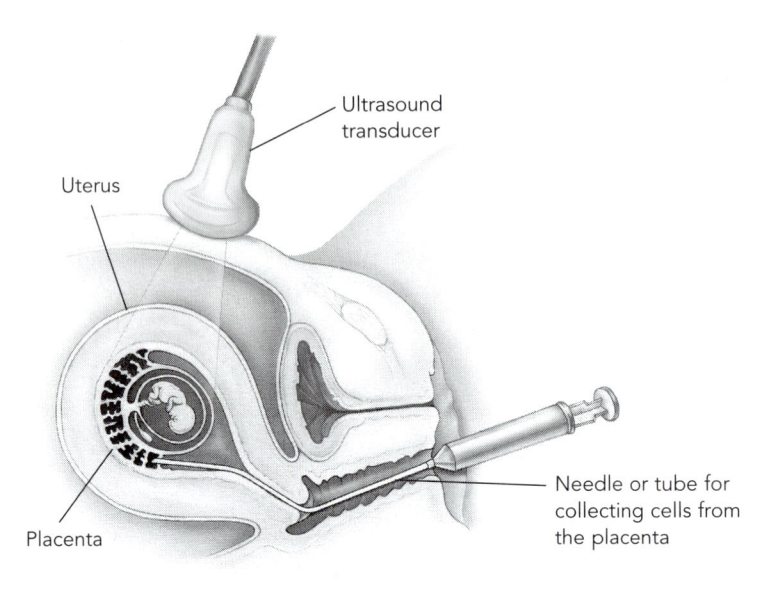

Chorionic villus sampling. In this procedure, a small sample of cells (chorionic villi) is removed from the placenta to be studied.

To do CVS, a small sample of tissue is taken from the placenta. The tissue contains cells with the same genetic makeup as the baby. The sample can be obtained in one of two ways. A small tube can be guided through the woman's ***vagina*** and ***cervix***, or a thin needle can be guided through the abdomen and wall of the uterus. The sample is sent to a lab. The cells are grown in a culture, which takes about 7 to 14 days. Then the cells are analyzed.

Complications from CVS may include

- vaginal bleeding
- leakage of amniotic fluid
- infection

The risk of miscarriage with CVS is 1 in 455 procedures.

CVS cannot be used to diagnose NTDs before birth. If you have CVS, you also may want to have the blood test for alpha-fetoprotein, a detailed ultrasound exam, or both to detect NTDs.

Preimplantation Genetic Testing

This testing may be offered to a couple who is using IVF to get pregnant and is at increased risk of having a baby with a disorder. Before an ***embryo*** is transferred to a woman's uterus, it is tested to see if it has a specific, known genetic disorder for which the couple is at risk.

How the Cells Are Analyzed

Different technologies are used in prenatal diagnostic testing. Each one is used to detect different kinds of genetic changes. Your ob-gyn or genetic counselor can recommend the test that is most appropriate for you.

Missing, extra, or damaged chromosomes can be detected by taking a picture of the baby's chromosomes and arranging them in order from smallest to largest. This is called a *karyotype*. A karyotype can show whether

- the number of chromosomes is abnormal
- the shape of one or more chromosomes is abnormal
- a chromosome is broken

A technique called *fluorescence in situ hybridization (FISH)* can be used to detect the most common aneuploidies, which involve chromosomes 13, 18, 21, and the X and Y chromosomes. Results are available more quickly than with traditional karyotyping because the cells do not need to be grown in a lab. A positive test result is confirmed with a karyotype.

Chromosomal *microarray* (CMA) is a technique that can look at the chromosomes in greater detail. CMA is designed to detect extra or missing parts of chromosomes (duplications or deletions) that may be associated with various genetic disorders. CMA may be done on samples from amniocentesis or CVS or on samples taken after something abnormal has been seen on an ultrasound exam. Sometimes an abnormality will be found but it will be unclear whether it will affect the pregnancy. This is called a "variant of unknown significance." You and your ob-gyn or genetic counselor should discuss results that show a variant of unknown significance.

Tests to find specific gene mutations also can be done. Testing for gene mutations must be specifically requested. Keep in mind that there is no one test that can find every possible gene mutation.

If Your Pregnancy Has a Disorder

If diagnostic testing shows that your pregnancy is affected by a disorder, you will need to think about your options. You may choose to continue the pregnancy, or you may end the pregnancy. Your health, values, beliefs, and situation all may play a role in the decision.

If you decide to continue the pregnancy, learn all that you can about the condition and what it will mean for your child's health. Some conditions are not serious or life-threatening and may require only minimal special health care. With other disorders, it is helpful to prepare for caring for a child with special needs. Your ob-gyn or hospital staff may be able to help you find this special care.

You also can seek out support groups for you and your partner. Ask whether the hospital where you are planning to deliver has **pediatricians** who can provide the best possible care for your baby. If it doesn't, talk with your ob-gyn about transferring your care to a hospital with pediatricians who can manage your baby's health condition.

Educating yourself about your child's condition is crucial. Look for resources in your area that can put you in contact with parents of children with similar disorders (see the "Resources" section below).

RESOURCES

Cystic Fibrosis Foundation
www.cff.org
National organization dedicated to research into cystic fibrosis and advocacy for people affected by this disorder.

Genetic Science Learning Center
http://learn.genetics.utah.edu
Website that offers basic information about genetics through videos, animations, and other learning aids.

Genetics Home Reference
https://ghr.nlm.nih.gov
Comprehensive, easy-to-read information about genes, chromosomes, and genetic health conditions from the U.S. National Library of Medicine.

Genomics and Medicine
http://genome.gov/27527652
Information from the National Human Genome Research Institute that covers many aspects of genetics and how it pertains to individual people and their families.

March of Dimes
www.marchofdimes.org
Comprehensive website that offers information about a wide variety of birth defects, including their causes, diagnosis, and treatment. Also explains the ongoing research being done to improve the outlook for children and adults born with certain disorders.

National Center on Birth Defects and Developmental Disabilities
www.cdc.gov/ncbddd
Provides information on birth defects, developmental disabilities, and hereditary blood disorders.

National Down Syndrome Society
www.ndss.org
National society that advocates for people with Down syndrome. Provides information for new and expecting parents about the health care needs for children with Down syndrome. Offers support for people with Down syndrome and families.

National Tay–Sachs & Allied Diseases
www.ntsad.org
Provides services, research, and education for Tay–Sachs, Canavan, and other related diseases.

Sickle Cell Disease Association of America
www.sicklecelldisease.org
National organization for education, awareness, and research on sickle cell disease.

Your Pregnancy and Childbirth
www.acog.org/MyPregnancy
Website from the American College of Obstetricians and Gynecologists (ACOG) with information on pregnancy, labor, delivery, and postpartum care. Includes the latest information from the experts in women's health care, questions answered by ACOG ob-gyns, pregnancy stories from real women, and an A–Z directory of health topics covering pregnancy and beyond.

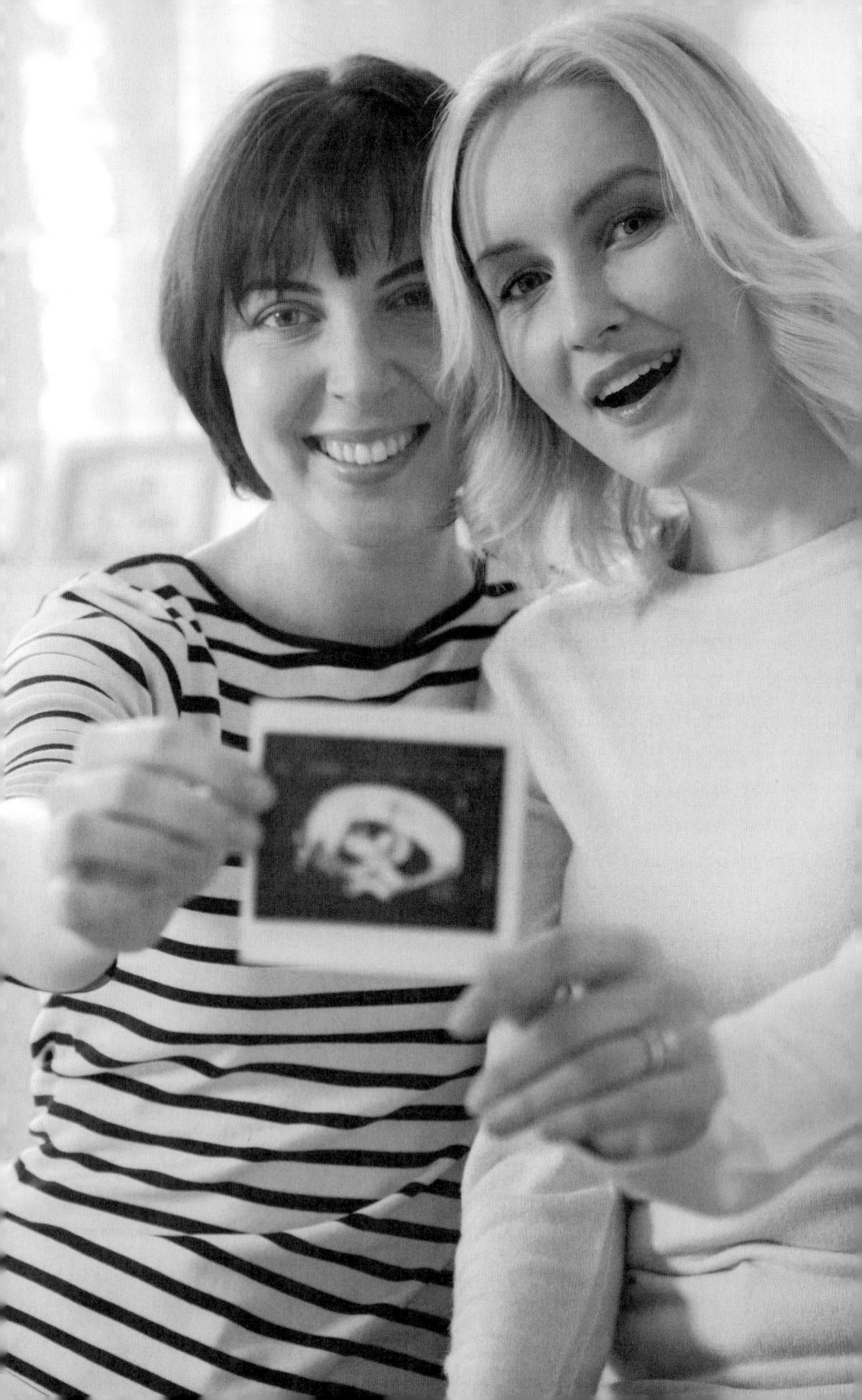

CHAPTER 34

Ultrasound Exams and Other Testing to Monitor Fetal Well-Being

Several types of testing can be done to check the well-being of the baby during pregnancy. The most common test is an **ultrasound exam**. There also are special tests that may help reassure you and your **obstetrician–gynecologist (ob-gyn)** that all is going well. Special tests may be done if

- a problem develops during the pregnancy
- you have a high-risk pregnancy
- you go past your due date

Ultrasound Exams

Most women have at least one ultrasound exam during pregnancy. Ultrasound is energy in the form of sound waves. These waves create pictures of the baby that can be seen on a video monitor.

Some women have an ultrasound exam in the first **trimester** of pregnancy. Common reasons for a first-trimester ultrasound exam include

- confirming the pregnancy
- estimating **gestational age**
- finding out if there is more than one baby
- screening for signs of certain **chromosome** problems or other problems in the baby

If you don't have an ultrasound exam in the first trimester, you likely will have what is called a standard ultrasound exam between 18 and 22 weeks of pregnancy. This exam may provide important information about your pregnancy, including

- estimated gestational age
- position of the **placenta**
- amount of **amniotic fluid** around the baby
- position, movement, and cardiac activity of the baby
- estimated weight of the baby
- whether certain parts of the baby are developing normally (heart, abdomen, face, head, and spine)
- sex of the baby

Other types of ultrasound exams may be done if problems are suspected. A limited ultrasound exam may be done to check a specific issue, such as vaginal bleeding or pelvic pain. If a problem with your baby's growth is suspected, several ultrasound exams may be done over time to check how the baby is growing. Sometimes ultrasound is used to evaluate your **cervix** if there are signs and symptoms of **preterm** labor. Ultrasound also can be used to help guide **chorionic villus sampling (CVS)** and **amniocentesis** testing.

A specialized ultrasound exam may be recommended based on

- your medical history
- a result of a laboratory test
- the results of a standard or limited ultrasound exam

Specialized exams may use extra technology. For example, a **Doppler ultrasound exam** (discussed later in this chapter) can evaluate blood flow through a blood vessel. A three-dimensional (3D) ultrasound exam can be used to show the baby's anatomy in more detail.

How It Is Done

Your ob-gyn or a technician will use a device called a **transducer** for your ultrasound exam. There are two types of transducers: 1) one that is moved over the abdomen (for a **transabdominal ultrasound exam**) and 2) one that is inserted into the **vagina** (for a **transvaginal ultrasound exam**).

For a transabdominal ultrasound exam, you will lie on your back with your belly exposed. A gel will be placed on your belly to improve the contact between the transducer and the skin. The transducer then is moved over your belly and records sound waves as they bounce off your baby. These sound waves create images that are shown on a screen.

For a transvaginal ultrasound exam, a vaginal transducer is inserted into the vagina to help view your pelvic organs and the baby. It works the same way as a transabdominal ultrasound, using sound waves to create images.

What the Results May Mean

Ultrasound cannot detect every problem. It is possible to have a "normal" ultrasound exam but still have a baby with a **birth defect** or other health problem. If something does not look normal on an ultrasound exam, you may have other tests to gather more information.

There is a type of business that creates baby portraits using ultrasound technology. You may have seen a business like this in a shopping mall. These businesses are not medical facilities. Employees may not be trained to interpret the ultrasound images for you. If you want an image of your baby, you can request one during a standard ultrasound exam arranged by your ob-gyn. Having an ultrasound exam without a medical reason—such as to create "keepsake" photos—is not recommended. An ultrasound exam is a medical tool that should be used only when there is a valid medical reason.

Testing to Monitor Fetal Well-Being

Special tests may be used to check the well-being of the baby during pregnancy. Testing may help reassure you and your ob-gyn that all is going well. If test results show a problem, more testing may be done. Your ob-gyn should carefully consider several factors when deciding how to manage your pregnancy after an abnormal test result, including

- your health
- the baby's gestational age
- the baby's health

Each situation is different. There is no "one size fits all" way to proceed.

Why Testing May Be Done

Special testing most often is done when there is a higher risk of pregnancy **complications** or **stillbirth**. Testing also may be done if a woman had a health condition before pregnancy (called a preexisting condition) that carries a risk for the baby. Preexisting conditions that may require special testing during pregnancy include

- *diabetes mellitus*
- *hypertension (high blood pressure)*
- *lupus* (systemic lupus erythematosus or SLE)
- *kidney disease*
- certain blood disorders
- *hyperthyroidism* that is not well controlled
- certain types of heart disease

Problems also can arise during pregnancy. Some pregnancy-related conditions may signal a need for special testing. These problems include

- *gestational hypertension*
- *preeclampsia*
- *gestational diabetes*

Frequently Asked Questions

Are these tests safe?
Most of these tests are noninvasive, meaning no medical equipment has to enter your body. The tests pose very few risks for you and the baby. Sometimes, an ultrasound exam may be done by placing the ultrasound probe in the vagina, but the probe does not go into the uterus. This procedure is safe when done by a trained technician or ob-gyn.

Will the tests hurt?
For most women, these tests are not painful. Some women may feel slight discomfort from insertion of the vaginal ultrasound probe, from staying in certain positions for a while, or from the contractions that are produced during a contraction stress test.

In what order will they happen?
There is no set order for the tests. Likewise, no test has been proved to be better than another. Your ob-gyn will follow the best order for your situation.

Why would the same test have to be repeated?
Tests to determine the well-being of the baby may be done once or at regular intervals, depending on the reason for the test. If your results are unclear or show a potential problem, tests are repeated more often to make sure the baby continues to do well for the rest of the pregnancy. Repeat tests also can help show your ob-gyn if the first results were accurate.

- too much or too little *amniotic fluid*
- growth problems for the baby
- *Rh sensitization*
- *multiple pregnancy* (if there are complications)
- decreased fetal movement (there is a change in how much the baby moves)
- *late term* or *postterm* pregnancy

These tests cannot find every complication that could happen during pregnancy. Some things can happen suddenly, such as *placenta* problems or problems with the *umbilical cord.* The tests discussed in this chapter cannot be used to predict these events.

When Tests Are Available

Special testing usually is done at 32 weeks of pregnancy or later. Testing may be started earlier than 32 weeks if there are serious problems or if there is more than one risk factor for problems. How often the tests are done may depend on

- the condition that prompted the testing
- whether the condition remains stable
- the results of the testing

If the condition that prompted the testing resolves and the test result is normal, more testing may not be needed.

Some tests are repeated every week. In certain situations, tests may be done twice a week. Testing twice a week may be needed

- for women with diabetes
- in a postterm pregnancy
- when there are growth problems for the baby

Interpreting Test Results

No test is 100 percent accurate. A test result that shows there is a problem when one does not exist is called a *false-positive* result. A false-positive result may lead to unnecessary interventions, including early delivery. For this reason, if you have a positive result from one of these tests, you may have further tests to find out whether a problem really exists.

A test result that shows there is no problem when one exists is called a *false-negative* result. A false-negative result from one of these tests means that a problem exists, but it was not found by the test. The rate of false-negative results with these tests is low. This means that if you have special testing and the result is negative, chances are good that the baby will remain stable until the next test is done.

Types of Special Tests

The tests used to monitor the baby's well-being include

- *kick counts*
- *nonstress test*
- *biophysical profile*
- *modified biophysical profile*
- *contraction stress test*
- Doppler ultrasound exam

Kick Counts

Kick counts (also called "fetal movement counting") can be done at home. You do not need special equipment.

Why It Is Done. Kick counts may be recommended if you have felt the baby move less often than what you think is normal. Feeling the same amount of movement from one day to the next may be a sign that the baby is doing well.

How It Is Done. To do this test, you track how long it takes for you to feel 10 movements. Choose a time when the baby usually is active. Often, a good time is after you've eaten a meal. Each baby has its own level of activity, and most have sleep cycles of 20 to 40 minutes.

Once you have felt 10 movements, you can stop counting for that day. If your ob-gyn has recommended kick counts, repeat the test every day.

What the Results May Mean. Call your ob-gyn if it takes longer than 2 hours for the baby to make 10 movements. If you do not feel enough movement, it does not necessarily mean that there is a problem. It could simply mean that the baby is sleeping. More tests usually may be needed to find out more information.

Nonstress Test

The nonstress test measures how the baby's heart rate responds to the baby's movement over a period of time. The term "nonstress" means that no stress is placed on the baby during the test.

Why It Is Done. The baby's heart normally beats faster when the baby moves. This is called an *acceleration.* During a nonstress test, the baby's heart rate is recorded. Your ob-gyn then notes the number of accelerations that happened during the test period.

How It Is Done. This test may be done in your ob-gyn's office or in a hospital. The test is done while you are leaning back or lying down. It usually takes at least 20 minutes, but it can take longer. A belt with a sensor is placed around your belly. The sensor measures the baby's heart rate, which is recorded by a machine. A second belt with a sensor typically is applied to monitor for contractions and to see how the baby's heart rate responds to the contractions.

What the Results May Mean. If two or more accelerations happen within 20 minutes, the result is considered reactive or "reassuring." A reactive result means that the baby is stable for now. Reactive results are slightly different if the gestational age is less than 32 weeks. Sometimes, the baby may be asleep and will not move two times in 20 minutes. If this happens, the test may last for 40 minutes or longer. In some cases, sound placed near the woman's belly may encourage the baby to move.

A nonreactive result is one in which not enough accelerations happened in 40 minutes. This may mean several things:

- It may mean that the baby was asleep during the test.
- It may mean that the baby is doing well but is too young for the test to be accurate.
- It can happen if the woman has taken certain medications.

But a nonreactive result also may mean that the baby is not getting enough *oxygen* or that the baby's nervous system is not functioning properly. If there is a nonreactive result, more testing may be done to gather more information. In some cases, delivery may be needed.

Biophysical Profile

The biophysical profile (BPP) combines two tests: 1) a nonstress test and 2) an ultrasound exam. Together these tests assess the baby's well-being in five areas.

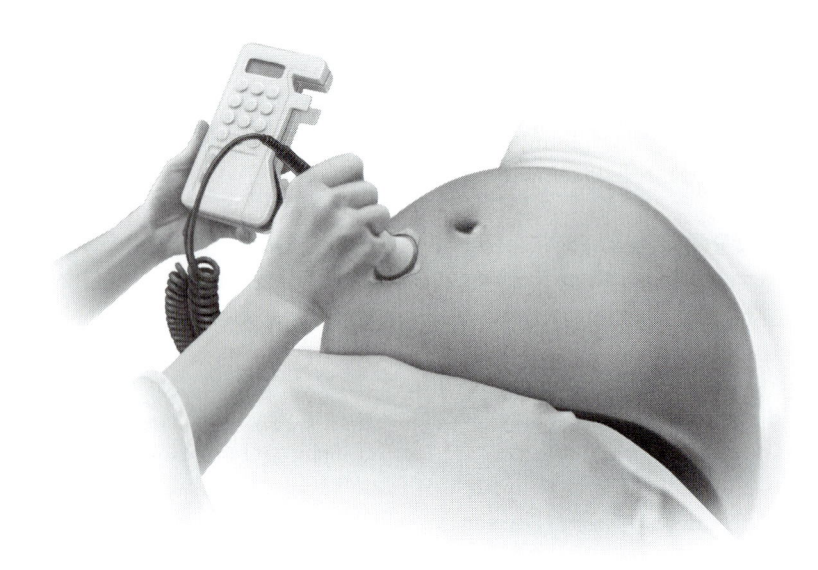

Listening to the baby's heart rate. Later in pregnancy, your ob-gyn may use a handheld Doppler device pressed against your belly to listen to the baby's heart rate. This is not the same as an ultrasound exam.

Why It Is Done. A BPP may be done when results of other tests are nonreassuring. The BPP assesses the following five areas:

1. Baby's heart rate (nonstress test)
2. Breathing movements
3. Body movements
4. Muscle tone
5. Amount of amniotic fluid

Each of the five areas is given a score of 0 or 2 points, for a possible total of 10 points.

How It Is Done. A BPP monitors the baby's heart rate (nonstress test) and checks the baby's movement and the amount of amniotic fluid (ultrasound exam).

What the Results May Mean. A score of 8 to 10 is reassuring. If there is a score of at least 8 with the ultrasound, the nonstress test may not be needed. A score of 6 is "equivocal" (neither reassuring nor nonreassuring). If you have an equivocal score, depending on how far along you are in your pregnancy, you may have another BPP within the next 12 to 24 hours, or your ob-gyn may recommend delivery. A score of 4 or less means that further testing is needed. Sometimes, it means that the baby should be delivered early or right away.

No matter what the score is, if there is not enough amniotic fluid, more testing should be done. In some cases, delivery may be needed.

Modified Biophysical Profile

The modified BPP checks only the baby's heart rate (nonstress test) and the amount of amniotic fluid (ultrasound exam). A modified BPP helps your ob-gyn assess whether the baby is getting enough oxygen and how well the placenta is working.

Why It Is Done. This test is done for the same reasons that a BPP is done.

How It Is Done. The baby's heart rate is monitored in the same way it is done for the nonstress test. The ultrasound exam is used to measure the amount of amniotic fluid.

What the Results May Mean. If the nonstress test results are nonreactive, it could mean that the baby is not getting enough oxygen. If the amniotic fluid level is low, it could mean that there is a problem with blood flow in the placenta. A full BPP or contraction stress test may be needed to clarify the result of the modified BPP.

Contraction Stress Test

The contraction stress test helps your ob-gyn see how the baby's heart rate reacts when the uterus contracts.

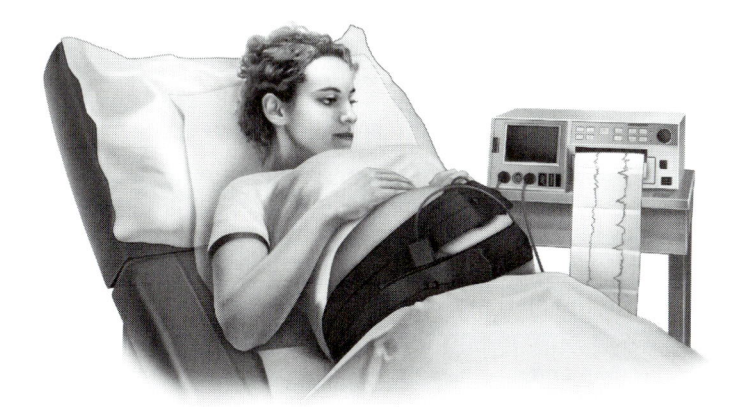

Contraction stress test. This test helps your ob-gyn see how the baby's heart rate reacts when the uterus contracts. Belts with sensors are placed across your belly. The sensors detect the baby's heart rate and measure the strength of your contractions.

Why It Is Done. The contraction stress test sometimes is used if other test results are positive or unclear.

How It Is Done. In this test, belts with sensors that detect the baby's heart rate and uterine contractions are placed across your belly. To make your uterus contract mildly, you may be asked to rub your nipples through your clothing or you may be given ***oxytocin***. Your uterus may contract on its own, especially if the test is done late in pregnancy.

What the Results May Mean. If the baby's heart rate does not slow down after a contraction, the result is "negative," providing reassurance that the baby is at low risk for complications for now. A slowing of the heart rate after most contractions is a "positive" result, which is a cause for concern. Results also can be equivocal (results were not clear) or unsatisfactory (there were not enough contractions to produce a meaningful result). If results are unclear, more tests may be needed. In some situations, the baby may need to be delivered right away.

Doppler Ultrasound Exam

A Doppler ultrasound exam is used with other tests when the baby shows signs of not growing well. This is called ***fetal growth restriction***.

Why It Is Done. The Doppler ultrasound exam is used to check the blood flow in the umbilical artery, a blood vessel located in the umbilical cord. Doppler ultrasound also may be used to look for signs of ***anemia*** in the baby. This is done by measuring blood flow through a blood vessel in the baby's brain.

How It Is Done. A Doppler ultrasound exam is done in the same way as a transabdominal ultrasound exam. A transducer is rolled over your abdomen to project sound waves. An image of the artery that is being examined is shown on a viewing screen.

What the Results May Mean. A normal Doppler ultrasound result is one that shows normal blood flow in the umbilical artery. If the test shows problems with the blood flow in the placenta, it may mean that less oxygen is being delivered to the baby. If there is a problem with blood flow in the placenta, your ob-gyn may recommend delivering your baby, depending how far along you are in your pregnancy. If the test shows the baby may have anemia, your ob-gyn may discuss possible treatment with you.

RESOURCES

Monitoring Your Baby Before Labor
https://medlineplus.gov/ency/patientinstructions/000485.htm
Webpage from the U.S. National Library of Medicine. Describes the special tests that can be done to assess the baby's well-being before labor.

Obstetric Ultrasound
www.radiologyinfo.org/en/info.cfm?pg=obstetricus
Website sponsored by the American College of Radiology and the Radiological Society of North America. Gives an overview of how an ultrasound exam is done during pregnancy, what it can tell you and your ob-gyn, and its risks and benefits.

Your Pregnancy and Childbirth
www.acog.org/MyPregnancy
Website from the American College of Obstetricians and Gynecologists (ACOG) with information on pregnancy, labor, delivery, and postpartum care. Includes the latest information from the experts in women's health care, questions answered by ACOG ob-gyns, pregnancy stories from real women, and an A–Z directory of health topics covering pregnancy and beyond.

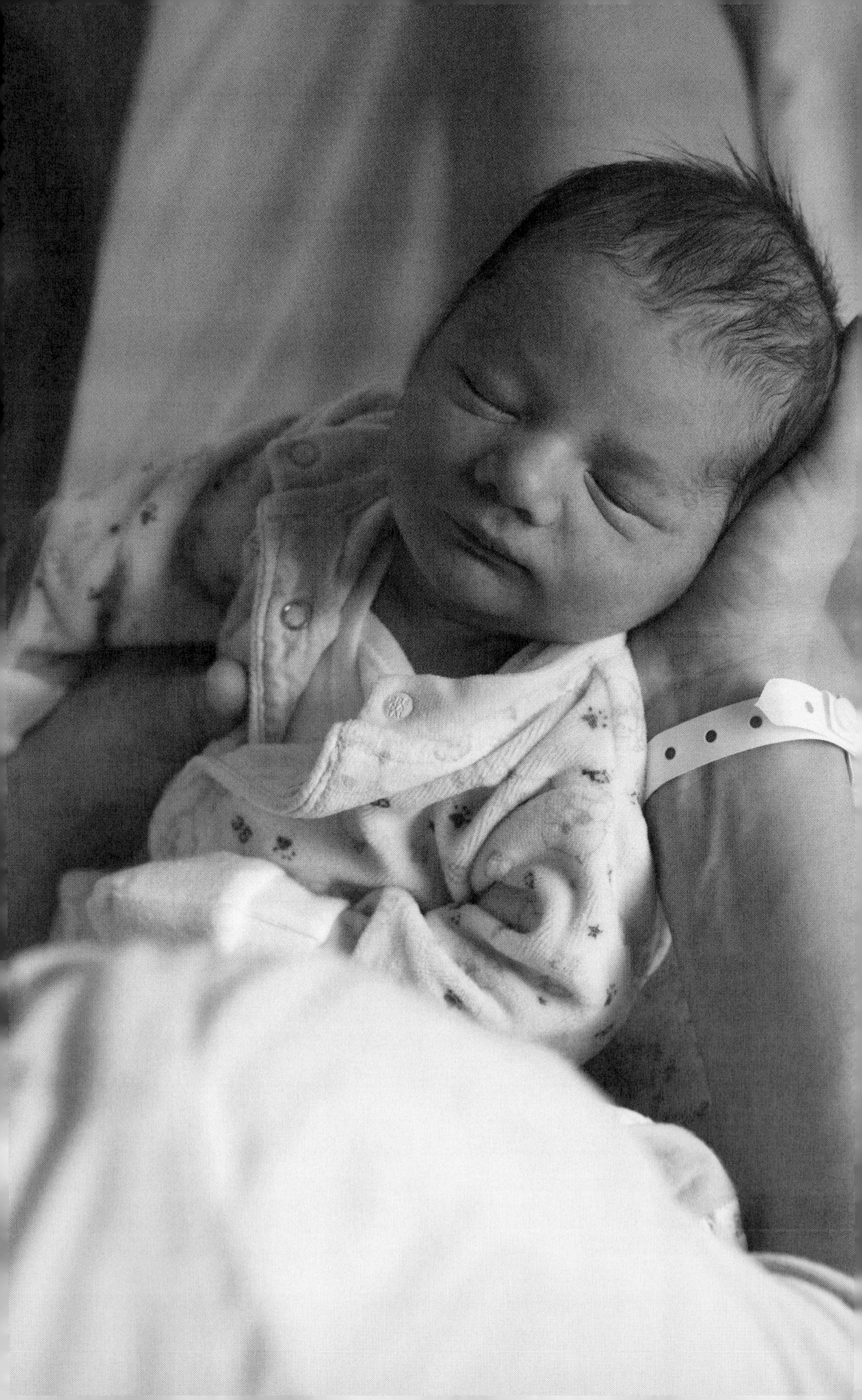

PART 8

Complications During Pregnancy and Childbirth

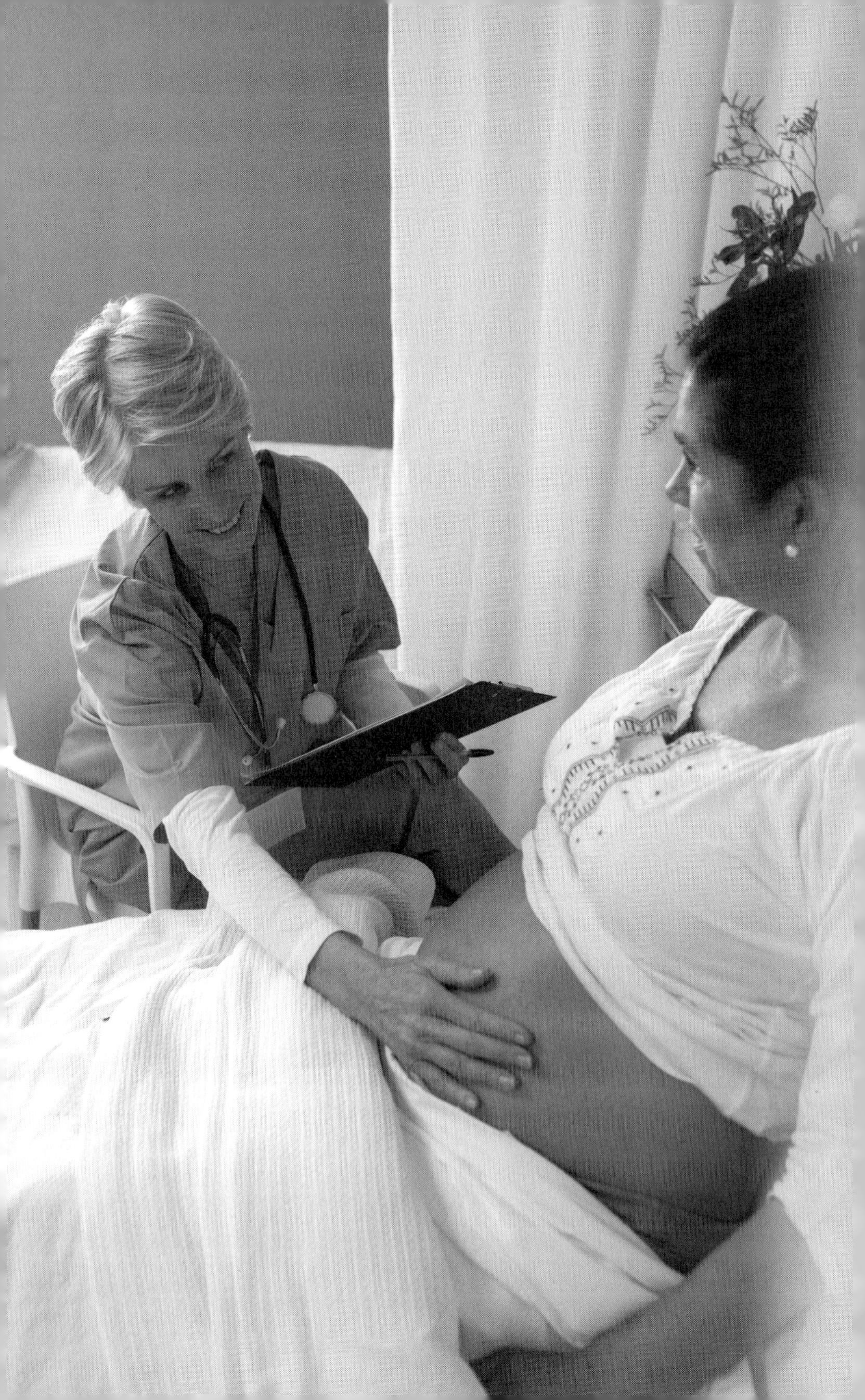

CHAPTER 35

When Labor Starts Too Soon
Preterm Labor, Prelabor Rupture of Membranes, and Preterm Birth

A normal pregnancy lasts about 40 weeks when measured from the first day of the **last menstrual period (LMP).** Sometimes labor starts while a baby is still developing in the **uterus**. **Obstetrician–gynecologists (ob-gyns)** use several terms to describe early labor and birth:

- **Preterm** labor is labor that starts before 37 weeks of pregnancy. Going into preterm labor does not automatically mean that a woman will have a preterm birth. But preterm labor needs medical attention right away.

- **Prelabor rupture of membranes (PROM)** happens when the **amniotic sac** breaks before labor has started. When the sac breaks before 37 weeks, it is called preterm PROM. PROM and preterm PROM also need immediate medical care.

- Preterm birth is the birth of a baby before 37 weeks. Preterm babies may be born with serious health problems. Some problems, like **cerebral palsy**, can be lifelong. Other problems, such as learning disabilities, may appear later in childhood or even in adulthood.

Preterm Labor

Preterm labor contractions lead to changes in the **cervix.** An ob-gyn can identify these changes during a **pelvic exam.** The changes include

- *effacement* (thinning of the cervix)
- *dilation* (opening of the cervix)

> ### What Do the Terms Mean?
>
> When ob-gyns talk about the length of pregnancy, they refer to weeks and days. There are different ways to explain preterm, which means less than 37 weeks of pregnancy. For example, you may hear these terms:
>
> - **Extremely preterm:** Less than 28 weeks and 0 days of pregnancy.
> - **Late preterm:** The period from 34 weeks and 0 days to 36 weeks and 6 days.
>
> As a woman gets closer to her due date, ob-gyns use different ways to refer to term, which include:
>
> - **Early term:** The period from 37 weeks and 0 days through 38 weeks and 6 days.
> - **Full term:** The period from 39 weeks and 0 days through 40 weeks and 6 days.
> - **Late term:** The period from 41 weeks and 0 days through 41 weeks and 6 days.
> - **Postterm:** The period equal to or greater than 42 weeks.
>
> Remember, the length of a pregnancy is measured from the date of the last menstrual period (LMP) or the first **ultrasound exam**.

For about 3 in 10 women, preterm labor stops on its own. If it does not stop, treatments may be given to try to delay birth. In some cases, these treatments may reduce the risk of **complications** if the baby is born. It's important to

- know if you have risk factors for preterm birth
- recognize the signs and symptoms of preterm labor
- get early care if you have signs and symptoms

Risk Factors

Preterm labor can happen to anyone without warning. But there are some factors that can increase the risk of preterm labor, including

- preterm birth in a past pregnancy
- past gynecologic conditions or surgeries
- current pregnancy complications, such as certain infections
- lifestyle factors (see the box "Risk Factors for Preterm Birth")

Risk Factors for Preterm Birth

Despite what is known about risk factors, doctors are still learning about preterm labor and preterm birth. Many women who have preterm births have no known risk factors. Some risk factors include the following:

Medical History
- Past preterm birth
- Short cervix (measured during a transvaginal ultrasound exam)
- Early cervical dilation (measured during a pelvic exam)
- Past procedures on the cervix, including **cone biopsy, loop electrosurgical excision procedure (LEEP)**, or mechanical dilation for **induced abortion**
- Injury during a past delivery

Pregnancy Complications
- *Multiple pregnancy*
- Vaginal bleeding during pregnancy
- Infections during pregnancy

Lifestyle Factors
- Low prepregnancy weight (a **body mass index [BMI]** lower than 19)
- Smoking during pregnancy
- Substance use during pregnancy
- Less than 18 months between pregnancies

Other Factors
- Younger than 17 or older than 35

Women who have had a past preterm birth are at highest risk. Women with a short cervix early in pregnancy also are at higher risk for preterm birth.

Diagnosis

Signs and symptoms of preterm labor are listed in the box "Warning Signs of Preterm Labor." If you have any of these signs or symptoms, call your ob-gyn right away, or go to the hospital.

Your ob-gyn should monitor your contractions and do a pelvic exam to see if your cervix has started to change. You may need to be examined several times over a few hours. Preterm labor is diagnosed when changes in the cervix are found after contractions start.

Your ob-gyn also may order tests:

- A standard ultrasound exam to estimate *gestational age* if this hasn't been done before, or to check the size of your baby
- A *transvaginal ultrasound exam* to measure the length of the cervix
- A vaginal swab to test for the presence of *fetal fibronectin*. This is a protein that acts like a glue, helping the amniotic sac stay connected to the inside of the uterus.

Having a short cervix or a positive fetal fibronectin test means you are at higher risk of delivering soon.

Management

Your ob-gyn should manage preterm labor based on what he or she thinks is best for your health and the baby's health. An important consideration is the gestational age. If the baby would benefit from a delay in delivery, medications may be given to

- help the baby's organs mature more quickly
- reduce the risk of certain complications
- attempt to delay delivery for a short time

See the section "Medications Before Preterm Birth" in this chapter for details on the medications that may be used during preterm labor. Sometimes, preterm labor is too far along and there isn't enough time to give these medications.

Warning Signs of Preterm Labor

Call your ob-gyn right away or go to the hospital if you notice any of these signs or symptoms:

- Mild abdominal cramps, with or without diarrhea
- Change in type of vaginal discharge—watery, bloody, or with mucus
- Increase in amount of discharge
- Pelvic or lower abdominal pressure
- Constant, low, dull backache
- Regular or frequent contractions or uterine tightening, often painless
- Ruptured membranes (your water breaks with a gush or a trickle of fluid)

Prelabor Rupture of Membranes

Usually, labor begins with contractions and is followed by your water breaking. If your water breaks before contractions start, it is called prelabor rupture of membranes (PROM). When this happens before 37 weeks of pregnancy, it is called preterm PROM.

Risk Factors for PROM

PROM happens in about 8 in 100 pregnancies. When it happens at full term, PROM is caused by

- the normal weakening of the amniotic sac as birth approaches
- the force of uterine contractions

In nearly all cases, labor begins within 28 hours after PROM occurs. The risks of PROM include:

- Infection in the uterus. The longer labor is delayed, the higher the risk of infection.
- Pressure on the **umbilical cord** that can keep **nutrients** and **oxygen** from getting to the baby.

Risk Factors for Preterm PROM

Preterm PROM usually happens when there is early weakening of the amniotic sac. This may be caused by infection or other factors. Preterm PROM poses more serious risks for the baby. Preterm PROM leads to about 1 in 4 cases of preterm birth.

Most cases of preterm PROM happen without any clear risk factors. But there are several factors that increase the chance of preterm PROM. Some of these risk factors include

- preterm birth in a past pregnancy
- **bladder** or **kidney** infections
- vaginal bleeding during the second or third **trimesters**
- smoking
- low weight before pregnancy (a body mass index [BMI] lower than 19)

Diagnosis

The main symptom of PROM is fluid leaking from your **vagina**. Call your ob-gyn or go to the hospital if you have any fluid leakage. Your ob-gyn will need to confirm if your water has broken. Sometimes you may have a discharge for other reasons, including **urine** leakage, cervical mucus, vaginal bleeding, or a vaginal infection. A physical exam and lab tests may be done to find out if there is amniotic fluid in your vagina.

Management

Once PROM is confirmed, your ob-gyn should assess

- the baby's gestational age
- if labor has begun
- if there are signs that the umbilical cord is being compressed (squeezed)

Your ob-gyn also will look for infection or **placental abruption**. Tests will be done, including

- physical exam
- ultrasound exam
- monitoring of your contractions and the baby's heart rate

Some or all of these tests may be done depending on how far along you are in your pregnancy. Putting together all the information, your ob-gyn should determine

- whether it is safe for you and your baby to go ahead with delivery, or
- whether to try to delay delivery to give your baby more time to mature

If you have conditions that put you or your baby's health in immediate danger, your baby should be delivered, regardless of gestational age. Also, preparations for delivery will need to be made if you are in the advanced stages of labor. If you have preterm PROM early in pregnancy, in some cases it may be possible to continue the pregnancy. When this is possible, it may give your baby a better chance of doing well whenever delivery happens.

If you are not in labor within a few hours after preterm PROM occurs, and a decision is made that delivery is best for you or your baby, your ob-gyn may recommend labor induction with **oxytocin** if

- the baby's heart rate suggests that he or she will tolerate labor
- your baby is in the correct position for delivery
- there is no significant placental bleeding
- you are otherwise considered to be a candidate for vaginal delivery

If the baby is not in the correct position (a **breech presentation,** for example), you most likely will have a **cesarean delivery** (see Chapter 17, "Cesarean Delivery and Vaginal Birth After Cesarean Delivery"). In either case, you likely will receive **antibiotics** to prevent infection.

If your ob-gyn thinks that continuing the pregnancy could improve your baby's chance of doing well after birth, you may have treatments to try to delay delivery and prepare the baby for delivery. These treatments may include

- staying in the hospital so you can be monitored
- receiving antibiotics to help prevent infection
- receiving **corticosteroids**, **magnesium sulfate**, or **tocolytics** (see the section "Medications Before Preterm Birth" in this chapter)

If you have preterm PROM before your baby is able to survive outside the uterus, your ob-gyn should explain

- the risks and benefits of trying to delay delivery
- the risks of having a very preterm baby

You may decide to have the baby right away. Or, if your condition is stable and there are no signs of infection, you may be able to wait and see what happens. If you are able to wait, you may go home. If you are sent home, you should return to the hospital if you have

- fever
- abdominal pain
- contractions
- vaginal bleeding

While at home, you should take your temperature daily to check for infection.

Once your pregnancy reaches 22 to 23 weeks, your ob-gyn likely will recommend that you return to the hospital. Being in the hospital means your health care team can closely monitor you and the baby. It also allows for quick evaluation and treatment if complications occur. Treatment at this point usually includes interventions to prepare the baby for preterm birth (see the section "Medications Before Preterm Birth" in this chapter).

Cervical Insufficiency

Sometimes preterm birth happens because the cervix is not strong enough to hold itself closed as the pregnancy grows. This is called **cervical insufficiency** or having an **incompetent cervix**. Weakness of the cervix is a risk factor for quick delivery, often with only mild contractions or "silent" dilation of the cervix. Silent dilation means the cervix begins to open without any pain or other signs. This is followed by the amniotic sac falling into the birth canal.

Fortunately, cervical insufficiency is rare. It affects only 1 to 2 in 100 pregnancies. It's not clear why cervical insufficiency happens, but risk factors may include past trauma to the cervix. This trauma may be caused by

- cone biopsy or loop electrosurgical excision procedure (LEEP)
- mechanical dilation for induced abortion
- injury during a past delivery

Diagnosis

Diagnosing cervical insufficiency can be difficult, especially during a first pregnancy. Tell your ob-gyn if you had a past pregnancy loss in the second trimester or if you had a past procedure on your cervix. Cervical insufficiency may be diagnosed if you have

- a history of painless cervical dilation and second trimester deliveries
- cervical dilation and effacement before 24 weeks of pregnancy without painful contractions, vaginal bleeding, water breaking, or infection

Sometimes cervical insufficiency is found with a transvaginal ultrasound exam or during a pelvic exam.

Evaluation

If your ob-gyn suspects cervical insufficiency, he or she may look for other problems, including **placental abruption**. If you are far along in your pregnancy, you may be monitored for labor contractions. A sample may be taken to check for infection. In some cases, **amniocentesis** may be used to look for infection.

Management

Your ob-gyn should determine if delivery is needed right away or if it is safe to delay delivery. If delivery can be delayed, your ob-gyn may recommend placing stitches around the cervix (**cerclage**). This helps the cervix hold the pregnancy in the uterus.

Indicated Preterm Birth

Sometimes preterm birth is best for the health of the woman and her baby. This is called an indicated preterm birth. Indicated preterm birth may be recommended when

- the woman has **preeclampsia,** poorly controlled **diabetes mellitus,** or **high blood pressure**

- there are pregnancy problems, including **placenta previa,** placental abruption, or **oligohydramnios** (a very low level of amniotic fluid)
- the baby has problems, including severe **fetal growth restriction** or some **birth defects**
- the woman is carrying more than one baby

If you have one or more of these conditions, you and your ob-gyn may discuss the risks of continuing the pregnancy versus the risks of preterm birth for your baby. The goal is to give you and your baby the best chance of being healthy.

Medications Before Preterm Birth

Whether preterm birth is planned or happens on its own, steps may be taken to improve the health of the baby before birth. If your hospital does not have the resources to care for preterm babies after birth, your ob-gyn may recommend transfer to another hospital with these resources. When possible, it is better to deliver a preterm baby at a facility that can handle his or her care rather than transfer the baby after birth. In addition, medications may be given to prepare the baby for preterm birth.

Corticosteroids

Corticosteroids are medications that can help speed up development of the baby's lungs, brain, and digestive organs. A single course of corticosteroids may be recommended between 24 and 34 weeks of pregnancy for

- women carrying one baby who are at risk of delivery within 7 days
- women carrying more than one baby, have ruptured membranes, and are at risk of delivery within 7 days

It may take 2 days after receiving corticosteroids for the most benefits to happen, but some benefits happen after 12 to 24 hours.

Magnesium Sulfate

When given before preterm birth, magnesium sulfate may reduce the risk of cerebral palsy and problems with physical movement. This medication may be given if you are less than 32 weeks pregnant and are at risk of delivery within the next 24 hours. Magnesium sulfate may cause minor side effects, including

- flushing
- hot flashes

- blurred vision
- weakness

Tocolytics

Tocolytics are medications used to delay delivery, sometimes for up to 48 hours. If delivery is delayed even a few hours, it can allow more time to give corticosteroids or magnesium sulfate. Tocolytics also may allow time for transfer to a hospital with specialized care for preterm babies.

Tocolytics can have side effects, some of which can be serious. They typically are not given when

- there are preterm labor symptoms but no changes in the cervix
- the ob-gyn thinks delivery would be better for the woman or her baby
- preterm labor has stopped
- corticosteroid treatment is completed or if corticosteroids have previously been given

When Preterm Birth Happens

In general, babies who are born before 23 weeks of pregnancy are not likely to survive. Survival rates increase with each week that delivery is delayed. More than 9 in 10 babies survive when they are delivered at or after 28 weeks. Still, babies who survive after preterm birth may have serious health problems and disabilities that can require lifelong care.

Breathing Support

Quick action may be needed to help the baby breathe after preterm birth. Your health care team will prepare for this possibility. For babies who are born very early, this may involve inserting a breathing tube and using a device called a *ventilator*. Sometimes all that is needed is extra oxygen or continuous pressure to help keep the baby's airways open. Open airways let oxygen get to the lungs and bloodstream more easily.

Surfactant Replacement Therapy

Surfactant is a substance that helps the air sacs in the lungs stay inflated. The lungs begin making surfactant at around 23 weeks of pregnancy. Babies who have breathing problems due to immature lungs may be given surfactant replacement therapy. Babies who need this therapy often are very sick and need highly specialized care. For this reason, surfactant therapy is offered only in hospitals where the staff is specially trained.

Neonatal Intensive Care

Preterm babies usually need to stay in a **neonatal intensive care unit (NICU)** for weeks or even months. A health care team cares for preterm babies in the NICU. The team may include a **neonatologist**, a doctor who specializes in treating problems in newborns.

What to Expect After Preterm Birth

If you are likely to give birth to a preterm baby, your ob-gyn and NICU team will help you know what you can expect. Information comes from studies of previous babies who have been born preterm. Also, there is an online calculator that lets you and your ob-gyn see a range of possible outcomes for babies born before 26 weeks of pregnancy. The calculator is at the website of the *Eunice Kennedy Shriver* National Institute of Child Health and Human Development. See the "Resources" section at the end of this chapter.

As useful as the calculator may be, remember that every baby is unique and every situation is different. Also, survival and complication rates change over time and differ from state to state and even from hospital to hospital. Your health care team may provide you with local and regional information about outcomes if it is available.

You may have a treatment plan before the baby is born, but you and your health care team may need to reconsider the plan based on new findings at birth and how the baby responds to treatment. Once the baby is born, the neonatologist may be able to give you a better idea of what you can expect. Ask questions if any information is unclear. Also, ask your family and friends for support as you decide what is best for your baby.

Caring for a Preterm Baby

After birth, your health care team will have a better idea of the baby's health. Even if your baby is healthy enough to overcome the challenges of being born preterm, he or she will still need special care during childhood. Find a doctor for your baby that you like and trust. This doctor will closely watch how your baby grows and watch to see if any problems develop over time.

You also can research how to care for a preterm baby. Learn as much as you can so you can give your baby the best care possible. See the "Resources" section at the end of this chapter for information about caring for a preterm baby.

Preventing Another Preterm Birth

A significant risk factor for preterm birth is a past preterm birth. Women with past preterm birth are 2 to 3 times more likely to deliver preterm in the future. This risk increases with each preterm birth. But some women will deliver preterm without any clear risk factors.

If you are at risk of preterm birth, talk with your ob-gyn about treatments that may help prevent it. Treatments may include:

- ***Progesterone*** shots—If you have had a preterm birth with a single baby, and you are pregnant with a single baby again, you may be offered progesterone shots starting at 16 to 24 weeks of pregnancy. This **hormone** may help prevent another preterm birth. These shots are usually continued weekly until 36 weeks, unless delivery happens sooner.

- Vaginal progesterone—This treatment may be given if you have not had a preterm birth before, but you have a very short cervix at 24 weeks of pregnancy or earlier. Vaginal progesterone is a gel or suppository that you place in your vagina every day until 37 weeks of pregnancy, unless delivery happens sooner.

Routine hospitalization and bed rest are not recommended for women at risk of preterm birth. Bed rest can increase the risk of blood clots, bone weakening, and loss of muscle strength. But hospitalization may be needed if a quick delivery is expected or if the woman and her baby need to be monitored closely.

Remember that not all women with a risk factor for preterm labor or preterm birth will deliver preterm. The goals of monitoring and treatment are to reduce the risk of preterm birth and protect the health of you and your baby.

RESOURCES

Extremely Preterm Birth Outcomes Tool
www.nichd.nih.gov/research/supported/EPBO/use
Calculator from the *Eunice Kennedy Shriver* National Institute of Child Health and Human Development. The calculator lets you see a range of possible outcomes for babies born before 26 weeks of pregnancy.

Premature Babies
https://medlineplus.gov/prematurebabies.html
Information from the U.S. National Library of Medicine about the short-term and long-term health and development of preterm babies.

Preterm Birth
www.cdc.gov/reproductivehealth/MaternalInfantHealth/PretermBirth.htm
Webpage from the Centers for Disease Control and Prevention. Provides an overview of preterm birth in the United States and the warning signs.

Preterm Labor and Birth
www.nichd.nih.gov/health/topics/preterm
Information from the *Eunice Kennedy Shriver* National Institute of Child Health and Human Development. This national organization studies health problems of children, provides information about preterm labor and preterm birth, and details how experts are studying ways to predict and prevent them.

Your Pregnancy and Childbirth
www.acog.org/MyPregnancy
Website from the American College of Obstetricians and Gynecologists (ACOG) with information on pregnancy, labor, delivery, and postpartum care. Includes the latest information from the experts in women's health care, questions answered by ACOG ob-gyns, pregnancy stories from real women, and an A–Z directory of health topics covering pregnancy and beyond.

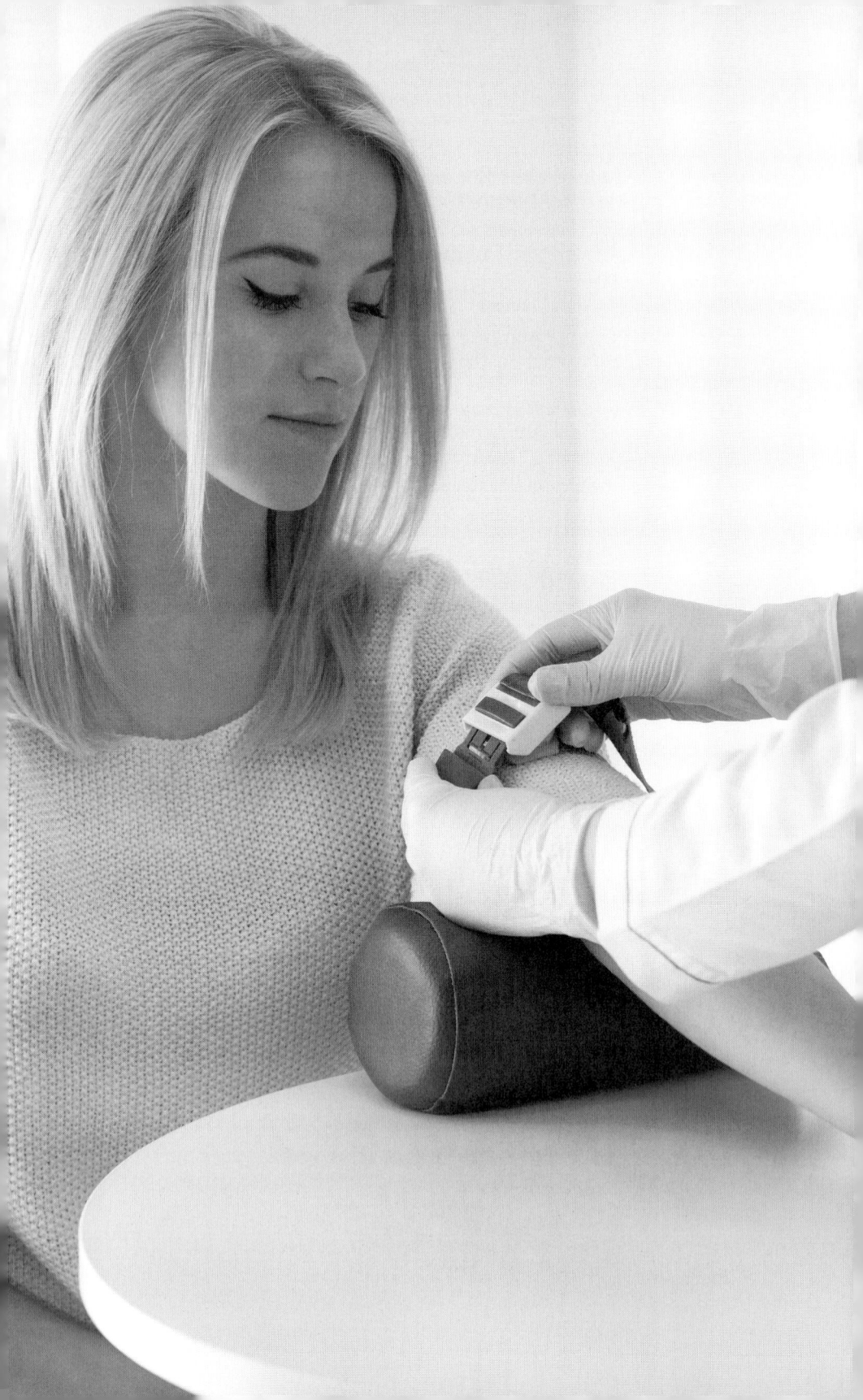

CHAPTER 36

Blood Type Incompatibility

There are four blood types: A, B, AB, and O. Blood types are determined by the types of ***antigens***—tiny proteins—on your blood ***cells***:

- Type A blood has only A antigens.
- Type B has only B antigens.
- Type AB has both A and B antigens.
- Type O has neither A nor B antigens.

There also is an antigen called the ***Rh factor***. If your blood has the Rh factor, you are Rh positive. If your blood does not have the Rh factor, you are Rh negative.

As part of your ***prenatal care***, you will have blood tests to find out your blood type and whether you are Rh positive or Rh negative. When a baby's blood type is different from the woman's, it is called blood type incompatibility. Blood type incompatibility can lead to ***complications*** that usually are mild. But sometimes complications can be more serious. With early testing and treatment, most complications may be prevented.

ABO Incompatibility

Although it happens very rarely, some pregnant women's blood types are incompatible with their babies' blood types. When this happens, the woman usually is type O and her baby is type A or type B. A woman with type O blood makes ***antibodies*** against the antigens that are found on the baby's type A and type B blood cells. If these antibodies cross the ***placenta***, they can attack the

607

baby's red blood cells. This is known as ABO incompatibility. The effects of ABO incompatibility can happen during any pregnancy, but they do not get worse with future pregnancies.

How It Affects the Baby

Babies born with ABO incompatibility can have mild *anemia* and high levels of *bilirubin* in the blood. When this happens, it is called **hemolytic disease of the newborn (HDN)**. Bilirubin is a substance that forms when old red blood cells break down. *Jaundice* (yellowish skin and eyes) is a sign of high levels of bilirubin. Too much bilirubin can be harmful, especially to the baby's nervous system, and can cause developmental problems. The anemia with ABO incompatibility usually is mild and rarely causes long-term or serious problems in a newborn.

Treatment

There is no preventive treatment that can be given during pregnancy. ABO incompatibility usually is diagnosed after the baby is born, and it usually is mild. If your baby has jaundice caused by HDN, the level of bilirubin in the baby's blood will be measured. If bilirubin is high, treatment, such as the use of special lights, will bring the level down. If this treatment does not lower the bilirubin level or there are other problems, the baby may need a blood *transfusion*.

Rh Incompatibility

More serious problems can happen if you are Rh negative and the baby is Rh positive. This is called Rh incompatibility. Problems with Rh incompatibility usually do not happen in a first pregnancy, but they can happen in future pregnancies.

What the Rh Factor Means for Pregnancy

The Rh factor is inherited, meaning it is passed from parent to child through *genes*. The baby can inherit the Rh factor from the father or the mother. Most people are Rh positive, meaning they have inherited the Rh factor from either their mother or father. If a baby does not inherit the Rh factor from either the mother or father, then he or she is Rh negative. When a woman is Rh negative and her baby is Rh positive, it is called Rh incompatibility.

During pregnancy, a woman and her baby usually do not share blood. But sometimes a small amount of blood from the baby can mix with the woman's blood. This can happen during labor and birth. It also can occur with

- **amniocentesis** or **chorionic villus sampling (CVS)**
- bleeding during pregnancy
- attempts to manually turn a baby so he or she is head-down for birth (move the baby out of a **breech presentation**)
- trauma to the abdomen during pregnancy

When the blood of an Rh-positive baby gets into the bloodstream of an Rh-negative woman, her body will recognize that the Rh-positive blood is not hers. Her body will try to destroy it by making anti-Rh antibodies. These antibodies can cross the placenta and attack the baby's blood cells. This can lead to serious health problems, even death, for the baby.

Health problems usually do not occur during an Rh-negative woman's first pregnancy with an Rh-positive baby. This is because her body does not have a chance to develop a lot of antibodies. But if the woman later gets pregnant with an Rh-positive baby, her body can make more antibodies, and this puts a future baby at risk.

An Rh-negative woman also can make antibodies after

- **miscarriage**
- **ectopic pregnancy**
- **induced abortion**

If an Rh-negative woman gets pregnant after one of these events and has not received treatment, a future baby may be at risk of problems if he or she is Rh positive.

How Rh Antibodies Can Cause Problems

During a pregnancy, Rh antibodies made in a woman's body can cross the placenta and attack the Rh factor on the baby's blood cells. This can cause a type of anemia called hemolytic disease of the newborn (HDN). This is the same type of anemia found with ABO incompatibility, but the anemia can be worse when Rh incompatibility is the cause.

When there are Rh antibodies, the baby's red blood cells are destroyed faster than the body can replace them. Red blood cells carry **oxygen** to all parts of the body. Without enough red blood cells, the baby will not get enough oxygen. In some cases, the baby can die from HDN before or after birth. Jaundice in the newborn is another common complication of Rh incompatibility.

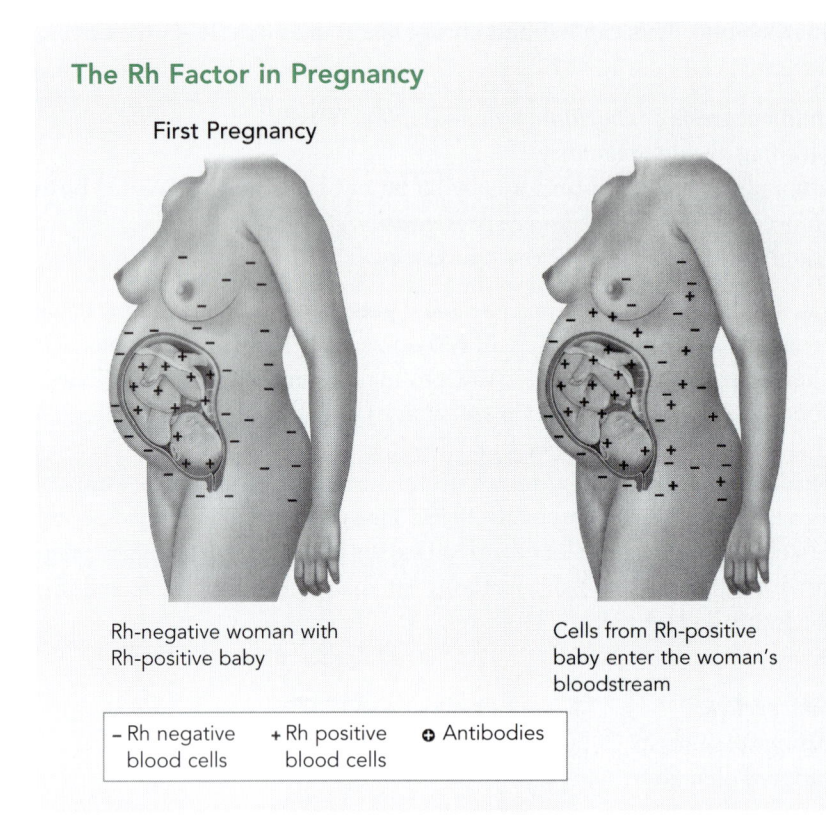

The Rh Factor in Pregnancy

First Pregnancy

Rh-negative woman with Rh-positive baby

Cells from Rh-positive baby enter the woman's bloodstream

- Rh negative blood cells   + Rh positive blood cells   ⊙ Antibodies

Preventing Rh Problems During Pregnancy

Problems during pregnancy caused by Rh incompatibility can be prevented. The goal of treatment is to stop an Rh-negative woman from making Rh antibodies in the first place. This is done by finding out if you are Rh negative early in pregnancy (or before pregnancy) and, if needed, giving you a medication to prevent antibodies from forming.

Blood Testing. A simple blood test can find out your blood type and Rh status. A blood sample can be taken in the office of your ***obstetrician–gynecologist (ob-gyn)***. This sample also can be drawn by an outside lab.

Another blood test, called an antibody screen, can show if an Rh-negative woman has made antibodies to Rh-positive blood. If so, this test can show how many antibodies have been made. If you are Rh negative and there is a possibility that your baby is Rh positive, your ob-gyn may request this test during your first ***trimester***. You may have this test again during week 28 of pregnancy. In some cases, you may be tested more often

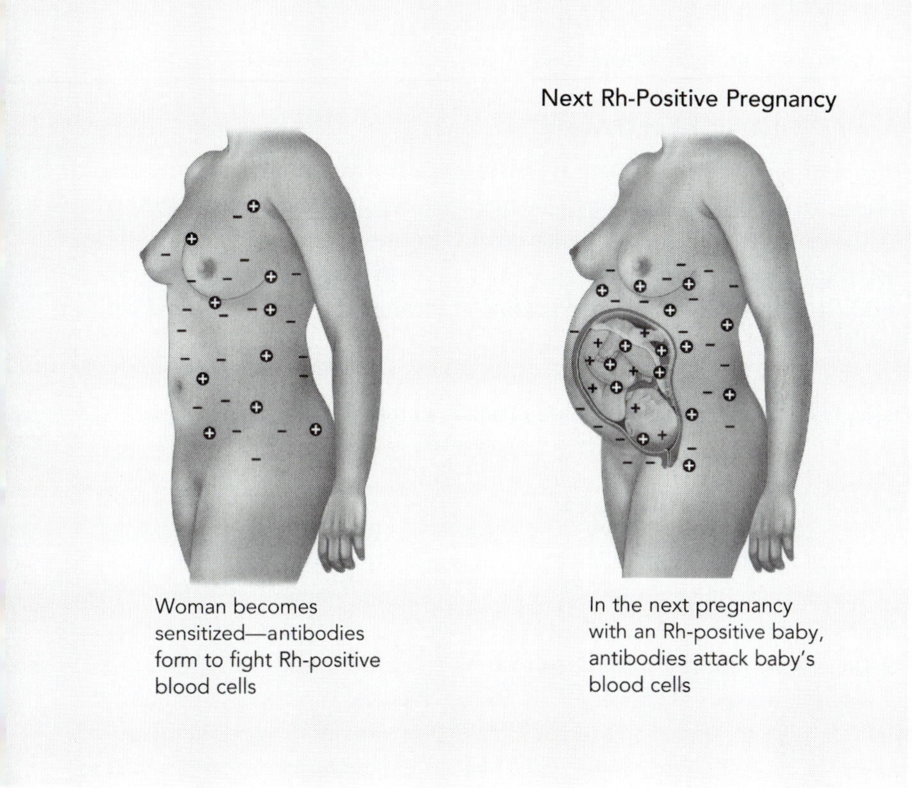

BLOOD TYPE INCOMPATIBILITY • 611

Next Rh-Positive Pregnancy

Woman becomes sensitized—antibodies form to fight Rh-positive blood cells

In the next pregnancy with an Rh-positive baby, antibodies attack baby's blood cells

Rh Immunoglobulin. When an Rh-negative woman has not already made antibodies, a medication called **Rh immunoglobulin (RhIg)** may be given. This medication also is known as RhoGAM. It prevents the woman's body from making antibodies. This may help prevent HDN, anemia, and jaundice in future pregnancies.

If you are in this situation, talk with your ob-gyn about whether you need RhIg and when you might be given this medication. It is not helpful if your body has already made Rh antibodies.

There are other times when a woman might need a dose of RhIg. The medication also may be needed after

- an ectopic pregnancy or a first-trimester miscarriage or abortion
- invasive procedures, such as amniocentesis, CVS, fetal blood sampling, or fetal surgery

Also, you may be given medication if you have had

- bleeding during pregnancy

- trauma to the abdomen during pregnancy
- attempts to manually turn a baby from a breech presentation

Treatment if Antibodies Develop

RhIg treatment does not help if an Rh-negative woman has already made antibodies. In this case, the well-being of the baby will be checked throughout the pregnancy, usually with **ultrasound exams**. If ultrasound exams show that the baby has severe anemia, early delivery may be needed. Another option may be to give a blood transfusion through the **umbilical cord** while the baby is still in the woman's **uterus**.

If the anemia is mild, the baby may be delivered at the normal time. After delivery, the baby may need a blood transfusion to replace blood cells.

Other Incompatibilities

ABO incompatibility and Rh factor incompatibility are the two most common causes of HDN. But there are some less common proteins on blood cells that may cause antibodies. An antibody screen early in pregnancy typically checks for these less common antibodies, too.

If you have one of the less common antibodies, your ob-gyn should tell you. Many of these antibodies act like ABO incompatibility and may not be major issues. But a few can be more like the Rh factor incompatibility. This means they may require closer management and treatment similar to the Rh factor treatment.

RESOURCES

Hemolytic Disease of the Newborn
https://medlineplus.gov/ency/article/001298.htm
Webpage from the U.S. National Library of Medicine. Describes hemolytic anemia, why it happens, and how it is treated.

Newborn Jaundice
www.marchofdimes.org/complications/newborn-jaundice.aspx
March of Dimes information that describes newborn jaundice, including signs and symptoms, possible causes, and treatment.

Rh Disease
www.marchofdimes.org/complications/rh-disease.aspx
March of Dimes information that describes Rh disease, risks, testing, complications, prevention, and treatment.

Rh Incompatibility
https://medlineplus.gov/rhincompatibility.html
Webpage from the U.S. National Library of Medicine that defines Rh incompatibility and discusses how this condition is prevented and treated.

Your Pregnancy and Childbirth
www.acog.org/MyPregnancy
Website from the American College of Obstetricians and Gynecologists (ACOG) with information on pregnancy, labor, delivery, and postpartum care. Includes the latest information from the experts in women's health care, questions answered by ACOG ob-gyns, pregnancy stories from real women, and an A–Z directory of health topics covering pregnancy and beyond.

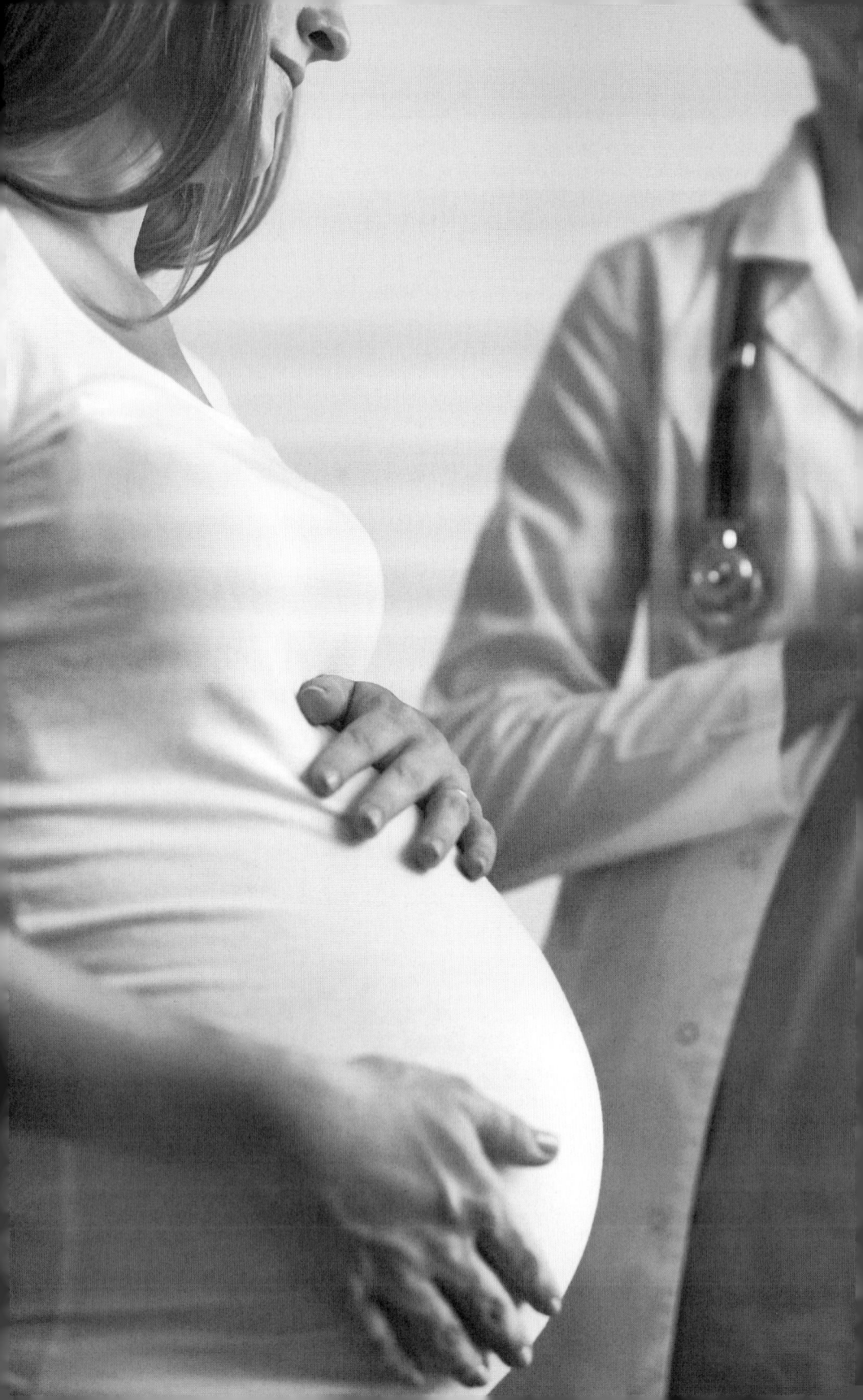

CHAPTER 37

Placenta Problems

The **placenta** is a unique organ that exists only during pregnancy. It delivers **nutrients** and **oxygen** to the baby. It also takes waste products away from the baby.

In a normal pregnancy, the placenta is attached high on the wall of the **uterus** away from the **cervix**. It remains attached until right after the baby is born. After delivery, contractions help the placenta come away from the wall of the uterus and pass down the birth canal. In most cases, it takes just one or two pushes from you for the placenta to come out of the vagina.

Certain problems with the placenta can happen during pregnancy. They can cause serious **complications** if they are not found early. Learn the signs and symptoms of these problems and tell your **obstetrician–gynecologist (ob-gyn)** right away if you think there is a problem.

Placenta Previa

With **placenta previa**, the placenta lies low in the uterus and covers part of the internal opening of the cervix (called the **internal os**). This can block the baby's exit from the uterus. Placenta previa happens in 1 in 200 pregnancies. The condition is more common in women who

- have had more than one child
- had a past **cesarean birth**
- have had surgery on the uterus
- are carrying twins or triplets

Smoking and cocaine use during pregnancy also may increase the risk of placenta previa.

If placenta previa is not diagnosed and managed, it can lead to serious complications, including **hemorrhage** (heavy bleeding) and infection in the woman. If there is heavy bleeding, blood **transfusions** may be needed. In some cases, an emergency **hysterectomy** (removal of the uterus) may be needed to stop bleeding.

Placenta previa also poses risks for the baby. **Preterm** delivery may be necessary. This means there is a higher risk that the baby will have problems from being born preterm, including

- *neurological* problems
- *respiratory system* problems
- long-term disabilities

Fortunately, most cases of placenta previa are diagnosed well before labor begins, so steps can be taken to reduce these risks.

Types

Placenta previa is described in different ways, depending on the location of the placenta and how much of the internal os is covered:

- Complete—The placenta completely covers the internal os.
- Partial—The placenta partially covers the internal os.
- Marginal—The placenta reaches the internal os but does not cover it.

A low-lying placenta is one that implants in the lower part of the uterus but does not reach the internal os.

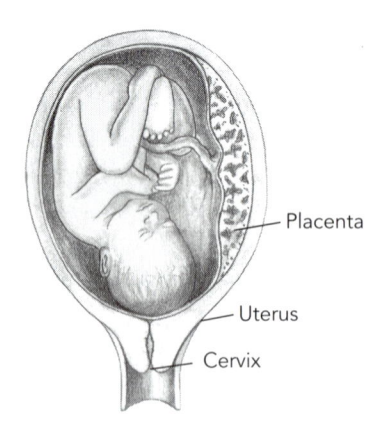

Normal position of placenta. The placenta normally attaches high on the uterine wall, away from the cervix.

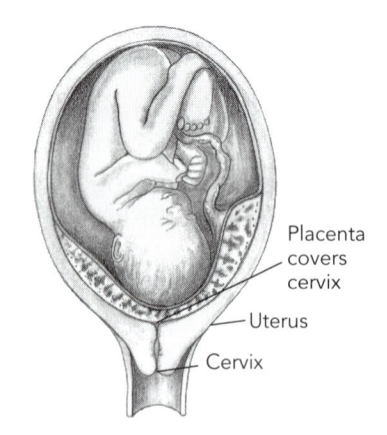

Placenta previa. The placenta lies low in the uterus and either partly or completely blocks the cervix.

Signs and Symptoms

There often are no signs or symptoms of placenta previa. Painless vaginal bleeding is the main sign of placenta previa. Not every woman with placenta previa will have bleeding. But for those that do, the bleeding usually happens near the end of the second **trimester** or at the start of the third trimester. At first, bleeding may be light and may stop on its own. Later, more severe bleeding may start. Call your ob-gyn right away if you have any bleeding in your second or third trimester, especially if you know you have placenta previa.

Diagnosis

Most cases of placenta previa are diagnosed during a routine **ultrasound exam** in the first or second trimester, before any bleeding happens. If you are diagnosed with placenta previa before 21 weeks of pregnancy, you may be monitored with periodic ultrasound exams.

Treatment

Most cases of partial placenta previa and low-lying placenta previa resolve on their own by 32 to 35 weeks of pregnancy. If this happens, labor and delivery can proceed normally.

If placenta previa does not go away by itself, treatment may be needed. The main goal is to give the baby more time to grow and develop. If you have episodes of bleeding, you may need to stay in the hospital, where your condition and the baby's condition can be watched closely. An ultrasound exam should be done to check the location of the placenta. You may be given **corticosteroids** to help the baby's lungs and other organs develop in case of a preterm birth. You may need blood transfusions.

If the bleeding stops on its own and you are less than 34 weeks pregnant, it may be possible to monitor your condition on an outpatient basis, meaning you don't have to stay in the hospital. But you will need to see your ob-gyn often and call him or her right away if you have any vaginal bleeding. You also need to be able to get to a hospital quickly in case of emergency.

If you have no other complications and the baby is doing well, a **cesarean delivery** may be recommended at 36 to 37 weeks of pregnancy. Delivery may be needed sooner than 36 weeks of pregnancy if

- you have other medical conditions
- there are complications with the baby
- there are other problems with the placenta

Your ob-gyn may refer you to a **neonatologist**, who can tell you what to expect when a baby is born preterm.

Placental Abruption

Placental abruption happens when the placenta separates from the wall of the uterus too early, meaning before or during birth. This can cause vaginal bleeding and severe pain in the abdomen. Placental abruption is dangerous for the woman and her baby. The baby may get less oxygen, and the woman may lose a large amount of blood. Prompt treatment is needed.

Only 1 percent of pregnant women have this problem. It usually happens in the last 12 weeks before birth. Placental abruption happens more often in women who have **high blood pressure**, smoke, or use illegal drugs during pregnancy. It also is more common in women who

- have already had children
- are older than 35
- have had placental abruption before
- have **sickle cell disease**

Types

Placental abruption is described in different ways, depending on the extent of the abruption and where the separation is located:

- Complete—The entire placenta separates from the wall of the uterus.
- Partial—Part of the placenta separates from the wall of the uterus.

Signs and Symptoms

The most common signs and symptoms are vaginal bleeding and abdominal or back pain. If the abruption is partial, there may only be bleeding. Some women do not have a lot of bleeding with placental abruption because the blood gets trapped inside the uterus behind the placenta.

Diagnosis

Diagnosis is based on a combination of your symptoms, a physical exam, and an ultrasound exam. It is not always possible to see an abruption with an ultrasound exam.

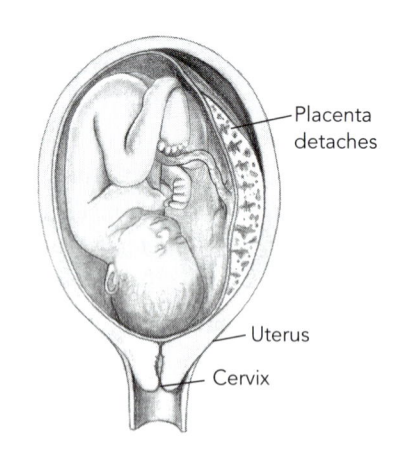

Placental abruption. The placenta detaches from the wall of the uterus.

Treatment

Treatment for placental abruption depends on your condition, your baby's condition, and how far along you are in your pregnancy. If you have lost a lot of blood, you may need a blood transfusion. After your condition is stabilized, your ob-gyn should check the baby's heart rate. You may have to stay in the hospital so doctors can monitor your condition.

If the abruption is small, and you are near your due date, there may be two options: 1) **labor induction** or 2) cesarean delivery. Sometimes bleeding stops on its own. In this case, you should be monitored closely to make sure the abruption does not get worse.

If your due date is still far off (you're between 24 and 34 weeks), you may be given corticosteroids to help the baby's lungs mature. After 34 weeks, the baby usually is delivered. Although there is a risk of the baby having health problems related to preterm birth, it may be safer to deliver the baby in some cases.

Placenta Accreta

In a normal pregnancy, the placenta attaches to the wall of the uterus. After the baby is born, it separates from the uterus and is delivered. With **placenta accreta**, the placenta (or part of it) attaches too firmly or too deeply in the wall of the uterus, and then does not fully separate after the baby is delivered. This can cause severe, life-threatening blood loss.

Placenta accreta has become more common over the past 40 years, possibly because the risk factors for this condition also have become more common. A major risk factor for placenta accreta is a past cesarean delivery. The more cesarean deliveries a woman has had, the higher her risk. Other risk factors include

- surgical removal of *fibroids* that are inside the wall of the uterus
- *endometrial ablation* performed with heat
- *uterine artery embolization*
- being older than 35
- carrying more than one baby
- placenta previa

Types

Placenta accreta is described in different ways, depending on how severe it is:

- Placenta accreta means that the placenta is attached too firmly to the wall of the uterus (***myometrium***), but it is still on the surface.
- When the placenta extends into the myometrium, it is called placenta increta.
- When the placenta extends through the entire wall of the uterus, it is called placenta percreta. In some cases of placenta percreta, the placenta also extends into nearby organs, such as the ***bladder***.

Signs and Symptoms

Placenta accreta may cause bleeding during the third trimester. But there may be no clear warning signs of this condition.

Diagnosis

Ob-gyns try to diagnose placenta accreta before delivery so they are prepared for heavy bleeding and complications. Your ob-gyn should be more watchful for this condition if you have risk factors.

In the past, placenta accreta often was not diagnosed until after the baby was delivered. This still happens sometimes, but an ultrasound exam can identify most cases of placenta accreta well before delivery. Your ob-gyn may use an ultrasound exam, which can show if the placenta is growing into or through the wall of the uterus. Some ob-gyns order a scan called ***magnetic resonance imaging (MRI)*** to get more information. MRI results also can help when ultrasound results are not clear.

Treatment

The treatment for placenta accreta is a planned cesarean delivery followed by a hysterectomy. If placenta accreta is suspected, you should give birth in a hospital with special facilities and staff who are experienced in managing this condition.

The recommended time for delivery is before labor starts and may be as early as 34 weeks. You and your ob-gyn should make this decision together. The goal is a planned cesarean delivery, but an emergency delivery may be necessary.

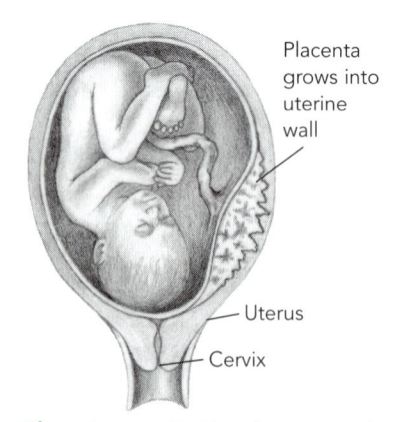

Placenta accreta. The placenta invades the wall of the uterus.

Women with placenta accreta are at risk of life-threatening bleeding during delivery. In some cases, a hysterectomy may be needed to save a woman's life. Blood for transfusion should be ordered so it is nearby if needed. In some cases, it may be possible to avoid hysterectomy, but there are significant risks with this approach, including heavy bleeding. You may need to have a hysterectomy in any case. But if you want to have more children, you may want to discuss this option with your ob-gyn. Together you can discuss the risks in detail.

RESOURCES

Placenta Accreta, Increta, and Percreta
www.marchofdimes.org/complications/placental-accreta-increta-and-percreta.aspx
March of Dimes page that offers basic information about these pregnancy complications.

Placenta Previa
https://medlineplus.gov/ency/article/000900.htm
Webpage from the U.S. National Library of Medicine. Covers all aspects of placenta previa, including signs and symptoms, diagnosis, and treatment.

Placental Abruption
www.marchofdimes.org/complications/placental-abruption.aspx
March of Dimes page that gives an overview of placental abruption, including signs and symptoms, causes, and treatment.

Your Pregnancy and Childbirth
www.acog.org/MyPregnancy
Website from the American College of Obstetricians and Gynecologists (ACOG) with information on pregnancy, labor, delivery, and postpartum care. Includes the latest information from the experts in women's health care, questions answered by ACOG ob-gyns, pregnancy stories from real women, and an A–Z directory of health topics covering pregnancy and beyond.

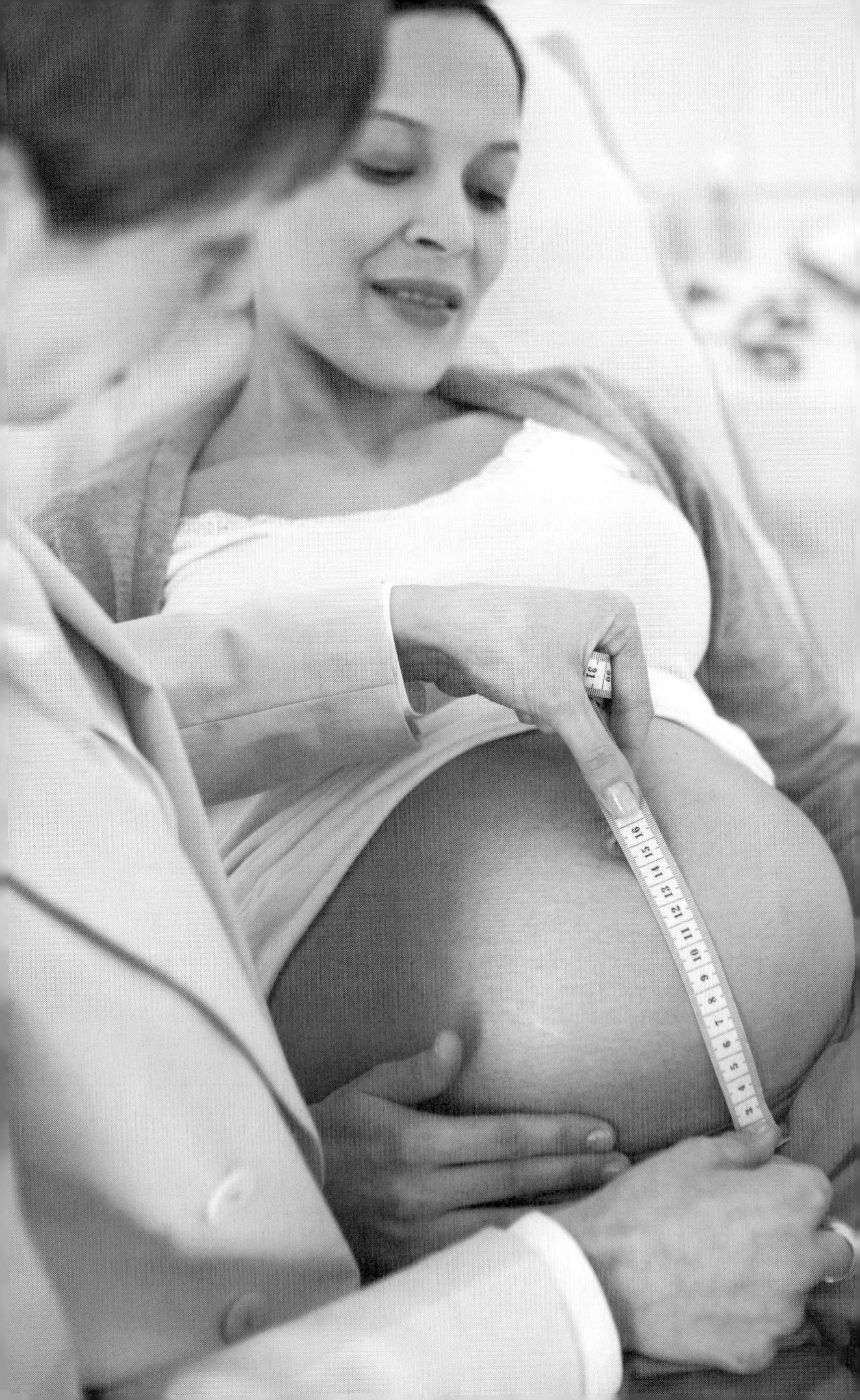

CHAPTER 38

Growth Problems

In some pregnancies, the baby does not grow as expected. Some babies are born smaller than average. Others are born larger than average. Either situation can cause problems for the woman and her baby.

Your *obstetrician–gynecologist (ob-gyn)* should monitor your baby's growth throughout your pregnancy. If a growth problem is suspected, your ob-gyn may take steps to reduce possible *complications*.

Fetal Growth Restriction

When babies are smaller than expected during pregnancy, they are considered small for gestational age (SGA). Some SGA babies are just destined to be smaller than usual. But other SGA babies have had difficulty growing in the *uterus*. This is called *fetal growth restriction*. Fetal growth restriction significantly increases the risk of

- fetal distress during labor and delivery
- health problems for the baby after birth
- health problems later in life for a small number of growth-restricted babies

Causes

Women with chronic health problems are at higher risk of having a baby with growth restriction. These health problems include

- **high blood pressure**

623

- *kidney disease*
- *diabetes mellitus*
- certain heart and lung diseases
- *antiphospholipid syndrome (APS)*
- *hemoglobinopathies* (such as *sickle cell disease*)

In addition to the health problems themselves, the use of certain drugs to treat some medical conditions may increase the risk of growth restriction. For example, medications for high blood pressure, *epilepsy*, and blood clots may increase the risk.

Other risk factors for fetal growth restriction include

- pregnancy with more than one baby *(multiple pregnancy)*

- problems with the *placenta*

- getting certain infections during pregnancy, such as *cytomegalovirus (CMV)*, *rubella* (German measles), and *varicella* (*chickenpox*)

- poor nutrition during pregnancy

- substance use during pregnancy, including smoking, drinking alcohol, and using marijuana or illegal drugs

In some cases, growth restriction may be a sign of a problem with the baby's health. Growth restriction is associated with certain conditions, including

- chromosomal abnormalities, such as *Patau syndrome (trisomy 13)* and *Edwards syndrome (trisomy 18)*

- *gastroschisis*, a birth defect that affects the baby's abdominal wall

Diagnosis

Many of the exams that you have during *prenatal care* visits are designed to find growth problems as early as possible:

- *Fundal height* measurement—Beginning at about 24 weeks of pregnancy, your ob-gyn should measure the fundal height at each prenatal visit. The fundal height is the distance from your pubic bone to the top of your uterus. Recording these measurements will help your ob-gyn track your baby's growth.

- *Ultrasound exam*—Most women have an ultrasound exam between 18 and 22 weeks of pregnancy. During this exam, the baby's measurements are taken and used to estimate weight.

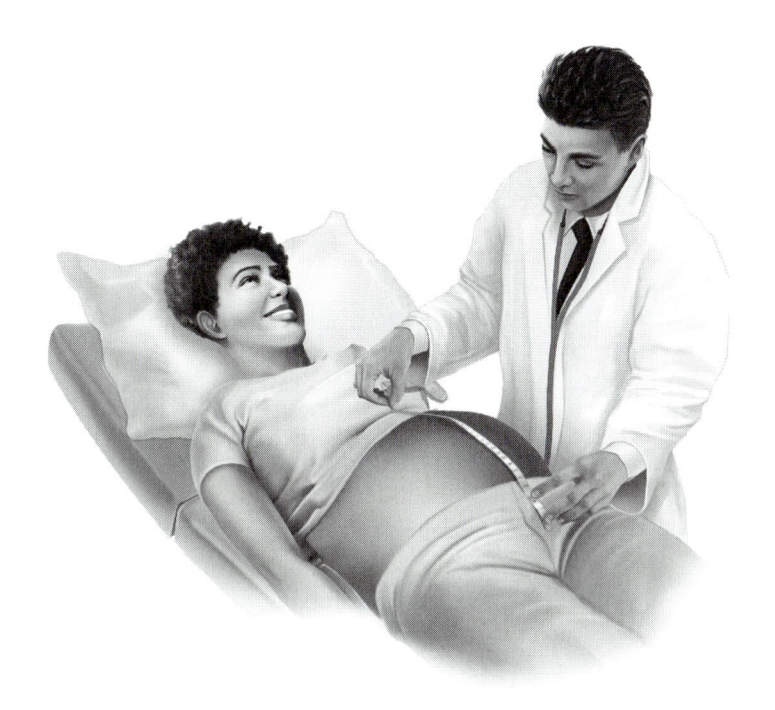

Measuring fundal height. Measuring fundal height can help your ob-gyn estimate the weight of your baby and track growth.

If your ob-gyn suspects growth problems, or if you have risk factors for fetal growth restriction, you may have ultrasound exams every 4 weeks or so. Results of these exams will be used to track the baby's growth.

If fetal growth restriction is suspected, special tests of the baby's health may be done on a weekly basis as your due date approaches. These tests may include

- *Doppler ultrasound exam*
- *nonstress test*
- *contraction stress test*
- *biophysical profile (BPP)*
- *modified biophysical profile*

See Chapter 34, "Ultrasound Exams and Other Testing to Monitor Fetal Well-Being," for details on these tests.

Management

Managing fetal growth restriction depends in part on what's causing it:

- If a medical condition is thought to be the cause, your ob-gyn should make sure that you are getting the proper treatment.
- If a *genetic disorder* is suspected, you may have tests to find out the type of disorder.

Even if a cause is found, there is little that can be done during pregnancy to reverse fetal growth restriction. Stopping smoking, though, has been shown to be helpful. Women who stop smoking before 16 weeks of pregnancy are the most likely to improve the weight of their babies. But even stopping as late as the seventh month can have a positive effect on the baby's weight.

The timing of delivery depends on how the baby is doing. If test results suggest the baby is doing well otherwise, you may be able to deliver at term. In some cases, *preterm* or *early term* delivery may be needed, especially if the baby is having problems or has stopped growing altogether. If early delivery is recommended, the following steps may be taken:

- You may be given medication to help the baby's organs mature.
- You may be given medication to reduce the baby's risk of **cerebral palsy.**
- You may be transferred to a hospital with a **neonatal intensive care unit (NICU)** that offers specialized care for preterm babies.

Prevention

You can improve your chances of having a normal-weight baby by eating healthy foods during pregnancy (see Chapter 22, "Nutrition During Pregnancy"). In addition, give up any lifestyle habits that can harm your baby. Do not smoke, drink alcohol, or use marijuana or illegal drugs while you are pregnant. Also, do not use prescription medication for a nonmedical reason. If you need help quitting, talk with your ob-gyn.

Macrosomia

When a baby grows more than expected before birth, the condition is called *macrosomia.* Babies with macrosomia often weigh more than 8 pounds and 13 ounces (4,000 grams). Several risk factors are associated with macrosomia, including

- *gestational diabetes*
- diabetes before pregnancy

> ## What Do the Terms Mean?
>
> When ob-gyns talk about the length of pregnancy, they refer to weeks and days. There are different ways to explain preterm, which means less than 37 weeks of pregnancy. For example, you may hear these terms:
>
> - **Extremely preterm:** Less than 28 weeks and 0 days of pregnancy.
> - **Late preterm:** The period from 34 weeks and 0 days to 36 weeks and 6 days.
>
> As a woman gets closer to her due date, ob-gyns use different ways to refer to term, which include:
>
> - **Early term:** The period from 37 weeks and 0 days through 38 weeks and 6 days.
> - **Full term:** The period from 39 weeks and 0 days through 40 weeks and 6 days.
> - **Late term:** The period from 41 weeks and 0 days through 41 weeks and 6 days.
> - **Postterm:** The period equal to or greater than 42 weeks.
>
> Remember, the length of a pregnancy is measured from the date of the **last menstrual period (LMP)** or the first ultrasound exam.

- macrosomia in a past pregnancy
- being overweight before pregnancy
- excessive weight gain during pregnancy
- having had more than one child
- having a male baby

Diabetes can lead to macrosomia if your **glucose** (blood sugar) level is high throughout pregnancy. When your blood sugar is too high, too much blood sugar reaches the baby. This causes the baby to grow too large.

Diagnosis

Macrosomia can be diagnosed with certainty only after the baby is born. Before birth, your ob-gyn may do some tests to assess your baby's size, including

- measuring fundal height

- ultrasound exams
- feeling your abdomen to gauge a baby's size

Complications

Macrosomia can cause complications for the woman and her baby, including problems with labor and delivery. Women who have large babies are more likely to have a prolonged labor and to need a ***cesarean delivery***. Large babies are more likely to need specialized care in the NICU.

Macrosomia also is a risk for a serious labor problem called ***shoulder dystocia***. This is a potentially life-threatening event that happens when the baby's shoulders get lodged in the woman's pelvis after the head has come out of the ***vagina***. Shoulder dystocia is diagnosed when the baby's shoulders do not come out with gentle downward pressure on the baby's head.

There is no way to predict a shoulder dystocia, and there is no way to prevent it. Shoulder dystocia is a labor emergency and requires immediate maneuvers to help deliver the baby.

When shoulder dystocia occurs, there may be injury to the baby. The most common injuries are to the collarbone, arm, and a group of nerves called the brachial plexus. Shoulder dystocia can cause theses nerves to be stretched or compressed. Damage to these nerves may cause weakness or paralysis in the arm and shoulder. This injury usually resolves on its own in the first year of the baby's life.

Also, during a shoulder dystocia, ***oxygen*** and blood do not get to the baby normally. In severe cases, this can result in permanent brain damage to the baby. Women who have deliveries complicated by shoulder dystocia have a higher risk of ***postpartum hemorrhage*** and tears of the ***perineum***.

Management

If macrosomia is suspected, you and your ob-gyn should discuss the risks and benefits of vaginal birth and ***cesarean birth***. Suspected macrosomia by itself does not always mean that a cesarean delivery should be done. This is because predicting macrosomia can be difficult. Also, your ob-gyn should weigh the possibility of macrosomia against the risks of cesarean delivery, which include

- heavy bleeding
- infection
- injury to the bowel or ***bladder***
- problems related to the ***anesthesia*** used
- longer recovery time than vaginal delivery

Cesarean delivery also increases risks in future pregnancies, including

- placenta problems
- rupture of the uterus
- *hysterectomy*

Still, cesarean delivery may be considered for women who do not have diabetes if the baby is estimated to weigh about 11 pounds. For women with diabetes, ob-gyns may recommend a cesarean birth if the baby is estimated to weigh 10 pounds or more.

Prevention

If you have diabetes, it's important to manage your blood sugar and follow your ob-gyn's advice to avoid hyperglycemia (high blood sugar). See Chapter 31, "Diabetes During Pregnancy," for more discussion.

For women without diabetes, there are no interventions that have been proven to reduce the risk of macrosomia. But there is some evidence that getting regular exercise during pregnancy may reduce the risk.

RESOURCES

Fetal Macrosomia
www.mayoclinic.org/diseases-conditions/fetal-macrosomia/symptoms-causes/syc-20372579
Information from the Mayo Clinic that explains macrosomia and its causes, diagnosis, and management.

Intrauterine Growth Restriction
https://medlineplus.gov/ency/article/001500.htm
Webpage from the U.S. National Library of Medicine that discusses fetal growth restriction.

Your Pregnancy and Childbirth
www.acog.org/MyPregnancy
Website from the American College of Obstetricians and Gynecologists (ACOG) with information on pregnancy, labor, delivery, and postpartum care. Includes the latest information from the experts in women's health care, questions answered by ACOG ob-gyns, pregnancy stories from real women, and an A–Z directory of health topics covering pregnancy and beyond.

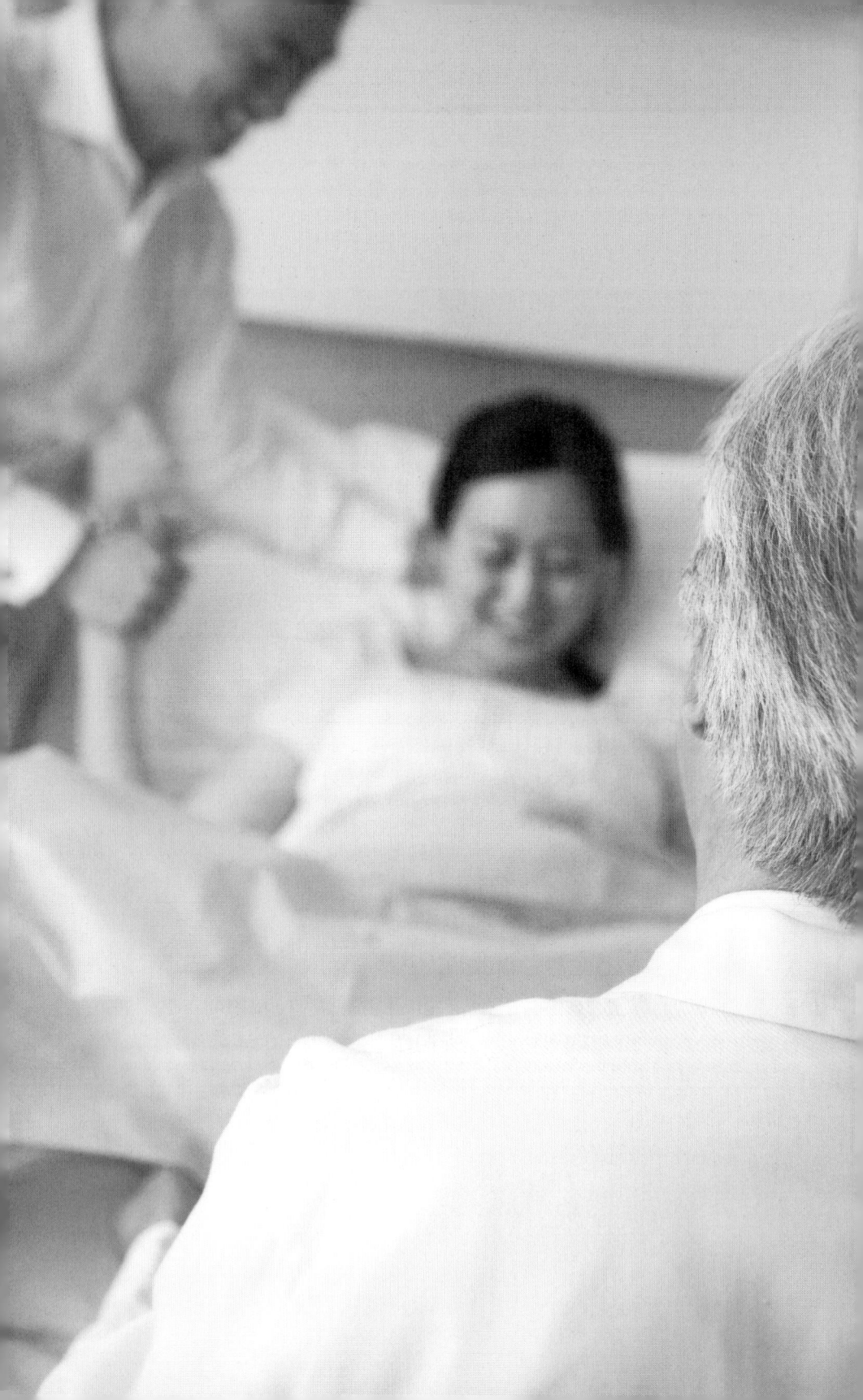

CHAPTER 39

Problems During Labor and Delivery

Most women go through labor and delivery without difficulty. But sometimes problems happen. Some women have risk factors that make these problems more likely. In some cases, **complications** can be anticipated, and actions can be taken beforehand to minimize risks. But sometimes unexpected things happen even if everything has gone well during pregnancy.

When you arrive at the hospital or birth center in labor, the health care team will monitor you and your baby to make sure that all is going well. Monitoring throughout labor and delivery and even after you give birth may help detect problems early. In most situations, the earlier a problem is found and managed, the better the outcome.

Abnormal Labor

When labor does not go as it should, it is called abnormal labor. You also may hear the term "failure to progress" or "labor arrest" when labor is going slowly or has stopped. Abnormal labor is the main reason for **cesarean delivery**.

Causes

Abnormal labor may be caused by the following:

- **Macrosomia**—Babies with macrosomia grow more than expected, often weighing more than 8 pounds and 13 ounces (4,000 grams). A large baby can make vaginal birth more difficult. If macrosomia is suspected, you and your **obstetrician–gynecologist (ob-gyn)** may discuss cesarean delivery.

- *Malpresentation*—Sometimes babies move into positions that make it difficult to deliver through the **vagina**. An example is **breech presentation**. This is when the baby's feet or buttocks are positioned to come out of the vagina first. When babies are in positions that complicate labor and delivery, you and your ob-gyn should talk about options for achieving a safe delivery (see Chapter 16, "Assisted Vaginal Delivery and Breech Presentation").

- Problems with the contractions—Sometimes the **uterus** does not contract strongly enough or frequently enough. When this happens, labor can take longer and may need to be helped along.

- Maternal **obesity**— Having too much body fat may block the passage of a baby through the pelvis. Also, being obese may increase the risk of a large baby. This in turn increases the risk of labor problems. See Chapter 29, "Weight During Pregnancy: Obesity and Eating Disorders," for more on how obesity affects pregnancy.

Risks

When problems happen with labor, it takes longer to deliver the baby. The main risk with a longer labor is **chorioamnionitis**. This is an infection of the membranes that surround the baby in the uterus. In most cases, **antibiotics** are used to treat the infection. But sometimes chorioamnionitis can lead to serious complications:

- For the woman, it can cause life-threatening conditions, such as **sepsis** or **endometritis** after delivery.

- For the baby, it can cause newborn infection, lung problems, and, in rare cases, developmental disabilities, **cerebral palsy**, or **stillbirth**.

Another risk of abnormal labor is that it may lead to a cesarean delivery. A cesarean delivery is a major surgical procedure. Like all surgeries, it has risks. These risks include, but are not limited to

- heavy bleeding
- infection
- injury to the bowel, **bladder**, or other organs
- problems with **anesthesia**
- longer recovery time than vaginal delivery

Cesarean delivery also increases risks in future pregnancies, including

- *placenta* problems
- rupture of the uterus
- *hysterectomy*

Assessment

Labor is divided into three stages (see Table 39–1, "Stages of Labor"):

- During the first stage, the *cervix* thins (effaces) and opens (dilates) as the uterus contracts.
- In the second stage, the woman pushes the baby out of the vagina.
- In the third stage, the *placenta* is delivered.

Ob-gyns closely follow how long each stage of labor takes to determine whether labor is progressing normally.

Many factors can affect how labor progresses. For example, first-time moms usually have longer labors. An *epidural block* is helpful for pain control, but it also may cause a longer labor.

Management

If your labor is going too slowly or has stopped, there are several options to help get your labor back on track. Decisions are made based on the risks and benefits of each option. Sometimes, the first option is simply to be patient and see if labor progresses on its own. For most stalled labors, **labor augmentation** is recommended. Augmentation means using medication to help your uterus contract the way it should to help dilate your cervix.

The medication used for labor augmentation is called **oxytocin**. This is the synthetic version of the **hormone** oxytocin that your body already makes. Oxytocin causes the uterus to contract. It can be used to begin labor or to speed up labor that started on its own. Oxytocin is given through an

TABLE 39–1 **Stages of Labor**

Stage	Description
Stage 1: Early Labor	Regular contractions; cervix effaces and dilates to 4 to 6 centimeters (cm)
Stage 1: Active Labor	Contractions get stronger and closer together; cervix dilates to 10 cm
Stage 2	Pushing and delivery of the baby
Stage 3	Delivery of the placenta

intravenous (IV) line in the arm. When oxytocin is given, the baby's heart rate is monitored.

In some cases, an ob-gyn may break your water. If your water has not broken on its own, rupturing the *amniotic sac* can make contractions stronger and more frequent. To rupture the amniotic sac, an ob-gyn makes a hole in the sac with a special device. This procedure is called an *amniotomy*.

In some cases, your ob-gyn may recommend delivery with the help of *forceps* or a *vacuum device*. This is called an *assisted vaginal delivery* (see Chapter 16, "Assisted Vaginal Delivery and Breech Presentation"). A cesarean delivery also may be recommended in some situations.

Shoulder Dystocia

Shoulder dystocia is a potentially life-threatening event that happens when the baby's shoulders get lodged in the woman's pelvis after the head has come out of the *vagina*. Shoulder dystocia is diagnosed when the baby's shoulders do not come out with gentle downward pressure on the baby's head. Shoulder dystocia is a labor emergency and requires immediate maneuvers to help deliver the baby.

There is no way to predict a shoulder dystocia, and there is no way to prevent it. But there are some known risk factors, including

- *diabetes mellitus*
- a large baby (macrosomia)
- maternal *obesity*
- an abnormal first or second stage of labor
- shoulder dystocia in past delivery

Most cases of shoulder dystocia happen without any risk factors and with normal size babies.

Risks

When shoulder dystocia occurs, there may be injury to the baby. The most common injuries are to the collarbone, arm, and a group of nerves called the brachial plexus. Shoulder dystocia can cause theses nerves to be stretched or compressed. Damage to these nerves may cause weakness or paralysis in the arm and shoulder. This injury usually resolves on its own in the first year of the baby's life.

Also, during a shoulder dystocia, *oxygen* and blood do not get to the baby normally. In severe cases, this can result in permanent brain damage to the baby. Women who have deliveries complicated by shoulder dystocia have a higher risk of **postpartum hemorrhage** and tears of the **perineum**.

Management

When shoulder dystocia is recognized, you will be told to stop pushing. Usually, an intervention called the McRoberts maneuver is tried first. Two nurses push the woman's legs up and alongside her abdomen, and the ob-gyn presses on her pubic bone. This position can help dislodge the baby's shoulders. Your ob-gyn may try other maneuvers as well.

Future Deliveries

If you've had this complication before, you and your ob-gyn should discuss the safest way to deliver your next baby. You may discuss the risks and benefits of vaginal birth versus **cesarean birth**. Factors that may affect your decision include

- the estimated weight of the baby
- whether your prior baby had an injury during delivery
- whether your blood sugar was well-controlled during pregnancy (if you have diabetes)

Umbilical Cord Compression

During labor, the **umbilical cord** can be compressed (squeezed) if it

- wraps around the baby's neck or other body parts
- gets tangled or knotted
- gets trapped between the baby and the wall of the uterus

Compression of the cord can reduce blood flow to the baby. A change in the baby's heart rate is usually the first sign of cord compression. When this happens, steps may be taken to prevent serious complications.

Risk Factors

Umbilical cord compression is more likely to happen if the level of **amniotic fluid** is low (**oligohydramnios**) or after your water has broken. The amniotic fluid provides a space for the umbilical cord to float freely. After your water breaks, this space is lost. Sometimes contractions during labor compress the umbilical cord.

Signs and Symptoms

Umbilical cord compression usually causes a decrease in the baby's heart rate called *deceleration*. This change in heart rate can be detected with *electronic fetal monitoring* during labor.

Management

If cord compression is suspected, you may be asked to change your position. This can relieve pressure on the cord. Another option may be amnioinfusion, which puts fluid back into the uterus. This is done by gently guiding a soft, flexible *catheter* through the cervix and into the uterus. Putting fluid back into the uterus may restore space for the cord and may reduce compression. The tube is removed before delivery. If the baby's heart rate is not normal after these things are tried, a cesarean delivery may be needed.

Umbilical Cord Prolapse

Although rare, the umbilical cord can slip out of the uterus and into the vagina before the baby is delivered. This is known as *umbilical cord prolapse*. When this happens, the cord gets compressed and the baby may not get enough oxygen. It can cause brain damage to the baby or death if it is not managed right away.

Risk Factors

Certain pregnancy conditions can increase the risk of umbilical cord prolapse:

- Rupture of membranes—When your water breaks, the cord may be carried along in the gush of amniotic fluid as it leaves the uterus. The risk is higher if there is a greater-than-normal amount of amniotic fluid (*polyhydramnios*).
- Baby's position—If the baby is not in a head-down position when your water breaks, the risk of cord prolapse is higher.
- *Low birth weight*—Smaller-than-normal babies, including *preterm* babies, have a higher risk of cord prolapse.
- Twin pregnancy—The risk of cord prolapse is higher for the second-born twin.

Signs and Symptoms

The first sign of cord prolapse often is a sudden drop in the baby's heart rate. An ob-gyn may be able to feel the cord in the vagina.

Management

Prompt delivery of the baby is needed if cord prolapse is diagnosed or suspected. This most often means a cesarean birth. But if your ob-gyn believes that a vaginal birth will be safer and quicker, the baby may be delivered through the vagina.

In the meantime, your ob-gyn may try to reduce the pressure on the umbilical cord by inserting a hand into the vagina and lifting the baby's head off the cord. You may be placed in a knee-to-chest position to further relieve pressure on the cord.

In most cases of cord prolapse, delivery is accomplished without problems and the baby is healthy. Success depends in part on how long it takes to deliver the baby after cord prolapse is found. Other factors that determine the outcome include

- how tightly the cord was compressed
- how long the cord was compressed
- the baby's well-being when the cord compressed

Postpartum Hemorrhage

When a woman bleeds heavily after delivery, it is called ***postpartum hemorrhage***. Severe blood loss can cause serious complications for the woman. Postpartum hemorrhage also can cause death if not treated right away.

Causes

Postpartum hemorrhage can happen within the first 24 hours of delivery (called "primary" or early hemorrhage). It also can happen between 1 day and 12 weeks after delivery (called "secondary" or late hemorrhage).

- Most cases of postpartum hemorrhage are caused by ***uterine atony***. Uterine atony happens when the muscles of the uterus do not contract normally. Without normal contractions, blood vessels do not tighten after delivery. This can lead to bleeding.

- Another cause of postpartum hemorrhage is ***placenta accreta***. In this condition, the placenta grows into the uterine wall and cannot be separated from it. This can cause hemorrhage during the third stage of labor when delivery of the placenta is attempted. Placenta accreta can be diagnosed during pregnancy in most cases, and steps may be taken before labor to help manage it (see Chapter 37, "Placenta Problems").

- **Uterine rupture** also can cause postpartum hemorrhage. This can happen when a cesarean scar tears during a ***trial of labor after cesarean delivery (TOLAC)***.

Other causes of postpartum hemorrhage may include

- cuts or tears to the uterus, cervix, vagina, or perineum
- blood clotting problems
- retained placental tissue (when part of the placenta stays inside the uterus)
- uterine inversion, a rare condition in which the uterus turns inside out after delivery
- amniotic fluid embolism, a rare condition in which amniotic fluid enters the mother's bloodstream
- infection, such as **endometritis** (see the section "Endometritis" later in this chapter)

Signs and Symptoms

The number one sign of postpartum hemorrhage is heavy bleeding after delivery. Other signs include a fast heartbeat and symptoms of low blood pressure (dizziness and lightheadedness).

After you leave the hospital, it's normal to have some bloody discharge (***lochia***) for a few weeks as your body sheds the blood and tissue that lined your uterus. But if your bleeding is heavy—you are soaking through two pads an hour for more than an hour or two—call your ob-gyn. This could be a sign of late postpartum hemorrhage.

Risk Factors

Postpartum hemorrhage often happens without warning to women who have no risk factors. But some conditions may increase the risk of heavy blood loss after delivery, including

- long labor
- augmented labor
- fast labor

- postpartum hemorrhage in the past
- *preeclampsia*
- chorioamnionitis
- larger uterus from having a large baby, twins, or polyhydramnios
- *episiotomy*
- cesarean birth
- *fibroid*
- bleeding disorders such as **hemophilia** or **von Willebrand disease**
- treatment for a blood clotting disorder (**thrombophilia**)

Management

Even if you do not have heavy bleeding, it is routine for ob-gyns to give oxytocin soon after delivery to prevent uterine atony. If heavy bleeding does happen, the health care team should respond quickly to stop the bleeding.

When postpartum hemorrhage is caused by uterine atony, the ob-gyn may massage the uterus with one hand on the abdomen and one hand in the vagina. Oxytocin, **prostaglandins**, and other medications may be given to make the uterus contract and reduce bleeding.

If these steps do not work, the ob-gyn may insert a gauze material or a balloon-like device into the uterus to stop the bleeding. **Uterine artery embolization** is a technique that can be done without an abdominal incision (cut). It involves inserting a device into an artery to stop bleeding. This procedure is done in the radiology department and only if the woman is stable.

Other procedures to stop heavy postpartum bleeding require abdominal surgery so the ob-gyn can get to the uterus. The arteries to the uterus may be tied off to stop the flow of blood. Or the uterus may be compressed with stitches to stop bleeding. If these techniques do not work, an emergency hysterectomy may be needed.

Depending on how much blood has been lost, you may need a blood **transfusion**. Once your condition is stable, your ob-gyn may recommend that you take iron tablets to replace the iron that was lost during heavy bleeding. Taking a prenatal vitamin along with iron tablets may help your body recover faster.

Endometritis

Endometritis is an infection of the lining of the uterus. When it happens after childbirth, it is called **postpartum endometritis**. The chance of getting endometritis is higher after a cesarean birth. For this reason, antibiotics are given before all cesarean deliveries.

Risk Factors

In addition to cesarean birth, there are other risk factors for postpartum endometritis. These risk factors include

- rupture of membranes more than 18 to 24 hours before delivery
- labor that lasts a long time and has required many **pelvic exams**
- having a fever during labor

Signs and Symptoms

Most cases of endometritis are diagnosed within a few days of delivery. Fever is an early sign. Other symptoms include

- a tender or painful abdomen
- tiredness
- feeling sick

Remember that after childbirth there is vaginal discharge called lochia. This discharge is normal, but if the lochia has a bad odor, this also could be a sign of infection. If you notice any of these symptoms, call your ob-gyn.

Management

Postpartum endometritis is treated with antibiotics. It usually takes 1 to 2 days for you to start feeling better and for your fever to go down. If you don't respond to the antibiotics, your ob-gyn may look for other causes of your infection.

If you have postpartum endometritis, your baby will be checked for infection. Blood tests may be done, and antibiotics may be given to the baby.

RESOURCES

Childbirth Problems
https://medlineplus.gov/childbirthproblems.html
Information from the U.S. National Library of Medicine about complications that can happen during and after labor and delivery.

Postpartum Care

www.marchofdimes.org/pregnancy/postpartum-care.aspx

Webpage from the March of Dimes about staying healthy after giving birth, including warning signs of postpartum hemorrhage and other potential health problems.

Your Pregnancy and Childbirth

www.acog.org/MyPregnancy

Website from the American College of Obstetricians and Gynecologists (ACOG) with information on pregnancy, labor, delivery, and postpartum care. Includes the latest information from the experts in women's health care, questions answered by ACOG ob-gyns, pregnancy stories from real women, and an A–Z directory of health topics covering pregnancy and beyond.

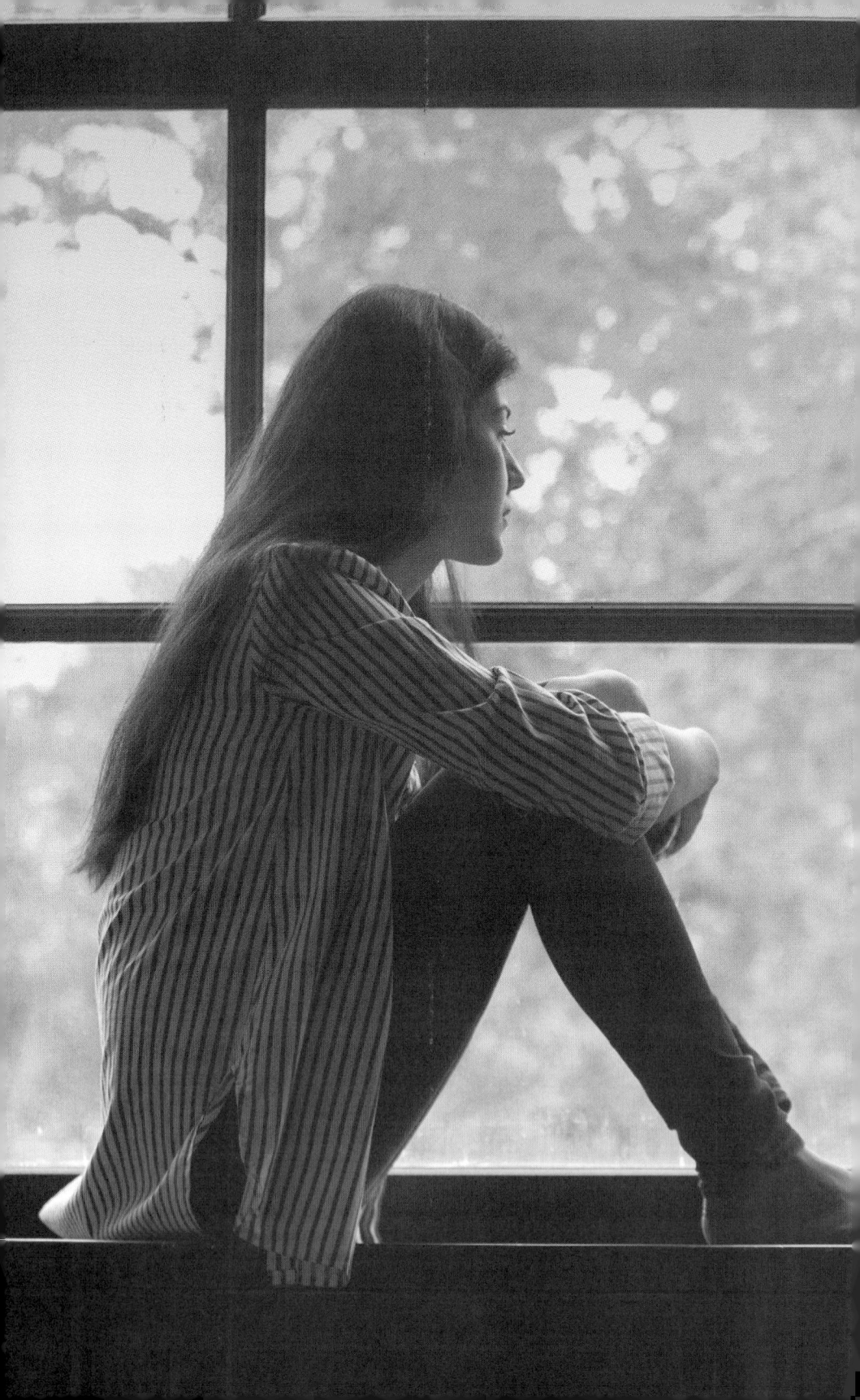

PART 9

Pregnancy Loss

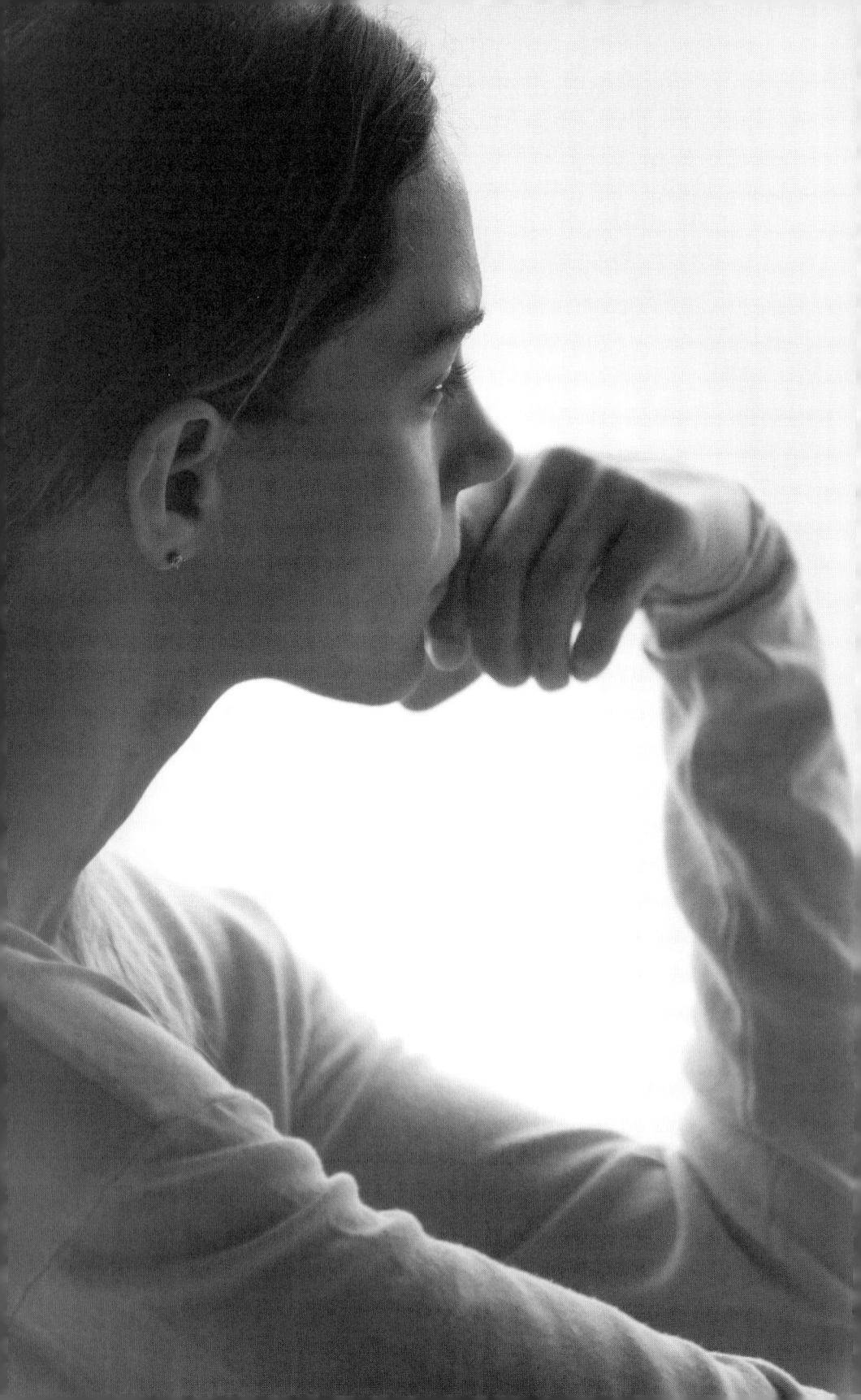

CHAPTER 40

Early Pregnancy Loss
Miscarriage, Ectopic Pregnancy, and Gestational Trophoblastic Disease

Most women have healthy pregnancies and babies. But sometimes problems happen that cause the loss of a pregnancy. Losing a pregnancy—no matter how early—can cause sadness and grief. Women need to heal physically and emotionally. For most women, emotional healing takes a lot longer than physical healing. Partners also need to heal when a pregnancy is lost.

Miscarriage

A normal pregnancy lasts about 40 weeks. The loss of a pregnancy before 20 completed weeks is called *miscarriage*. Miscarriages happen in about 15 in 100 known pregnancies.

Causes

In almost every case, miscarriage is not a woman's fault. This is important to understand. Miscarriage usually is a random event. Working, exercising, stress, arguments, having sex, or having used **birth control** pills before getting pregnant do not cause miscarriage. Few medications can cause miscarriage. Morning sickness—the nausea and vomiting that is common in early pregnancy—also does not cause miscarriage.

Some women who have had a miscarriage believe that it was caused by a recent fall, blow, fright, or stress. In most cases, this is not true. It may simply be that these things happened to occur around the same time and are fresh in the memory.

About half of early miscarriages happen when the **embryo** does not develop properly. This often is due to an abnormal number of **chromosomes**. Chromosomes are in each **cell** of the body and carry the blueprints (**genes**) for how we develop and function. During **fertilization**, when the **egg** and **sperm** join, two sets of chromosomes come together. If an egg or sperm has more or fewer chromosomes than normal, the embryo also will have an abnormal number. This can lead to miscarriage.

The chance of these problems increases as a woman gets older. For women over age 40, about 1 in 3 pregnancies end in miscarriage. Most end because of a chromosome abnormality. There also is some evidence that chromosome abnormalities in the embryo increase as men get older. But it is not clear at what age this begins for men.

Signs and Symptoms

Bleeding is the most common sign of miscarriage. Call your **obstetrician–gynecologist (ob-gyn)** if you have signs or symptoms of miscarriage, including

- vaginal spotting or bleeding with or without pain
- a gush of fluid from your vagina, even if you do not have pain or bleeding
- passage of tissue from the vagina

A small amount of bleeding early in pregnancy is common and does not necessarily mean that you will have a miscarriage. If your bleeding is heavy or happens with a pain like menstrual cramps, contact your ob-gyn right away.

Diagnosis

If you have bleeding or cramping, your ob-gyn may do an **ultrasound exam**. This exam can check whether the pregnancy is growing normally. If your pregnancy is far enough along, the ultrasound exam may detect cardiac activity. Finding cardiac activity is reassuring. It suggests a much higher chance that the pregnancy will continue.

If cardiac activity isn't found, it may be too early to detect it. But in some cases, not finding cardiac activity means the embryo has stopped developing.

Your ob-gyn also may do a **pelvic exam** to see if your **cervix** has begun to dilate (open). **Dilation** of the cervix means that a miscarriage may be more likely.

If your ob-gyn thinks your pregnancy is not growing normally, he or she may suggest you rest and avoid **sexual intercourse**. Although these measures have not been proved to prevent miscarriage, they may help reduce discomfort and anxiety.

Treatment

It is rarely possible to prevent or stop a miscarriage. After a miscarriage, some of the pregnancy tissue may be left in the ***uterus***. This is called an incomplete miscarriage. There are options to remove this tissue. The choice depends on many factors, including how large the pregnancy has grown.

If you do not show any signs of an infection, your ob-gyn may recommend waiting and letting the tissue pass naturally. This usually takes up to 2 weeks, but it may take longer in some cases. Another option is to take medication that helps expel the tissue.

With both options, you will have bleeding, some of which may be heavy. Cramping pain, diarrhea, and nausea also can happen. You may pass tissue as well. With an early miscarriage, the tissue may look like a blood clot mixed with grey-white material or a clear, fluid-filled sac.

If needed, your ob-gyn also may suggest one of the following procedures to remove the remaining tissue:

- ***Vacuum aspiration*** removes the contents of the uterus with a suction device. The device is inserted through the cervix and into the uterus. This procedure often can be done in your ob-gyn's office.

- If the pregnancy is large or if you are bleeding heavily, your ob-gyn may recommend a procedure called a ***dilation and curettage (D&C)***. A D&C usually is done in the hospital. The cervix is dilated and an instrument is used to remove the remaining tissue from the uterus.

The risks of these procedures include bleeding, infection, and injury to internal organs. Before any procedure, your ob-gyn should explain how it is done. He or she also should explain the risks and benefits.

If your blood type is Rh negative, you may get a shot of ***Rh immunoglobulin***. This can prevent problems with the ***Rh factor*** in a future pregnancy. See Chapter 36, "Blood Type Incompatibility."

Recovery

To help prevent infection, you should not put anything in your vagina for 1 to 2 weeks. This includes not using tampons, not having sexual intercourse, and not having sex with ***penetration*** (using fingers or sex toys). You should see your ob-gyn for a follow-up visit a few weeks after your miscarriage. Call your ob-gyn right away if you have

- heavy bleeding
- fever
- chills
- severe pain

Trying Again

You can *ovulate* and get pregnant as soon as 2 weeks after an early miscarriage. If you do not wish to get pregnant again now, use birth control. If you want to get pregnant, talk with your ob-gyn about the best timing for trying again.

Take time to recover before trying again. Most women who have a miscarriage go on to have successful pregnancies. Repeated miscarriages are rare. Testing can be done to try to find a cause if you have had two or more miscarriages. Even if no cause is found, most women will have successful pregnancies after repeated miscarriages.

Ectopic Pregnancy

In a typical pregnancy, a fertilized egg moves through the *fallopian tube* and implants in the lining of the uterus, where it starts to grow. When a fertilized egg grows outside of the uterus, it is called an *ectopic pregnancy*. Almost all ectopic pregnancies occur in a fallopian tube.

Because it is outside of the uterus, an ectopic pregnancy cannot grow into a healthy baby. An ectopic pregnancy cannot be moved to the uterus. As the pregnancy grows, it can cause the fallopian tube to rupture (burst). A rupture can cause major internal bleeding. This can be a life-threatening emergency that needs immediate surgery. If the fallopian tube has not burst, the ectopic pregnancy often can be treated with medication.

Risk Factors

Any woman having sexual intercourse who is of childbearing age is at risk of ectopic pregnancy. But women who have had certain conditions or procedures are at higher risk. These include

- past ectopic pregnancy
- past fallopian tube surgery
- past pelvic or abdominal surgery
- certain *sexually transmitted infections (STIs)*
- *pelvic inflammatory disease*
- *endometriosis*

Some of these conditions create scar tissue in the fallopian tubes. This may keep a fertilized egg from reaching the uterus.

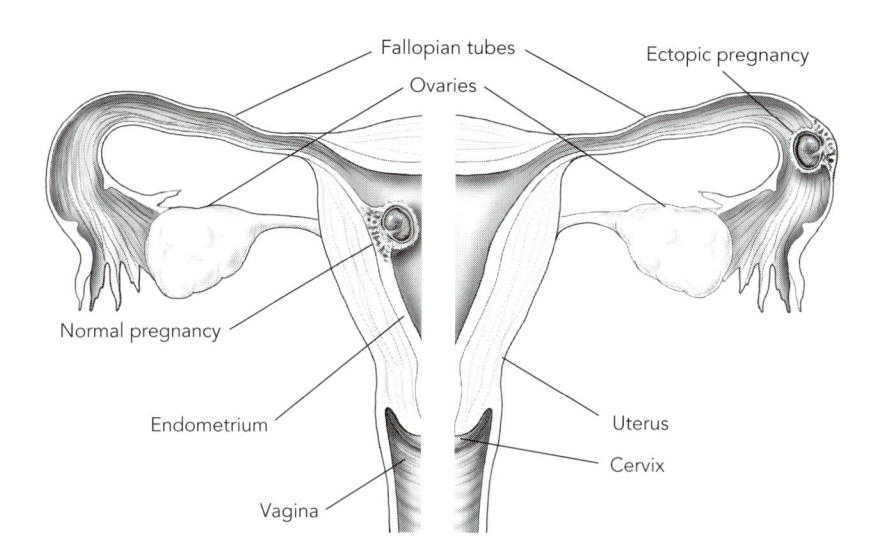

Ectopic pregnancy. In a typical pregnancy (*left*), the fertilized egg grows in the uterus. In an ectopic pregnancy (*right*), the fertilized egg grows in the fallopian tube. In rare cases, an ectopic pregnancy can grow in other parts of the body, including the cervix, an ovary, or another organ in the abdomen.

Other factors that may increase a woman's risk of ectopic pregnancy include
- cigarette smoking
- being over 35
- history of infertility

About half of all women who have an ectopic pregnancy do not have known risk factors. This means that women should be alert to changes in their bodies, especially if they have symptoms of an ectopic pregnancy.

Signs and Symptoms

At first, an ectopic pregnancy may feel like a typical pregnancy with some of the same signs, such as a missed period, tender breasts, or an upset stomach. Other signs may include

- abnormal vaginal bleeding
- low back pain
- mild pain in the abdomen or pelvis
- mild cramping on one side of the pelvis

At this stage, it may be hard to know if you are experiencing a typical pregnancy or an ectopic pregnancy. Call your ob-gyn if you have abnormal bleeding and pelvic pain.

As an ectopic pregnancy grows, more serious symptoms may develop, especially if a fallopian tube ruptures. Symptoms may include

- sudden, severe pain in the abdomen or pelvis
- shoulder pain
- weakness, dizziness, or fainting

A ruptured fallopian tube can cause life-threatening internal bleeding. If you have sudden, severe pain, shoulder pain, or weakness, go to an emergency room.

Diagnosis

If you do not have the symptoms of a fallopian tube rupture but your ob-gyn suspects you may have an ectopic pregnancy, he or she may

- perform a pelvic exam
- perform an ultrasound exam to see where the pregnancy is developing
- test your blood for a pregnancy **hormone** called **human chorionic gonadotropin (hCG)**

The hCG test may be repeated to check the levels again. If the level does not increase as it would during a typical pregnancy, you may be at risk of an ectopic pregnancy or a miscarriage.

Tests to find an ectopic pregnancy may take time. Results may not be clear right away. More tests may be needed. If the fallopian tube is not in danger of rupture, medication may be an option. But if your ob-gyn thinks you have a ruptured fallopian tube, you will need to have surgery right away.

Treatment

An ectopic pregnancy cannot be moved to the uterus, so it always requires treatment. There are two ways used to treat an ectopic pregnancy: 1) medication and 2) surgery. If your ob-gyn thinks you have an ectopic pregnancy, he or she should explain the benefits and risks of treatment based on your

- medical condition
- test results
- plans for future pregnancies

Several weeks of follow-up care are required with each treatment.

Medication

If the pregnancy has not ruptured a fallopian tube, medication may be used to treat ectopic pregnancy. The drug used is called methotrexate. This drug stops cells from growing, which ends the pregnancy. The pregnancy then is absorbed by the body over 4 to 6 weeks. This does not require the removal of the fallopian tube.

There are many factors that go into the decision to use methotrexate. One of the most important factors is your ability to follow up with blood tests that check your blood levels of hCG. If you are breastfeeding, you will not be able to use methotrexate. Women with certain health problems also cannot use this medication.

Taking Methotrexate. Methotrexate often is given by injection in one dose. In some cases, it may be given in more than one dose over several days. Your ob-gyn should take a sample of your blood before the first dose. Blood tests will be done to measure the level of hCG and the functions of certain organs. If levels have not decreased enough, another dose of methotrexate may be recommended. You will have careful follow-up over time until hCG is no longer found in your blood.

Side Effects and Risks. Taking methotrexate can have some side effects. Most women have some abdominal pain. Other side effects may include

- vaginal bleeding or spotting
- nausea
- vomiting
- diarrhea
- dizziness

It is important to follow up with your ob-gyn until your treatment with methotrexate is complete. The risk of a fallopian tube rupture does not go away until your treatment is over. Seek care right away if you have symptoms of a rupture, including sudden abdominal pain, shoulder pain, or weakness.

Guidelines. During treatment with methotrexate you should avoid

- heavy exercise
- sexual intercourse
- alcohol

- vitamins and foods that contain **folic acid**, including fortified cereal, enriched bread and pasta, peanuts, dark green leafy vegetables, orange juice, and beans
- prescription pain medication and **nonsteroidal anti-inflammatory drugs (NSAIDs),** which can affect the way methotrexate works in the body
- foods that produce gas, which can cause discomfort and mask the pain of a possible rupture of a fallopian tube
- prolonged exposure to sunlight, as methotrexate can cause sun sensitivity

Talk with your ob-gyn about when it is safe to go back to normal activities and foods. You also can talk with your ob-gyn about when it is safe to try to get pregnant again.

Surgery

If the fallopian tube has not ruptured but surgery is needed, there are two options:

1. The ectopic pregnancy can be removed from the tube.
2. The entire tube with the pregnancy can be removed.

Surgery typically is done with **laparoscopy**. This procedure uses a slender, lighted camera that is inserted through small cuts in the abdomen. It is done in a hospital with **general anesthesia**. If the ectopic pregnancy has ruptured a tube, emergency surgery is needed.

Side effects and risks. You and your ob-gyn should talk about the possible side effects and risks of surgery for ectopic pregnancy. Side effects may include pain, fatigue, bleeding, and infection.

It is important that all of the ectopic pregnancy is removed. If any tissue is left, it may cause internal bleeding. Blood tests for hCG may be needed for a few weeks after surgery to ensure that the pregnancy has been removed completely.

If you have had surgery and one or both fallopian tubes have been left in place, there is a good chance that you can have a normal pregnancy in the future. Talk with your ob-gyn about when it is safe for you to try again.

Recovery and Trying Again

Whether you were treated with methotrexate or surgery, you may feel tired for several weeks while you recover. You may have abdominal discomfort or pain. If you have pain that does not respond to over-the-counter pain relievers, talk with your ob-gyn.

It can take time for the level of hCG in your body to drop after treatment for an ectopic pregnancy. You may still feel pregnant for a while. It may take a few cycles for your periods to return to normal. Repeat blood tests may be needed until hCG is no longer found in your body.

Once you have had an ectopic pregnancy, you are at higher risk of having another one. During future pregnancies, be alert for signs and symptoms of ectopic pregnancy until your ob-gyn confirms that the pregnancy is growing in the right place.

Gestational Trophoblastic Disease

Gestational trophoblastic disease (GTD) is a rare group of disorders in which abnormal tissue grows in the uterus during pregnancy. The most common form of GTD is called a **hydatidiform mole** or **molar pregnancy**. A hydatidiform mole happens when a sperm fertilizes an egg that does not contain any genetic material. This condition cannot result in a successful pregnancy. There are two types:

1. A complete hydatidiform mole contains no fetal tissue.
2. A partial hydatidiform mole contains some fetal tissue, but it is not able to grow because it has abnormal genetic material.

Signs, Symptoms, and Diagnosis

Most cases of GTD cause symptoms that signal a problem. The most common symptom is vaginal bleeding during the first trimester. Your ob-gyn also may find other signs of molar pregnancy, such as a uterus that is too large for the stage of the pregnancy.

If your ob-gyn suspects a molar pregnancy, he or she may order an hCG test. An abnormally high level of hCG for the stage of pregnancy suggests molar pregnancy.

Your ob-gyn also may do an ultrasound exam. If a molar pregnancy is found, a series of tests will be done to check for other medical problems that sometimes happen along with it. These problems may include

- *high blood pressure*
- *anemia*
- *hyperthyroidism*

Many of these problems go away when the molar pregnancy is removed.

Treatment

If you have a molar pregnancy, the tissue must be removed. This usually is done with a D&C, similar to the procedure that is sometimes performed for a miscarriage (see the section "Miscarriage" earlier in this chapter). Nearly all women whose molar pregnancies are removed do not need any further treatment. But careful follow-up is needed. Regularly scheduled tests of hCG levels are done for at least 6 months and up to 1 year.

Sometimes abnormal cells remain after a molar pregnancy has been removed. This is called persistent GTD. It is indicated by hCG levels that rise or stay the same. Some forms of persistent GTD are ***malignant*** (cancerous). In a small number of women, malignant cells travel to other parts of the body. Persistent GTD is treated with medication and sometimes ***hysterectomy*** (removal of the uterus). Treatment is successful in most cases.

Trying Again

If you have had a molar pregnancy, your ob-gyn may recommend you wait 6 months to 1 year before trying to get pregnant again. It is safe to use birth control pills during this time. The chances of having another molar pregnancy are very low.

Coping With the Loss

After the loss of a pregnancy, you need to heal physically and emotionally. For many women, emotional healing takes longer than physical healing. The feelings of loss can be intense. Even if the pregnancy ended very early, the sense of bonding between a woman and her pregnancy can be strong. The loss of a pregnancy—no matter how early—can cause deep sadness.

Grief can involve a wide range of feelings. You may find yourself searching for the reason your pregnancy ended. You may wrongly blame yourself. You may have headaches, lose your appetite, feel tired, or have trouble concentrating and sleeping. If you develop ***depression***, talk with your ob-gyn.

Your feelings of grief may differ from those of your partner. You are the one who has felt the physical changes of pregnancy. Your partner also may grieve but may not express feelings in the same way you do. If either of you is having trouble handling the feelings that go along with a pregnancy loss, talk with your ob-gyn. It also may help to talk with a counselor.

RESOURCES

Ectopic Pregnancy
https://medlineplus.gov/ectopicpregnancy.html
Webpage from the U.S. National Library of Medicine that discusses causes, risk factors, and treatment of ectopic pregnancy.

Hydatidiform Mole
https://medlineplus.gov/ency/article/000909.htm
Webpage from the U.S. National Library of Medicine that provides information about molar pregnancy.

Miscarriage or Recurrent Pregnancy Loss
www.reproductivefacts.org/topics/topics-index/miscarriage-or-recurrent-pregnancy-loss/
Webpage from the American Society for Reproductive Medicine. Offers an expert discussion about recurrent pregnancy loss, including possible causes and information about new research. Also explains how recurrent pregnancy loss may be evaluated and the chances of successful pregnancy after recurrent pregnancy losses.

SHARE: Pregnancy and Infant Loss Support
www.nationalshare.org
Organization that provides support for families who have lost a baby through miscarriage, stillbirth, or newborn death.

Your Pregnancy and Childbirth
www.acog.org/MyPregnancy
Website from the American College of Obstetricians and Gynecologists (ACOG) with information on pregnancy, labor, delivery, and postpartum care. Includes the latest information from the experts in women's health care, questions answered by ACOG ob-gyns, pregnancy stories from real women, and an A–Z directory of health topics covering pregnancy and beyond.

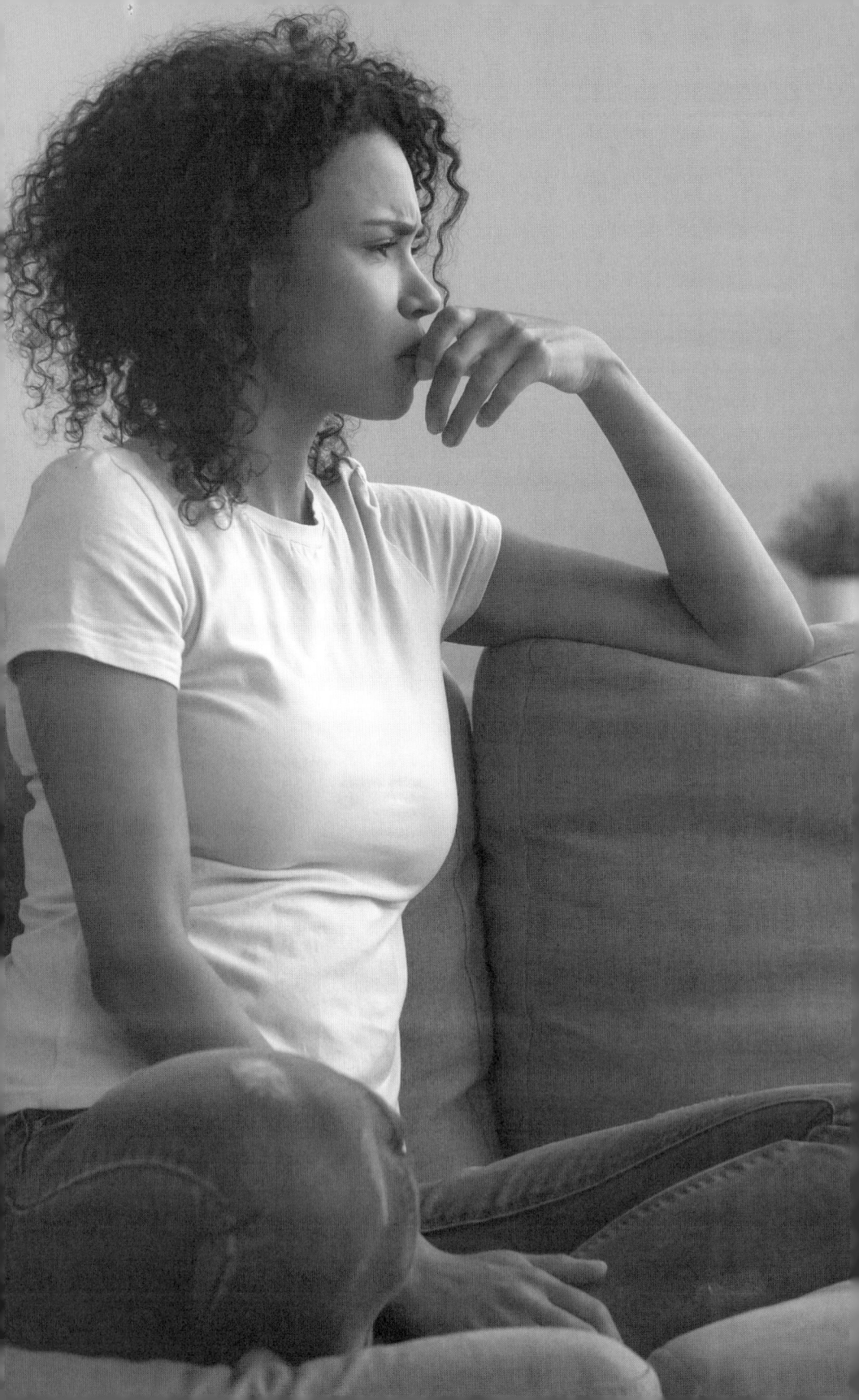

CHAPTER 41

Late Pregnancy Loss
Stillbirth

When a baby dies in the **uterus** after 20 weeks of pregnancy, it is called **stillbirth**. Many women who experience stillbirth have intense feelings of sadness and shock. It helps women to grieve for as long as needed and to have the support of a partner and loved ones. It may help to understand what went wrong, but sometimes it isn't possible to find a complete answer.

How Stillbirth Is Diagnosed

Sometimes stillbirth happens before labor begins. A woman may notice that the baby has stopped moving, or an **obstetrician–gynecologist (ob-gyn)** may not find the baby's heartbeat at a prenatal visit. Stillbirth also can happen during labor, but this is rare, especially when **electronic fetal monitoring** is used. Continuous monitoring of the baby during labor can help find problems so an ob-gyn can take steps to help the baby.

If there are concerns about your baby, an **ultrasound exam** may be done. If a heartbeat cannot be found, it means the baby has died in the uterus. Your ob-gyn should talk with you about the best options for delivery. In the second **trimester**, a procedure called **dilation and evacuation (D&E)** can be considered. Later in the second trimester and in the third trimester, **labor induction** also may be an option for delivery after stillbirth. The decision depends on your health and the stage of your pregnancy.

What Went Wrong?

Perhaps the most difficult question to answer is what happened. Unfortunately, the reasons for most stillbirths are unknown. Death may be caused by a **birth defect** or a **genetic disorder**. Sometimes a baby has trouble growing in the uterus. Growth problems can happen when there are problems with the **placenta** or the pregnant woman's circulation.

Some infections can cause illness in a pregnant woman and increase the risk of fetal death. For some illnesses, a baby's life can be at risk even if the woman has mild symptoms or no symptoms at all. Examples of infections that can cause fetal death include

- *parvovirus*
- *cytomegalovirus (CMV)*
- *syphilis*
- *listeria*
- *malaria*

See Chapter 25, "Protecting Yourself From Infections," for more on infections and how to protect yourself during pregnancy.

Problems with **chromosomes** are found in about 1 in 10 stillbirths. Some medical conditions in the woman can be a factor in stillbirth, including

- **high blood pressure**
- **kidney disease**
- **diabetes mellitus**
- **lupus** (systemic lupus erythematosus or SLE)
- **antiphospholipid syndrome (APS)**
- **intrahepatic cholestasis of pregnancy**

Some **complications** during labor and delivery also can cause stillbirth. These complications may include

- problems with the placenta or **umbilical cord**
- lack of **oxygen** to the baby
- infection

These problems are unlikely to happen if labor is monitored closely. Stillbirth almost never happens because of something a woman has done or because of a medication she has taken.

Tests and Evaluations

After a stillbirth, it is normal to want to find a cause. This is not always possible, but results from exams and tests usually are gathered to try to find the most likely cause or to rule out a suspected cause. A team of health care practitioners may be involved, including your ob-gyn and others with special expertise.

A physician with expertise in genetics (**geneticist**), a **pediatrician**, or a **neonatologist** may examine the baby's body to look for signs of a genetic condition or syndrome. A **pathologist** may do tests to look for birth defects, abnormal placenta development, or infections. You may also be referred to a **maternal–fetal medicine (MFM) specialist** to discuss how to take care of a future pregnancy.

Your ob-gyn should take a history of your pregnancy and document problems or illnesses that you had, if this hasn't already been done. A family history also may be taken to look for possible **inherited disorders**. Depending on your family and medical history, more laboratory tests may be recommended to check for inherited disorders. The baby's measurements and weight will be recorded. Photographs may be taken.

When searching for an explanation for a stillbirth, the most useful tests are an evaluation of the placenta, an **autopsy**, and genetic testing. During an autopsy, the baby's organs are examined to look for birth defects or abnormalities. A genetic test called a **microarray** may be offered. To do this test, a small piece of tissue is taken from the placenta, the umbilical cord, or the baby's thigh. The microarray can provide more genetic information than what is found looking at the baby's chromosomes.

If you do not want an autopsy, other exams and tests may be available. These include

- a physical exam of the baby and the placenta
- taking samples of tissue for testing
- **magnetic resonance imaging (MRI)**
- X-rays

With these options, the baby's organs are left intact.

Although the exact reason why your baby died may not be found, an autopsy or other tests may help answer some questions about what happened. This information could be useful to you and your ob-gyn in planning future pregnancies.

Grieving

The death of a baby is a profoundly painful event. Grief is a normal, natural response. Mourn your loss for as long as you need (see the box "Honoring Your Loss"). It's best to go through the complete grieving process to help you cope and move ahead. Remember that everyone grieves in a different way. It is important to talk with your partner or another person you trust about what you are feeling.

The Stages of Grief

Grieving includes a wide range of feelings. Just as each pregnancy is unique, ways to react to a stillbirth also are unique. The way you grieve may be affected by

- your religious beliefs and customs
- your role in the family

Honoring Your Loss

Grieving your loss will take time. There are things that may make it easier to deal with the pain:

- Saying goodbye—It may be helpful to hold your baby to say goodbye. The hospital staff may take pictures of your baby or give you keepsakes, such as the baby's cap, a handprint or footprint, an identification bracelet, or a crib card. If these things are not offered, ask for them.

- Express yourself—Talk about your feelings with your partner, family, and friends. It often helps to write down your thoughts in a journal or in letters to the baby and others.

- Reach out—Tell your family and friends what they can do to help, whether it's cooking a meal, doing house chores, running errands, or just spending time with you.

- Take care of yourself—Eat well, try to get enough sleep, and stay physically active. Avoid using alcohol or drugs to cope with grief.

- Choose a name—Naming the baby gives your child an identity. A name allows you, your friends, and your family to refer to a specific child, not just "the baby you lost."

- Plan a funeral or memorial service—For many parents, it's a great comfort to have family and friends acknowledge the life and death of their baby and to express their sorrow at a special service. You may wish to contact a funeral home for burial or cremation.

- your experiences with death
- what you think others expect of you

Your grief may last for weeks, months, or years. The grieving process involves certain stages that can overlap and repeat. But the process often seems to follow a pattern that includes

- shock, numbness, and disbelief
- searching and yearning
- anger or rage
- *depression* and loneliness
- acceptance

Shock, Numbness, and Disbelief

When faced with news of their baby's death, parents often think that it is not really happening or that it can't be true. You may have trouble grasping the news or feel nothing at all. You may deny that the loss has happened. Even though you and your partner may be together physically, you each may feel a very private sense of being alone or empty.

Searching and Yearning

These feelings tend to overlap with the initial shock and get stronger over time. You may look for a reason for your baby's death. It is common during this stage to feel guilty. You may think that you somehow brought about your baby's death. You may blame yourself for things you did or did not do. You may have dreams about the baby and yearn for what might have been.

Anger or Rage

"What did I do to deserve this?" and "How could this happen to me?" are common questions after losing a baby. In this stage of grief, you may feel angry with your partner, your health care team, the hospital staff, or even other women whose babies were born healthy. This is all a normal part of the grieving process.

Many parents feel angry if the cause of the stillbirth cannot be determined. It's good to accept your anger, express it, and try to get it out of your system. If you or your partner feel angry toward each other, it may be hard for you to comfort each other. Anger becomes unhealthy if you direct it toward yourself.

Depression and Loneliness

In this stage, the reality sinks in that you have lost your baby. You may feel tired, sad, and helpless. You may have trouble getting back into your normal routine. The support from friends and family may not be as intense as it was in the early weeks of your loss. Slowly, you will start to get back on your feet and work through your loss.

Acceptance

In this final stage of grieving, you come to terms with what has happened. Your baby's death no longer rules your thoughts. You start to have renewed energy. Although you will never forget your loss, you begin to think of your baby less often and with less pain. You pick up your normal daily routine and social life. You make plans for the future. Some families find that holding a memorial service or funeral service provides comfort and honors their baby.

As you come to terms with your baby's death, you may feel guilty about moving through the worst of your grief. But it's OK to accept what has happened. A normal part of life is planning for the future. Moving on does not mean that you will forget your baby. It just means that you are healing and ready to accept what life has to offer next.

You and Your Partner

Your relationship with your partner may be affected by the stress of the loss of your child. You may have trouble getting your thoughts and feelings across to each other. You may find it hard to be intimate again or do other things together that you used to enjoy. This is normal. Try to be patient with each other. Let your partner know what your needs are and what you are feeling. Take time to be tender, caring, and close. Make an extra effort to be open and honest.

Throughout the grieving process, your partner may not respond in the same way as you do. Your partner may feel differently from you and may be able to move on before you are ready. Your partner may not want to talk about the loss when you do. Each person should grieve in their own way. Try to understand and respond to your partner's needs as well as your own.

Seeking Support

Surround yourself with your partner, family, and friends for support during the coming months. Know that you are not alone. Ask your ob-gyn to direct you to support systems in your community. These can include childbirth educators, self-help groups, social workers, and religious leaders (see the "Resources" section in this chapter).

Many grieving parents find it helpful to get involved with groups of parents who have gone through the same loss. Members of such support groups respect your feelings, understand your stresses and fears, and have a good sense of the kindness you need.

Professional counseling also can help to relieve your pain, guilt, and depression. Talking with a counselor can help you understand and accept what has happened. You may wish to get counseling for only yourself, for you and your partner, or for your entire family.

The Future

The pain of losing your baby may never vanish completely, but it will not always be the main focus in your life and thoughts. At some point, you will be able to talk and think about the baby more easily and with less pain. One day you'll find yourself doing more of the things you used to do, such as enjoying favorite activities, renewing friendships, and looking forward to the future.

Another Pregnancy

In time, you may feel ready to start planning another pregnancy. Before thinking about getting pregnant again, allow time for you and your partner to work through your feelings. After losing a baby, some couples feel a need to have another baby right away. They think it will fill the empty feeling or take away the pain. A new baby cannot replace the baby that was lost. That baby needs to be mourned before you can move on.

Should you choose to have another pregnancy, keep in mind that the chances of losing another baby are very small in most cases. If the cause of the stillbirth is not known, and you do not have a medical condition, the chance of stillbirth happening again is very low. Even so, you may be anxious and worried during your next pregnancy. There may be things that you can do to be in the best health possible before pregnancy, including

- weight loss if you are obese
- genetic counseling if a genetic disorder is suspected
- prepregnancy counseling with your ob-gyn or an MFM specialist
- tests and evaluations if you have a medical condition

Some dates may be painful when they come around again. These may include the due date or the date when you lost your baby. These dates may bring sadness for many years and can be particularly stressful during a future pregnancy. Throughout your next pregnancy, emotional support and reassurance are vital. Your ob-gyn may be able to recommend counseling or a support group if you feel this would be helpful to you.

RESOURCES

CLIMB: Center for Loss in Multiple Birth, Inc.
www.climb-support.org
Offers support for families who have experienced loss during a multiple pregnancy or during infancy and childhood.

The Compassionate Friends
www.compassionatefriends.org
Offers support for families experiencing grief following the death of a child of any age.

Now I Lay Me Down to Sleep
www.nowilaymedowntosleep.org
Organization that coordinates volunteer photographers who will take memorial portraits of babies who have died.

SHARE: Pregnancy and Infant Loss Support
www.nationalshare.org
Organization that provides support for families who have lost a baby through miscarriage, stillbirth, or newborn death.

Your Pregnancy and Childbirth
www.acog.org/MyPregnancy
Website from the American College of Obstetricians and Gynecologists (ACOG) with information on pregnancy, labor, delivery, and postpartum care. Includes the latest information from the experts in women's health care, questions answered by ACOG ob-gyns, pregnancy stories from real women, and an A–Z directory of health topics covering pregnancy and beyond.

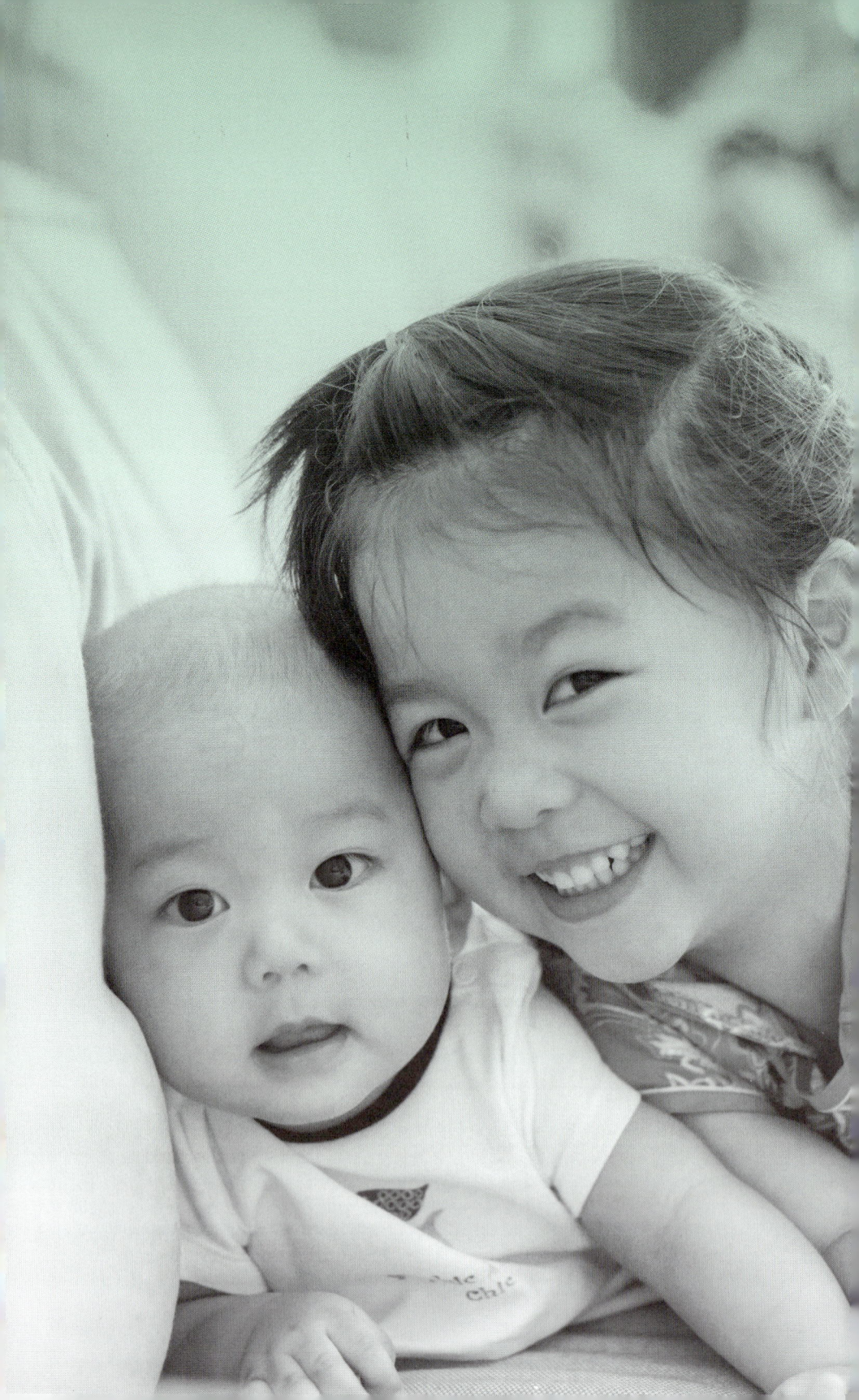

PART 10

Looking Ahead

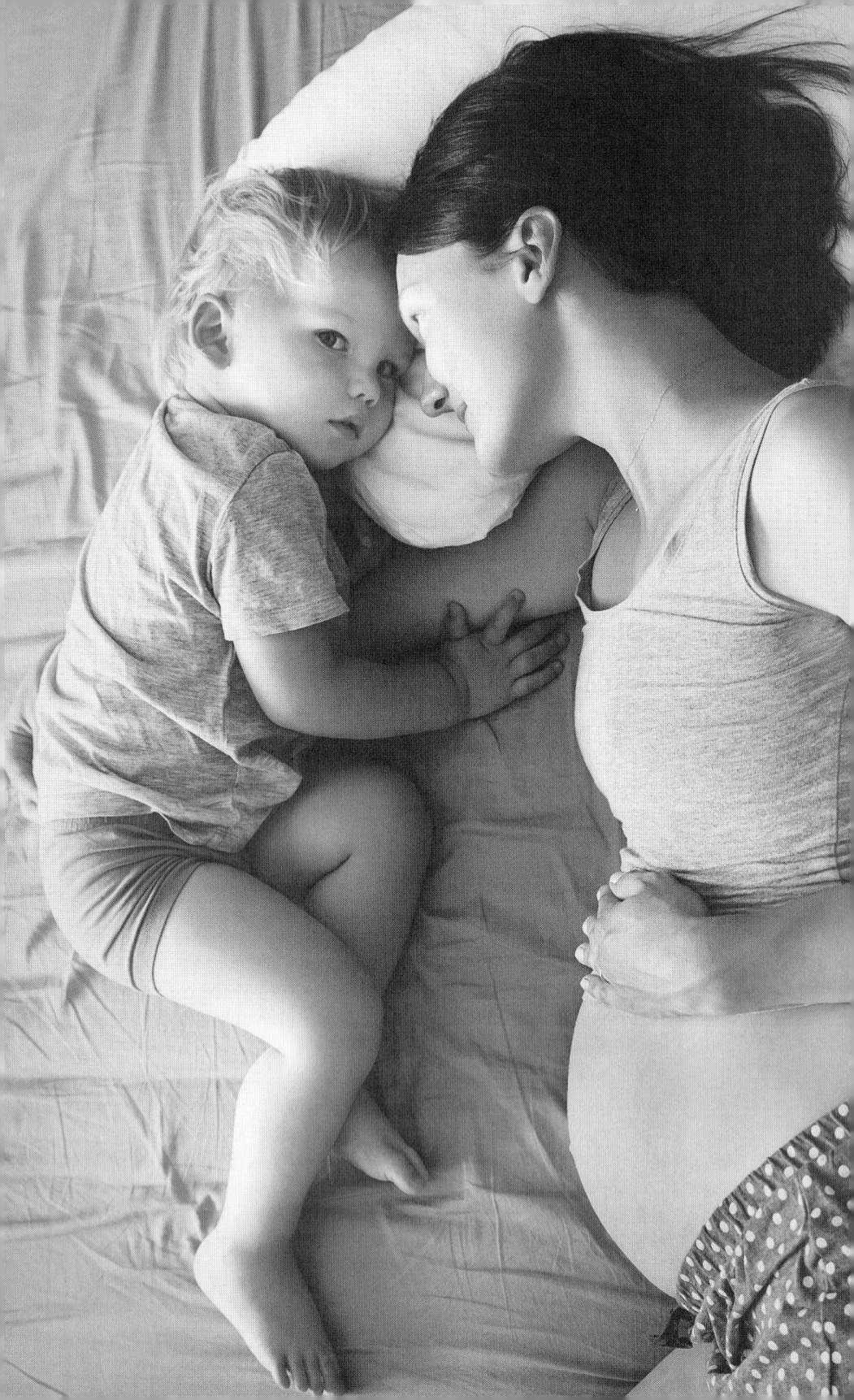

CHAPTER 42

Having Another Baby
What to Expect the Next Time Around

Once you've been through pregnancy and childbirth, you know a lot about what to expect if you get pregnant again. But every pregnancy is different. Whether you are just thinking about having another baby or you are already pregnant, there are a few things to think about.

Timing for Another Baby

Some parents think it is important to have children close in age. Others think it is important for their first child to be near school age before having another.

The timing of your next pregnancy is your decision. Only you can decide what you are ready to handle—physically, emotionally, and financially. But there are some health concerns you should keep in mind when deciding to have another baby. You can schedule a **prepregnancy** checkup with your **obstetrician–gynecologist (ob-gyn)** to talk about the following concerns.

How Long Should You Wait?

Ideally, pregnancies should be spaced at least 18 months apart. This offers the best health outcomes for both mom and baby. There may be a greater risk of certain **complications** when the time between pregnancies is less than 18 months. These complications may include

- *gestational diabetes*
- *preterm* birth
- *low birth weight*

There are a few theories about why these problems may happen. Some experts believe having children too close together doesn't give your body enough time to build up your stores of *folate* and iron. Other theories suggest that a woman's body needs enough time to heal before another pregnancy. This is especially important after a **cesarean birth.**

If you feel the need to attempt another pregnancy sooner than 18 months, talk with your ob-gyn about the risks and benefits in your situation. Together you should review your age and medical history when talking about how to space your children.

It also is helpful to wait for your **menstrual cycle** to return to normal. Having regular periods will help you detect pregnancy earlier. This also will help your ob-gyn estimate your due date.

Is Your Body Ready?

Think about whether you have the energy to parent another baby. You are likely to be more tired than the first time. There are a few reasons for this:

- You will be older than you were during your first pregnancy.
- You may not have had a chance to get back in shape after giving birth.
- You'll have another child (or children) to take care of while you are pregnant.

During your prepregnancy visit, you and your ob-gyn should talk about how you can be as healthy as possible:

- You should talk about getting back to your weight before your last pregnancy. Gaining too much weight between pregnancies may lead to complications. These complications may include **high blood pressure** and gestational diabetes.

- You should talk about taking a daily prenatal vitamin with *folic acid* to help prevent **neural tube defects (NTDs)**. The vitamin should have at least 400 micrograms (mcg) of folic acid. The label may show this amount as 667 mcg dietary folate equivalents (DFE).

- You should talk about your **vaccinations** to be sure they are up to date (see Chapter 25, "Protecting Yourself From Infections").

As you plan your next pregnancy, follow the same healthy habits you did the first time around. Review Chapter 1, "Getting Ready for Pregnancy."

You're Pregnant Already

While every pregnancy is different, there are a few things you can expect. The changes your body goes through won't be such a surprise this time around. And you may not have the roller coaster of emotions that you did with your last pregnancy.

How Will It Be Different?

Some things about your next pregnancy will be different this time around:

- You'll show earlier—In fact, you may need to start wearing maternity clothes before your fourth month. That's because your abdominal muscles were stretched by your last pregnancy and may not have regained strength. As a result, these muscles may not hold the **uterus** in or up as well as they did during the last pregnancy.

- You'll feel the baby move sooner—You may feel this baby move a few weeks earlier than you felt your first baby move. The baby isn't really moving sooner. You just know what it feels like this time.

- You'll notice **Braxton Hicks contractions** sooner—Braxton Hicks contractions may happen during the second **trimester** rather than the third trimester, for example.

- Your breast changes are different—Your breasts may not be as tender or grow as much as they did before. If you breastfed your first baby, your breasts may begin to leak earlier in pregnancy.

Possible Problems

Even though every pregnancy is different, you'll likely have some of the same discomforts you had the first time. Knowing this can help you prepare for them. For example, if you had constipation or **hemorrhoids** last time, you can try to prevent these problems early on by eating plenty of fiber, drinking plenty of water, and exercising regularly.

If you're healthy and had no serious problems the last time, your risk of complications now is low. But if you have certain medical conditions (called "preexisting conditions"), they can cause problems during pregnancy. These conditions include high blood pressure and **diabetes mellitus**. Your ob-gyn can help you make sure these conditions are under control.

If you had any serious complications during or after your last pregnancy, you may be at higher risk of these problems again. If you had one of the following complications, schedule a visit with your ob-gyn as soon as you know you're pregnant. You can find out how to recognize symptoms earlier. There also may be steps you can take to reduce your risks:

- Preterm birth—Women who've had a preterm birth are two to three times more likely to have another one. Your ob-gyn may tell you to avoid heavy physical activity and watch for the signs of preterm labor. You may be offered additional testing, such as an **ultrasound exam** to measure the length of your **cervix**. Certain treatments may be suggested depending on your situation (see Chapter 35, "When Labor Starts Too Soon: Preterm Labor, Prelabor Rupture of Membranes, and Preterm Birth").

- Preterm **prelabor rupture of membranes (PROM)**—Preterm PROM can happen even when there are no known risk factors. But the risk of preterm PROM happening in another pregnancy is higher if you have had it before. Your ob-gyn may recommend certain treatments and monitoring if you have a history of preterm PROM (see Chapter 35, "When Labor Starts Too Soon: Preterm Labor, Prelabor Rupture of Membranes, and Preterm Birth").

- **Postpartum depression**—Talk with your ob-gyn about what you can do to reduce your risk of postpartum depression this time around. Your ob-gyn may recommend that you take an **antidepressant** right after you give birth to prevent postpartum depression. If you were taking an antidepressant before pregnancy, your ob-gyn can help you decide whether to continue taking medication during your pregnancy. If you do continue taking medication, changes may be made to the type or dosage. For more information, see Chapter 19, "Your Postpartum Care."

- Gestational diabetes—If you had gestational diabetes in your first pregnancy, you are more likely to have it again. Also, up to half of women with gestational diabetes develop diabetes later in life. This means you should have your **glucose** (blood sugar) level tested beginning 4 to 12 weeks after giving birth and then at least once every 1 to 3 years. Your ob-gyn may discuss ways to lower your diabetes risk through diet, exercise, and possibly medication (see Chapter 31, "Diabetes During Pregnancy").

- **Preeclampsia**—If you had preeclampsia or **eclampsia** in an earlier pregnancy, you have a higher risk of having it again. You should see your ob-gyn early in pregnancy, and ideally before pregnancy, to discuss it. Your ob-gyn can assess whether you have other risk factors (such as **obesity**, high blood pressure, or type 2 diabetes), do certain tests, and give you advice about staying healthy. You also should be familiar with the signs and symptoms of preeclampsia and know how to reach your ob-gyn right away if you have any of them (see Chapter 30, "Hypertension and Preeclampsia").

- **Fetal growth restriction**—Women who have given birth to a smaller-than-normal baby are at increased risk of having a smaller baby the next time. Your ob-gyn may order a series of ultrasound exams during your second pregnancy to monitor your baby's growth (see Chapter 38, "Growth Problems").

Telling Your Other Children

When is the best time to tell your other children that you're having another baby? You know your children best, so it's really your decision when to tell them. It depends on how old your children are and how you think they will handle the news.

Some experts suggest that you wait until sometime after your first trimester, when the risk of **miscarriage** decreases. You may want to wait until after a healthy pregnancy is confirmed by listening for the baby's cardiac activity or by ultrasound exam. With very young children, it may be good to wait until you start to show. Young children may have a hard time imagining you are carrying a baby if your body still looks the same. It can be easier to explain once you have a bump.

Whenever you share the news, remind your children that you love them and that the new baby won't change that. Involve your children in your pregnancy as much as you can. The relationship between siblings is one of the longest and most important ones in life. These tips can help encourage the bond right from the start:

- Involve children in choosing the baby's name.
- Tell your children about the role they can play in helping you with the new baby.
- Read books together about pregnancy and on being a big brother or sister.
- Show your children their own baby pictures.
- Take your children shopping and ask them to pick out items for the new baby.

You may want to set up the baby's room early. If you need to move your children out of a crib or into a different room, do it as early as possible so that they don't feel displaced by the new baby. You can ask them to help decorate the room. You might even suggest that they pick a few of their old toys to give to the baby.

Remember that welcoming another baby into the family may bring both happiness and anxiety for your other children. Do your best to plan for the new arrival to help make the transition as easy as possible.

RESOURCES

Before Pregnancy: Planning for Pregnancy
www.cdc.gov/preconception/planning.html
Prepregnancy care information from the Centers for Disease Control and Prevention that's relevant to all parents-to-be, whether they're having their first baby or their second and beyond.

Birth of a Second Child
https://kidshealth.org/en/parents/second-child.html
Tips and advice from KidsHealth for getting your kids ready for a new baby.

Your Pregnancy and Childbirth
www.acog.org/MyPregnancy
Website from the American College of Obstetricians and Gynecologists (ACOG) with information on pregnancy, labor, delivery, and postpartum care. Includes the latest information from the experts in women's health care, questions answered by ACOG ob-gyns, pregnancy stories from real women, and an A–Z directory of health topics covering pregnancy and beyond.

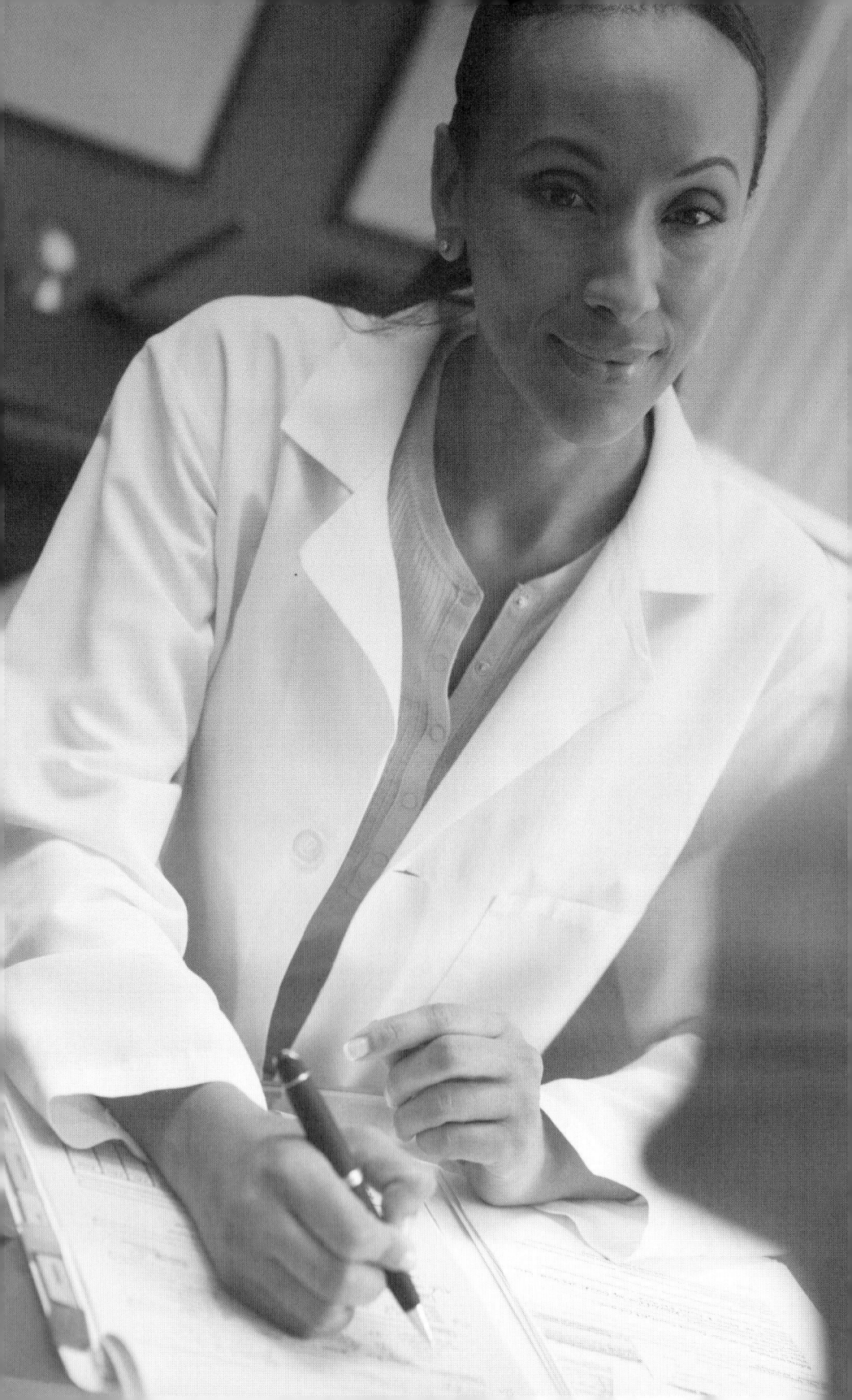

PART 11

Resources and Tools

Terms You Should Know

A

Acceleration: An increase in the heart rate of a fetus.
Accidental Bowel Leakage: Involuntary loss of control of the bowels. This condition can lead to leakage of solid stool, liquid stool, mucus, or gas. Also called fecal incontinence.
Acquired Immunodeficiency Syndrome (AIDS): A group of signs and symptoms, usually of severe infections, in a person who has human immunodeficiency virus (HIV).
Adjuvants: Substances used in vaccines that help the body create a stronger immune response to the vaccine.
Alpha-fetoprotein (AFP): A protein made by a fetus. AFP can be found in amniotic fluid and in a pregnant woman's blood.
Amniocentesis: A procedure in which amniotic fluid and cells are taken from the uterus for testing. The procedure uses a needle to withdraw fluid and cells from the sac that holds the fetus.
Amnionicity: The number of amniotic (inner) membranes that surround fetuses in a multiple pregnancy. When multiple fetuses have only one amnion, they share an amniotic sac.
Amniotic Fluid: Fluid in the sac that holds the fetus.
Amniotic Sac: Fluid-filled sac in a woman's uterus. The fetus develops in this sac.
Amniotomy: Artificial rupture (bursting) of the amniotic sac.
Anal Incontinence: Involuntary loss of solid stool, liquid stool, mucus, or gas through the anus. Also called accidental bowel leakage.
Analgesia: Relief of pain without loss of muscle function.
Analgesic: A drug used to ease pain.
Anemia: Abnormally low levels of red blood cells in the bloodstream. Most cases are caused by iron deficiency (lack of iron).
Anencephaly: A type of defect that happens when the fetus's head and brain do not develop normally.

Anesthesia: Relief of pain by loss of sensation.

Anesthesiologist: A doctor who is an expert in pain relief.

Anesthetic: A drug used to prevent pain.

Aneuploidy: Having an abnormal number of chromosomes. Types include trisomy, in which there is an extra chromosome, or monosomy, in which a chromosome is missing. Aneuploidy can affect any chromosome, including the sex chromosomes. Down syndrome (trisomy 21) is a common aneuploidy. Others are Patau syndrome (trisomy 13) and Edwards syndrome (trisomy 18).

Anorexia Nervosa: An eating disorder that causes a person to severely restrict food so they lose weight. People with this disorder fear weight gain and have a distorted body image.

Antibiotics: Drugs that treat certain types of infections.

Antibodies: Proteins in the blood that the body makes in reaction to foreign substances, such as bacteria and viruses.

Antidepressants: Drugs that are used to treat depression.

Antigen: A substance that can trigger an immune response and cause the body to make an antibody.

Antiphospholipid Syndrome (APS): A disorder that can lead to abnormal blood clotting and pregnancy problems.

Anus: The opening of the digestive tract through which bowel movements leave the body.

Apgar Score: A measurement of a baby's response to birth and life on its own, taken 1 minute and 5 minutes after birth.

Areola: The darker skin around the nipple.

Arteries: Blood vessels that carry oxygen-rich blood from the heart to the rest of the body.

Assisted Reproductive Technology (ART): Treatments or procedures that are done to start a pregnancy. This may include handling eggs and sperm or embryos.

Assisted Vaginal Delivery: The use of forceps or a suction device to help guide the fetal head out of the birth canal.

Aura: A sensation or feeling experienced just before the onset of certain disorders like migraine attacks or epileptic seizures. These sensations may be flashing lights, a particular smell, dizziness, or seeing spots.

Autoimmune Disorder: A condition in which the body attacks its own tissues.

Autopsy: An exam done on a dead body to learn the cause of death.

Autosomal Dominant Disorder: Genetic disorder caused by one defective gene. The defective gene is located on one of the chromosomes that is not a sex chromosome.

Autosomal Recessive Disorder: Genetic disorder caused by two defective genes, one inherited from each parent. The defective genes are located on one of the pairs of chromosomes that are not the sex chromosomes.

Autosomes: Any of the chromosomes that are not the sex chromosomes. In humans, there are 22 pairs of autosomes.

B

Baby Blues: Feelings of sadness, fear, anger, or anxiety occurring about 3 days after childbirth and usually ending within 1 to 2 weeks.

Bacteria: One-celled organisms that can cause infections in the human body.

Bacterial Vaginosis (BV): A condition in which the normal balance of bacteria is changed by an overgrowth of other bacteria. Symptoms may include vaginal discharge, fishy odor, pain, itching, and burning.

Bariatric Surgery: Surgical procedures that cause weight loss. These procedures are used to treat obesity.

Barrier Methods: Birth control that stops sperm from entering the uterus, such as condoms.

Basal Body Temperature (BBT): The temperature of the body at rest.

Bilirubin: A yellow substance that is formed when red blood cells break down. High levels of bilirubin in the blood cause jaundice in newborns.

Biophysical Profile (BPP): A test that uses ultrasound to measure a fetus's breathing, movement, muscle tone, and heart rate. The test also measures the amount of fluid in the amniotic sac.

Birth Control: Devices or medications used to prevent pregnancy.

Birth Control Implant: A small, single rod that is inserted under the skin in the upper arm. The implant releases a hormone to prevent pregnancy.

Birth Defect: A physical problem that is present at birth.

Bladder: A hollow, muscular organ in which urine is stored.

Blastocyst: The stage of embryo development that occurs 4 to 5 days after fertilization.

Body Mass Index (BMI): A number calculated from height and weight. BMI is used to determine whether a person is underweight, normal weight, overweight, or obese.

Bone Loss: The gradual loss of calcium and protein from bone, making it brittle and more likely to break.

Braxton Hicks Contractions: False labor pains.

Breakthrough Bleeding: Vaginal bleeding that happens in between regular periods.

Breech Presentation: A position in which the feet or buttocks of the fetus appear first during birth.

Bulimia Nervosa: An eating disorder in which a person binges on food and then forces vomiting or abuses laxatives.

C

Calcium: A mineral stored in bone that gives it hardness.

Calorie: A unit of heat used to express the fuel or energy value of food.

Canavan Disease: An inherited disorder that causes ongoing damage to brain cells.

Cardiologist: A doctor with special training in diagnosing and treating diseases of the heart and blood vessels.

Cardiovascular Disease: Disease of the heart and blood vessels.

Carpal Tunnel Syndrome: A condition that causes numbness, tingling, and pain in the fingers and hand.

Carrier: A person who shows no signs of a disorder but could pass the gene to his or her children.

Carrier Screening: A test done on a person without signs or symptoms to find out whether he or she carries a gene for a genetic disorder.

Catheter: A tube used to drain fluid from or give fluid to the body.

Cell: The smallest unit of a structure in the body. Cells are the building blocks for all parts of the body.

Cell-Free DNA: DNA from the placenta that moves freely in a pregnant woman's blood. Analysis of this DNA can be done as a noninvasive prenatal screening test.

Cephalic Presentation: A head-down position of a fetus before birth.

Cerclage: A procedure in which the cervical opening is closed with stitches to prevent or delay preterm birth.

Cerebral Palsy: A disorder of the nervous system that affects movement, posture, and coordination. This disorder is present at birth.

Certified Lactation Consultants: Counselors who have taken a training course in breastfeeding education.

Cervical Insufficiency: A condition in which the cervix is unable to hold a pregnancy in the uterus in the second trimester.

Cervical Ripening: When the cervix softens to prepare for labor.

Cervix: The lower, narrow end of the uterus at the top of the vagina.

Cesarean Birth: Birth of a fetus from the uterus through an incision (cut) made in the woman's abdomen.

Cesarean Delivery: Delivery of a fetus from the uterus through an incision (cut) made in the woman's abdomen.

Chancre: A sore caused by syphilis that is found at the place of infection.

Chemotherapy: Treatment of cancer with drugs.

Chickenpox: A contagious disease caused by a virus that results in small, fluid-filled blisters on the skin. Also called varicella.

Chlamydia: A sexually transmitted infection caused by bacteria. This infection can lead to pelvic inflammatory disease and infertility.

Cholesterol: A natural substance that is a building block for cells and hormones. This substance helps carry fat through the blood vessels for use or storage in other parts of the body.

Chorioamnionitis: A condition during pregnancy that can cause unexplained fever with uterine tenderness, a high white blood cell count, rapid heart rate in the fetus, rapid heart rate in the woman, and/or foul-smelling vaginal discharge.

Chorion: The outer membrane that surrounds the fetus.

Chorionic Villus Sampling (CVS): A procedure in which a small sample of cells is taken from the placenta and tested.

Chorionicity: The number of chorionic (outer) membranes that surround the fetuses in a multiple pregnancy.

Chromosomes: Structures that are located inside each cell in the body. They contain the genes that determine a person's physical makeup.

Circumcision: The surgical removal of a fold of skin called the foreskin that covers the glans (head) of the penis.

Cleft Lip: A birth defect that causes an opening or split in the upper lip or roof of the mouth.

Cleft Palate: A birth defect that causes an opening or split in the roof of the mouth.

Clubfoot: A birth defect in which the foot is misshaped and twisted out of position.

Colostrum: A fluid that comes out of the breasts at the beginning of milk production.

Combined Spinal–Epidural (CSE) Block: A form of pain relief. Pain medications are injected into the spinal fluid (spinal block) and given through a thin tube into a space at the base of the spine (epidural block).

Complete Blood Count (CBC): A blood test that measures and describes different cell types in the blood.

Complications: Diseases or conditions that happen as a result of another disease or condition. An example is pneumonia that occurs as a result of the flu. A complication also can occur as a result of a condition, such as pregnancy. An example of a pregnancy complication is preterm labor.

Computed Tomography (CT): A type of X-ray that shows internal organs and structures in cross section.

Cone Biopsy: Surgical removal of cone-shaped wedges of cervical tissue.

Congenital: A condition that a person has from birth.

Congenital Rubella Syndrome (CRS): A condition that can be found in a newborn after a fetus has been infected with the rubella virus (German measles) during the first trimester of pregnancy. Long-term complications can include heart and eye problems, deafness, and being mentally slow.

Congenital Varicella Syndrome: A condition that can be found in a newborn after a fetus has been infected with varicella (chickenpox), usually during the first or second trimester of pregnancy. Long-term complications can include eye problems, brain damage, and misshaped limbs.

Conjunctivitis: Inflammation or infection of the tissue that covers the inside of the eyelids and the outer surface of the eye.

Contraction Stress Test: A test to measure a fetus's heart rate during mild contractions of a woman's uterus.

Contrast Agents: Substances that are injected into a vein or artery during certain X-ray procedures. Contrast agents make it easier to see structures or tissues.

Corticosteroids: Drugs given for arthritis or other medical conditions. These drugs also are given to help fetal lungs mature before birth.

Crowning: One of the last phases of childbirth when a large part of the fetus's scalp is visible at the vaginal opening.

Cystic Fibrosis (CF): An inherited disorder that causes problems with breathing and digestion.

Cytomegalovirus (CMV): A virus that can be transmitted to a fetus if a woman becomes infected during pregnancy. CMV can cause hearing loss, mental disability, and vision problems in newborns.

D

Deceleration: A decrease in the heart rate of a fetus.

Deep Vein Thrombosis (DVT): A condition in which a blood clot forms in veins in the leg or other areas of the body.

Dehydration: A condition that happens when the body does not have as much water as it needs.

Dental Dam: A thin piece of latex or polyurethane used between the mouth and the vagina or anus during oral sex. Using a dental dam can help protect against sexually transmitted infections (STIs).

Depression: Feelings of sadness for periods of at least 2 weeks.

Diabetes Mellitus: A condition in which the levels of sugar in the blood are too high.

Diagnostic Tests: Tests that look for a disease or cause of a disease.

Diamnionic–Dichorionic: Describes twin embryos in which each twin has its own gestational sac surrounded by a layer of membranes (the inner amnion and the outer chorion) and two separate placentas. These twins are usually fraternal (non-identical, with different genetic material), but sometimes can be identical (have the same genetic material).

Diamnionic–Monochorionic: Describes twin embryos formed from the same egg in which each twin has its own gestational sac surrounded by its own inner layer of membranes (the amnion), but a single outer layer of membranes (the chorion) that surrounds both sacs together. These twins share a single placenta and are identical (have the same genetic material).

Diastolic Blood Pressure: The force of the blood in the arteries when the heart is relaxed. It is the lower reading when blood pressure is taken.

Dilation: Widening the opening of the cervix.

Dilation and Curettage (D&C): A procedure that opens the cervix so tissue in the uterus can be removed using an instrument called a curette.

Dilation and Evacuation (D&E): A procedure that can be used after 12 weeks of pregnancy. The cervix is opened and the contents of the uterus are removed using instruments and a suction device.

Discordant: A large difference in the size of fetuses in a multiple pregnancy.

DNA: The genetic material that is passed down from parent to child. DNA is packaged in structures called chromosomes.

Dominant Disorder: A genetic disorder caused by one gene.

Doppler Ultrasound Exam: A type of ultrasound in which sound waves can tell how fast an object is moving. Doppler ultrasound can be used to find the heartbeat of a fetus or how fast blood is moving through a vein or artery.

Doula: A birth coach who gives continual emotional and physical support to a woman during labor and childbirth.

Down Syndrome (Trisomy 21): A genetic disorder that causes abnormal features of the face and body, medical problems such as heart defects, and mental disability. Most cases of Down syndrome are caused by an extra chromosome 21 (trisomy 21).

E

Early Term: In pregnancy, the period from 37 weeks and 0 days through 38 weeks and 6 days.

Eclampsia: Seizures occurring in pregnancy or after pregnancy that are linked to high blood pressure.

Ectopic Pregnancy: A pregnancy in a place other than the uterus, usually in one of the fallopian tubes.

Edwards Syndrome (Trisomy 18): A genetic condition that causes serious problems. It causes a small head, heart defects, and deafness.

Effacement: Thinning out of the cervix.

Egg: The female reproductive cell made in and released from the ovaries. Also called the ovum.

Ejaculates: The release of semen from the penis at the time of orgasm.

Elective Delivery: A delivery that is done for a nonmedical reason.

Elective Procedure: A planned, nonemergency procedure that is chosen by a patient or health care professional. The procedure is seen as positive for the patient but not absolutely necessary.

Electronic Fetal Monitoring: A test in which instruments are placed on a woman's abdomen and used to record the heartbeat of the fetus and contractions of the woman's uterus.

Embryo: The stage of development that starts at fertilization (joining of an egg and sperm) and lasts up to 8 weeks.

Emergency Contraception (EC): Methods that are used to prevent pregnancy after a woman has had sex without birth control, after the method has failed, or after a rape.

Endometrial Ablation: A minor surgical procedure in which the lining of the uterus is destroyed to stop or reduce menstrual bleeding.

Endometriosis: A condition in which tissue that lines the uterus is found outside of the uterus, usually on the ovaries, fallopian tubes, and other pelvic structures.

Endometritis: Infection of the lining of the uterus.

Endometrium: The lining of the uterus.

Epidural Block: A type of pain medication that is given through a tube placed in the space at the base of the spine.

Epilepsy: A group of disorders in which the normal activity in the brain suddenly becomes abnormal. This can lead to seizures.

Episiotomy: A surgical cut made in the area between the vagina and the anus to widen the vaginal opening for delivery.

Erection: A lengthening and hardening of the penis.

Estimated Due Date (EDD): The estimated date that a baby will be born.

Estrogen: A female hormone produced in the ovaries.

Exclusive Breastfeeding: Feeding a baby only breast milk and no other foods or liquids, unless advised by the baby's doctor.

Expanded Carrier Screening: A blood test to screen for a large number of genetic disorders.

External Cephalic Version (ECV): A technique, performed later in pregnancy, in which the doctor attempts to manually move a breech baby into the head-down position.

F

Factor V Leiden: A genetic disorder that can increase the chance of developing blood clots.

Fallopian Tubes: Tubes through which an egg travels from the ovary to the uterus.

False-Negative: A test result that says you do not have a condition when you do.

False-Positive: A test result that says you have a condition when you do not.

Fecal Incontinence: Involuntary loss of control of the bowels. This condition can lead to leakage of solid stool, liquid stool, mucus, or gas. Also called accidental bowel leakage.

Fertility Awareness: A collection of ways to track a woman's natural body functioning and determine when she is most likely to get pregnant.

Fertilization: A multistep process that joins the egg and the sperm.

Fetal Alcohol Spectrum Disorder (FASD): A group of physical, mental, behavioral, and learning disabilities that can occur in a person whose mother drank alcohol during pregnancy.

Fetal Alcohol Syndrome (FAS): The most severe disorder resulting from alcohol use during pregnancy. FAS can cause abnormalities in brain development, physical growth, and facial features of a baby or child.

Fetal Blood Sampling: A procedure in which a sample of blood is taken from the fetus's umbilical cord and tested.

Fetal Fibronectin: A protein that is produced by fetal cells. It helps the amniotic sac stay connected to the lining of the uterus.

Fetal Growth Restriction: A condition in which a fetus has an estimated weight that is less than 90 percent of other fetuses of the same pregnancy age.

Fetus: The stage of human development beyond 8 completed weeks after fertilization.

Fibroids: Growths that form in the muscle of the uterus. Fibroids usually are noncancerous.

Fluorescence in Situ Hybridization (FISH): A screening test for common chromosome problems. The test is done using a tissue sample from an amniocentesis or a chorionic villus test.

Folate: A B vitamin that women need before and during pregnancy. When found in prenatal vitamins it is called folic acid.

Folic Acid: A vitamin that reduces the risk of certain birth defects when taken before and during pregnancy.

Follicle: The sac-like structure in which an egg develops inside the ovary.

Follicle-Stimulating Hormone (FSH): A hormone made by the pituitary gland in the brain that helps an egg to mature.

Forceps: An instrument placed around the fetus's head to help guide it out of the birth canal during birth.

Foreskin: A layer of skin covering the end of the penis.

Fragile X Syndrome: A genetic disease of the X chromosome that is the most common inherited cause of mental disability.

Fraternal Twins: Twins that have developed from two different fertilized eggs.

Full Term: The period of pregnancy from 39 weeks and 0 days through 40 weeks and 6 days.

Fundal Height: The distance from your pubic bone to the top of your uterus. When measured throughout pregnancy, the fundal height helps determine the size and growth rate of the fetus.

G

Gastroschisis: A birth defect in which a hole in the abdominal wall of the fetus lets the bowel stick out. This defect can be diagnosed during pregnancy with ultrasound and treated with surgery after birth.

General Anesthesia: The use of drugs that create a sleep-like state to prevent pain during surgery.

Genes: Segments of DNA that contain instructions for the development of a person's physical traits and control of the processes in the body. The gene is the basic unit of heredity and can be passed from parent to child.

Genetic Counselor: A health care professional with special training in genetics who can provide expert advice about genetic disorders and prenatal testing.

Genetic Disorders: Disorders caused by a change in genes or chromosomes.

Geneticist: A specialist in the study of genes, genetic variation, and heredity.

Genital Herpes: A sexually transmitted infection (STI) caused by a virus. Herpes causes painful, highly infectious sores on or around the vulva and penis.

Genitals: The sexual or reproductive organs.

Gestational Age: How far along a woman is in her pregnancy, usually reported in weeks and days.

Gestational Diabetes: Diabetes that starts during pregnancy.

Gestational Hypertension: High blood pressure that is diagnosed after 20 weeks of pregnancy.

Gestational Trophoblastic Disease (GTD): A rare disorder of pregnancy in which cells from the placenta grow abnormally.

Gingivitis: Inflammation of the gums.

Glucose: A sugar in the blood that is the body's main source of fuel.

Gonadotropin-releasing Hormone (GnRH): A hormone made in the brain that tells the pituitary gland when to produce follicle-stimulating hormone (FSH) and luteinizing hormone.

Gonorrhea: A sexually transmitted infection that can lead to pelvic inflammatory disease, infertility, and arthritis.

Granuloma Gravidarum: A growth on the gums that can develop during pregnancy.

Group B Streptococcus (GBS): A type of bacteria that many people carry normally and can be passed to the fetus at the time of delivery. GBS can cause serious infection in some newborns. Antibiotics are given to women who carry the bacteria during labor to prevent newborn infection.

Gynecology: The branch of medicine that involves care of the female reproductive system and breasts.

H

HELLP Syndrome: A severe type of preeclampsia. HELLP stands for **h**emolysis, **el**evated **l**iver enzymes, and **l**ow **p**latelet count.

Hematologist: A doctor with special training in diagnosing and treating diseases of the blood.

Hemoglobinopathies: Any inherited disorder that affects the number or shape of red blood cells in the body. Examples include sickle cell disease and the different forms of thalassemia.

Hemolytic Disease of the Newborn (HDN): A type of anemia that can affect a fetus or newborn. HDN is caused by the breakdown of the fetus's red blood cells by antibodies in a woman's blood.

Hemophilia: A disorder caused by a mutation on the X chromosome. Affected people are usually males who lack a substance in the blood that helps clotting. People with hemophilia are at risk of severe bleeding from even minor injuries.

Hemorrhage: Heavy bleeding.

Hemorrhoids: Swollen blood vessels located in or around the anus.

Hepatitis: Infection of the liver that can be caused by several types of viruses.

Hepatitis A: An infection caused by a virus that can be spread by contaminated food or water.

Hepatitis B: An infection caused by a virus that can be spread through blood, semen, or other body fluid infected with the virus.

Hepatitis B Immune Globulin (HBIG): A substance given to provide temporary protection against infection with hepatitis B virus.

Hepatitis C: An infection caused by a virus that can be spread by sharing needles used to inject drugs.

Herpes Zoster (Shingles): A disease caused by re-awakening of the varicella zoster (chickenpox) virus in people who have had chickenpox. Shingles cause a painful rash and blisters.

Heterozygous: A term to describe when a person has one defective copy and one normal copy of a gene.

High Blood Pressure: Blood pressure above the normal level. Also called hypertension.

Homozygous: A term to describe when a person has two defective copies of a gene.

Hormone: A substance made in the body that controls the function of cells or organs.

Human Chorionic Gonadotropin (hCG): A hormone made during pregnancy. Checking for this hormone is the basis for most pregnancy tests.

Human Immunodeficiency Virus (HIV): A virus that attacks certain cells of the body's immune system. If left untreated, HIV can cause acquired immunodeficiency syndrome (AIDS).

Human Papillomavirus (HPV): The name for a group of related viruses, some of which cause genital warts and some of which are linked to cancer of the cervix, vulva, vagina, penis, anus, mouth, and throat.

Hydatidiform Mole: An abnormal pregnancy that happens when a sperm fertilizes an egg that does not contain any genetic material. This type of pregnancy may be precancerous and must be treated. Also called a molar pregnancy.

Hydramnios: A condition in which there is an excess amount of amniotic fluid in the sac surrounding the fetus.

Hyperemesis Gravidarum: Severe nausea and vomiting during pregnancy that can lead to loss of weight and body fluids.

Hypertension: High blood pressure.

Hyperthyroidism: A condition in which the thyroid gland makes too much thyroid hormone.

Hysterectomy: Surgery to remove the uterus.

Hysteroscopy: A procedure in which a lighted telescope is inserted into the uterus through the cervix to view the inside of the uterus or perform surgery.

I

Identical Twins: Twins that have developed from a single fertilized egg and that are usually genetically identical.

Immune: Protected against infectious disease.

Immune System: The body's natural defense system against viruses and bacteria that cause disease.

Implantation: The stage of pregnancy when the blastocyst attaches to the wall of the uterus.

Implantation Bleeding: A small amount of spotting or bleeding that happens early in pregnancy, about 2 weeks after ovulation. This may be a sign that a fertilized egg has attached to the lining of the uterus.

In Vitro Fertilization (IVF): A procedure in which an egg is removed from a woman's ovary, fertilized in a laboratory with the man's sperm, and then transferred to the woman's uterus to achieve a pregnancy.

Incompetent Cervix: A cervix that begins to dilate (open) earlier than it should in pregnancy without uterine contractions.

Induced Abortion: An intervention to end a pregnancy so that it does not result in a live birth.

Infertility: The inability to get pregnant after 1 year of having regular sexual intercourse without the use of birth control.

Inflammatory Bowel Disease (IBD): The name for a group of diseases that cause inflammation of the intestines. Examples include Crohn's disease and ulcerative colitis.

Influenza: An infection with the flu virus that most commonly affects the mouth, throat, nose, and lungs. Symptoms include fever, headache, muscle aches, cough, nasal congestion, and extreme fatigue. Complications can occur in severe cases, including pneumonia and bronchitis.

Influenza Vaccine: A shot given to protect against the flu.

Inherited Disorders: Disorders caused by a change in a gene that can be passed from parents to children.

Insulin: A hormone that lowers the levels of glucose (sugar) in the blood.

Internal Os: The internal opening of the cervix into the uterus.

International Board-Certified Lactation Consultant (IBCLC): A health care professional who specializes in managing the medical aspects of breastfeeding. IBCLCs are certified by the International Board of Lactation Consultant Examiners.

Intimate Partner Violence: The use of physical, sexual, or emotional threats or actions against a current or former romantic partner. This type of violence is aimed at establishing control over the other person.

Intrahepatic Cholestasis of Pregnancy: A liver condition that develops during pregnancy.

Intrauterine Device (IUD): A small device that is inserted and left inside the uterus to prevent pregnancy.

Intravenous (IV) Line: A tube inserted into a vein and used to deliver medication or fluids.

Irritable Bowel Syndrome (IBS): A digestive disorder that can cause gas, diarrhea, constipation, and belly pain.

Isotretinoin: A prescription drug with vitamin A that is used to treat acne. The drug can cause severe birth defects and should not be taken during pregnancy.

J–K

Jaundice: A buildup of bilirubin (a brownish yellow substance formed from the breakdown of red cells in the blood) that causes the skin to have a yellowish appearance.

Karyotype: An image of a person's chromosomes, arranged in order of size.

Kegel Exercises: Pelvic muscle exercises. Doing these exercises helps with bladder and bowel control as well as sexual function.

Kick Count: A record kept during late pregnancy of the number of times a fetus moves over a certain period.

Kidney: An organ that filters the blood to remove waste that becomes urine.

Kidney Disease: A general term for any disease that affects how the kidneys function.

L

Labia: Folds of skin on either side of the opening of the vagina.

Labor Augmentation: Steps taken to stimulate the uterus to have more contractions that are longer and closer together. Labor augmentation is done after labor has started on its own but contractions have slowed or stopped.

Labor Induction: The use of medication or other methods to start labor.

Laborists: Obstetrician–gynecologists (ob-gyns) who work only in a hospital to care for women in labor and to deliver babies.

Lactation: Production of breast milk.

Lactational Amenorrhea Method (LAM): A temporary method of birth control that is based on the natural way the body prevents ovulation when a woman is breastfeeding.

Lactose: A sugar found in many dairy products.

Lactose Intolerance: Being unable to digest lactose, a sugar found in many dairy products.

Laminaria: Slender rods made of natural or synthetic material that expand when they absorb water. Laminaria are inserted into the opening of the cervix to widen it.

Lanugo: Soft, downy hair that covers the fetus's body.

Laparoscope: A thin, lighted telescope that is inserted through a small incision (cut) in the abdomen to view internal organs or to perform surgery.

Laparoscopy: A surgical procedure in which a thin, lighted telescope called a laparoscope is inserted through a small incision (cut) in the abdomen. The laparoscope is used to view the pelvic organs. Other instruments can be used with it to perform surgery.

Last Menstrual Period (LMP): The date of the first day of the last menstrual period before pregnancy. The LMP is used to estimate the date of delivery.

Late Term: In pregnancy, the period from 41 weeks and 0 days through 41 weeks and 6 days.

Laxatives: Products that are used to help empty the bowels.

Ligaments: Bands of tissue that connect bones or support large internal organs.

Linea Nigra: A line running from the belly button to pubic hair that darkens during pregnancy.

Listeria: A type of bacteria that causes foodborne illness.

Listeriosis: A type of illness you can get from bacteria found in unpasteurized milk, hot dogs, luncheon meats, and smoked seafood.

Live, Attenuated Influenza Vaccine: An influenza (flu) vaccine with live viruses that have been changed to not cause disease. It is given as a nasal spray. It is not recommended for pregnant women.

Local Anesthesia: The drugs that stop pain in a part of the body.

Lochia: Vaginal discharge that happens after delivery.

Long-Acting Reversible Contraception (LARC): Birth control methods that are highly effective in preventing pregnancy and can be used for several years. These include the intrauterine device (IUD) and the birth control implant.

Loop Electrosurgical Excision Procedure (LEEP): A procedure that removes abnormal tissue from the cervix using a thin wire loop and electric energy.

Low Birth Weight: Weighing less than 5 1/2 pounds (2,500 grams) at birth.

Lupus: An autoimmune disorder that affects the connective tissues in the body. The disorder can cause arthritis, kidney disease, heart disease, blood disorders, and complications during pregnancy. Also called systemic lupus erythematosus or SLE.

Luteinizing Hormone (LH): A hormone made in the pituitary gland that helps an egg to be released from the ovary.

M

Macrosomia: A condition in which a fetus grows more than expected, often weighing more than 8 pounds and 13 ounces (4,000 grams).

Magnesium Sulfate: A drug that may help prevent cerebral palsy when it is given to women in preterm labor who may deliver before 32 weeks of pregnancy.

Magnetic Resonance Imaging (MRI): A test to view internal organs and structures by using a strong magnetic field and sound waves.

Malaria: A disease caused by a parasite that is spread through mosquito bites.

Malignant: A way to describe abnormal cells or tumors that are able to spread to other parts of the body.

Malpresentation: Any time the fetus is not in a head-down position.

Mastitis: Infection of the breast tissue that can occur during breastfeeding.

Maternal–Fetal Medicine (MFM) Specialist: An obstetrician–gynecologist with additional training in caring for women with high-risk pregnancies. Also called a perinatologist.

Measles–Mumps–Rubella (MMR) Vaccine: A shot given to protect against measles, mumps, and rubella. The shot contains live viruses that have been changed to not cause disease. The shot is not recommended for pregnant women.

Melanin: A dark pigment that gives color to the skin and hair.

Melasma: A common skin problem that causes brown to gray-brown patches on the face. Also known as the "mask of pregnancy."

Meningitis: Inflammation of the covering of the brain or spinal cord.

Meningococcal Disease: Inflammation of the coverings of the brain and spinal cord caused by a bacteria called meningococcus.

Menopause: The time when a woman's menstrual periods stop permanently. Menopause is confirmed after 1 year of no periods.

Menstrual Cycle: The monthly process of changes that occur to prepare a woman's body for possible pregnancy. A menstrual cycle is defined as the first day of menstrual bleeding of one cycle to the first day of menstrual bleeding of the next cycle.

Menstrual Period: The monthly shedding of blood and tissue from the uterus.

Menstruation: The monthly shedding of blood and tissue from the uterus that happens when a woman is not pregnant.

Metabolism: The physical and chemical processes in the body that maintain life.

Microarray: A technology that examines all of a person's genes to look for certain genetic disorders or abnormalities. Microarray technology can find very small genetic changes that can be missed by the routine genetic tests.

Microcephaly: A birth defect in which a baby's head and brain are smaller than normal. Babies with microcephaly may have seizures, developmental delays, mental disability, vision and hearing problems, and problems with balance and movement.

Milk Ducts: Small tubes that bring milk from milk lobules to the nipple.

Milk Lobules: Small structures in the breast that make and store milk when a woman is breastfeeding.

Miscarriage: Loss of a pregnancy that is in the uterus.

Modified Biophysical Profile: A different version of the biophysical profile that is used to check fetal well-being. This profile includes checking the amount of amniotic fluid and the fetal heart rate.

Molar Pregnancy: An abnormal pregnancy that happens when a sperm fertilizes an egg that does not contain any genetic material. This type of pregnancy may be precancerous and must be treated. Also called a hydatidiform mole.

Monoamniotic–Monochorionic: Describes twins formed from the same egg that are both in one sac, instead of two separate sacs. These twins share a single placenta and are identical (have the same genetic material).

Monosomy: A condition in which there is a missing chromosome.

Multifetal Pregnancy Reduction: A procedure used to reduce the number of fetuses in a multiple pregnancy.

Multiple Pregnancy: A pregnancy where there are two or more fetuses.

Multiple Sclerosis (MS): A disease of the nervous system that leads to loss of muscle control.

Mutation: A change in a gene that can be passed from parent to child.

Myometrium: The muscular layer of the uterus.

N

Neonatal Abstinence Syndrome (NAS): A group of problems that happen to a newborn who was exposed to addictive substances before birth. A common cause of NAS is opioid use disorder.

Neonatal Intensive Care Unit (NICU): A special part of a hospital in which sick newborns receive medical care.

Neonatologist: A doctor who specializes in the diagnosis and treatment of disorders that affect newborn infants.

Neural Tube Defect (NTD): A birth defect that results from a problem in development of the brain, spinal cord, or their coverings.

Neurological: Related to the nervous system.

Nitrous Oxide: A gas with no odor that when inhaled causes you to feel relaxed and calm. Also known as laughing gas.

Nonsteroidal Anti-Inflammatory Drug (NSAID): A drug that relieves pain by reducing inflammation. Many types are available over the counter, including ibuprofen and naproxen.

Nonstress Test: A test in which changes in the fetal heart rate are recorded using an electronic fetal monitor.

Nuchal Translucency Screening: A test to screen for certain birth defects, such as Down syndrome, Edwards syndrome, or heart defects. The screening uses ultrasound to measure fluid at the back of the fetus's neck.

Nutrients: Nourishing substances found in food, such as vitamins and minerals.

O

Obesity: A condition characterized by excessive body fat.

Obstetrician–Gynecologist (Ob-Gyn): A doctor with special training and education in women's health.

Obstetrics: The branch of medicine that involves caring for patients that are pregnant or are in labor.

Obstructive Sleep Apnea: A serious sleep disorder that causes a person to have brief pauses in breathing during sleep.

Oligohydramnios: A small amount of fluid around the fetus in pregnancy.

Opioid Use Disorder: A treatable disease that can be caused by frequent opioid use. It is sometimes called opioid addiction.

Opioids: Drugs that decrease the ability to feel pain.

Orgasm: The feelings of physical pleasure that can happen during sexual activity.

Ovarian Cancer: Cancer that affects one or both of the ovaries.

Ovary: Organs in women that contain the eggs necessary to get pregnant and make important hormones, such as estrogen, progesterone, and testosterone.

Ovulate: The act of an ovary releasing an egg.

Ovulation: The time when an ovary releases an egg.

Oxygen: An element that we breathe in to sustain life.

Oxytocin: A hormone made in the body that can cause contractions of the uterus and release of milk from the breast.

P

Parvovirus: A virus that can be passed to the fetus during pregnancy and cause harm.

Patau Syndrome (Trisomy 13): A genetic condition that causes serious problems. It involves the heart and brain, cleft lip and palate, and extra fingers and toes.

Pathogens: Any small life forms that can cause disease.

Pathologist: A doctor that looks at tissues and laboratory tests to diagnose disease.

Pediatrician: A doctor who cares for infants and children.

Pelvic Exam: A physical examination of a woman's pelvic organs.

Pelvic Inflammatory Disease (PID): An infection of the upper female genital tract.

Pelvic Organ Prolapse (POP): A condition in which a pelvic organ drops down. This condition is caused by weakening of the muscles and tissues that support the organs in the pelvis, including the vagina, uterus, and bladder.

Penetration: The act of inserting a penis, finger, or other object into the vagina.

Penis: The male sex organ.

Perineal Tear: A tear that occurs in the area between the vagina and the anus. A tear can happen at the time of vaginal delivery.

Perineum: The area between the vagina and the anus.

Peritoneum: The membrane that lines the abdominal cavity and surrounds the internal organs.

Pertussis: A contagious respiratory infection. Also known as whooping cough.

Pica: The urge to eat things that are not food.

Pituitary Gland: A gland located near the brain that controls growth and other changes in the body.

Placenta: An organ that provides nutrients to and takes waste away from the fetus.

Placenta Accreta: A condition in which part or all of the placenta attaches abnormally to the uterus.

Placenta Previa: A condition in which the placenta covers the opening of the uterus.

Placental Abruption: A condition in which the placenta has begun to separate from the uterus before the fetus is born.

Platelets: Small cells found in the blood that help to stop bleeding.

Pneumococcal Disease: A disease caused by a bacterial infection that can affect the lungs, ears, or brain.

Pneumonia: An infection of the lungs.

Polycystic Ovary Syndrome (PCOS): A condition that leads to a hormone imbalance that affects a woman's monthly menstrual periods, ovulation, ability to get pregnant, and metabolism.

Polyhydramnios: A large amount of fluid surrounding the fetus in pregnancy.

Postpartum: Related to the weeks following the birth of a child.

Postpartum Depression: A type of depressive mood disorder that develops in the first year after the birth of a child. This type of depression can affect a woman's ability to take care of her child.

Postpartum Endometritis: Infection of the lining of the uterus following childbirth.

Postpartum Hemorrhage: Heavy bleeding that occurs after the birth of a baby and the placenta.

Postpartum Sterilization: A permanent procedure that prevents a woman from becoming pregnant, done soon after the birth of a child.

Postterm: In pregnancy, the period equal to or longer than 42 weeks.

Preeclampsia: A disorder that can occur during pregnancy or after childbirth in which there is high blood pressure and other signs of organ injury. These signs include an abnormal amount of protein in the urine, a low number of platelets, abnormal kidney or liver function, pain over the upper abdomen, fluid in the lungs, or a severe headache or changes in vision.

Pre-Exposure Prophylaxis (PrEP): Daily medication taken to help prevent infection with human immunodeficiency virus (HIV). Along with other preventive measures, such as using condoms, PrEP may reduce the risk of getting HIV.

Pregestational Diabetes Mellitus: Diabetes that existed before pregnancy.

Preimplantation Genetic Testing: A type of genetic testing that can be done during in vitro fertilization. Tests are done on the fertilized egg before it is transferred to the uterus.

Prelabor Rupture of Membranes (PROM): Rupture of the amniotic membranes that happens before labor begins. Also called premature rupture of membranes.

Premenstrual Dysphoric Disorder (PMDD): A severe form of premenstrual syndrome (PMS) that interferes with a woman's daily life. Symptoms may include sharp mood swings, irritability, hopelessness, anxiety, problems concentrating, changes in appetite, sleep problems, and bloating.

Premenstrual Syndrome (PMS): A term used to describe a group of physical and behavioral changes that some women experience before their menstrual periods every month.

Prenatal Care: A program of care for a pregnant woman before the birth of her baby.

Prepregnancy: Before pregnancy.

Prepregnancy Care: Medical care that is given before pregnancy to improve the chances of a healthy pregnancy. This care includes a physical exam; counseling about nutrition, exercise, and medications; and treatment of certain medical conditions.

Presentation: A term that describes the part of the fetus that is lowest in the vagina during labor.

Preterm: Less than 37 weeks of pregnancy.

Progesterone: A female hormone that is made in the ovaries and prepares the lining of the uterus for pregnancy.

Progestin: A synthetic form of progesterone that is similar to the hormone made naturally by the body.

Prostaglandins: Chemicals that are made by the body that have many effects, including causing the muscles of the uterus to contract, usually causing cramps.

Proteinuria: The presence of an abnormal amount of protein in the urine.

Pyelonephritis: A kidney infection caused by bacteria.

Q–R

Quickening: The pregnant woman's first feeling of movement of the fetus.

Radiation: A type of energy that is transmitted in the form of rays, waves, or particles.

Recessive Disorder: Genetic disorder caused by two genes, one inherited from each parent.

Rectum: The last part of the digestive tract.

Regional Analgesia: The use of drugs to relieve pain in a region of the body.

Regional Anesthesia: The use of drugs to block sensation in a region of the body.

Respiratory Distress Syndrome (RDS): A condition in which a newborn's lungs are not mature, which causes breathing difficulties.

Rh Factor: A protein that can be found on the surface of red blood cells.

Rh Immunoglobulin (RhIg): A substance given to prevent an Rh-negative person's antibody response to Rh-positive blood cells.

Rheumatoid Arthritis (RA): A chronic disease that causes pain, swelling, redness, and irritation of the joints and changes in the muscles and bones. The condition can become more severe with time.

Rubella: A virus that can be passed to the fetus if a woman becomes infected during pregnancy. The virus can cause miscarriage or severe birth defects.

S

Sciatica: Pain or numbness anywhere along the sciatic nerve. Pain often is felt from the buttock down the back of the leg.

Screening Tests: Tests that look for possible signs of disease in people who do not have signs or symptoms.

Scrotum: The external genital sac in the male that contains the testicles.

Sedative: An agent or drug that eases nervousness or tension.

Seizure Disorders: Any condition that causes seizures, which cause changes in movement, consciousness, mood, or emotions. Epilepsy is one kind of seizure disorder.

Selective Serotonin Reuptake Inhibitors (SSRIs): A type of medication used to treat depression.

Semen: The fluid made by male sex glands that contains sperm.

Sepsis: A condition in which infectious toxins (usually from bacteria) are in the blood. It is a serious condition that can be life threatening. Symptoms include fever, rapid heart rate, breathing difficulty, and mental confusion.

Sex Chromosomes: The chromosomes that determine a person's sex. In humans, there are two sex chromosomes, X and Y. Females have two X chromosomes and males have an X and a Y chromosome.

Sex-Linked Disorders: Genetic disorders caused by a change in a gene located on the sex chromosomes.

Sexual Abuse: Sex acts that are forced on one person by another.

Sexual Intercourse: The act of the penis of the male entering the vagina of the female. Also called "having sex" or "making love."

Sexually Transmitted Infection (STI): An infection that is spread by sexual contact. Infections include chlamydia, gonorrhea, human papillomavirus (HPV), herpes, syphilis, and human immunodeficiency virus (HIV, the cause of acquired immunodeficiency syndrome [AIDS]).

Shoulder Dystocia: A situation during labor when one or both of a fetus's shoulders get stuck inside the woman's body after the fetus's head has come out. Extra steps may be needed to deliver the baby.

Sickle Cell Disease: An inherited disorder in which red blood cells have a crescent shape. The disorder causes chronic anemia and episodes of pain.

Sperm: A cell made in the male testicles that can fertilize a female egg.

Spermicide: Chemical (creams, gels, foams) that inactivate sperm.

Sphincter Muscle: A muscle that can close a bodily opening, such as the sphincter muscle of the anus.

Spina Bifida: A type of birth defect that happens when the spine of the fetus does not completely close during pregnancy. This leads to an exposed spinal cord or membranes, which causes paralysis or weakness of the lower limbs.

Spinal Block: A type of regional anesthesia or analgesia in which pain medications are injected into the spinal fluid.

Spinal Muscular Atrophy (SMA): An inherited disorder that causes wasting of the muscles and severe weakness. SMA is the leading genetic cause of death in infants.
Stem Cells: Cells with the ability to become specialized cells.
Sterilization: A permanent method of birth control.
Stillbirth: Birth of a dead fetus.
Stroke: A sudden interruption of blood flow to all or part of the brain, caused by blockage or bursting of a blood vessel in the brain. A stroke often results in loss of consciousness and temporary or permanent paralysis.
Sudden Infant Death Syndrome (SIDS): The unexpected death of an infant in which the cause is unknown.
Surfactant: A substance made by cells in the lungs. This substance helps keep the lungs elastic and keeps them from collapsing.
Symptothermal Method: A fertility awareness method used to predict when a woman might be fertile. The method uses body temperature and other signs and symptoms of ovulation.
Syphilis: A sexually transmitted infection (STI) that is caused by an organism called Treponema pallidum. This infection may cause major health problems or death in its later stages.
Systolic Blood Pressure: The force of the blood in the arteries when the heart is contracting. It is the higher reading when blood pressure is taken.

T

Tay–Sachs Disease: An inherited disorder that causes mental disability, blindness, seizures, and death, usually by age 5.
Teratogen: An agent that can cause birth defects when a woman is exposed to it during pregnancy.
Testicles: Paired male organs that make sperm and the male sex hormone testosterone. Also called "testes."
Tetanus Toxoid, Reduced Diphtheria Toxoid, and Acellular Pertussis (Tdap) Vaccine: A shot that protects again tetanus, diphtheria, and pertussis (whooping cough).
Thalassemia: A group of inherited anemias.
Thrombophilia: A condition in which the blood does not clot correctly.
Thyroid Gland: A butterfly-shaped gland located at the base of the neck in front of the windpipe. This gland makes, stores, and releases thyroid hormone, which controls the body's metabolism and regulates how parts of the body work.
Thyroid Hormone: The hormone that is made by the thyroid gland.
Tocolytic: A drug used to slow contractions of the uterus.
Toxin: A substance made by bacteria that is poisonous to other living organisms.
Toxoplasmosis: An infection caused by Toxoplasma gondii, an organism that may be found in raw meat, garden soil, and cat feces (stool). This infection can harm a fetus.
Transabdominal Ultrasound Exam: A type of ultrasound in which a device is moved across the abdomen.
Transducer: A device that sends out sound waves and translates the echoes into electrical signals.

Transfusion: Injection of blood, plasma, or platelets into the blood.

Transvaginal Ultrasound Exam: A type of ultrasound in which the device is placed in your vagina.

Trial of Labor After Cesarean Delivery (TOLAC): Labor in a woman who has had a cesarean birth before. The goal is to achieve vaginal birth.

Trichomoniasis: A type of vaginal infection caused by a parasite. This infection is passed through sex.

Triglycerides: A form of body fat found in the blood and tissues. High levels can cause heart disease.

Trimester: A 3-month time in pregnancy. It can be first, second, or third.

Trisomy: A problem where there is an extra chromosome.

Tuberculosis (TB): A disease that affects the lungs and other organs in the body. TB is caused by bacteria.

Turner Syndrome: A problem that affects women when there is a missing or damaged X chromosome. This syndrome causes a webbed neck, short height, and heart problems.

Twin–Twin Transfusion Syndrome (TTTS): A condition of identical twins in which one twin gets more blood than the other during pregnancy.

U

Ultrasound Exam: A test in which sound waves are used to examine inner parts of the body. During pregnancy, ultrasound can be used to check the fetus.

Umbilical Cord: A cord-like structure containing blood vessels. It connects the fetus to the placenta.

Umbilical Cord Prolapse: A problem that causes the umbilical cord to come out of the vagina before delivery. This is an emergency situation during childbirth.

Urethra: A tube-like structure. Urine flows through this tube when it leaves the body.

Urinary Incontinence: Involuntary loss of urine.

Urinary Tract Infection (UTI): An infection in any part of the urinary system, including the kidneys, bladder, or urethra.

Urine: A liquid that is excreted by the body and is made up of wastes, water, and salt removed from the blood.

Uterine Artery Embolization: A procedure to block the blood vessels to the uterus. This procedure is used to stop bleeding after delivery. It is also used to stop other causes of bleeding from the uterus.

Uterine Atony: A condition in which muscles of the uterus do not contract after the birth of a baby and the placenta. The condition is a common cause of bleeding after delivery.

Uterine Rupture: A condition in which the uterus tears during labor.

Uterus: A muscular organ in the female pelvis. During pregnancy, this organ holds and nourishes the fetus.

V

Vaccination: Giving a vaccine to help the body's natural immune system develop protection from a disease.

Vaccine: A substance that helps the body fight disease. Vaccines are made from very small amounts of weak or dead agents that cause disease (bacteria, toxins, and viruses).

Vacuum Aspiration: Removal of the contents of the uterus using a suction device.

Vacuum Device: A suction cup that is applied to the fetus's head to help with birth.

Vagina: A tube-like structure surrounded by muscles. The vagina leads from the uterus to the outside of the body.

Vaginal Birth After Cesarean Delivery: A vaginal birth in a woman who has had a previous cesarean birth.

Varicella: A contagious disease caused by a virus. The disease causes chickenpox and shingles.

Varicella Vaccine: A shot given to protect against chickenpox. The shot is not recommended for pregnant women.

Varicella Zoster Virus: The virus that causes chickenpox and shingles.

Varicose Veins: Swollen, twisted veins often caused by poor blood flow.

Vas Deferens: One of two small tubes that carries sperm from each male testicle to the prostate gland.

Vasectomy: A permanent birth control method for men. In this procedure, a portion of the tube that carries sperm is removed.

Veins: Blood vessels that carry blood from various parts of the body back to the heart.

Ventilator: A machine that blows air into the lungs to help a person breathe.

Vernix: The greasy, whitish coating of a newborn.

Viruses: Agents that cause certain types of infections.

Von Willebrand Disease: A disorder in which the blood does not clot well.

Vulva: The external female genital area.

X–Z

X Chromosome: One of two chromosomes that determine a person's sex. Egg cells carry only the X chromosome.

X-linked Disorders: Genetic disorders caused by defective genes. The genes are located on the X chromosome.

Y Chromosome: One of two chromosomes that determine a person's sex. Sperm cells can carry a Y chromosome or an X chromosome.

Yeast Infection: An infection caused by an overgrowth of a fungus. Symptoms may include itching, burning, and irritation of the vulva or vagina and a thick, white discharge.

Zika: A disease caused by the Zika virus, which is spread through mosquito bites.

Zygote: The single cell formed from the joining of the egg and sperm.

Body Mass Index Chart

To calculate your body mass index (BMI), find your height in inches in the left column. Then look across the line to find your weight in pounds. The number at the top of that column is your BMI.

	NORMAL						OVERWEIGHT					OBESE				
BMI	19	20	21	22	23	24	25	26	27	28	29	30	31	32	33	34	35
HEIGHT (Inches)	BODY WEIGHT (Pounds)																
58	91	96	100	105	110	115	119	124	129	134	138	143	148	153	158	162	167
59	94	99	104	109	114	119	124	128	133	138	143	148	153	158	163	168	173
60	97	102	107	112	118	123	128	133	138	143	148	153	158	163	168	174	179
61	100	106	111	116	122	127	132	137	143	148	153	158	164	169	174	180	185
62	104	109	115	120	126	131	136	142	147	153	158	164	169	175	180	186	191
63	107	113	118	124	130	135	141	146	152	158	163	169	175	180	186	191	197
64	110	116	122	128	134	140	145	151	157	163	169	174	180	186	192	197	204
65	114	120	126	132	138	144	150	156	162	168	174	180	186	192	198	204	210
66	118	124	130	136	142	148	155	161	167	173	179	186	192	198	204	210	216
67	121	127	134	140	146	153	159	166	172	178	185	191	198	204	211	217	223
68	125	131	138	144	151	158	164	171	177	184	190	197	203	210	216	223	230
69	128	135	142	149	155	162	169	176	182	189	196	203	209	216	223	230	236
70	132	139	146	153	160	167	174	181	188	195	202	209	216	222	229	236	243
71	136	143	150	157	165	172	179	186	193	200	208	215	222	229	236	243	250
72	140	147	154	162	169	177	184	191	199	206	213	221	228	235	242	250	258
73	144	151	159	166	174	182	189	197	204	212	219	227	235	242	250	257	265
74	148	155	163	171	179	186	194	202	210	218	225	233	241	249	256	264	272
75	152	160	168	176	184	192	200	208	216	224	232	240	248	256	264	272	279
76	156	164	172	180	189	197	205	213	221	230	238	246	254	263	271	279	287

Source: National Heart, Lung, and Blood Institute. Clinical guidelines on the identification, evaluation, and treatment of overweight and obesity in adults. U.S. Department of Health and Human Services, 1998 June: 139.

BODY MASS INDEX CHART

									EXTREME OBESITY									
36	37	38	39	40	41	42	43	44	45	46	47	48	49	50	51	52	53	54
172	177	181	186	191	196	201	205	210	215	220	224	229	234	239	244	248	253	258
178	183	188	193	198	203	208	212	217	222	227	232	237	242	247	252	257	262	267
184	189	194	199	204	209	215	220	225	230	235	240	245	250	255	261	266	271	276
190	195	201	206	211	217	222	227	232	238	243	248	254	259	264	269	275	280	285
196	202	207	213	218	224	229	235	240	246	251	256	262	267	273	278	284	289	295
203	208	214	220	225	231	237	242	248	254	259	265	270	278	282	287	293	299	304
209	215	221	227	232	238	244	250	256	262	267	273	279	285	291	296	302	308	314
216	222	228	234	240	246	252	258	264	270	276	282	288	294	300	306	312	318	324
223	229	235	241	247	253	260	266	272	278	284	291	297	303	309	315	322	328	334
230	236	242	249	255	261	268	274	280	287	293	299	306	312	319	325	331	338	344
236	243	249	256	262	269	276	282	289	295	302	308	315	322	328	335	341	348	354
243	250	257	263	270	277	284	291	297	304	311	318	324	331	338	345	351	358	365
250	257	264	271	278	285	292	299	306	313	320	327	334	341	348	355	362	369	376
257	265	272	279	286	293	301	308	315	322	329	338	343	351	358	365	372	379	386
265	272	279	287	294	302	309	316	324	331	338	346	353	361	368	375	383	390	397
272	280	288	295	302	310	318	325	333	340	348	355	363	371	378	386	393	401	408
280	287	295	303	311	319	326	334	342	350	358	365	373	381	389	396	404	412	420
287	295	303	311	319	327	335	343	351	359	367	375	383	391	399	407	415	423	431
295	304	312	320	328	336	344	353	361	369	377	385	394	402	410	418	426	435	443

Medical History Form

During your first prenatal care visit, you and your obstetrician–gynecologist (ob-gyn) will talk a lot about your health. It's important to answer all questions honestly and with as much detail as you can. Use this form to help you prepare. You can fill out this form before your visit and bring the book with you, or you can just read it through to see some of the questions that will be asked.

Your Menstrual History

What was the first day of your last menstrual period? _____

Was it a normal period for you in number of days and amount of bleeding? ❏ Y ❏ N

What symptoms have you had since your last menstrual period? _____

Your Past Pregnancies

Total number of pregnancies ____

Number of pregnancies that were:

    Full term ____

    Premature ____

    Miscarriages ____

    Induced abortions ____

    Ectopic pregnancies ____

    Multiple births ____

    Number of living children ____

Fill in the following information for each of your past live births.

Date of Birth	Gestational Age at Birth (Weeks)	Length of Labor (Hours)	Birth Weight	Sex	Type of Delivery (Vaginal, Cesarean, Assisted)	Anesthesia	Place of Delivery	Complications, Including Preterm Labor, High Blood Pressure, Diabetes

Your Medical History

Check all that apply.

____ Medication allergies/reactions
____ Latex allergy/reaction
____ Food/seasonal/environmental allergies
____ Neurologic disease or epilepsy
____ Thyroid dysfunction
____ Breast disease or surgery
____ Lung disease, such as asthma
____ Heart disease
____ Hypertension (high blood pressure)
____ Cancer
____ Hematologic (blood) disorders
____ Anemia
____ Gastrointestinal disorders
____ Hepatitis or liver disease
____ Kidney disease or infection
____ Blood clots in the legs (deep vein thrombosis [DVT])
____ Diabetes mellitus (type 1 or type 2)
____ Gestational diabetes mellitus
____ Autoimmune disorders (lupus, multiple sclerosis, inflammatory bowel disease)
____ Dermatologic (skin) disorders
____ Operations/hospital stays
      If checked, list dates and reasons _____
____ Gynecologic surgery
      If checked, list dates and reasons _____

_____ Uterine abnormality
_____ Anesthetic complications
_____ History of blood transfusions
_____ Infertility
_____ Assisted reproductive technology treatment (IVF, FET)
_____ History of abnormal Pap test results
_____ History of sexually transmitted infection (STI)
_____ Psychiatric illness
_____ Depression, including postpartum depression
_____ Trauma or violence
_____ Polycystic ovary syndrome
_____ Other

Your Lifestyle

Smoking
Do you smoke when you are not pregnant? ❏ Y ❏ N
If yes, how much?_____
Do you currently smoke? ❏ Y ❏ N
If yes, how much?_____

E-cigarettes
Do you vape when you are not pregnant? ❏ Y ❏ N   If yes, how much? _____
Do you currently vape? ❏ Y ❏ N   If yes, how much? _____

Chewed Tobacco, Snuff, Gel Strips
Do you use any of these forms of tobacco when you are not pregnant? ❏ Y ❏ N
If yes, which ones and how much? _____
Do you currently use these forms of tobacco? ❏ Y ❏ N   If yes, which ones and how much? _____

Alcohol
Do you drink alcohol when you are not pregnant? ❏ Y ❏ N
If yes, how much?_____
Do you drink alcohol now? ❏ Y ❏ N
If yes, how much?_____

Drugs (illegal and prescription)
Do you use drugs (including opioids) when you are not pregnant? ❏ Y ❏ N
If yes, what type and how much? _____
Do you use drugs (including opioids) now? ❏ Y ❏ N   If yes, what type and how much?_____

Marijuana (medical or recreational)

Do you use marijuana when you are not pregnant? ❏ Y ❏ N   If yes, what type and how much? _____

Do you use marijuana now? ❏ Y ❏ N   If yes, what type and how much? _____

Your Home Life

Do you feel safe in your current living situation? ❏ Y ❏ N

Do you feel safe with your current partner? ❏ Y ❏ N

If you answered "no" to either question, do not leave this form where your partner may see it. It is important that you protect yourself and your baby by finding a safe place.

Your Genetic Background

Note whether you, your baby's father, or anyone in either of your families has had any of the following conditions:

Condition	Yes	No
Neural tube defect (NTD) (spina bifida, anencephaly)		
Congenital heart defect		
Down syndrome		
Tay–Sachs disease		
Canavan disease		
Familial dysautonomia		
Sickle cell disease or trait		
Hemophilia, thalassemia, or other blood disorder		
Muscular dystrophy		
Cystic fibrosis		
Spinal muscular atrophy (SMA)		
Huntington disease		
Intellectual disability or autism		
Other inherited genetic or chromosomal disorder		
Birth defects not listed above		
Recurrent pregnancy loss or a stillbirth		

Have you or your baby's father had a child with a birth defect not listed above? ❏ Y ❏ N

If yes, what type? _____

Your Medication History

List all medications you take (include supplements, vitamins, herbs, and over-the-counter drugs). Note the strength and dosage. Include recent medications you may have stopped.

Medication (including opioids)	Strength (example: milligrams)	Dosage (how often)	Start date	Stop date, if it applies

Your Infection History

Do you live with someone with tuberculosis (TB) or have you been exposed to TB? ❑ Y ❑ N

Do you or your sexual partner have oral or genital herpes? ❑ Y ❑ N

Have you had a rash or viral illness since your last menstrual period? ❑ Y ❑ N

Have you had a previous child with group B streptococcus (GBS) infection? ❑ Y ❑ N

Have you ever had an STI, such as
    Gonorrhea ❑ Y ❑ N
    Chlamydia ❑ Y ❑ N
    Human immunodeficiency virus (HIV) infection ❑ Y ❑ N
    Syphilis ❑ Y ❑ N
    Human papillomavirus (HPV) infection ❑ Y ❑ N

Do you have hepatitis B virus or hepatitis C virus infection? ❑ Y ❑ N

Have you been exposed to Zika virus? ❑ Y ❑ N

Have you or your partner traveled outside the country recently? ❑ Y ❑ N

Your Vaccination History

Vaccine	Yes (month/year)	No
Tdap (tetanus, diphtheria, and pertussis [whooping cough])		
Influenza (flu)*		
Varicella (chickenpox)*		
Measles–Mumps–Rubella (MMR)*		
Human Papillomavirus (HPV)		
Hepatitis A		
Hepatitis B		
Meningococcal		
Pneumococcal		

*Some vaccines should not be given during pregnancy, including the flu nasal spray (but the flu shot is OK), MMR, and varicella. All women who will be pregnant during flu season (October through May) should get the flu shot at any point during pregnancy. MMR and varicella should be given after pregnancy if needed.

Your Questions

List any questions that you would like to ask your ob-gyn.

_____

_____

_____

_____

_____

_____

_____

_____

Adapted from the Antepartum Record (2017) from the American College of Obstetricians and Gynecologists (ACOG).

Sample Birth Plan

A birth plan is a written outline of what you would like to happen during labor and delivery. This plan lets your obstetrician–gynecologist (ob-gyn) and other health care practitioners know your wishes for your labor and delivery.

Go over your plan with your ob-gyn well before your due date. But keep in mind that having a birth plan does not guarantee that your labor and delivery will go according to that plan. Unexpected things can happen.

Remember that you and your ob-gyn have a common goal: the safest possible delivery for you and your baby. A birth plan is a great starting point, but you should be prepared for changes as the situation dictates.

Birth Plan

Your name: _____

Name of your ob-gyn: _____

Name of your baby's doctor: _____

Type of childbirth preparation:_____

Labor (choose as many you wish)

❏ I would like to be able to move around as I wish during labor.
❏ I would like to be able to drink fluids during labor.

I prefer:

❏ An intravenous (IV) line for fluids and medications
❏ A heparin or saline lock (this device provides access to a vein but is not hooked up to a fluid bag)

❏ I don't have a preference

I would like the following people with me during labor (check hospital or birth center policy on the number of people who can be in the room):

_____

_____

_____

_____

❏ It's OK ❏ not OK for people in training (e.g., medical students or residents) to be present during labor and delivery.

I would like to try the following options if they are available (choose as many as you wish):
❏ A birthing ball
❏ A birthing stool
❏ A birthing chair
❏ A squat bar
❏ A warm shower or bath during labor. I understand that a bath would be used only for the first stage of labor, not during delivery.

Anesthesia Options (choose one):
❏ I do not want anesthesia offered to me during labor unless I specifically request it.
❏ I would like anesthesia. Please discuss the options with me.
❏ I do not know whether I want anesthesia. Please discuss the options with me.

Delivery

I would like the following people with me during delivery (check hospital or birth center policy):

_____

_____

_____

_____

❏ I prefer to avoid an episiotomy unless it is necessary.
❏ I have made prior arrangements for storing umbilical cord blood.

For a vaginal birth, I would like (choose as many as you wish):
❏ To use a mirror to see the baby's birth
❏ For my labor partner to help support me during the pushing stage
❏ For the room to be as quiet as possible

- ❏ For one of my support people to cut the umbilical cord
- ❏ For the lights to be dimmed
- ❏ To be able to have one of my support people take a video or pictures of the birth. (Note: Some hospitals have policies that prohibit videotaping or taking pictures. Also, if it is allowed, the photographer needs to be positioned in a way that does not interfere with performing medical care.)
- ❏ For my baby to be put directly onto my chest immediately after delivery
- ❏ To begin breastfeeding my baby as soon as possible after birth

In the event of a cesarean delivery, I would like the following person to be present with me:

_____

- ❏ I would like to see my baby before he or she is given eye drops.
- ❏ I would like one of my support people to hold the baby after delivery if I am not able to.
- ❏ I would like one of my support people to go with my baby to the nursery.
- ❏ I would like my support person to know what shots my newborn will receive.

Baby Care Plan

Feeding the Baby

I would like to (check one):
- ❏ Breastfeed exclusively
- ❏ Bottle-feed
- ❏ Combine breastfeeding and bottle-feeding

It's OK to offer my baby (check as many as you wish):
- ❏ A pacifier
- ❏ Sugar water
- ❏ Formula
- ❏ None of the above

Nursery and Rooming-In

If available at my hospital or birth center, I would like my baby to stay (check one):
- ❏ In my room with me at all times
- ❏ In my room with me except when I am asleep
- ❏ In the nursery but be brought to me for feedings
- ❏ I don't know yet. I will decide after the birth.

Circumcision

- ❏ If my baby is a boy, I would like him circumcised at the hospital or birth center.

My Postpartum Care Checklist

The postpartum period—the 12 weeks following the birth of a child—is an important time for your health. As you recover from childbirth and learn to care for your baby, your postpartum checkups will help make sure you are

- healing physically, mentally, and emotionally
- feeling good about your health and your baby's care
- feeling that you can ask for help if you need it

Use this checklist to keep track of the things you want to talk about with your obstetrician–gynecologist (ob-gyn).

My Self-Care

- ❏ I am not getting enough sleep and rest
- ❏ I have enough support at home but would like more help
- ❏ I do not have enough support at home

My Health and Lifestyle

- ❏ I would like to learn more about healthy eating and exercise
- ❏ I have questions about managing my health conditions (such as high blood pressure, diabetes)
- ❏ I want to stop smoking and need help
- ❏ I would like to drink less alcohol and need help
- ❏ I need help with my drug use
- ❏ I am concerned about keeping myself and my family safe

My Bleeding

❏ I am concerned about the amount, color, or odor of my bleeding

My Incision/Tear

❏ My incision/tear has been healing well, but I have questions
❏ I am concerned that my incision/tear is not healing well

My Bladder

❏ I have pain or other problems when emptying my bladder
❏ I leak urine with activity or after feeling an urge to urinate

My Bowel Movements

❏ I have problems moving my bowels (pain, constipation)
❏ I have trouble holding my gas or stool

My Feelings

In the past 7 days, I have
❏ felt anxious or worried for no clear reason
❏ been sad, scared, or panicky
❏ been so unhappy that I can't sleep
❏ been crying a lot
❏ had thoughts of harming myself or my baby

My Family Planning

❏ I want to talk about timing for future pregnancies
❏ I want to talk about birth control

My Sex Life

❏ I am interested in having sex but have questions
❏ I am not interested in having sex and would like to talk about it

My Breastfeeding and Baby Care

❏ Breastfeeding is going well, but I have questions
❏ I am having a hard time breastfeeding (nipple pain, problems with latching)
❏ I have concerns about going back to work/school and maintaining my milk supply
❏ I have questions about caring for my baby

Environmental Exposure History Form

Before you get pregnant, or as soon as you learn you are pregnant, talk with your obstetrician–gynecologist (ob-gyn) about agents that you may be exposed to at home or work. This is called an environmental exposure history.

Use this form to review the places and situations in which you may be exposed to toxic substances. Share the results with your ob-gyn.

Assessment	Check All That Apply
Questions About Your Home or Apartment	
Do you live in a house or apartment building built before 1978?	
Do you live next door to or near an industrial plant, commercial business, dump site, or nonresidential property?	
Have you or anyone living with you ever been treated for lead poisoning?	
Do you plan to remodel your living space?	
Have you recently added new furniture, refurnished furniture, or new carpeting?	
Have you ever lived outside the United States?	
Have you ever moved because of a health problem?	
Do you use a mercury thermometer at home?	
Where does your drinking water come from?	
Private well	
City water supply	
Are you exposed to secondhand smoke at home?	

Assessment	Check All That Apply
Do any people living in your home have unusual symptoms?	
Has the health or behavior of your pets changed?	
Do you or your family members use imported pottery, ceramics, china, or crystal for cooking, eating, or drinking?	
Do you or your landlord use insect sprays and powders, weed killer, or rat or mouse poison?	
Inside your house or apartment	
Outside your house or apartment	
To control bugs on your pets (flea and tick sprays/powders)	
Questions About What You Use and Eat	
Have you ever used any home remedies such as azarcon, greta, or pay-loo-ah?	
Have you ever eaten candy or canned food imported from foreign countries?	
Have you ever eaten any of the following?	
Clay	
Soil or dirt	
Pottery	
Paint chips	
Do you wear jewelry that may contain lead (including jewelry purchased from large-volume stores or from vending machines)?	
Do you eat any of the following types of fish?	
Bigeye tuna	
King mackerel	
Marlin	
Orange roughy	
Shark	
Swordfish	
Tilefish (from Gulf of Mexico)	
Do you eat any locally caught fish?	
Questions About Your Workplace	
Have you been exposed to any of the following at work, now or in the past?	
Metals	
Dust or fibers	
Chemicals	

Assessment	Check All That Apply
Fumes	
Radiation	
Biologic agents	
Loud noise or vibration	
Extreme heat or cold	
If you are exposed to metals, dusts, fibers, or chemicals at work, do you get the material on your skin?	
Do you wash your work clothes at home?	
Do you shower at work?	
Do you use safety equipment such as gloves, masks, or respirators?	
Does anyone in your house have contact with metals, dust, fibers, chemicals, fumes, radiation, or biologic agents?	
Questions About Your Hobbies	
Do you do any of the following in your spare time?	
Painting	
Darkroom processing for making prints	
Sculpting	
Welding	
Woodworking	
Restoring old cars	
Shooting firearms	
Creating stained glass	
Creating ceramics	
Gardening	

Sources: Consortium for Reproductive Environmental Health in Minority Communities; U.S. Department of Health and Human Services, Agency for Toxic Substances and Diseases Registry; U.S. Food and Drug Administration, Advice About Eating Fish: What Pregnant Women and Parents Should Know.

My Postpartum Care Team Chart

When you plan your postpartum care, you should think about who you want on your care team. This is a group of family, friends, and health care practitioners who can help with medical care, emotional support, child care, pet care, and household tasks.

Talk with your obstetrician–gynecologist (ob-gyn) about your postpartum care team before you give birth. After you give birth, review and update your plan as needed. Fill in this chart with the names and contact information for everyone on your postpartum care team.

Care Team Member	What They Do	Name(s)	Contact Information
Your family and friends	• Offer emotional support • Help with child care, pet care, breastfeeding support, meals, chores, transportation		
Your maternal care practitioner	• Takes care of your health during the postpartum period		
Your baby's doctor	• Takes care of your baby's health		
Other professionals	• Help with medical conditions • Help with breastfeeding • Other special needs		

Index

Page numbers followed by italicized letters *b*, *f*, and *t* indicate boxes, figures, and tables, respectively.

A

Abdomen
　defects, prenatal screening for, 564
　physical exam, 28
Abdominal binder, 288
Abdominal muscles, postpartum exercises for, 289
Abdominal pain. *See also* Lower abdominal pressure
　ectopic pregnancy and, 63, 64
　foodborne illness and, 368*b*, 369
　lower, calling ob-gyn about, 91*b*
　lower, ligaments and, 86–87
　miscarriage and, 63
　placental abruption and, 618
　PROM and, 599
　second trimester aches and, 86
　severe, calling ob-gyn about, 140*b*, 160*b*
　upper, calling ob-gyn about, 168*b*
　upper, preeclampsia and, 117, 502*b*, 508
Abdominal support garments, 100
Abortion. *See also* Induced abortion
　RhIg after, 611
Acceleration, of baby's heart rate, 585
Accidental bowel leakage, 286–287
Accreditation Association for Ambulatory Health Care, 93, 183
Accredited freestanding birth centers, 93, 183
ACE. *See* Angiotensin-converting enzyme inhibitors
Acesulfame-K (Sunett), 75, 366
Acetaminophen, 114, 277
Aches and pains, 114. *See also* Backache; Headache; Pain or pains
Acid reflux, 112–113
Acne, 70–71, 337

Acquired immunodeficiency syndrome (AIDS), 79, 425–426
Active labor, 232, 234*f*, 235, 237–238, 633*t*
Activity restriction, 146
Addiction, 544–545
Adjuvants, 411
Administration for Children and Families, U.S. Department of Health and Human Services, 200
Adoption, 8
Aerobic activities, 380–381
Affordable Care Act, 322, 328, 443, 449
African descent, carrier screening, 9*t*, 554*t*, 567*t*
After the baby is born. *See also* Postpartum period
　the first few hours, 269–273
　frequently asked questions on, 463–464
　getting to know your baby, 272–273
　going home, 277–279, 278*b*
　multiple sclerosis and, 533
　preeclampsia and, 508
　preterm birth and, 603
　resources, 279
　your baby's health, 270–272
　your recovery after delivery, 275–277
Afterbirth pains, 289, 309
Afterpains, 307
AFP. *See* Alpha-fetoprotein
Age of father, 562, 563*b*, 646
Age of mother
　another baby and, 670
　cesarean delivery on request and, 255
　Down syndrome risk and, 561
　ectopic pregnancy and, 649
　genetic disorder risks and, 563*b*

717

Age of mother (continued)
   miscarriage and, 646
   multiple pregnancy and, 469
   placenta accreta and, 619
   placental abruption and, 618
   preeclampsia and, 507
   preterm birth risk and, 595b
   screening or diagnostic testing and, 562
   TOLAC and, 263
AIDS. *See* Acquired immunodeficiency syndrome
Air travel, 404, 446–447
Airline staff, hazards for, 405b
Albuterol, 532
Alcohol
   avoiding or limiting, 364, 520
   birth defects and, 400–401
   breastfeeding and, 313–314
   fetal growth restriction and, 624
   methotrexate for ectopic pregnancy and, 651
   pregnancy complications and, 56–57
   prepregnancy care and, 13
   T-ACE test, 57b
   as teratogen, 396
Allergic reactions, 205, 259
Allergy remedies, 60, 454
Alpha-fetoprotein (AFP), 92, 570t, 571, 574
Alpha-thalassemia, 9t, 567t
American Academy of Family Physicians, 31, 251
American Academy of Pediatrics (AAP)
   baby's doctor choices and, 107, 193
   on birth centers within hospital complexes, 92, 183
   on breastfeeding, 159, 306
   on car seats, 161, 200, 201
   on circumcision, 200
   on skin-to-skin care, 279
American Association of Birth Centers, 93, 183
American College of Allergy, Asthma, and Immunology, 547
American College of Cardiology, 503, 503b
American College of Nurse–Midwives (ACNM), 31
American College of Obstetricians and Gynecologists (ACOG)
   on bed rest, 146–147
   on birth centers within hospital complexes, 92, 183
   on coronavirus, pregnancy, and breastfeeding, 437, 464
   on COVID and pregnancy, 439, 453
   on eating during labor, 170
   on episiotomy, 463
   on exclusive breastfeeding, 306
   Find an Ob-Gyn tool, 25b, 31, 65, 445, 449
   on home births, 93, 183
   on opioid use disorder, 13, 210
   on postpartum office visits, 282–283, 283f
American College of Radiology, 589
American Dental Association, 93
American Diabetes Association, 526
American Heart Association, 503, 503b, 547
American Medical Association DoctorFinder tool, 445, 448

American Midwifery Certification Board (AMCB), 25
American Psychiatric Association, 547
American Society for Reproductive Medicine, 482, 655
Amniocentesis
   cervical insufficiency and, 600
   diagnostic testing with, 92, 564, 572–573, 573f
   month 5, 103
   multiple pregnancy and, 479
   as prenatal diagnostic testing, 81t
   Rh incompatibility and, 609
   RhIg after, 611
   TTTS treatment with, 476
   ultrasound guidance of, 580
Amnioinfusion, 636
Amnionicity, 472, 473f
Amniotic fluid
   for amniocentesis, 572, 573f
   amount, ultrasound exam of, 580
   baby's warmth after birth and, 272
   biophysical profile of, 519, 586–587
   breech presentation and, 247
   chorioamnionitis of, 225
   decrease, labor induction and, 219, 220
   delivery before 39 weeks and, 171
   embolism, 638
   fetal well-being tests of, 583
   gestational hypertension or preeclampsia and, 509
   infections, 425
   low level of, 601, 635
   month 5, 102
   postterm pregnancy and, 175
   pregestational diabetes mellitus and, 521
   problems, 134
   umbilical cord prolapse and, 636
   in vagina, PROM and, 598
   water intake and, 359, 459
   weeks 9 to 12 and, 68
   weight of, 55b
   weight of mother and, 488
Amniotic sac. *See also* Rupture of membranes
   baby at week 38 in, 163
   multiple pregnancy and, 472, 476
   prelabor rupture of, 146
   PROM or preterm PROM and, 593
   sex during pregnancy and, 458
   sexual activity and, 111
   stripping the membranes of, 174, 176, 224, 634
   weeks 1 to 5 and, 62
   weeks 17 to 20 and, 95
Amniotomy, 224–225, 634
Anal incontinence, 246
Anal sex, 422
Analgesia, 204, 207–208
Analgesics, 144, 185, 204
Anemia. *See also* Hemolytic disease of the newborn
   ABO incompatibility and, 608

INDEX • 719

Anemia (continued)
    blood tests for, 74*b*, 76, 78, 130, 357
    celiac disease and, 539
    craving nonfood items and, 91, 402, 497–498
    delayed cord clamping and, 190
    delivery before 39 weeks and, 173*b*, 174, 222*b*, 256
    Doppler ultrasound exam for, 588
    exercise and, 376
    molar pregnancy and, 653
    RhIg and, 611
    Rh-negative woman with antibodies and, 612
Anencephaly, 12*b*, 53*b*, 356
Anesthesia. *See also* Anesthetics
    for cesarean delivery, 256
    complications, cesarean delivery and, 226
    consent forms, 236
    general, 144, 256, 343, 652
    during labor, ob-gyn views on, 26
    local, 205, 206, 275, 454
    problems, cesarean delivery and, 173, 244, 255, 628
    problems, obesity and, 492
    recovery from, 275
    regional, 144, 205–208
    solid food restrictions before, 170
    spinal block for, 207–208
    von Willebrand disease and, 538
Anesthesiologists, 144, 204, 206, 256, 493, 538
Anesthetics, 144, 185, 204–205, 256
Aneuploidy, 479, 560, 561
Anger, 290, 661
Angiotensin-converting enzyme inhibitors (ACE inhibitors), 398
Animal care workers, hazards for, 405*b*
Anorexia nervosa, 496–497, 544–545
Another baby
    already pregnant with, 671–673
    resources, 674
    telling your other children about, 673–674
    timing for, 669–670
Antacids, 113
Antibiotics
    for baby's eyes, 274
    for cesarean delivery, 257, 493, 639
    for chlamydia, 425
    for chorioamnionitis, 632
    for GBS, 155, 156, 431–432
    for gonorrhea, 425
    for listeriosis, 369
    for mastitis, 318
    for postpartum endometritis, 640
    PROM management and, 598, 599
    for urinary tract infections, 78, 90
Antibodies
    ABO incompatibility and, 607–608
    antiphospholipid syndrome and, 537–538
    breastfeeding and, 302, 463
    in colostrum, 306
    in cord blood, 189, 463

Antibodies (continued)
    expressed milk and, 324
    flu shot during pregnancy and, 414, 415*f*
    infections and, 409–410
    against Rh factor, 78, 130
    Rh incompatibility and, 609
    Tdap vaccine and, 7
Antibody screen, 130, 610, 612
Antidepressants, 127, 291–292, 398, 672
Anti-epilepsy drugs, 53*b*
Antigens, 607
Antihistamines, 454
Antiphospholipid syndrome (APS), 532, 537–538, 624, 658
Antithrombin deficiency, 536–537
Anus
    genital warts around, 418
    hemorrhoids near, 141
    HPV and cancer of, 418
    injuries, assisted vaginal delivery and, 246
    midline episiotomy and, 463
    nerves, accidental bowel leakage and, 286–287
    perineum and, 276
Anxiety, 91*b*, 127, 133*b*, 290–292
Anxiety disorders, 544–545
Apgar score, 271–272, 271*t*
Appetite loss, 489
APS. *See* Antiphospholipid syndrome
Aqua aerobics, 380
Arab descent, carrier screening, 9*t*, 554*t*, 567*t*
Areolas, 72, 308, 308*f*
Arsenic, workplace, 60
ART. *See* Assisted reproductive technology
Arteries, 501
Artery disease, 508
Arthritis, 297*t*
Arthritis Foundation, 547
Artists, hazards for, 405*b*
Asian Americans, 514
Asian descent, genetic disorders and, 554*t*
Asian Indian descent, genetic disorders and, 554*t*
Aspartame (Equal and NutraSweet), 75, 366
Aspiration, general anesthesia and, 208
Aspirin, 114, 511, 525, 543
Assisted reproductive technology (ART), 8
Assisted vaginal delivery
    abnormal labor and, 239, 634
    labor not going as planned and, 243
    ob-gyn views on, 26
    overview, 243–244, 462
    risks, 245–246
    types, 245, 245*f*
    von Willebrand disease and, 538–539
Association of Women's Health, Obstetric and Neonatal Nurses, 176
Asthma
    birth defects with medications for, 398
    flu shot during pregnancy and, 415
    during pregnancy, 529, 530–532, 531*f*
    resources, 547
    severity and control, 532*t*

Attenuated, defined, 6
Aura, migraines with, 337
Autism, vaccines and, 415
Auto shop workers, hazards for, 405b
Autoimmune conditions or disorders, 507, 529
Autopsy, 659
Autosomal dominant disorders, 557, 560f
Autosomal recessive disorders, 557–558, 560f
Autosomes, 555
Avoidant restrictive food intake disorder (ARFID), 497
Azelaic acid, 71

B

B vitamins, 358. *See also* under vitamin B
Babies, 433. *See also* After the baby is born; Another baby; Fundal height measurement; Newborns; specific months
    ABO incompatibility and, 608
    body language, 310, 311b
    breastfeeding technique, 308, 308f, 310
    development of, 33–41f, 580
    doctor for. *See* Doctor, baby's
    fetal growth restriction. *See* Fetal growth restriction
    fetal well-being tests. *See* Fetal well-being monitoring tests
    flu vaccine and, 414
    genital herpes and, 423
    growth problems. *See* Growth problems for baby
    hepatitis B infection and, 417
    hepatitis C infection and, 433
    large. *See* Macrosomia
    mother's eating disorders and, 496
    mother's gestational diabetes and, 491, 515–516
    movement. *See* Baby's movement
    position. *See* Baby's position
    sex, learning of, 101–102, 103, 580
    ultrasound portraits of, 457, 581
    weight of mother and, 487, 491
Baby blues, 278b, 290, 481. *See also* Depression; Feelings
Baby-Friendly USA, 161, 306, 328
    hospitals or birth centers designated as, 158–159, 305b
Baby-led latch, 308
Baby's clothes, washing and organizing, 166b
Baby's movement
    biophysical profile of, 586–587
    feeling, 85–86, 671
    fetal well-being tests and, 583
    go to hospital, 168b, 232
    less than normal, 98b
    normal, 96–97
    ultrasound exams of, 580
Baby's position. *See also* Turning the baby
    feeling baby's movements and, 96
    locating, 247–248
    moving to head-down position for birth, 159

Baby's position (continued)
    preparing for delivery, 171
    ultrasound exams of, 580
    umbilical cord prolapse and, 636
Baby's size. *See also* Fetal growth restriction; Growth problems for baby; Macrosomia
    postterm pregnancy and, 175, 220
    TOLAC and, 262
Back labor, 462
Back problems, pain relief during childbirth and, 203
Backache (pain). *See also* Lower back pain
    calling ob-gyn about, 113b, 133b, 140b, 160b
    exercise and, 55
    preterm labor and, 117, 133, 145, 159, 475b, 596b
    tips to lessen, 100
    UTIs and, 90
Bacteria. *See also* Infections
    bottles and nipples and, 324b
    dental care and, 454
    digestive system, IBD and, 540
    disease-causing, vaccines and, 6, 410–411
    eye infection in newborns and, 274
    foodborne illness and, 362, 368–370, 368b
    infections and, 409, 410
    safe food preparation and, 370–371
    in sushi and sashimi, 458
    urine culture for, 78
Bacterial vaginosis (BV), 90, 428
Baking soda mouth rinse, 88
Balance, 114–115, 379, 381–382
Ball shoulder stretch, 385, 385f
Ball wall squat, 385, 385f
Bariatric surgery, 493, 494–495
Barrier methods of birth control, 332, 334–335t, 339–341, 342–343
Basal body temperature (BBT), 19–20, 19f, 342–343
Baths
    during active labor, 238
    cornstarch in, for itchy skin, 141
    for hemorrhoid relief, 141, 287
    for pain relief, 114
    pain relief during early labor and, 185
    pelvic pressure and, 152
    sleep and, 69
    for urination problems, 285
Battery-operated breast pumps, 322
BBT. *See* Basal body temperature
Beauty salon hazards, 405b
Bed. *See also* Birthing beds; Sleep
    raising head of, heartburn and, 113
    waterproof sheet or mattress for, 166b
Bed rest, 146–147, 457, 480, 604
Bedroom, relaxing for sleep and, 70
Behavioral problems, 105, 174, 256
Behavioral therapy, 59
Bending, workplace accommodations for, 440b, 441
Benzoyl peroxide, 71

INDEX • 721

Beta-thalassemia, carrier screening, 9t, 567t
Bilirubin, 608
Binge eating disorder, 497, 544–545
Biophysical profile (BPP)
    fetal growth restriction and, 625
    fetal well-being monitoring with, 584, 585–587, 586f
    gestational diabetes and, 519
    gestational hypertension or preeclampsia and, 509
    multiple pregnancy and, 479
    postterm pregnancy and, 175
    pregestational diabetes mellitus and, 525
Bipolar disorder, 544–545
Birth, giving. *See* Delivery
Birth, preparing for. *See also* Birth plan; Childbirth; Childbirth classes
    birth places, 26, 92–93, 131, 182–183
    birth plan, 182–186
    child care, 197–199
    childbirth classes, 186–187
    choosing your baby's doctor, 191, 193
    decisions about your baby's health, 187–191
    heart disease and, 543
    overview, 181
    packing for the hospital, 191, 192b
    preparing your home for the baby, 193–195, 196b, 197f
    resources, 200–201
Birth centers within hospital complexes, 92, 183, 189
Birth control. *See also* Reversible birth control; specific methods
    after childbirth, 131, 132, 181, 288–289, 295–296, 331, 334–335t, 464
    after miscarriage, 648
    breastfeeding and, 302
    choosing a method for, 331–332
    emergency contraception, 346–347
    fertility awareness, 342–343
    lactational amenorrhea method, 341–342
    permanent, 343–346
    resources, 347
    reversible, 332–341
    stopping, pregnancy and, 20
Birth control implant, 332, 334–335t, 334–336, 464
Birth control injection, 20, 334–335t, 336–337
Birth control patch, 20, 334–335t, 337–339, 338f
Birth control pills, 334–335t, 337–339, 338f, 464, 494, 645. *See also* Combined hormonal birth control methods
Birth control ring, 334–335t, 337–339, 338f
Birth defects. *See also* Genetic disorders
    alcohol and, 400–401
    antidepressants and, 127
    approved vaccines and, 415
    breech presentation and, 247
    delivery before 39 weeks and, 171
    diabetes mellitus and future risk of, 297t
    diagnostic tests, 79
    elevated core body temperature and, 405
    environmental toxins and, 401–403

Birth defects (continued)
    exposure history and, 396–397
    folic acid and, 52, 53b
    hair dye and, 451
    indicated preterm birth and, 601
    infections and, 403
    medications and, 397–400
    mercury in fish and, 365
    multiple pregnancy and, 478–479
    normal ultrasound exam and, 581
    NSAIDs in third trimester and, 114
    overview, 395, 553
    as preexisting health condition, 4
    pregestational diabetes mellitus and, 521
    pseudoephedrine for allergies and, 454
    resources, 407, 577
    screening tests, 79, 92, 564
    stillbirth and, 658
    substance use and, 59
    teratogens and, 395–396
    toxoplasmosis and, 434
    unhealthy substances and, 13
    vitamin A in high doses and, 354
    workplace hazards, 405–406, 405b
    X-rays and other radiation, 403–404
    Zika virus and, 435–436
Birth injuries
    assisted vaginal delivery and, 246
    cesarean delivery and, 80, 173, 244, 255, 259
    gestational diabetes and risk of, 515, 516
    macrosomia and, 628
    shoulder dystocia, 491, 515, 628, 634–635
Birth places, 26, 92–93, 131, 182–183
Birth plan
    components, 182–186
    drafting, 131
    frequently asked questions on, 461
    sample, 182, 187, 189, 708–710
    on your baby's hospital stay, 189
Birthing balls, 185, 212, 214f
Birthing beds, 157, 185, 212
    with squatting bar, 215f
Birthing chairs, 157, 185, 212, 215f
Birthing positions
    alternative, ob-gyn views on, 26
    discussions with your ob-gyn on, 157
    pain management and, 185, 210–211, 235
    pushing and delivery and, 240
    umbilical cord prolapse and, 637
Birthing stools, 157, 185, 212, 214f
Bishop score, 223
Bladder
    empty, active labor and, 238
    infection, preterm PROM and, 597
    injury, cesarean delivery and, 173, 244, 255, 259, 628
    injury, multiple cesarean births and, 80
    Kegel exercises and, 286b, 383
    placenta percreta and, 620
    postpartum problems, 278b, 285
    pregnancy and, 46, 150, 166
    urinary tract infections and, 428–430, 429f

Blastocysts, 43–44
Bleeding. *See also* Hemorrhage; Postpartum hemorrhage; Vaginal bleeding
   in brain, early preterm birth and, 116
   in brain, preterm multiples and, 473
Bleeding disorders, 529, 535–539
Bloating, 46, 55
Blood
   hepatitis C virus transmission and, 432
   HIV transmission and, 425
   hypertension during pregnancy and, 505f
   loss, VBAC and, 80
   shoulder dystocia and, 628
   weight gain during pregnancy and, 55b
Blood clots and clotting. *See also* Deep vein thrombosis
   cesarean delivery and, 259, 492
   drugs for, fetal growth restriction and, 624
   HELLP syndrome and, 507
   lupus and, 534
   obesity, delivery and, 492–493
   symptoms, 535b
Blood clotting disorders
   antiphospholipid syndrome, 532, 537–538, 624, 658
   inherited, 536–537
   postpartum hemorrhage and, 639
   pregnancy and, 529, 535
   resources, 548
Blood disorders
   banked cord blood and, 132
   fetal well-being tests with, 582
   genetic, testing for, 92, 569, 570t, 571
Blood patch, epidural block or spinal block and, 207b
Blood pressure. *See also* High blood pressure; Hypertension
   about, 501–503
   after delivery, 275
   epidural block or spinal block and, 207b
   home monitoring, 29b, 509
   measuring/monitoring, 502, 503b, 506
   medication, pregnancy and, 505
   preeclampsia and, 117, 508
   preeclampsia with severe features and, 510
   prenatal care testing, 28, 62, 155
   readings, 502b
Blood sugar. *See also* Diabetes mellitus; Glucose
   after delivery, pregestational diabetes and, 526
   controlling gestational diabetes and, 516–517
   glucose meter for tracking, 517
   hypoglycemia and, 523
   insulin and absorption of, 513
   low, mother's gestational diabetes and, 515
   during pregnancy, macrosomia and, 627
   testing, diabetes medications and, 519
   testing, gestational diabetes and, 516
   tracking log, 517, 522, 525
Blood tests
   anemia, 74b

Blood tests (continued)
   antibodies, 409–410
   blood type and Rh status, 78, 610
   complete blood count, 76, 78
   cord blood, 240
   Down syndrome, 76, 92, 569
   genetic disorders, 92, 564, 570t, 571
   lead levels, 105
   listeriosis, 433
   newborns, 274–275
   preeclampsia monitoring, 509
   pregnancy, 47
   prenatal care and, 62
   syphilis, 427
Blood transfusion. *See* Transfusion, blood
Blood type incompatibility
   ABO incompatibility, 607–608
   other incompatibilities, 612
   overview, 607
   resources, 612–613
   Rh incompatibility, 608–612
Blood types, 78, 607
Blood vessels
   blood pressure and, 501
   breastfeeding and, 315
   Doppler ultrasound of, 580, 588
   maternal, as connection between mother and baby, 58f
   in placenta, hypertension and, 505f
   sleeping positions and, 99
   uterus contraction and, 241
Blood volume, 542
BMI. *See* Body mass index
Body aches, mastitis and, 318
Body fluids
   hepatitis B transmission and, 417
   salmonellosis and, 369
   STI transmission and, 422, 425, 430
   TB transmission and, 435
   weight gain during pregnancy and, 55b
Body image
   eating disorders and, 487, 495, 498, 499
   during pregnancy, 111, 122
Body mass index (BMI)
   cesarean delivery on request and, 255
   chart for calculating, 700–701
   excessive weight gain during pregnancy and, 297t
   higher, TOLAC and, 263
   low prepregnancy, preterm birth risk and, 595b, 597
   MyPlate food-planning guide on, 360f
   obesity subcategories based on, 490
   preeclampsia and, 507
   VBAC and, 263
   weight gain during pregnancy and, 53–54, 54t, 73, 91, 101, 112, 122, 363t, 456
   weight loss after pregnancy and, 493
Bone loss, 336
Booster seats, 161
Bottle-feeding, 158, 320f, 326
Bottles and nipples, 320, 324b

INDEX • 723

Bowel injury, 80, 173, 255, 259, 628
Bowel problems, postpartum, 285–287
BPP. *See* Biophysical profile
Bradley Method of Natural Childbirth, 144, 186, 216, 217
Brain
    bleeding in, early preterm birth and, 116
    congenital varicella syndrome and, 421
    development, marijuana and, 58
    fetal development of, 41f
    lupus and, 534
    preeclampsia and, 117
    problems, cesarean delivery and, 254
    problems, preterm multiples and, 473
Bras, 72, 189, 289, 325, 377
BRATT diet, 50–51, 167
Braxton Hicks contractions
    another baby and, 671
    as practice contractions, 124, 126
    strength of, as due date nears, 146, 150–151
    true labor compared with, 168, 169, 170t, 229, 231, 232, 233t
    uterus growth and, 133
Break Time for Nursing Mothers Law, 443
Breakthrough bleeding, 338
Breast cancer, 302, 317, 339
Breast implants, 317
Breast milk. *See also* Expressed milk; Human milk; Milk
    delayed lactogenesis, 315–316
    nutrients in, 481
    storing and using, 323
Breast pumps. *See also* Expressed milk
    delayed milk production and, 316
    expressing milk using, 319, 322–323, 323f
    flat or inverted nipples and, 316–317
    health insurance and, 443
    sore nipples and, 314
    workplace types, 325
Breastfeeding. *See also* Expressed milk
    after delivery, 464
    antidepressants and, 292
    babies with NAS and, 210
    baby getting enough milk? 311b
    baby's technique, 308, 310
    benefits, 301–302, 463–464
    birth control implant and, 336
    blocked ducts and, 317–318, 318f
    breast surgery and, 317
    challenges, 314–319
    combined hormonal birth control and, 338
    counselors, postpartum care team and, 284
    decisions on, 158–159, 188–189
    eating disorders and, 496
    engorgement and, 315
    estrogen in birth control pills and, 464
    exclusive, 306
    expressed milk as alternative to, 323–324
    in the first hour, 270
    food and drinks while, 312–314
    genital herpes and, 424

Breastfeeding (continued)
    getting started, 306–308
    health insurance and, 443
    HIV transmission and, 425
    how long? 310, 327
    HPV vaccination and, 419
    infections and, 304b
    information, 304–306, 465
    inverted or flat nipples and, 316–317
    IUDs and, 333
    lactational amenorrhea method and, 341–342
    LARC methods and, 332
    latching on, 308, 308f
    laws, by U.S. states and territories, 328
    let-down reflex, 307, 307f
    low milk supply and, 316
    mastitis and, 318–319
    medications during, 312, 313, 407, 533, 651
    menstrual periods and, 288
    multiple babies, 481
    multiple sclerosis and, 533
    positions, 288, 309b
    pregestational diabetes mellitus and, 526
    pregnancy risk during, 295
    problems, postpartum depression and, 291
    resources, 299, 464–465
    signs that baby wants, 310
    skin-to-skin contact and, 270
    sore nipples and, 314–315
    support, contact information for, 278b
    systemic pain medication and, 204
    thinking about, 115, 181
    twins, 319
    uterine contraction and, 284, 302, 307f
    vaginal bleeding and, 284
    vitamin D and iron supplements, 310, 312
    when to avoid, 303–304
    Zika virus and, 436
Breasts
    changes during pregnancy, 72, 72f, 671
    injuries, delayed milk production and, 316
    lumps, painful new, 282b
    painful, after delivery, 276
    postpartum care for, 278b
    postpartum engorgement, 289
    red streaks on, 282b, 318
    surgery, breastfeeding and, 158, 317
    tender and swollen, pregnancy and, 46
    tenderness, combined hormonal birth control and, 337
    tenderness, ovulation and, 15
    weight gain during pregnancy and, 55b
Breath, baby's first, 270–271
Breathing
    after cesarean delivery, 260, 261b
    Apgar score of, 271t
    baby's, 270, 271–272, 274
    baby's, biophysical profile of, 519, 586–587
    deep, fear of needles and, 411b
    delivery before 39 weeks and, 174, 256
    early preterm birth and, 116

724 • INDEX

Breathing (continued)
    exercises, practicing, 167
    in later weeks of pregnancy, 138
    mother's gestational diabetes and, 515
    for pain relief during labor, 144, 184, 185, 235, 237
    preeclampsia and, 113b, 117, 133b, 502b, 508
    problems, calling ob-gyn about, 112, 140b, 160b, 168b, 282b
    pulmonary embolism and, 535b
    shortness of, exercise and, 377b
    support, preterm birth and, 602
    systemic pain medication and, 204
    tubes, general anesthesia and, 208
Breech presentation. *See also* Birthing positions; Turning the baby
    abnormal labor and, 632
    baby moving to head-down position from, 159
    cesarean delivery and, 254
    delivery options, 250–251
    image of, 231b
    labor induction as unsafe with, 222
    options, 243
    overview, 160–161, 246–247
    PROM and, 598
    resources, 251
    TOLAC and, 262
Bulimia nervosa, 497, 544–545
Buprenorphine, 59, 209

C

Caffeine, 114, 364, 458
Cajun descent, carrier screening, 9t, 563b, 567t
Calcium
    in balanced diet, 351
    breastfeeding and, 312
    celiac disease and, 539
    deficiency, weight-loss surgery and, 494–495
    lactose intolerance and, 459
    during pregnancy, 354, 355t
    vegetarian diets and, 368
Calf pain, 125, 133b, 139–140, 377b. *See also* Deep vein thrombosis
Calories
    breastfeeding and, 302
    empty, active labor and, 362
    healthy pregnancy weight and, 9, 351, 487
    hot flashes and, 113
    IBD and, 540
    restrictions, mental skills and, 495
    weight control and, 363, 493
Campylobacteriosis, 369
Canavan disease, 563b
Cancer. *See also* specific types of
    future risks, 297t
    HIV and AIDS and, 425
    HPV types and, 418
    multifactorial genetic disorders and, 559
Carbamazepine, 398

Carbohydrates, 351, 352–353, 517–518, 522, 524
Cardiac activity
    checking on, 102, 145
    elective labor induction and, 221
    listening to, 76f, 95
    miscarriage diagnosis and, 646
    ultrasound exams, 580
    weeks 1 to 8 and, 62
Cardio activities, 380–381
Cardiologists, 542
Cardiovascular disease, 337, 339
Carpal tunnel syndrome, 152
Carriers, of genetic disorders, 560f
    autosomal recessive disorders, 557–558
    expanded carrier screening, 457, 564, 566–568
    results and what to do next, 568
    screening recommendations, 8, 9t, 554t, 563b, 567t
Cars
    car seat buying and installing tips, 161, 196b, 200
    pain getting out of, 133b
    preparing for the baby and, 154, 193–195, 194f, 201, 278
    travel and safety in, 200, 447b, 448
Catheters
    for amnioinfusion, 636
    for cesarean delivery anesthesia, 256
    for epidural block, 205, 206
    for pain relief medications, 277
    ripening the cervix and, 224
    urinary, cesarean delivery and, 257, 260
Cats, toxoplasmosis and, 434, 461
CBC. *See* Complete blood count
Celiac disease
    as autoimmune disorder, 532
    pregnancy and, 10, 366, 529, 539
    resources, 372, 548
Cell-free DNA test, 92, 479, 570t, 571
Cells
    chromosomes in, 646
    zygote formation, 43
Centers for Disease Control and Prevention (CDC)
    on breastfeeding with Zika virus, 436
    on COVID-19, 406, 437, 439, 453, 464
    on formula safety, 326–327
    on hepatitis C testing, 79, 433
    on HPV vaccination, 419
    on infant feeding, 328
    on lead exposure, 401
    on preconception planning, 20, 674
    on preterm birth, 604
    on STIs, 437
    Travelers' Health website, 446, 449
    on vaccines, 410, 411, 437
    on Zika virus and pregnancy, 437, 465
Central European Jewish descent, carrier screening, 9t, 554t, 563b, 567t
Cephalic presentation, 160–161, 231b
Ceramic pottery, lead-glazed, 106
Cerclage, 376, 600

Cerebral palsy, 116, 473, 593, 626, 632
Certified lactation consultants, 299, 481
Certified midwives (CMs), 24, 25, 26
Certified nurse–midwives (CNMs), 24–25, 26
Certified professional midwives (CPMs), 25
Cervical cancer, 418
Cervical cap, 296, 334–335t, 340, 341f, 464
Cervical insufficiency, 376, 599–600
Cervical mucus. See also Vaginal discharge
  birth control implant and, 334
  birth control injection and, 336
  combined hormonal birth control and, 337
  fertility awareness method, 342–343
  as fluid leakage from vagina, 146, 597
  hormonal IUDs and, 333
  monitoring, 19
  plug, 169, 229, 232
  progestin-only pills and, 339
Cervix. See also Dilation; Effacement
  assisted vaginal delivery and, 244
  Braxton Hicks contractions and, 126
  breech presentation and, 250
  changes during labor, 230b, 236, 633
  changes during pregnancy, 90
  checking for preterm labor, 479, 595
  chlamydia or gonorrhea infections and, 424
  chorionic villus sampling and, 574, 574f
  HPV and cancer of, 418
  inflamed, vaginal bleeding and, 133
  nipple stimulation and, 462, 588
  pelvic exam, 30f
  placenta previa and, 615
  preparing for birth, 145
  preterm labor and, 593–594
  ripening, 223–224
  short, 595, 595b, 596, 604
  sperm through, 17
  stripping the membranes and, 174
  tears, postpartum hemorrhage and, 638
  ultrasound exam of, 580
Cesarean birth
  asthma during pregnancy and, 530
  calling ob-gyn after, 261b
  chronic hypertension and, 504–505
  consent forms, 236
  delayed milk production and, 315
  eating during labor and, 170, 238
  elective delivery and, 171
  endometritis and, 639–640
  exercise and, 375
  GBS and, 156
  gestational diabetes and risk of, 516
  hepatitis C virus and, 433
  incision pain, 288
  inducing labor before 39 weeks and, 172, 221b
  IUD insertion after, 333
  large babies and, 514, 628
  multiple pregnancy with umbilical cord complications, 476
  obesity and, 491, 492–493
  partners and, 145

Cesarean birth (continued)
  placenta previa and, 134, 615
  postpartum hemorrhage and, 639
  postpartum sterilization and, 343
  pregestational diabetes mellitus and, 525
  previous, delivery before 39 weeks and, 171
  previous, ECV and, 248
  previous, ob-gyn discussions on, 80
  previous, placenta previa and, 615
  previous, subsequent deliveries after, 253
  regional analgesia and anesthesia, 205
  side-lying breastfeeding and, 309b
  skin-to-skin contact and, 270
  time between pregnancies and, 331, 670
Cesarean delivery. See also Incisions
  abnormal labor and, 631, 632–633
  after labor induction attempt, 226
  after the baby is born, 269
  breech presentation and, 250
  continuous labor support and, 213
  epidural block and, 206
  genital herpes and, 424
  going home after, 277
  HIV and, 426
  labor induction failure and, 221b
  labor not going as planned and, 243
  long second stage of labor and, 239
  macrosomia and, 628
  obesity during pregnancy and, 491, 492
  past, placenta accreta and, 619
  placenta accreta and, 620
  placenta previa and, 617
  placental abruption and, 619
  postterm pregnancy and, 175, 220
  preeclampsia and, 509
  preparing for, 257
  reasons for, 253–254
  on request, 173, 255–256
  resources, 265
  risks, 244, 259
  skin-to-skin contact after, 306
  spinal block for, 207–208
  what happens during? 256–259
Cetirizine, 454
Chairs
  lower back pain and, 100
  pain getting up from, calling ob-gyn about, 133b
Chalk, craving to eat, 91, 91b. See also Pica
Chancre, 427
Chaperones, during pelvic exams, 30, 75
Chat rooms, pregnancy, 455
Chat with an Expert, Postpartum Support International's Helpline, 465
Checklists
  for after the baby is born, 278, 283, 711–712
  before delivery, 143, 462
Chemical exposure, 14–15, 98b, 396
Chemicals, in vaccines, 411
Chemotherapy, 61

Chest pain
  calling ob-gyn about, 138, 140b, 160b, 282b
  go to hospital with, 168b
  postpartum, 282b
  pulmonary embolism and, 535b
Chickenpox. See also Varicella vaccine
  breastfeeding and, 303
  exposure, 461
  infections, 421–422
  as teratogen, 396, 403
  vaccine, 412
Child care, 29b, 197–199, 198–199b
Childbirth. See also After the baby is born; Birth control; Childbirth classes; Delivery; Labor
  checklist of tasks before, 143, 462
  complications, obesity and, 492
  doula hired for, 184
  education, 147
  exercise after, 387–388
  getting ready for, 166b
  physical health after, 284–288
  progestin-only pills and, 339
  recovery, FMLA and, 442–443
  resources, 241
  stages, 232–241, 234f
Childbirth classes
  choosing, 147, 181, 213, 216–217
  components of, 144
  labor partner and, 115–116, 184
  multiple pregnancy and, 481
  purpose for, 186–187
Childbirth educators, 26
Childbirth Without Fear (Dick-Read), 216
Children
  another baby to care for and, 670
  other, involving in your pregnancy, 118, 673–674
  wanting more, cesarean delivery on request and, 255
Chills, after delivery, 261b, 278b
Chlamydia, 7, 79, 156, 424–425
Chlorpheniramine, 454
Chocolate, 113
Cholesterol, 297t, 337, 353
Choline, 355t, 356
Chorioamnionitis, 225, 232, 304b, 632, 639
Chorion, 472
Chorionic villi, 58f
Chorionic villus sampling (CVS)
  diagnostic testing with, 564, 572, 573–574, 574f
  multiple pregnancy and, 479
  prenatal, 81t
  Rh incompatibility and, 609, 611
  ultrasound guidance of, 580
Chorionicity, 472, 473f
Chromosomal disorders, 560–562, 563b, 565t, 579. See also Genetic disorders
Chromosomal microarray (CMA), 575
Chromosomes
  abnormalities, 81t, 92, 553, 646

Chromosomes (continued)
  analysis of, 575
  genes and, 555–556, 556f
  problems, miscarriage and, 63
  stillbirth and, 658
Chronic conditions
  asthma, 530–532
  autoimmune disorders, 532–534
  blood clotting and bleeding disorders, 535–539
  digestive disorders, 539–540
  epilepsy and other seizure disorders, 541–542
  heart disease, 542–543
  kidney disease, 543–544
  lupus, 534
  mental illness, 544–545
  multiple sclerosis, 533
  overview, 529–530
  physical disabilities, 545
  resources, 547–548
  rheumatoid arthritis, 533
  thyroid disease, 545–547
Chronic hypertension, 220, 504–506, 507
Cigarettes, 56. See also Smoking; Tobacco
Circumcision, 115, 181, 187–188, 188f, 200, 275
Cirrhosis (liver damage), 432
Clay, craving to eat, 91, 91b. See also Pica
Cleft lip, 395, 541
Cleft palate, 541, 559
CLIMB: Center for Loss in Multiple Birth, Inc., 664
Closed loop glucose monitoring system, 522
Clubfoot, 395
CMV. See Cytomegalovirus
Cocaine, 13, 303–304, 616
Codeine, 209–210
Cold medications, 60, 399
Cold sores, 304b
Collaborative practice ob-gyns, 25, 26
Colon cancer, 337
Color blindness, 553, 555t, 559
Colostrum, 306
Combined estrogen–progestin birth control pills, 347
Combined hormonal birth control methods, 334–335t, 337–339, 338f
Combined screening for genetic disorders, 570t
Combined spinal–epidural (CSE) block, 208, 256
Compassionate Friends, 664
Complete blood count (CBC), 76
Complete breech presentation, 247f
Complex carbohydrates, 352–353, 517, 518
Complications
  abnormal labor, 631–634
  alcohol and, 56–57
  amniocentesis, 573
  another baby and, 671–672
  assisted vaginal delivery, 246
  autoimmune disorders and, 532–533
  birth place choices and, 93, 183
  blood type incompatibility and, 607
  circumcision and, 188

Complications (continued)
    depression after birth, 127
    diagnostic tests and, 572
    endometritis, 639–640
    exercise and, 375
    external cephalic version, 250
    fetal well-being tests and, 581
    food in stomach, cesarean birth and, 238
    gluten-free diet and, 366
    hypertension and, 506
    infections and, 6, 369
    kidney disease, 544
    labor in water and, 211
    large babies and, 514–515, 628
    marijuana and, 58
    monitoring after delivery for, 275
    multiple pregnancy, 472–477
    obesity and, 490
    ob-gyn training for, 23–24
    placenta problems and, 615
    postpartum hemorrhage, 637–639
    prenatal care visits and, 75
    preterm birth, 594, 595*b*
    resources, 640–641
    sexual activity and, 112, 458
    shoulder dystocia, 634–635
    smoking or vaping, 56
    stillbirth and, 658
    substance use, 59
    thrombophilias and, 536–537
    time between pregnancies and, 331, 669
    umbilical cord compression, 635–636
    umbilical cord prolapse, 636–637
    vaginal birth and, 219
    waiting until 39 weeks for delivery and, 173*b*
    workplace accommodations for, 441
Compression belt, 288
Compression stockings, 445*b*
Computed tomography (CT), 404
Condoms, 336, 339, 340, 340*f*, 422
Cone biopsy, 595*b*, 600
Congenital conditions, 542. *See also* Genetic disorders
Congenital rubella syndrome (CRS), 419
Congenital varicella syndrome, 421
Conjunctivitis, 425
Consent forms, at hospital, 236
Constipation
    another baby and, 671
    breastfed babies and, 302
    exercise and, 55
    fiber near end of pregnancy and, 460
    iron supplements and, 74*b*
    postpartum, 285–286
    pregnancy and, 73
    travel and, 445
    water and fiber and, 359
Contingent sequential screening for genetic disorders, 570*t*, 572
Continuous glucose monitoring systems, 522
Continuous labor support, 212–213

Contraction stress test
    fetal growth restriction and, 625
    fetal well-being monitoring and, 584, 587–588, 587*f*
    frequently asked questions, 582*b*
    postterm pregnancy and, 175
    pregestational diabetes mellitus and, 525
Contractions. *See also* Preterm labor; Uterine contraction after delivery
    abnormal labor and, 632
    active labor, 235, 237–238
    after sex with penetration, 112
    Braxton Hicks, 126, 133, 146, 150, 168, 169
    calling ob-gyn about, 113*b*, 133*b*, 140*b*, 159, 160*b*, 168*b*
    continuous labor support and, 213
    early labor, 233–234, 235
    labor, 169, 232
    placenta delivery and, 240
    placental abruption and, 134
    preterm labor and, 117, 133, 475*b*
    PROM and, 599
    transition to stage 2 and, 239
    true labor, 150–152, 168–169
    uterine atony and, 637
Contrast agents, 404
Copper IUDs, 20, 333, 347
Cord blood
    about, 134
    banking, 132, 187, 190–191, 240–241
    delayed clamping, 189–190
    information, 200, 465
Core muscles, 388, 671
Coronavirus (COVID-19)
    breastfeeding and, 303
    CDC guidelines, 406, 464
    frequently asked questions, 453
    health crisis, telehealth and, 29*b*
    safest place for birth and, 461
    travel and, 439, 444
Corticosteroids
    for asthma, 532
    multiple pregnancy and preterm labor and, 474
    nasal spray containing, 454
    placenta previa and, 617
    placental abruption and, 619
    preeclampsia and, 510
    pregestational diabetes mellitus and, 525
    before preterm birth, 601
    PROM management and, 599
    tocolytics and, 475, 602
Cosmetics, lead containing, 106
Cough
    calling ob-gyn about, 138, 140*b*, 160*b*, 282*b*
    go to hospital with, 168*b*
    sudden, pulmonary embolism and, 535*b*
    tuberculosis and, 434
Counseling, opioid use disorder, 59
COVID-19. *See* Coronavirus.
Cow's milk formulas, 326

Cradle hold, 309b
Cramps or cramping
    afterbirth pains, 289, 307
    amniocentesis and, 573
    breastfeeding after cesarean delivery and, 261
    calling ob-gyn about, 113b, 168b
    ectopic pregnancy and, 63, 649–650
    foodborne illness and, 368b
    legs, 139–140
    let-down reflex and, 306–307
    miscarriage and, 63
    preterm labor and, 117, 133, 145, 475b, 596b
    sexual activity and, 111
Cribs, 154
Criss-cross hold, 321b
Crohn's and Colitis Foundation of America, 547
Crohn's disease, 540
Cross-cradle hold, 309b
Crowning, 231b
Crown–rump length, 62
Cruise ships, 437, 448
Crying, baby's, 271, 307
CVS. *See* Chorionic villus sampling
Cycling, 381
Cyclophosphamide, 533
Cystic fibrosis
    as autosomal recessive disorder, 558
    carrier screening, 8, 9t, 566, 567t
    family history of, 554t, 563b
    prenatal diagnostic tests for, 81t
Cystic Fibrosis Foundation, 566, 576
Cytomegalovirus (CMV), 304b, 403, 430–431, 624, 658

D

Dairy products
    digesting, 10
    five food groups and, 10, 360–362, 361t
    lactose intolerance and, 367, 459
    morning sickness and, 51
    unpasteurized milk, 370
Days, in gestational age calculations, 49
Death. *See also* Early pregnancy loss; Stillbirth; Sudden infant death syndrome
    autosomal recessive disorders and, 558
    of baby, thyroid disease and, 546
    infections and, 416, 417, 420, 426
    newborn screening tests against, 274
    postpartum hemorrhage and, 637
    preeclampsia and, 491, 507
    Rh incompatibility and, 609
    thyroid disease and, 546
    umbilical cord prolapse and, 636
Deceleration, 636
Deep vein thrombosis (DVT)
    blood clotting disorders and, 535
    combined hormonal birth control and, 335t, 337, 338
    lupus and, 534
    massaging sleeves during surgery and, 257

Deep vein thrombosis (DVT) (continued)
    multiple pregnancy and, 480
    progestin-only pills and, 339
    sciatica and, 125
    surgery and obesity and, 492
    symptoms, 535b
    traveling and, 445, 445b
    walking after delivery and, 276
DEET, Zika virus and, 436
Dehydration, 50, 312, 448, 458
Delayed cord clamping, 189–190, 191, 463
Deletion, chromosomal disorders and, 562
Delivery. *See also* After the baby is born; Birthing positions; Cesarean delivery; Complications; Labor; Presentation
    before 39 weeks, 171
    birth plan for, 131, 182
    breech presentation and, 161
    checklist, 143, 462
    complications, obesity and, 492
    delay, PROM and, 599
    elective, 171–172
    equipment for, 212, 214–215f
    estimated due date and, 49
    first prenatal questions on, 26
    genital herpes and, 424
    gestational diabetes and, 519
    getting ready for, 142–145, 153–154
    heart disease and, 543
    hypertension and, 506
    injury, preterm birth risk and, 595b
    multiple pregnancy, 480
    obesity and, 492–493
    planning for, 115–116
    preeclampsia and, 507
    pregestational diabetes mellitus and, 525
    as stage 2 of childbirth, 232, 233f
    trauma, large babies and, 515
    umbilical cord prolapse and, 637
    waiting until 39 weeks for, 172, 173b, 176
    in water, 186, 211
Delivery nurses, 236
Delivery room, other people in, 186
Dental care, 454. *See also* Teeth
Dental changes, 87–88, 93
Dental dams, 7
Dental X-rays, 454
Depression. *See also* Postpartum depression
    calling ob-gyn about, 91b, 133b
    early pregnancy loss and, 654
    eating disorders and, 496
    getting help for, 93
    grieving stillbirth and, 662
    normal sadness or, 456–457
    as preexisting health condition, 4
    during pregnancy, 89, 126–127, 135, 544–545
    resources, 93, 135
    screening test, 128–129b
Despair, postpartum depression and, 290–292
Developmental delays or disabilities, 431, 577, 632

Dexchlorpheniramine, 454
DFE. *See* Dietary folate equivalents
Diabetes educators, 517
Diabetes mellitus. *See also* Gestational diabetes;
 Pregestational diabetes mellitus
  another baby and, 671
  breastfeeding and, 302
  combined hormonal birth control and, 337
  exercise and, 387
  fetal growth restriction and, 624
  fetal well-being tests with, 582
  future, gestational diabetes and, 297t, 515,
   520
  genetic disorder risk and, 563b
  glucose and, 78
  indicated preterm birth and, 600–601
  labor induction and, 220
  low-glycemic foods and, 353
  macrosomia, cesarean delivery and, 629
  multifactorial genetic disorders and, 559
  obesity during pregnancy and, 491
  overview, 513
  pneumococcal pneumonia vaccine and, 421
  preeclampsia and, 507, 511
  as preexisting health condition, 4
  before pregnancy, macrosomia and, 626
  pregnancy and, 529
  resources, 526
  shoulder dystocia and, 634
  stillbirth and, 658
  as teratogenic, 396
  your future health and, 296
Diabetic ketoacidosis (DKA), 523
Diagnostic tests. *See also* Screening tests
  analysis of cells, 575
  for genetic disorders, 8, 79, 81t, 553–555,
   564, 569
  methods, 572–574, 573f, 574f
  multiple pregnancy and, 479
  prenatal, 81, 81t
  screening tests compared with, 565t, 566
  of specific problems, 553
Diamniotic–dichorionic twins, 472, 473f
Diamniotic–monochorionic twins, 472, 473f
Diaphragms, 334–335t, 340, 341f, 464
Diarrhea, 133, 145, 368b, 369
Diastolic blood pressure, 502, 502b, 503
Dick-Read, Grantly, 216
Dick-Read, Grantly childbirth classes, 144, 186,
   216
Diet. *See* Nutrition
Dietary folate equivalents (DFE), 11, 313,
   355–356, 355t, 362, 521, 559, 670. *See also*
   Folate; Folic acid
Dietitians, 517
Digestive disorders, 529, 539–540
Digestive system development, 36f
Dilation. *See also* Cervix
  active labor and, 235
  breech presentation and, 250
  defined, 230b
  early labor contractions and, 233

Dilation (continued)
  labor induction and, 176, 223–224
  mechanical, cervical insufficiency and, 600
  mechanical, preterm birth risk and, 595b
  miscarriage diagnosis and, 646
  pelvic exam to check for, 152, 155
  preterm labor and, 593–594
  silent, 599–600
  spotting and, 167
  as stage 1 of childbirth, 233f, 633, 633t
Dilation and curettage (D&C), 647, 654
Dilation and evacuation (D&E), 657
Diphtheria, 415–416
Disabilities, long-term, placenta previa and, 616
Discordant twins, 477
Discrimination, pregnancy and, 64
Dizziness
  ectopic pregnancy and, 64, 650
  epidural block or spinal block and, 207b
  nitrous oxide and, 205
  pain relief medications and, 204
  in second trimester, 98
  as warning to stop exercises, 377b
  working during early pregnancy and, 60
DKA (diabetic ketoacidosis), 523
DMPA (medroxyprogesterone acetate), 336
DNA, 555, 556f
Doctor, baby's. *See also* Family medicine doctors;
 Pediatricians
  choosing, 104, 181, 191, 193
  on feeding your baby methods, 301
  newborn's rest results sent to, 275
  postpartum care and, 279, 284
  weighing baby, 311b
Doctor, mother's. *See* Maternal–fetal medicine
  (MFM) specialists; Obstetrician–
  gynecologists
DoctorFinder tool, AMA, 445, 448
Domestic abuse, 454–455, 465
Dominant genetic disorders, 554t. *See also*
  Autosomal dominant disorders
DONA International, 184, 200, 217
Doppler ultrasound exam, 237, 580, 584, 588,
   625
Double electric breast pumps, 322, 325
Double-clutch hold, 321b
Double-cradle hold, 321b
Doulas, 184, 213
Down syndrome (trisomy 21)
  as aneuploidy, 561
  diagnostic tests, 573, 573f
  family history of, 563b
  multiple pregnancy and, 479
  prenatal screening for, 564
  resources, 577
  screening tests, 76, 81t, 82, 569, 570t, 571,
   572
Doxylamine, 51
Dreams, strange, 86, 89–90
Drinking fluids. *See* Fluids, drinking
Drinking problem quiz, 57b. *See also* Alcohol
Drugs. *See* Illegal drugs; Medications; Prescription
  drugs

730 • INDEX

Dry-cleaning facilities, hazards at, 15, 405b
Duchenne muscular dystrophy, 555t, 559
Dull heavy feeling in chest, pulmonary embolism and, 535b
Duplication, chromosomal disorders and, 562
DVT. See Deep vein thrombosis

E

Early labor, 232, 233–235, 234f, 633t
    pain relief during, 185, 210–212
Early pregnancy loss
    coping with, 654
    ectopic pregnancy, 648–653
    gestational trophoblastic disease, 653–654
    miscarriage, 645–648
    resources, 655
Early preterm babies, 116
Early term
    defined, 163, 172b, 594b, 627b
    fetal growth restriction and, 626
Eastern European Jewish descent, carrier screening, 9t, 554t, 563b, 567t
Eating. See also Food or foods; Meals; MyPlate food-planning guide; Nutrients; Nutrition
    during active labor, 238
    after delivery, 275
    gestational diabetes and, 516, 517–518, 520
    healthy, tips for, 362–363
    heartburn and, 112–113
    during labor, 170
    morning sickness and, 50
    nausea in final weeks and, 167
    obesity and, 490
    partners' role, 14b
    postpartum diet, 293
    pregestational diabetes mellitus and, 524
    during pregnancy, 153
    prepregnancy care and, 9–10
    problems, preeclampsia and, 508
Eating disorders
    anorexia nervosa, 496–497
    avoidant restrictive food intake disorder, 497
    binge eating disorder, 497
    bulimia nervosa, 497
    dealing with comments about weight and, 488b
    effects for mothers, 495–496
    effects for your baby, 496
    getting help for, 498–499
    pica, 91, 106, 402, 497–498
    as preexisting health condition, 4
    pregnancy and, 489, 495–499, 544–545
    prepregnancy care and, 10
    risk factors and warning signs, 498
    rumination disorder, 498
    telling ob-gyn about, 453
    types, 496–498
    weight gain during pregnancy and, 54
E-cigarettes, 56. See also Smoking
Eclampsia, 171, 220, 491, 507, 672–673. See also Preeclampsia

Ectopic pregnancy
    about, 648, 649f
    diagnosis, 650
    PID and, 424
    recovery and trying again, 652–653
    resources, 655
    Rh incompatibility and, 609
    RhIg after, 611
    risks, 648–649
    signs and symptoms, 63–64, 649–650
    treatment, 650–652
ECV. See External cephalic version
EDD. See Estimated due date
Edinburgh Postnatal Depression Scale, 128–129b
Edwards syndrome (trisomy 18)
    as aneuploidy, 561
    fetal growth restriction and, 624
    screening tests, 92, 479, 570t, 571, 572
Effacement, 176. See also Cervix
    active labor and, 236
    defined, 230b
    labor induction and, 176
    preterm labor and, 593–594
    as stage 1 of childbirth, 633, 633t
Eggs
    chromosomes in, 555–556, 646
    IUDs preventing fertilization of, 333
    maturation and release of, 48
    menstrual cycle and, 16f, 17
    ovulation and, 15, 17f
    postpartum release of, 288–289
    twins formation and, 470, 471f
    week 2 development, 43
Eggs, chicken, 370
Ejaculation, 17, 345
Elective delivery, 171–172
Elective procedures, 187
Electric breast pumps, 322
Electronic fetal monitoring, 210, 223, 223f, 236, 657
Electronics workers, hazards for, 405b
Elemental iron, 74b, 357
Elevated blood pressure, 503b. See also, High blood pressure; Hypertension
Embryo. See also Babies
    assisted reproductive technology and, 470b
    crown–rump length, 62
    development problems, 646
    end of week 8, 45f
    multiple, 469–471
    pelvic exam, 30f
    preimplantation genetic testing of, 574
    week 5 development, 44, 62
    weeks 1 to 8 and, 33f
    weeks 9 to 12 and, 67–68
Emergencies
    after-hours phone numbers for, 26
    recognizing, 278
Emergency contraception (EC), 346–347
Emotional changes, 73. See also Depression; Feelings

INDEX • 731

Ending a pregnancy, 82, 555, 566
Endometrial ablation, 619
Endometriosis, 337, 648
Endometritis, 304b, 632, 639–640
Endometrium, 15, 16f, 44
Endurance, exercise and, 55
Engorgement, 289, 315, 320, 327
Environmental exposure history, 14–15, 396–397, 713–715
Environmental toxins, 56, 401–403, 559
Epidural blocks
    for cesarean delivery, 256
    labor induction and, 226
    longer labors and, 633
    monitoring after delivery, 275
    observation after baby is born, 241
    as regional anesthesia, 144, 205–206, 206f
    side effects, 207b
    spinal block combined with, 208
    transition to stage 2 and, 239
    von Willebrand disease and, 538
Epilepsy, 12b, 529, 541–542, 624
Epilepsy Foundation, 548
Episiotomy
    caring for, 276
    frequently asked questions on, 462–463, 463f
    local anesthesia and, 205
    ob-gyn views on, 26
    perineal tears compared with, 287
    postpartum hemorrhage and, 639
    redness, discharge, or pain from, 282b
    repair, 240
Equal (aspartame), 75, 366
Erection, 345
Escherichia coli (*E. coli*), 369–370
Estimated due date (EDD), 43, 48–49, 49b, 62, 164, 360
Estrogen
    in birth control pills, milk supply and, 464
    in combined hormonal birth control, 337
    cream, for vaginal dryness, 294
    menstrual cycle and, 16f
    pregnancy and, 15
    role in reproduction, pregnancy, and birth, 48
    skin color changes and, 71
Ethnicity, genetic disorders and, 9t, 554t, 562, 567
Eunice Kennedy Shriver National Institute of Child Health and Human Development, 265, 603, 604, 605
Exercise
    activities to avoid, 378–379
    aerobic activities, 380–381
    after childbirth, 387–392
    ball shoulder stretch, 385, 385f
    ball wall squat, 385, 385f
    4-point kneeling, 383, 383f, 389, 389f
    gestational diabetes and, 516, 518
    heel touches, 391, 391f
    home regimen, 382–387
    Kegel exercises, 285, 286b, 383

Exercise (continued)
    knee raises, 390, 390f
    kneeling heel touch, 386, 386f
    leg extensions, 392, 392f
    leg slides, 389, 389f
    lower back pain and, 100
    methotrexate for ectopic pregnancy and, 651
    multiple pregnancy and, 478
    MyPlate food-planning guide and, 360
    obesity and, 490
    obesity during pregnancy and, 492
    overview, 375
    postpartum, 289, 293
    pregestational diabetes mellitus and, 522, 524
    during pregnancy, 54–55, 114–115, 142, 167
    during pregnancy, guidelines for, 376–379, 377b, 458
    pregnancy changes affecting, 379
    pregnancy-related stress and, 89
    regular routine, 11
    resources, 393
    safe and healthy tips for, 377–378
    seated leg raises, 384, 384f
    seated overhead triceps extension, 384, 384f
    seated side stretch, 386, 386f
    sleep and, 70
    standing back bend, 387, 387f
    starting during pregnancy, 379–380
    warning signs to stop, 377b
    weight gain during pregnancy and, 101
    weight loss after pregnancy and, 493
Expanded carrier screening, 457, 564, 566–567
Exposures. *See* Environmental exposure history
Expressed milk (expressing milk)
    ability for, 158
    as baby's primary feeding method, 323–324
    blocked ducts and, 318
    bottles and nipples for, 324b
    breast pump for, 319, 322–323, 323f
    engorgement and, 289, 315
    by hand, 319, 320, 322
    methods, 319–320, 322–323
    sore nipples and, 314
    at work, 325
External cephalic version (ECV), 160, 248, 249f
Extremely preterm, 594b, 604, 627b
Eyes. *See also* Vision problems
    high blood sugar and, 513
    preeclampsia and, 117

F

Face
    defects of, prenatal screening for, 564, 571, 580
    fetal alcohol syndrome and, 400
    newborn's, 273
Face, mother's swelling
    calling ob-gyn about, 140b, 160b, 168b

Face, mother's swelling (continued)
    postpartum, 282b
    preeclampsia and, 117, 133b, 502b
FACOG, meaning of, 23
Factor V Leiden, 536–537
Factory work, hazards with, 15, 405b
Fainting, 64, 411b, 650
Fallopian tubes
    chlamydia or gonorrhea infections and, 424
    ectopic pregnancy and, 63–64, 648, 649f
    menstrual cycle and, 16f, 17f
    pregnancy and, 15, 17
    sterilization and, 343–345, 344f, 345f
    week 2 development and, 43
Falls, 60, 115, 204, 441, 541
False labor. See Braxton Hicks contractions
False-negative results, 47, 555, 565t, 566, 583–584
False-positive results, 47, 555, 565t, 566, 583
Family. See also Partners
    after the baby comes and, 154, 166b
    baby blues and, 290
    bottle-feeding by, 320f, 324
    as chaperones during pelvic exams, 30
    continuous labor support by, 213
    in delivery room, 186
    extra hands for multiple babies and, 481
    postpartum care team and, 166b, 283
    prenatal care visits and, 27b
Family and Medical Leave Act (FMLA), 442–443, 448
Family doctors, 31. See also Family medicine doctors
Family health history
    CDC information on, 20
    genetic disorders and, 562
    preeclampsia and, 507
    prenatal care and, 62
    prepregnancy screening, 4–5
    targeted carrier screening and, 567
Family medicine doctors (family practice doctors)
    choosing, 104, 107, 191, 193
    finding, 31
    postpartum care team and, 284
Farms and farmers, hazards for, 15, 405b
Fasting, 10
Fat. See also Fats
    maternal stores of, 55b
Fatigue
    caring for multiples and, 481
    lack of interest in sex and, 294
    mastitis and, 318
    postpartum period, 292–293
    sleep apnea and, 491
    weeks 1 to 8 and, 46, 51–52
    weeks 9 to 12 and, 68–70
    working during early pregnancy and, 60
Fats
    in balanced diet, 10, 351, 353–354, 361t
    omega-3 fatty acids, 357–358
Fecal incontinence, 286–287

Feedback, for telehealth visits, 29b
Feeding your baby. See also Breastfeeding
    Baby-Friendly hospitals and, 305b
    decisions on, 158–159, 188–189
    delivery before 39 weeks and, 174, 256
    expressed or pumped breast milk, 319–320, 322–325
    final thoughts on, 327
    food, drinks, and medication while breastfeeding, 312–314
    with formula, 325–327
    HIV and, 426
    overview, 301
    resources, 328–329
Feelings
    after childbirth, 289–292
    baby blues, 278b, 290
    of hopelessness, calling doctor about, 282b
    mood swings during pregnancy, 46
    postpartum depression, 278b, 290–292
    during pregnancy, 126–127
    sadness or depression? 456–457
Fees, telehealth, 29b
Feet
    increased size of, 96
    numbness, leg pain with, calling ob-gyn about, 133b
    numbness and tingling, 152
Fentanyl, 209–210
Ferrous fumarate, 74b, 357
Ferrous gluconate, 74b, 357
Ferrous sulfate, 74b, 357
Fertility
    birth control implant and, 335
    birth control injection and, 337
    IUDs and, 333
    timing (awareness), 15, 17, 18b, 19–20, 19f, 342–343
    treatments, multiple pregnancy and, 469, 470b
    weight loss and, 494
Fertilization, 43, 67, 333, 646
Fetal alcohol spectrum disorders (FASD), 57, 400
Fetal alcohol syndrome (FAS), 400
Fetal blood sampling, 564, 611
Fetal development. See also specific months
    illustrations of, 32–41f
    ultrasound exams of, 580
Fetal fibronectin, 596
Fetal growth restriction
    another baby and, 673
    causes, 623–624
    diagnosis, 624–625, 625f
    Doppler ultrasound exam and, 588
    hypertension and, 504
    indicated preterm birth and, 601
    management, 626
    overview, 623
    prevention, 626
    resources, 629
Fetal movement counting, 584. See also Kick counts

INDEX • 733

Fetal position, newborn appearance and, 272
Fetal surgery, 555
   RhIg after, 611
Fetal tissue
   miscarriage and, 63
   sampling, 564
Fetal well-being monitoring tests. *See also* Ultrasound exams
   frequently asked questions, 582*b*
   interpreting results of, 583–584
   overview, 579
   resources, 589
   risk of complications and, 155
   types, 584–588
   when available, 583
   why testing may be done, 581–583
Fetus. *See also* Babies
   crown–rump length, 62
   defined, 67–68
   prenatal screening tests and, 81*t*
Fever
   after cesarean delivery, 261*b*
   calling ob-gyn about, 140*b*, 160*b*
   engorgement and, 315
   epidural block or spinal block and, 207*b*
   foodborne illness and, 368*b*, 369
   go to hospital with, 168*b*
   during labor, 639
   mastitis and, 318
   postpartum care for, 278*b*, 282*b*
   PROM and, 599
   Zika virus and, 435
Fiber
   in balanced diet, 351, 352–353
   constipation and, 73, 286, 445
   dietary, hemorrhoids and, 141
   dietary, information on, 135
   in third trimester, 460
   travel during pregnancy and, 445
Fibroids
   breech presentation and, 247
   combined hormonal birth control and, 337
   delivery before 39 weeks and, 171
   placenta accreta and, 619
   postpartum hemorrhage and, 639
   surgery, labor induction as unsafe after, 222
Fifth disease, 433
Find an Ob-Gyn tool, ACOG's, 25*b*, 31, 65, 445, 449
Fingers, extra, 554*t*
Firefighters, hazards for, 405*b*
First trimester
   chorionic villus sampling during, 81*t*
   defined, 49
   fatigue during, 46
   multiple pregnancy signs in, 472
   pregestational diabetes mellitus in, 523
   recommended weight gain during, 488
   Rh antibody screen during, 610
   screening tests during, 81*t*, 82, 569, 570*t*
   sexual desire during, 111
   ultrasound exams during, 76, 579

Fish
   to avoid or limit, 365, 370
   breastfeeding and, 313
   healthy eating and, 10, 362
   heme iron in, 74*b*
   mercury exposure and, 402–403
   nutrients in, 357–358
   safe consumption of, 372, 407
   sushi, 365, 370, 458
Fitness apps, 381*b*
Five food groups, 10, 360–362, 361*t*
Flexibility exercises, 381–382
Flu. *See* Influenza; Influenza vaccination
Fluid, retained, 488
Fluids, drinking
   Braxton Hicks contractions and, 126
   breastfeeding and, 312
   constipation and, 286
   DVT prevention and, 445*b*
   exercise and, 377
   healthy eating and, 362
   heartburn and, 112–113
   hemorrhoids and, 141
   itchy skin and, 141
   month 10 and, 166
   morning sickness and, 50
   nasal congestion or nosebleeds and, 98
   travel and, 445
   working during early pregnancy and, 61
Flu-like symptoms, foodborne illness and, 368*b*
Fluorescence in situ hybridization (FISH), 575
FMLA. *See* Family and Medical Leave Act
Folate, 331, 362, 477, 670. *See also* Dietary folate equivalents (DFE); Folic acid
Folic acid. *See also* Dietary folate equivalents (DFE); Folate
   another baby and, 670
   in balanced diet, 351
   breastfeeding and, 313
   deficiency, weight-loss surgery and, 494–495
   focus on, 12*b*, 53*b*
   methotrexate and, 652
   multiple pregnancy and, 477
   NTDs and, 559
   pregestational diabetes mellitus and, 521
   prepregnancy care and, 11, 52
   recommendations and sources, 355*t*, 356–357
   seizure medications and, 541
   supplements, 354
Follicles, 15
Follicle-stimulating hormone (FSH), 48
Follow-up care, 278*b*, 279. *See also* Postpartum care
Food or foods. *See also* Eating; Meals; Pica
   acid reflux and, 112–113
   allergies, pregnancy and, 10, 366, 367
   to avoid or limit, 364–366, 369–370
   cravings, 91, 91*b*
   heartburn and, 113
   international travel and, 446
   lead containing, 106

Food or foods (continued)
    safe preparation of, 368, 370–371, 409
Foodborne illness, 368–370, 368b, 372, 437
Football position, 288
Football position or hold, 309b, 321b
Footling breech presentation, 247f
Forceps
    abnormal labor and, 634
    assisted vaginal delivery and, 239, 243, 245, 245f, 462
    continuous labor support and, 213
Foremilk, 307
Foreskin, 187, 188f
Formula feeding
    as breastfeeding alternative, 325–327
    decisions on, 158, 188–189
    postpartum engorgement and, 289
    twins or triplets, 319
    vitamin D and, 312
    4-point kneeling exercise, 383, 383f, 389, 389f
Fourth trimester. See Postpartum care
Fragile X syndrome, 559, 563b
Frank breech presentation, 247f
Fraternal twins, 469–470, 471f
French Canadian descent, carrier screening, 9t, 554t, 563b, 567t
Frequently asked questions
    after the baby is born, 463–464
    allergy medications, 454
    assisted vaginal delivery, 462
    bed rest, 457
    birth control after childbirth, 464
    birth plan, 461
    breastfeeding, 463–464
    caffeine, 458
    calcium and not eating dairy products, 459
    cats, 461
    chickenpox exposure, 461
    childbirth readiness, 462
    COVID-19, 453, 461
    delayed cord clamping, 463
    dental care, 454
    dental X-rays, 454
    douching, 452
    eating disorders, 453
    episiotomy, 462–463, 463f
    exercise, 458
    expanded carrier screening, 457
    fetal well-being monitoring tests, 582b
    fiber in third trimester, 460
    hair dye, 451
    health and health care, 453–455
    home births, 461
    hot tubs, 452
    keepsake ultrasounds, 457, 581
    labor, how to start, 462
    labor and delivery, 461–463
    lactose intolerance, 459
    massage, 451–452
    nausea during pregnancy, 456
    nutrition, 458–460

Frequently asked questions (continued)
    partner as controlling and jealous, 454–455
    pedicures, 452
    personal care, 451–453, 452f, 453f
    potentially harmful substances, 460–461
    pregnancy, 456–458
    resources, 464–465
    sadness or depression? 456–457
    saunas, 452
    secondhand smoke, 460
    sex during pregnancy, 458
    smartphone pregnancy apps, 455
    smell of prenatal vitamins, 458
    stretch marks, 452–453, 453f
    surgery while pregnant, 453
    sushi, 458
    teeth, care after vomiting, 456
    ultrasound exams, 457, 582b
    varicose veins, 452
    vitamin D deficiency, 459
    vomiting during pregnancy, 456
    water drinking, 459
        weight gain during pregnancy? 456
    Zika virus, 460–461
Friends. See also Partners
    after the baby comes and, 154, 166b
    continuous labor support by, 213
    in delivery room, 186
    extra hands for multiple babies and, 481
    postpartum care team and, 166b, 283
    prenatal care visits and, 27b
    talking about feelings with, 290
Front V hold, 321b
Fruits, 10, 101, 353, 361, 361t, 362
Full term
    defined, 164, 171, 172b, 594b, 627b
    reasons to go, 173b, 176
Full-body pillows, 69, 70f, 99, 99f
Full-term babies, 189–190, 247, 463, 473
Fundal height measurement
    baby's growth and, 102, 115, 130, 155, 624, 625f
    macrosomia diagnosis and, 627
    obesity and, 491
    prenatal care visit and, 103f
Fungi, 409
Future pregnancies, 173, 226, 255, 259, 262, 635

G

Gas, painful, 73, 286, 447, 652
Gasping for air, 282b
Gastric band surgery, 495
Gastroschisis, 624
GBS. See Group B streptococcus
General anesthesia, 144, 256, 343, 652
Genes. See also Genetic disorders
    abnormalities, 553
    chromosomes and, 555–556, 556f
    in cord blood, 190
    inherited, 557f
    Rh factor in, 608
Genetic Alliance, 82

INDEX • 735

Genetic counseling, 14b, 82
Genetic counselors, 5, 82, 555, 562, 564
Genetic disorders. *See also* Birth defects; Genes
    chromosomal, 560–562
    common, 554t
    cord blood and, 190
    deciding whether to be tested, 564–566, 565t
    decisions if pregnancy has, 575–576
    expanded carrier screening, 457
    fetal growth restriction and, 626
    inherited, 557–560, 557f, 560f
    overview, 553
    prenatal carrier screening, 5, 8, 9t, 564, 566–569
    prenatal screening and diagnosis, 79, 81–82, 81t, 92
    prenatal screening tests, 569, 570t, 571–572
    resources, 576–577
    risk assessment, 562, 563b, 564
    screening, ob-gyn discussions on, 4, 80
    stillbirth and, 658
    types of tests for, 564
    ultrasound exams for, 76
Genetic Science Learning Center, 576
Geneticists, 659
Genetics Home Reference, 576
Genital herpes
    breastfeeding and, 304b
    cesarean delivery and, 254
    labor induction as unsafe with, 222
    lack of cure for, 7
    as viral infection, 422–424, 423f
Genital warts, 418
Genitals
    baby's development of, 68, 85, 101–102
    genital herpes and, 422–424
    newborns,' 273
    physical exam of, 28
    postpartum care for, 285
    Turner syndrome and, 561
Genomics, medicine and, 576
German measles. *See* Rubella
Gestational age
    calculating, 49, 62
    elective labor induction and, 221
    fetal well-being tests and, 581
    PROM management and, 598
    ultrasound exam to estimate, 579, 580, 596
Gestational diabetes
    another baby and, 672
    care after pregnancy, 520
    controlling, 516–517
    defined, 513
    delivery before 39 weeks and, 171
    eating disorders and, 496
    effect on baby, 515–516, 515f
    exercise and, 375, 518
    fetal well-being tests with, 582
    future health risks and, 494, 515–516
    labor and delivery, 519
    labor induction and, 220

Gestational diabetes (continued)
    macrosomia and, 626
    medications for, 518–519
    multifetal pregnancy reduction and, 470b
    multiple pregnancy and, 476
    obesity during pregnancy and, 491
    overview, 514
    past pregnancies and, 5
    resources, 526
    risk factors, 514
    special tests, 519
    testing, 130, 492, 516
    time between pregnancies and, 669
    type 2 diabetes risks and, 297t
    weight gain between pregnancies and, 670
    weight gain during pregnancy and, 364
Gestational hypertension
    chronic hypertension and, 504
    fetal well-being tests with, 582
    hypothyroidism and, 546
    inducing labor before 39 weeks and, 172, 221b
    obesity during pregnancy and, 490
    risks, 506
    treatment, 509
Gestational trophoblastic disease (GTD), 653–654
Ginger, morning sickness and, 51
Gingivitis, 88
Glucagon pens, 523
Glucose. *See also* Blood sugar; Diabetes mellitus
    as body's fuel, 513
    carbohydrates and, 352
    challenge test, 130, 516
    continuous glucose monitoring systems, 522
    diabetes mellitus and, 4
    obesity during pregnancy and, 491
    during pregnancy, macrosomia and, 627
    urinalysis for, 78, 92
Glucose challenge test, 130, 516
Glucose meter, 517
Gluten, 366
Gluten-free diet, 366, 539
Glycolic acid, 71
Golden hour, 270. *See also* Skin-to-skin care or contact
Gonadotropin-releasing hormone (GnRH), 48
Gonorrhea, 7, 79, 156, 424–425
Grains, 10, 360–361, 361t, 362
Granuloma gravidarum, 88
Greek descent, carrier screening, 9t, 567t
Greenhouse hazards, 405b
Group B Strep International, 161
Group B streptococcus (GBS), 155–156, 161, 171, 431–432
Group practice ob-gyns, 25, 26
Growth problems for baby. *See also* Baby's size; Fetal growth restriction; Low birth weight; Macrosomia
    antiphospholipid syndrome and, 537–538
    asthma and, 398, 530, 531f
    chlamydia or gonorrhea infections and, 424
    chronic hypertension and, 506

Growth problems for baby (continued)
    delivery before 39 weeks and, 171
    diet or exercise plan and, 489
    eating disorders and, 496
    fetal alcohol syndrome and, 400
    fetal growth restriction, 623–626
    labor induction and, 219
    lupus and, 534
    maternal depression and, 127
    mother's eating disorder and, 496
    multiple pregnancy and, 476–477
    obesity and, 491
    opioid use disorder and, 59
    preeclampsia and, 491
    special tests of, 583
    stillbirth and, 658
    ultrasound exam to determine, 580
GTD (gestational trophoblastic disease), 653–654
Gums, changes, 86, 87–88, 93
Gynecology, 23

H
Hair
    changes during pregnancy, 82
    combined hormonal birth control and, 337
    fetal development of, 36f, 96
Hair dye, 451
Hand washing, 7, 409, 448
Hands
    mother's, postpartum swelling, 282b
    swelling. see Preeclampsia
    tingling, late pregnancy and, 152
Harmful substances. See also Lead
    environmental exposure history, 14–15, 396–397, 713–715
    environmental toxins, 56, 401–403, 559
    pregnancy complications and, 56
    at work, 14, 60–61, 405–406, 405b
hCG. See Human chorionic gonadotropin
Headache
    calling ob-gyn about, 140b, 160b, 168b
    combined hormonal birth control and, 337
    postpartum, 282b
    preeclampsia and, 117, 502b, 508
    relief for, 114
    severe, 112, 113b, 114, 168b, 207b, 508
    as warning to stop exercises, 377b
Head-down position, of fetus, 40f
Health and health care, 453–455, 481. See also Health insurance
Health care workers, hazards for, 405b, 432
Health history. See Family health history; Medical history
Health insurance
    baby's doctor choices and, 104, 193
    birth place choices and, 93, 183
    circumcision and, 187
    cord blood banking and, 191
    doulas and, 184
    follow-up care and, 279
    genetic disorder testing and, 565t
    multiple babies and, 481

Health insurance (continued)
    for obstetric care, 26
    options, 443–444
    for telehealth, 29b
Health insurance marketplace, 443, 449
Health problems for baby. See also Complications
    delivery before 39 weeks and, 173b
    normal ultrasound exam and, 581
Health records, travel during pregnancy and, 444, 446
Healthcare.gov, 449
Healthy eating. See Eating
Healthy lifestyles. See also Eating; Exercise
    eating, 9–10
    environmental toxin safety, 14–15
    exercise, 11
    folic acid and, 11, 12b
    postpartum period, 292–293
    preterm labor risks and, 594
    stopping use of unhealthy substances, 13–14
    tips for partners, 14b
    weight, 11–13
Hearing problems or loss
    CMV and, 430–431
    delivery before 39 weeks and, 174, 256
    preeclampsia and, 508
    prenatal care visits and, 27b
    testing newborns for, 274
Heart. See also Heart disease; Heart rate, baby's; Heart rate, mother's
    blood circulation and, 501
    defects, 491, 559
    defects of, prenatal screening for, 564
    high blood sugar and, 513
    problems, 205, 219, 254, 491
Heart attack, 337, 491, 508, 535
Heart disease
    birth control injection and, 336
    chronic hypertension and, 504
    congenital, 542, 563b
    exercise and, 55, 387
    fats and, 354
    fetal well-being tests with, 582
    future, gestational diabetes and, 520
    future risks of, 297t
    gestational diabetes and, 514
    high blood pressure during pregnancy and, 296
    low-glycemic foods and, 353
    preeclampsia and, 476
    pregestational diabetes mellitus and, 521
    pregnancy and, 529, 542–543
    resources, 547
Heart failure, 508, 546
Heart rate, baby's
    abnormal, cesarean delivery and, 254
    Apgar score of, 271–272, 271t
    biophysical profile of, 586–587, 586f
    contraction stress test and, 587–588, 587f
    external cephalic version and, 250
    modified biophysical profile of, 587

INDEX • 737

Heart rate, baby's (continued)
    placental abruption and, 619
    umbilical cord compression and, 635, 636
    umbilical cord prolapse and, 637
Heart rate, mother's, 207b, 379, 535b
Heartbeat, baby's, 237, 270, 271t, 274, 462, 657
Heartbeat, mother's, 113b, 114, 638
Heartburn, 112–113, 113b
Heating pads, 100, 114, 315
Heavy metals, as workplace hazards, 441
Heel touches, 391, 391f
Height, mother's, 62, 360
HELLP syndrome, 507
Hematologists, 539
Heme iron, 74b, 357
Hemoglobin A$_{1C}$, 516, 522
Hemoglobinopathies, 566, 624
Hemolysis, HELLP syndrome and, 507
Hemolytic disease of the newborn (HDN), 608, 609, 611, 612
Hemophilia, 553, 555t, 559, 563b, 639
Hemorrhage, 226, 259, 275, 616. See also Postpartum hemorrhage
Hemorrhoids, 141, 147, 285, 287, 671
Heparin, 537, 538
Hepatitis A virus
    infections, 416–417
    vaccine, 412, 413t
Hepatitis B immune globulin (HBIG), 304b, 418
Hepatitis B virus
    breastfeeding and, 304b
    infections, 416, 417–418
    lack of cure for, 7
    newborn vaccination, 274
    screening tests, 8, 79
    vaccine, 79, 274, 412, 413t, 417
Hepatitis C virus, 7, 79, 304b, 416, 432–433
Hepatitis D virus, 416
Hep-lock, 236
Herbal medications or remedies, 5, 106, 399, 460
Heroin, 13, 59, 303–304
Herpes, 303. See also Genital herpes
Herpes zoster (shingles), 421, 422
Heterozygous mutations, 536, 537
High blood pressure. See also Blood pressure; Hypertension; Preeclampsia
    activity restriction and, 146
    another baby and, 671
    breastfeeding and, 302
    chronic, future health risks and, 297t
    combined hormonal birth control and, 337
    delivery before 39 weeks and, 171
    exercise and, 376
    fetal growth restriction and, 623, 624
    fetal well-being tests with, 582
    future health risks and, 297t
    gestational diabetes and, 514, 515
    indicated preterm birth and, 600–601
    kidney disease and, 543
    molar pregnancy and, 653
    multiple pregnancy and, 476
    obesity during pregnancy and, 490
    past pregnancies and, 5

High blood pressure (continued)
    placental abruption and, 618
    preeclampsia and, 508
    preexisting, 4
    pregestational diabetes mellitus and, 521
    pregnancy and, 529
    progestin-only pills and, 339
    resources, 511
    risks, 516
    as silent disease, 501
    sleep apnea and, 491
    stillbirth and, 658
    as teratogenic, 396
    weight gain and, 364, 670
    your future health and, 296
Hispanic descent, carrier screening, 9t, 514, 567t
HIV. See Human immunodeficiency virus
Hobbies, pregnancy risks with, 15, 61, 106, 397, 402
Home, preparing, for baby, 154, 181, 193–195, 196b, 197f
Home births, 93, 183, 461
Home pregnancy tests, 47
Home renovators, hazards for, 405b
Homozygous mutations, 536, 537
Hopelessness feelings, 282b, 290–292
Hormonal birth control, 20, 49, 332, 337–339, 343, 346
Hormonal IUDs, 20, 333
Hormones. See also Estrogen; Insulin; Oxytocin; Progesterone; Progestin; Relaxin
    in acne treatments, 71
    baby's development and, 44
    blood sugar and, 513
    breastfeeding and, 302, 307f
    constipation and, 73
    delayed milk production and, 315
    hot flashes and, 112, 113
    insulin resistance and, 521
    lack of interest in sex and, 294
    loosening joints and, 96
    looser teeth and, 88
    pregnancy and, 15, 46
    preventing another preterm birth and, 604
    reproduction, pregnancy, and birth, 48
    uterine contraction and, 307f, 463–464, 633
    in uterus, newborns' genitals and, 273
Hospitals or hospitalization
    Baby-Friendly, 305b, 306
    baby's stay in, 157–158, 189
    as birth places, 26, 92, 182–183
    checking into, 235–237
    multiple pregnancy and, 480
    packing for, 153, 191, 192b
    preventing another preterm birth and, 604
    PROM and, 599
    for psychiatric illness during pregnancy, 545
    resources of, VBAC and, 80–81
    stay, after cesarean delivery, 260
    tours, 144–145, 183
    type of, early preterm birth and, 116
    type of, TOLAC and, 262
    when to go to, 168b, 169, 232, 234

Hot flashes, 112, 113
Hot tubs, 452
HPV. *See* Human papillomavirus
Human chorionic gonadotropin (hCG)
    ectopic pregnancy and, 650, 652, 653
    fetal development and, 44
    molar pregnancy and, 653, 654
    pregnancy tests and, 47, 48
Human immunodeficiency virus (HIV)
    breastfeeding and, 158, 303
    circumcision and, 187
    infections, 7, 425–426
    meningococcal meningitis and, 420
    testing, 7–8, 79, 156
Human milk, 302, 310. *See also* Breastfeeding; Milk
Human Milk Banking Association of North America, 328
Human milk banks, 316, 328
Human papillomavirus (HPV), 418–419
    vaccine, 412, 413*t*, 418–419
Humidifiers, 98
Hunger, baby's signaling of, 310
Huntington disease, family history of, 563*b*
Hydatidiform mole, 653–654, 655
Hydramnios, 521
Hydration. *See* Fluids, drinking
Hydrocodone or hydromorphone, 209–210
Hydroxyzine, 454
Hyperemesis gravidarum, 51
Hyperglycemia, 523
Hypertension
    chronic, 220, 504–506, 505*f*
    fetal well-being tests with, 582
    labor induction and, 220
    as preexisting health condition, 4
    as silent disease, 501
    types, 503*b*, 504
    white coat, 503
Hypertensive crisis, 503*b*
Hyperthyroidism, 545, 582, 653
HypnoBirthing, 216, 217
Hypnosis, 216
Hypoglycemia, 522
Hypothyroidism, 545
Hysterectomy
    cesarean delivery and, 173, 244, 255, 259, 629, 633
        multiple cesarean births and, 80
        persistent GTD and, 654
        placenta accreta and, 620, 621
        placenta previa and, 616
        postpartum hemorrhage and, 639
Hysteroscopy, 343

I
IBD. *See* Inflammatory bowel disease
Ibuprofen, 114, 277, 287, 289, 307, 318
Identical twins, 469–470, 471*f*
Illegal drugs
    breastfeeding and, 303–304
    fetal growth restriction and, 624

Illegal drugs (continued)
    needle sharing, hepatitis C transmission and, 432
    needle sharing, HIV transmission and, 425
    placental abruption and, 618
    prepregnancy care and, 13
    teratogenic, 396
Immune system
    baby's, flu vaccine and, 414
    disorders, cord blood and, 132, 190
    HIV and AIDS and, 425
    infections and, 408–409
Immunity (to be immune), 78, 419
Implantation, 44
Implantation bleeding, 48
In vitro fertilization (IVF), 14*b*, 343, 568, 574
Incisions
    cesarean delivery, 253, 257–258, 258*f*, 259, 260, 261, 264
    drainage, postpartum care for, 278*b*
    drainage or leakage from, 261*b*
    episiotomy, 463, 463*f*
    infection, cesarean delivery and, 259
    learning care for, 276
    pain from, 277, 288
    previous cesarean delivery, 254
    uterine, VBAC and, 262
Incompetent cervix, 599–600. *See also* Cervical insufficiency
Incomplete miscarriage, 647
Indicated preterm birth, 600–601
Indigestion medications, 399
Induced abortion, 595*b*, 600, 609
Induced labor. *See* Labor induction
Infant-only car seats, 194
Infections. *See also* Sexually transmitted infections; Urinary tract infections
    amniocentesis and, 573
    in the baby, labor induction and, 225
    bacterial vaginosis, 428
    birth defects and, 403
    breastfeeding and, 303
    cesarean delivery and, 173, 226, 244, 255, 261
    chorionic villus sampling and, 574
    cord blood and, 191
    COVID-19, 29*b*, 303, 406
    cytomegalovirus, 430–431
    diphtheria, 415–416
    endometritis, 639–640
    group B streptococcus, 431–432
    hepatitis A and B virus, 416–418
    hepatitis C virus, 432–433
    human papillomavirus, 418–419
    influenza, 412, 414–415, 415*f*
    IUD insertion after birth and, 333
    listeriosis, 433
    mastitis, 318–319
    measles, 419
    meningitis, 420
    mumps, 419
    norovirus, 448

Infections (continued)
  obesity, cesarean delivery and, 492
  overview, 409
  parvovirus, 433
  pertussis, 415–416
  placenta previa and, 616
  pneumococcal pneumonia, 420–421
  during pregnancy, 6, 595b
  pyelonephritis, 430
  resources, 437
  rubella, 419
  sexually transmitted, 422–427
  stillbirth and, 658
  tetanus, 415–416
  toxoplasmosis, 434
  tuberculosis, 434–435
  uterine, 171, 219, 597
  vaccine-preventable, 412, 413–414t, 414–422
  vaginal, 146
  vaginal, PROM and, 598
  varicella, 421–422
  VBAC and, 80, 263
  what happens during, 409–410
  as workplace hazards, 441
  yeast infection, 90, 428
  Zika virus, 435–436
Infertility, 14b, 424, 649
Inflammatory bowel disease (IBD), 529, 532, 540
Influenza (flu), 412, 414–415
Influenza vaccination
  after delivery, 276
  live, attenuated, 6, 411
  in postpartum period, 298
  pregnancy and, 131, 413t
  prenatal care and, 155
Inherited genetic disorders, 557–560, 557f, 565t, 659. See also Genetic disorders
Inherited thrombophilias, 536–537
Insulin, 513, 518–519, 521, 522, 526. See also Diabetes mellitus
Insulin pumps, 522, 524
Insure Kids Now, 449
Integrated screening for genetic disorders, 570t, 572
Intellectual disabilities or problems, 400, 434, 554t, 561, 563b
Internal os, 615, 616
International Association for Medical Assistance to Travelers, 446, 449
International board-certified lactation consultants (IBCLCs), 158, 299
International Childbirth Education Association, 147, 217
International Lactation Consultant Association, 299, 305, 328
International travel, 446
Interpreters, for prenatal care visits, 27b
Intimate partner violence, 455
Intrahepatic cholestasis of pregnancy, 658
Intrauterine devices (IUDs), 20, 332, 333f, 334–335t, 464

Intravenous (IV) line
  for antibiotics, 155, 257, 431
  for fluids, 51, 448
  for general anesthesia, 208
  for insulin during labor, 525
  for labor induction medications, 226
  for oxytocin, 224, 633–634
  for pain relief medications, 185, 277
  placement at hospital, 236
  for systemic analgesics, 204
Iodine, 355t, 404
IR3535, Zika virus and, 436
Iranian, southern, descent, carrier screening, 9t
Iron
  in balanced diet, 351
  constipation and, 73
  in cord blood, 189, 463
  deficiency, pica and, 91, 497
  deficiency, weight-loss surgery and, 494–495
  focus on, 74b
  as prenatal supplement, 52
  recommendations and sources, 355t, 357
  stores of, time between pregnancies and, 331, 670
  supplements, 310, 312, 354, 639
  vegetarian diets and, 368
Irritable bowel syndrome (IBS), 529, 540, 548
Ischial spines, station measurements and, 231b
Isotretinoin, 71, 398, 460
Italian descent, carrier screening, 9t, 567t
Itching, 91b, 141
IUDs. See Intrauterine devices
IVF. See In vitro fertilization

J

Jaundice
  ABO incompatibility and, 608
  CMV and, 430
  delayed cord clamping and, 190
  delivery before 39 weeks and, 173b, 174, 222b, 256
  mother's gestational diabetes and, 515
  resources, 612
  Rh incompatibility and, 609
  RhIg and, 611
  vacuum-assisted delivery and, 246
Jewish descent, Eastern or Central European, carrier screening, 9t, 554t, 563b, 567t
Jogging, 381
Joint Commission, 93, 183
Joints
  exercise and pregnancy changes affecting, 379
  loosening, hormones and, 96
  lupus and, 534
  parvovirus and, 433
  sacroiliac, 124, 124f
  Zika virus and, 435
Journal, writing in, 166b

K

Karyotypes, 575
Keepsake ultrasounds, 457, 581
Kegel exercises, 285, 286b, 383
Ketones, 523
Kick counts, 175, 509, 519, 525, 584. *See also* Baby's movement
Kidney disease
    blood clotting disorders and, 535
    chronic hypertension and, 504
    fetal growth restriction and, 624
    fetal well-being tests with, 582
    future risks of, 297t
    preeclampsia and, 507
    pregestational diabetes mellitus and, 521
    pregnancy and, 529, 543–544
    resources, 548
    stillbirth and, 658
Kidney failure, 543
Kidneys
    chronic hypertension and, 504, 510
    fetal growth restriction and, 624
    future risks of, 297t
    high blood sugar and, 513
    infections, preterm PROM and, 597
    lupus and, 534
    preeclampsia and, 117, 476, 490–491, 509
    pregnancy and, 46
    problems, labor induction and, 219
    urinary tract infections and, 428–430, 429f
KidsHealth, 118, 674
Knee raises, 390
Kneeling
    heel touch exercise, 386, 386f
    pain relief during early labor and, 185, 210–211
Kohl, 106

L

La Leche League International, 159, 161, 189, 200, 299, 305, 328, 465
Lab tests, 75, 76, 78. *See also* Diagnostic tests; Screening tests
Labia, 273
Labor. *See also* Braxton Hicks contractions; Contractions; Pain relief; Preterm labor; Rupture of membranes
    abnormal, 631–634
    amniotic sac rupture and, 146
    back labor, 462
    birth plan for, 131, 182
    body changes signaling, 168–169, 168b, 229, 231
    common terms, 230b
    continuous support for, 212–213
    difficulties, large babies and, 514
    eating disorders and, 496
    eating during, 170
    epidural block during, 205–206, 206f
    equipment for, 212, 214–215f
    estimated due date and, 49
    failure, cesarean delivery and, 253

Labor (continued)
    false labor compared with, 170t, 233t
    as first stage of childbirth, 232
    gestational diabetes and, 519
    HIV transmission during, 425
    how do I start? 462
    long or fast, 638
    methods, 222–224
    natural, TOLAC and, 262
    obesity and, 492
    overview, 229
    pain relief during, 143–144, 184–185, 210–212
    planning for, 115–116
    positions for, 157, 210–211, 235, 237
    prolonged, macrosomia and, 628
    as stage 1 of childbirth, 232–239, 234f
    as stage 2 of childbirth, 239-240, 234f
    as stage 3 of childbirth, 240-241, 234f
    stillbirth during, 657
    undigested food and, 208
    in water, 186, 211
    your partner in, 115–116, 184, 235, 238, 240
Labor augmentation, 238, 633–634, 638
Labor induction
    decisions, 175–176
    delivery before 39 weeks and, 171
    elective reasons for, 171–172, 220–221
    failure of, 225–226
    gestational hypertension or preeclampsia and, 509
    medical reasons for, 219–220
    overview, 219
    placental abruption and, 619
    postterm pregnancy and, 174
    pregestational diabetes mellitus and, 525
    procedure, 222–225
    PROM management and, 598
    resources, 227
    risks, 225
    situations unsafe for, 221–222
    stillbirth delivery and, 657
    at 39 weeks, 221b
    what to understand about, 226
Labor nurses, 236
Labor partner, 115–116, 184, 235, 238, 240
Laboratory technicians, hazards for, 405b
Laborists, 26
Lactaid, 459
Lactation, 115, 181, 304
Lactation consultants, international board-certified, 158
Lactation specialists, 189, 304–305, 526
Lactational amenorrhea method (LAM), 341–342
LactMed, 313
Lactose, 326
Lactose intolerance, 366, 367, 372, 459
Lamaze, Fernand, 213
Lamaze childbirth classes, 144, 186, 213
Lamaze International, 213, 217
Laminaria, 224

Lanugo, 36f, 96, 138, 163
Laparoscope, 344
Laparoscopic sterilization, 335t, 344–345, 345f
Laparoscopy, 344, 652
Large baby. See Macrosomia
Laser surgery, TTTS treatment with, 476
Last menstrual period (LMP)
    estimated due date and, 43, 48–49, 49b
    measuring pregnancy from, 456, 593, 594b, 627b
LATCH system, for car seats, 196b
Latching on, 308, 308f, 314. See also Breastfeeding
Late pregnancy loss. See Stillbirth
Late preterm, 594b, 627b
Late term
    defined, 172b, 220, 594b, 627b
    fetal well-being tests and, 583
    reasons for, 174–175
Latent labor, 233. See also Early labor
Latent TB, 435
Laughing gas, 205
Laundry starch, craving to eat, 91. See also Pica
Laxatives, 60
Lead
    as environmental toxin, 14–15, 401–402
    EPA information on, 107, 407
    prenatal exposure to, 105–106
    screening tests, 104
    workplace exposure, 60, 92, 98b
Learning disabilities, 116
Learning problems, 105, 174, 256
Leg extensions, 392, 392f
Leg slides exercise, 389, 389f
Legs. See also Calf pain; Deep vein thrombosis
    blood clots in, 259
    cramps, 139–140
    pain, 133b, 152, 261b, 278b
    postpartum pain in, 282b
    seated leg raises, 384, 384f
    swelling, 140–141, 152
Let-down reflex, 307, 307f, 319
Leukemia, cord blood and, 190
Levothyroxine, 546
Lifestyle habits. See Healthy lifestyles
Lifting, 100, 440b, 441
Ligaments, 86–87, 124, 124f, 152. See also Joints
Lightening, 169, 229
Linea nigra, 71
Lipoproteins, 353
Liquid concentrated formula, 326
Liquids. See Fluids, drinking
Listeria, 658
Listeriosis, 369, 433
Live, attenuated influenza vaccines, 6, 411, 419, 421
Liver
    HELLP syndrome and, 507
    hepatitis C infection and, 432–433
    preeclampsia and, 117, 476, 491, 509
LMP. See Last menstrual period
Local anesthesia, 205, 206, 275, 454

Lochia, 278b, 284, 638, 639
Long-acting reversible contraception (LARC), 332
Loop electrosurgical excision procedure (LEEP), 595b, 600
Loratadine, 454
Low birth weight
    CMV and, 431
    eating disorders and, 496
    lead exposure and, 105
    maternal depression and, 127
    secondhand smoke and, 13
    smoking and, 56
    thyroid disease and, 546
    time between pregnancies and, 331, 669
    trichomoniasis and, 427
    umbilical cord prolapse and, 636
    unhealthy substances and, 13
Lower abdominal pressure, 117, 133, 145, 596b
Lower back pain, 98, 100, 113b. See also Backache
Low-glycemic foods, 353
Low-lying placenta, 616, 616f, 617
Lubricants, sex after childbirth and, 294
Lungs
    fluid in, preeclampsia and, 117
    function, asthma and, 530
    problems, 219, 491, 632
    surfactant replacement therapy for, 602–603
Lupus (systemic lupus erythematosus or SLE)
    fetal well-being tests with, 582
    preeclampsia and, 507
    during pregnancy, 529, 532, 534
    progestin-only pills and, 339
    stillbirth and, 658
Lupus Foundation of America, 548
Luteinizing hormone (LH), 19, 48

M

Macrosomia
    abnormal labor and, 631–632
    cesarean delivery and, 254
    complications and, 628
    diagnosis, 627–628
    gestational diabetes and, 514–515, 515f, 516
    management, 628–629
    obesity and, 491
    postpartum hemorrhage and, 639
    pregestational diabetes mellitus and, 521
    prevention, 629
    resources, 629
    risks, 626–627
    shoulder dystocia and, 634
    weight gain during pregnancy and, 364
Magnesium sulfate, 475, 599, 601–602
Magnetic resonance imaging (MRI), 404, 620, 659
Malabsorptive surgery, for weight loss, 494, 495
Malaria, 436, 658
Male babies, macrosomia and, 627
Males, X-linked genetic disorders and, 555t
Malignant persistent GTD, 654
Malpresentation, 632

Manual breast pumps, 322, 323f
March of Dimes
   on birth defects and research, 576
   on depression during pregnancy, 93, 135
   on newborn jaundice, 612
   parent support networks and, 566
   on placenta problems, 621
   on postpartum care, 641
   on Rh disease, 612
Marijuana, 13, 58, 304, 624
Marketplace, health insurance, 443, 449
Massage, 114, 185, 212, 213, 318, 451–452
Mastitis, 318–319
Masturbation, 295
Maternal care practitioner, 284. *See also* Obstetrician–gynecologists
Maternal serum alpha-fetoprotein (MSAFP), 570t, 571
Maternal–fetal medicine (MFM) specialists
   chronic conditions and, 530
   heart disease and, 542
   high-risk pregnancy roles, 24
   kidney disease and, 543
   lupus and, 534
   multiple pregnancy and, 474b
   resources, 31, 482
   stillbirth evaluation by, 659
   Zika virus and referral to, 436
Maternity care, health insurance and, 443
Mayo Clinic, 629
McRoberts maneuver, 635
Meals. *See also* Eating; Food or foods; Nutrients; Nutrition
   constipation and, 73, 125
   heartburn and, 112–113
   preparing for birth and, 166b
   small, morning sickness and, 50
Measles infections, 419. *See also* Rubella
Measles–mumps–rubella (MMR) vaccine
   after delivery, 276
   as live, attenuated vaccine, 411–412, 419
   in postpartum period, 298
   pregnancy and, 6, 79, 414t
Mechanical dilation, 595b
Medicaid, 444
Medical bracelet or necklace, 524
Medical history. *See also* Family health history
   environmental exposure, 14–15
   form, 702–707
   preterm birth risk and, 595b
   reviews, 29b, 62
   ultrasound exams specific to, 580
Medical students, 237
Medications. *See also* Prescription drugs; Supplements
   acne treatment, 70–71
   after childbirth, 298
   antiphospholipid syndrome, 538
   asthma, 530, 531
   blood clotting disorders and, 537
   blood pressure, 510
   breastfeeding and, 158, 304, 313

Medications (continued)
   for chronic conditions, 530
   continuous labor support and, 213
   delayed milk production and, 315
   early preterm birth and, 116
   eating disorders and, 496
   ectopic pregnancy and, 650, 651–652
   fetal growth restriction and, 624, 626
   formula feeding and, 325
   gestational diabetes and, 517, 518–519
   heart disease and, 543
   hypertension, 505, 506
   incomplete miscarriage and, 647
   infections, 410
   kidney disease and, 543
   mental illness, 544–545
   methadone or buprenorphine effects and, 209
   multiple sclerosis, 533
   pain relief, 144, 184, 185, 203, 204
   pregestational diabetes mellitus and, 524–525
   pregnancy and, 60
   prepregnancy care and, 5
   preterm birth and, 599, 601–602
   seasickness, 448
   seizure disorders, 541–542
   telehealth reviews of, 29b
   telling ob-gyn about, 460
   thyroid disease, 546
   weight loss and, 493, 494
Meditation, 70
Mediterranean descent, carrier screening, 9t, 554t, 563b, 567t
Medroxyprogesterone acetate (DMPA), 336
Melanin, 71
Melasma, 71
Membranes. *See* Amniotic sac; Rupture of membranes
Memory changes, 99
Men. *See also* Sperm
   CDC pregnancy planning information for, 20
   X-linked genetic disorders and, 555t
Meningitis, 420
Meningococcal disease vaccine, 412, 414t
Meningococcal meningitis, 420
Menopause, 343, 563b
Menstrual blood, 16f, 538
Menstrual cramps, 288
Menstrual cycle
   breastfeeding and, 302
   charting, 17, 18b
   estrogen and, 48
   events during, 16f
   fertility awareness and, 343
   pregnancy and, 15
   time between pregnancies and, 670
Menstrual periods (menstruation)
   anorexia nervosa and, 497
   birth control implant and, 335
   combined hormonal birth control and, 337
   fertility awareness methods, 343

Menstrual periods (menstruation) (continued)
    getting pregnant before return of, 132, 331
    heavier, calling ob-gyn about, 282b
    IUDs and changes in, 333
    menstrual cycle and, 15
    pregnancy risk and, 295
    return of, 288–289
    vaginal bleeding heavy as, 167
Mental health during pregnancy, 126–127, 128–129b
Mental illness, 529, 544–545, 548
Mercury, 14–15, 60, 358, 402–403
Metabolic disorders, genetic disorder risk and, 563b
Metabolism, 51, 113, 132, 190
Metals, heavy, as workplace hazards, 441
Methadone, 59, 209
Methamphetamines, 13, 303–304, 396
Methimazole, 546
Methotrexate, 651–652
MFM. See Maternal–fetal medicine (MFM) specialists
Microarray, 659. See also Chromosomal microarray
Microcephaly, 435
Middle Eastern descent, genetic disorders and, 554t
Midwives, 24, 25–26, 31, 213
Migraines, 337
Milk. See also Breastfeeding; Dairy products; Expressed milk; Human milk
    'coming in,' 306
    continuous making of, 307
    delayed production, 315–316
    digesting, 10
    low supply of, 316
    production, suckling and, 308
Milk ducts, 72, 72f, 307f, 317–318, 318f
Milk glands, 72, 72f
Milk lobules, 307
Minerals, 354, 355t, 356–359. See also Supplements
Miscarriage
    amniocentesis and, 81t, 573
    aneuploidy and, 560
    antiphospholipid syndrome and, 537–538
    bleeding disorders and, 535
    caffeine and, 364, 458
    causes, 645–646
    chorionic villus sampling and, 574
    CVS and, 81t
    diagnosis, 646
    eating disorders and, 496
    genetic disorder risk and, 563b
    gonorrhea and, 425
    hypothyroidism and, 546
    kidney disease and, 543
    lead exposure and, 105
    listeriosis and, 369, 433
    lupus and, 534
    multiple, blood clots and, 537
    pregestational diabetes mellitus and, 521

Miscarriage (continued)
    resources, 655
    Rh incompatibility and, 609
    RhIg after, 611
    rubella and, 419
    second trimester and, 86
    signs, 63, 646
    subsequent pregnancies and, 6
    substance use and, 59
    telling your other children about another baby and, 673
    thrombophilias and, 536
    treatment, 647
    when to share the news and, 64
MMR vaccine. See Measles–mumps–rubella (MMR) vaccine
Modified biophysical profile, 584, 587, 625
Molar pregnancy, 653–654
Monoamniotic–monochorionic twins, 472, 473f
Monosodium glutamate (MSG), 365
Monosomy, 561
Month 1. See Months 1 and 2
Month 2. See Months 1 and 2
Month 3
    baby's development, 67–68
    discomforts and how to manage them, 68–73
    discussions with your ob-gyn, 80–82
    mother and baby, 34f, 69f
    nutrition, 73–75
    prenatal care visits, 75–79
    resources, 82–83
    your changing body, 68
Month 4
    baby's development, 85–86
    discomforts and how to manage them, 86
    discussions with your ob-gyn, 92–93
    mother and baby, 35f, 87f
    nutrition, 90–91
    prenatal care visits, 92
    resources, 93
    when to call your ob-gyn, 91b
    your changing body, 86
Month 5
    baby's development, 95–96
    discomforts and how to manage them, 97–100
    discussions with your ob-gyn, 103–104
    mother and baby, 36f, 96–97
    nutrition, 100–101
    prenatal care visits, 101–103
    resources, 107
    special concerns, 104–106
    when to call your ob-gyn, 98b
    your changing body, 96–97
Month 6
    baby's development, 109–110
    discomforts and how to manage them, 112–114
    discussions with your ob-gyn, 115–116
    exercise, 114–115
    involving your other children in your pregnancy, 118

Month 6 (continued)
   mother and baby, 110f
   prenatal care visits, 115
   resources, 118
   special concerns, 116–117
   when to call your ob-gyn, 113b
   your changing body, 111–112
Month 7
   baby's development, 121–122
   discomforts and how to manage them, 124–126
   discussions with your ob-gyn, 131–132
   mental health, 126–127, 128–129b
   mother and baby, 38f, 123f
   prenatal care visits, 130–131
   resources, 134–135
   special concerns, 132–134
   when to call your ob-gyn, 133b
   your changing body, 122–123
Month 8
   baby's development, 137–138
   discomforts and how to manage them, 138–141
   exercise, 142
   getting ready for delivery, 142–145
   mother and baby, 39f, 139f
   nutrition, 142
   prenatal care visits, 145
   resources, 147
   special concerns, 145–147
   when to call your ob-gyn, 140b
   your changing body, 138
Month 9
   baby's development, 149–150
   discomforts and how to manage them, 150–152
   discussions with your ob-gyn, 157–159
   exercise, 153
   getting ready for delivery, 153–154
   mother and baby, 40f, 151f
   nutrition, 153
   prenatal care visits, 155–156
   resources, 161
   special concerns, 159–161
   when to call your ob-gyn, 160b
   your changing body, 150
Month 10
   baby's development, 163–164
   deciding to induce labor, 175–176
   discomforts and how to manage them, 166–167
   discussions with your ob-gyn, 171–174
   false labor and true labor differences, 170t
   late term and postterm pregnancy, 174–175
   length of pregnancy terms, 172b
   mother and baby, 41f, 165f
   prenatal care visits, 170–171
   preparing for delivery, 167–169
   resources, 176
   thing to do to get ready, 166b
   waiting until 39 weeks, 173b
   when to call your ob-gyn, 168b
   your changing body, 164–166

Months 1 and 2
   baby's development, 43–44
   discomforts and how to manage them, 50–52
   exercise, 54–55
   healthy lifestyle decisions, 55–60
   mother and baby, 33f, 45f
   nutrition, 52–54
   prenatal care visits, 61–62
   resources, 65
   special concerns, 63–64
   when to share the news, 64
   workplace safety, 60–61
   your changing body, 46–49
Moodiness, 46, 55. *See also* Emotional changes
Morning sickness, 50–51, 73, 442, 472, 523
Morning-after pill, 347
Mosquitoes
   Malaria and, 436
   Zika virus and, 435–436
MotherToBaby, 328, 398, 407
Motion sickness, 448
Motivation, for exercise, 380
Mouth
   changes during pregnancy, 86, 87–88, 93
   HPV and cancer of, 418
Moving about, 141, 185, 260. *See also* Exercise; Walking
MS. *See* Multiple sclerosis
Mucus plug, loss of, 169, 229, 232
Multidrug therapy, for TB, 435
Multifactorial genetic disorders, 559
Multifetal pregnancy reduction, 470b
Multiple pregnancy. *See also* Twins
   activity restriction and, 146, 480
   average birth weight, 474t
   average length of, 474t
   bed rest, 480
   birth place choices and, 93
   cesarean delivery and, 254
   delivery, 480
   delivery before 39 weeks and, 171
   early preterm birth and, 116
   everyday health during, 477–478
   exercise and, 376, 478
   feeding your baby decisions and, 158
   fertility treatments and, 469, 470b
   fetal growth restriction and, 624
   fetal well-being tests with, 583
   genetic screening and diagnosis, 478–479
   gestational diabetes and, 476
   getting ready for, 480–481
   growth problems for baby, 476–477
   health care and, 478–480
   healthy weight during, 351
   high blood pressure and, 476
   hospitalization, 480
   indicated preterm birth and, 601
   macrosomia and, 627
   nutrition, 477
   overview, 469
   placenta accreta and, 619
   placenta previa and, 615–616

INDEX • 745

Multiple pregnancy (continued)
　　placenta problems, 476
　　preeclampsia and, 476, 507
　　prenatal care during, 479
　　prenatal genetic testing, 478–479
　　preterm birth risk and, 473–475, 595b
　　process of, 469–471
　　resources, 482
　　risks with, 472–477
　　signs of, 471–472
　　terms to know, 472
　　three or more, 471
　　twins, 469–471, 471t
　　ultrasound exam to determine, 579
　　umbilical cord problems, 476
　　weight gain during, 477–478, 478t
Multiple sclerosis (MS), 529, 532, 533, 548
Mumps, 419. See also Measles–mumps–rubella (MMR) vaccine
Muscle tone
　　another baby and, 671
　　Apgar score of, 271t
　　baby's, biophysical profile of, 586–587
　　baby's Apgar score of, 271–272, 271t
　　exercise and, 55
Muscular dystrophy, 563b
Musculoskeletal system, fetal development of, 41f
Music, pain management or relief and, 185, 212, 234
Mutations, 536–537, 557, 575. See also Genetic disorders
My Family Health Portrait tool, 20
My Postpartum Care Checklist, 283. See also Postpartum care
Myometrium, 620. See also Uterus
MyPlate food-planning guide
　　healthy diet planning and, 359–360, 360f, 372
　　postpartum diet, 293, 299
　　prepregnancy care and, 10, 20
MyPregnancy website, ACOG's
　　on after the baby is born, 279
　　on another baby, 674
　　on assisted vaginal delivery, 251
　　on birth control, 347
　　on birth defects, 407
　　on blood type incompatibility, 613
　　on breech presentation, 251
　　on cesarean birth, 265
　　on childbirth, 241
　　on chronic diseases, 548
　　on delivery, 31
　　on diabetes and pregnancy, 526
　　on early pregnancy loss, 655
　　on eating disorders, 499
　　on exercise and physical fitness, 393
　　on feeding your baby, 329
　　on fetal growth restriction, 629
　　on fetal well-being before labor, 589
　　on frequently asked questions, 465
　　on genetic disorders, screening, and testing, 578

MyPregnancy website, ACOG's (continued)
　　on getting ready for pregnancy, 21
　　on healthy eating on a budget, 363
　　on high blood pressure, 511
　　on infections, 437
　　on labor, 31
　　on labor induction, 227
　　on macrosomia, 629
　　on multiple pregnancy, 482
　　on nutrition, 372
　　on obesity, 499
　　on placenta problems, 621
　　on postpartum care, 31, 299, 641
　　on preeclampsia, 511
　　on pregnancy, 31, 65, 83, 93, 107, 135, 147, 161, 176
　　on preparing for birth, 201, 217
　　on preterm birth, 118
　　on preterm labor and birth, 605
　　on stillbirth, 664
　　on travel safety, 449
　　on ultrasound exams, 589
　　on VBAC, 265
　　on workplace safety and health, 449

N

Nasal congestion, 97–98. See also Nosebleeds
Nasal spray flu vaccine, 6, 411, 413t, 415
National Academy of Medicine, 488
National Alliance on Mental Illness, 548
National Blood Clot Alliance, 548
National Bone Marrow Donor Program, 200
National Cancer Institute, 21, 65
National Center on Birth Defects and Developmental Disabilities, 576
National Conference of State Legislatures, 328
National Cord Blood Program, 135, 200, 465
National Domestic Violence Hotline, 455, 465
National Down Syndrome Society, 566, 576
National Eating Disorders Association, 465, 499
National Foundation for Celiac Awareness, 372, 548
National Highway Traffic Safety Administration, 161, 200
National Human Genome Research Institute, 576
National Institute for Occupational Safety and Health (NIOSH)
　　on workplace accommodations, 440b
　　on workplace hazards, 61, 406, 442
　　on workplace safety and health, 65, 407, 449
National Institute of Diabetes and Digestive and Kidney Diseases, 372, 526, 548
National Kidney Foundation, 548
National Multiple Sclerosis Society, 548
National Sexual Assault Telephone Hotline, 30, 31
National smoking "quit line," 56
National Tay–Sachs & Allied Diseases, 577
Native Americans, gestational diabetes and, 514
Natural childbirth, 115, 181

Nausea
　active labor and, 237
　calling ob-gyn about, 168b
　combined hormonal birth control and, 337
　epidural block or spinal block and, 207b
　excessive salivation and, 88
　final weeks of pregnancy and, 167
　managing, 50–51, 68
　multiple pregnancy and, 477
　nitrous oxide and, 205
　postpartum care for, 282b
　preeclampsia and, 117, 502b
　pregnancy and, 46, 456
　systemic pain medication and, 204
　weight gain during pregnancy and, 489
　working during early pregnancy and, 60
Needles, coping with fear of, 411b
Needles sharing, 425, 432
Neonatal abstinence syndrome (NAS), 210
Neonatal intensive care unit (NICU)
　delivery before 39 weeks and, 173b, 174, 222b, 256
　expressed milk feeding in, 319
　fetal growth restriction and, 626
　macrosomia and, 628
　mother's gestational diabetes and, 515
　multiple pregnancy and, 474
　postpartum depression and, 291
　preeclampsia and, 510
　preterm birth and, 603
Neonatologists, 603, 617, 659
Nervous system, fetal development of, 38f, 41f
Nesting instinct, 165–166
Neural tube defects (NTDs). See also Folic acid
　another baby and, 670
　diagnostic tests, 573, 574
　family history of, 563b
　folic acid and, 11, 12b, 53b, 356
　as multifactorial disorder, 559
　obesity during pregnancy and, 491
　pregestational diabetes mellitus and, 521
　quad screen for, 92
　screening tests, 81t, 564, 570t, 571, 572
　seizure disorders and, 541
Neurofibromatosis, 554t
Neurological problems, 116, 430, 616
Newborns. See also After the baby is born; Babies
　appearance of, 272–273
　assisted vaginal delivery risks for, 246
　choosing doctors for, 104, 181
　delivery before 39 weeks and, 174
　flu shot during pregnancy and, 414, 415f
　FMLA and caring for, 442
　general anesthesia and, 208
　keeping warm after birth, 272
　mother's opioid use disorder and, 210
　preparing your home for, 154, 181
　preterm, caring for, 603
　systemic pain medication and, 204
NICU. See Neonatal intensive care unit
Night sweats, 434

Nipple shields, 316–317
Nipples
　bottles and, 320, 324b
　changes during pregnancy, 72
　contraction stress test and, 588
　flat or inverted, 158, 316–317
　sore, breastfeeding and, 314–315
　stimulation, labor and, 462
Nitrous oxide ("laughing gas"), 205
Nonfood items, craving to eat, 91, 497–498. See also Pica
Non-heme iron foods, 74b, 357
Non-opioid pain medications, 209
Nonsteroidal anti-inflammatory drugs (NSAIDs), 114, 277, 652
Nonstress test
　biophysical profile and, 585–587
　fetal growth restriction and, 625
　fetal well-being monitoring with, 584, 585
　gestational diabetes and, 519
　gestational hypertension or preeclampsia and, 509
　modified biophysical profile and, 587
　multiple pregnancy and, 479
　postterm pregnancy and, 175
　pregestational diabetes mellitus and, 525
Normal blood pressure, defined, 503b
Normal weight, 54t, 490
Norovirus infection, 448
North American Registry of Midwives (NARM), 25
Northern European descent, genetic disorders and, 554t
Nosebleeds, 98
Now I Lay Me Down to Sleep, 664
NSAIDs. See Nonsteroidal anti-inflammatory drugs
NTDs. See Neural tube defects
Nuchal translucency screening, 81t, 569
Numbing spray or cream, 288
Numbness
　carpal tunnel syndrome and, 152
　cesarean birth incision, 260
　in feet or legs, 125, 133b
Nurse practitioners, 26
Nursery, hospital, 157, 187, 189, 273, 274
Nurses, 26, 213, 284
NutraSweet (aspartame), 75, 366
Nutrients
　deficiency, craving for nonfood items and, 402
　digestive disorders and, 539
　for healthy lifestyle, 9
　healthy pregnancy weight and, 351, 487
　hypertension during pregnancy and, 504, 505f
　in lactose-free products, 459
　major, 352–353
　maternal stores, weight gain during pregnancy and, 55b
　mother's delivery to baby of, 114, 137, 153
　in mother's milk, 307, 324, 481
　placenta and, 615

Nutrients (continued)
    pressure on umbilical cord and, 597
    problems, multiple pregnancy and, 476–477
    vitamins and minerals, 354, 355t, 356–359
    weight gain during pregnancy and, 91
    weight loss surgery and, 495
Nutrition. See also Diet; Eating; Food or foods; Meals; Weight gain during pregnancy
    balancing your diet, 351
    breastfeeding and, 312–313
    food safety, 368–371, 368b
    foods to avoid or limit during pregnancy, 364–366
    healthy eating tips, 362–363
    major nutrients for, 352–353
    multiple pregnancy and, 477
    overview, 351
    planning healthy meals, 359–363
    poor, fetal growth restriction and, 624
    postpartum, 278b, 293
    resources, 372
    special diets and food restrictions, 366–368
    weeks 1 to 8 and, 52–54
    weeks 9 to 12 and, 73–75
    weeks 13 to 16, 90–91
    weeks 17 to 20, 100–101
    weeks 29 to 32, 142
    weeks 33 to 36, 153
    weight gain during pregnancy and, 363–366, 363t, 489
Nutrition Facts label, 362, 372
Nutritional counseling, 495
Nuts, 51

O

Obesity. See also Overweight; Weight of mother
    abnormal labor and, 632
    another baby and, 672–673
    BMI before pregnancy and, 54t
    dealing with comments about weight and, 488b
    defined, 490
    fundal height measurements and, 102
    future health risks and, 297t
    gestational diabetes and, 514
    pregnancy and, 489–490
    shoulder dystocia and, 634
Obsessive–compulsive disorder, 544–545
Obstetrician–gynecologists (ob-gyns). See also Maternal–fetal medicine (MFM) specialists; Prenatal care visits
    board-certification for, 23–24
    calling, after cesarean delivery, 261b
    calling, in labor, 151–152
    calling, in month 4, 91b
    calling, in month 5, 96–97, 98b
    calling, in month 6, 113b
    calling, in month 7, 133b
    calling, in month 8, 140b
    calling, in month 9, 160b
    calling, in month 10, 168b
    calling, lack of interest in sex, 295

Obstetrician–gynecologists (ob-gyns) (continued)
    calling, on feeding your baby, 301
    calling, on influenza, 415
    calling, on postpartum depression, 291b
    on coronavirus and travel, 439
    how often to see, 28
    how to talk with, 27b
    pelvic exam by, 30–31, 30f
    questions to ask, 26
    types of practices, 25–26
Obstetricians, 275
Obstetrics, 23
Obstructive sleep apnea, 167, 491
Occupational Safety and Health Act (OSH Act), 406, 442
Occupational Safety and Health Administration (OSHA), 61, 65, 406, 407, 449
Odors
    fishy, bacterial vaginosis and, 428
    fishy, trichomoniasis and, 427
    healthy vagina, 452
    of lochia, endometritis and, 640
    morning sickness and, 50
    of prenatal vitamins, 458
    of urine, hyperemesis gravidarum and, 51
    vaginal discharge, 90, 91b
Office on Women's Health, 347
Oil of lemon eucalyptus, Zika virus and, 436
Oils, dietary, 10, 353, 354, 361t. See also Fats
Oligohydramnios, 601, 635
Omega-3 fatty acids, 353, 357–358
Online pregnancy chat rooms, 455
Opioid use disorder, 13, 59, 209–210
Opioids, 13, 58–59, 204, 277
Oral sex, 7, 295
Organ damage, future risks of, 297t
Organization of Teratology Information Specialists (OTIS), 328
Orgasm, 111, 112, 345
Ovarian cancer, 302, 337
Ovaries
    FSH and, 48
    postpartum egg release by, 288–289
    pregnancy and, 15, 16f, 17f
    ultrasound exam of, 76
    week 2 development and, 43
Overheating, exercise and, 377
Over-the-counter medications
    acne treatment, 70–71
    birth defect risks with, 399–400
    prenatal care and, 62
    telling ob-gyn about, 5, 460
    teratogenic, 396
Overweight
    BMI before pregnancy and, 54t
    dealing with comments about weight and, 488b
    defined, 490
    gestational diabetes and, 514
    preeclampsia prevention and, 510
    prepregnancy, macrosomia and, 627

Overweight (continued)
  resources, 499
  weight gain during pregnancy and, 364
  weight loss after pregnancy and, 493
Ovulation
  after miscarriage, 648
  birth control implant and, 334
  birth control injection and, 336
  breastfeeding and, 302
  combined hormonal birth control and, 337
  lactational amenorrhea method and, 341–342
  menstrual cycle and, 15
  peak day for, 19
  progestin-only pills and, 339
  week 2 development and, 43
  weight loss and, 494
Ovulation predictor kits, 19
Oxycodone, 13, 209–210
Oxygen
  asthma during pregnancy and, 530, 531f
  blood circulation and, 501
  cesarean delivery and, 257
  exchange, week 16 and, 86
  hypertension during pregnancy and, 504, 505f
  lack of, stillbirth and, 658
  mother's delivery to baby of, 114, 138, 270
  nitrous oxide mixed with, 205
  nonreactive nonstress test and, 585
  pinched umbilical cord and, 254
  placenta and, 615
  placental abruption and, 618
  pressure on umbilical cord and, 597
  Rh incompatibility and, 609
  seizure disorders and, 541
  shoulder dystocia and, 628, 634
  umbilical cord prolapse and, 636
Oxytocin
  after delivery, 639
  breastfeeding and, 302, 463–464
  contraction stress test and, 588
  labor augmentation and, 238, 633–634
  labor induction and, 176, 221b, 224, 225
  PROM management and, 598
  uterine atony prevention and, 639

P

Pacific Islanders, gestational diabetes and, 514
Pacifiers, 195, 302, 305b, 312
Pain or pains. *See also* Abdominal pain; Backache; Chest pain
  aches and, 114
  after cesarean delivery, 261b
  breastfeeding, 315
  calf pain, 125, 133b, 139–140, 377b
  ectopic pregnancy and, 63, 649–650
  fear of, lack of interest in sex and, 294
  lower back, 98, 100, 113b
  with no relief between contractions, 168b, 232
  pelvic, ultrasound exam to determine, 580

Pain or pains (continued)
  perineal, 287–288
  placental abruption and, 134
  postpartum, 277, 282b
  shoulder, 117, 502b
  sore nipples, 314–315
  vaginal area, 91b
Pain relief
  after cesarean delivery, 260
  after delivery, 276–277
  childbirth classes, 213, 216–217
  equipment for labor and delivery, 212, 214–215f
  during labor, 115, 143–144, 181, 184
  labor induction and, 226
  medications, 60, 185, 204–208, 652
  non-medication options, 185
  opioid use disorder and, 209–210
  overview, 203
  pacifiers and, 312
  resources, 217
  techniques, 210–212
Panic disorder, 544–545
Parallel hold, 321b
Para-menthane-diol, Zika virus and, 436
Parasites, 409, 422, 427, 434, 458
Parent support networks, 566
Parents with genetic disorders, 562
Partners. *See also* Men
  childbirth and, 115–116, 145
  continuous labor support by, 213
  as controlling and jealous, 454–455
  feeding duties and, 320f, 324
  FMLA for, 442
  with HIV, pre-exposure prophylaxis and, 426
  labor, 115–116, 184, 235, 238, 240
  multiple sexual, STIs and, 7
  pelvic exams and, 30
  postpartum care team and, 283–284
  prenatal care visits and, 27b
  role of, 13–14, 14b
  stillbirth and, 662
  talking about feelings with, 290, 295
Parvovirus, 433, 658
Past pregnancies
  asthma and, 530
  gestational diabetes and, 514
  macrosomia in, 627
  postpartum hemorrhage and, 639
  prepregnancy review of, 5–6
  preterm birth in, 594, 595
  problems, news of new pregnancy and, 64
  shoulder dystocia and, 634
Patau syndrome (trisomy 13)
  as aneuploidy, 561
  fetal growth restriction and, 624
  multiple pregnancy and, 479
  screening tests, 570t, 571,
Patch, birth control. *See* Birth control patch
Pathogens, 409, 410–412
Pathologists, 659
Patient-controlled analgesia, 204, 206
Peak day, for ovulation, 19

Pediatric care services, 443. *See also* Child care
Pediatric sub-specialist, 200
Pediatric surgical specialist, 200
Pediatricians
    baby's genetic disorder and, 576
    choosing, 104, 107, 191, 193, 200
    newborn's test results sent to, 275
    postpartum care team and, 284
    stillbirth evaluation by, 659
Pedicures, 452
Pelvic bone pain, 125
Pelvic exams
    cervical insufficiency and, 600
    to check for dilation, 145, 152, 155, 176, 236, 593–594
    ectopic pregnancy and, 650
    endometritis diagnosis, 640
    many, long labor and, 639
    miscarriage diagnosis and, 646
    prenatal care and, 62
    what happens during? 28, 30, 30f
Pelvic inflammatory disease (PID), 424, 648
Pelvic organ prolapse (POP), 246
Pelvic pressure, 117, 133, 145, 152, 596b
Penetration, 111, 294, 295, 458, 647
Penicillin, 156, 432
Penis, 187, 188f, 275, 340, 340f, 418
Perinatologists, 474b. *See also* Maternal–fetal medicine (MFM) specialists
Perineal pain, 287–288
Perineal tears
    assisted vaginal delivery and, 246
    calling ob-gyn about, 282b
    large babies and, 515, 628
    learning care for, 276
    pain from, 285, 287–288
    postpartum hemorrhage and, 638
    shoulder dystocia and, 628, 635
Perineum, 205, 240, 277, 278b
Peritoneum, 257
Permanent birth control, 332
Permethrin, Zika virus and, 436
Persistent GTD, 654
Personal care, frequently asked questions on, 451–453, 452f, 453f
Personal protective equipment (PPE), 406
Personality, newborn's, 273
Personality disorders, 544–545
Pertussis (whooping cough), 7, 415–416. *See also* Tetanus toxoid, reduced diphtheria toxoid, and acellular pertussis (Tdap) vaccine
Pesticides, 14–15, 60, 403, 441
Petroleum jelly, 98
Phenylketonuria, 563b
Phobias, 544–545
Phone, telehealth visits by, 29b
Physical activity. *See also* Exercise
    gestational diabetes and, 514
    postpartum, 278b
Physical disabilities, 529, 545
Physical exams
    comfort with ob-gyn and, 27
    making more comfortable, 28, 30

Physical exams (continued)
    for newborn, 274
    pregnancy and, 47
    prenatal care and, 62, 75
    PROM management and, 598
Physician assistants, 26
Pica, 91, 106, 402, 497–498
Picaridin, Zika virus and, 436
Pictures of the birth, 145
PID (pelvic inflammatory disease), 424, 648
Pilates, 382
Pillows, full-body, 69, 70f, 99, 99f
Pills. *See* Birth control pills
Pins-and-needles feeling, let-down reflex and, 307
Pituitary gland, 48
Placenta. *See also* Placenta problems
    ABO incompatibility and, 607–608
    agents passing through, 396
    asthma and oxygen delivery to, 530
    chorionic villus sampling of, 81t, 574, 574f
    cord blood from, 132, 190
    delivery, as third stage of childbirth, 232, 233f, 240–241, 633, 633t
    delivery, cesarean delivery and, 259
    delivery before 39 weeks and, 171
    diagnostic tests of, 564
    fats and, 354
    hypertension and, 504, 505f
    insulin and, 518, 524
    lead exposure through, 105
    medications crossing, 304
    multiple pregnancy and, 472, 473f
    nutrients for baby through, 114
    oxygen for baby through, 114, 270
    position, feeling baby's movements and, 96
    position, normal, 616f
    position, ultrasound exam of, 580
    postterm pregnancy and, 175, 220
    preeclampsia and, 117
    retained tissue, 638
    stillbirth and evaluation of, 659
    syphilis transmission through, 426
    TB transmission through, 435
    teratogens and, 396
    weight gain during pregnancy and, 55b
    weight of mother and, 487
Placenta accreta, 619–621, 620f, 637–638
Placenta increta, 620, 621
Placenta percreta, 620, 621
Placenta previa
    about, 615–616, 616f
    breech presentation and, 247
    cesarean delivery and, 254
    delivery before 39 weeks and, 171
    discordant twins and, 477
    exercise and, 376
    external cephalic version and, 248
    fetal growth restriction and, 624
    incision for cesarean delivery and, 258
    indicated preterm birth and, 601
    labor induction as unsafe with, 221
    placenta accreta and, 619
    resources, 621

750 • INDEX

Placenta previa (continued)
    signs, symptoms, and treatment, 617
    types, 616
    vaginal bleeding and, 134
Placenta problems
    cesarean delivery and, 173, 226, 244, 254, 255, 259, 629, 633
    delivery before 39 weeks and, 171
    fetal growth restriction and, 624
    fetal well-being tests and, 583
    labor induction and, 219
    multiple cesarean births and, 80
    multiple pregnancy and, 476
    overview, 615
    preeclampsia and, 491
    resources, 621
    stillbirth and, 658
    testing and, 583
    TOLAC and, 262
Placental abruption
    about, 618, 618f
    cervical insufficiency and, 600
    chronic hypertension and, 504
    delivery before 39 weeks and, 171
    diagnosis, 618
    external cephalic version and, 248, 250
    indicated preterm birth and, 601
    labor induction and, 219
    opioid use disorder and, 59
    PROM management and, 598
    resources, 621
    thrombophilias and, 536
    treatment, 619
    types, 618
    vaginal bleeding and, 134
Platelets, 78, 117, 507, 508
Pneumococcal disease vaccine, 412, 414t
Pneumococcal pneumonia and vaccine, 420–421
Pneumonia, 369–370, 414, 425
Polycystic ovary syndrome (PCOS), 514
Polydactyly, isolated, 554t
Polyhydramnios, 636, 639
POP (pelvic organ prolapse), 246
Positions. See Birthing positions
Postpartum care. See also After the baby is born; Postpartum period
    doula hired for, 184
    lifestyle habits, 292–293
    physical health after childbirth, 284–288
    plan (checklist), 278, 283, 711–712
    planning, 281–284, 283f
    resources, 299
    sex and family planning, 293–296
    when to call your doctor, 282b
    your changing body, 288–289
    your feelings after childbirth, 289–292
    your future health, 296, 297t, 298
Postpartum care team, 269, 278, 278b, 283–284, 545, 716

Postpartum depression
    another baby and, 672
    exercise and, 387
    mental health during pregnancy and, 544, 545
    multiple babies and, 481
    resources, 299
    risk factors and treatment, 291–292
    screening test, 128–129b
    symptoms, 278b, 290
    warning signs, 291b
Postpartum endometritis, 639–640
Postpartum exercises, 388–392
Postpartum hemorrhage
    bleeding disorders and, 535
    causes, 637–638
    large babies and, 514, 628
    management, 639
    risk factors, 638–639
    shoulder dystocia and, 635
    signs and symptoms, 638
Postpartum period. See also After the baby is born; Postpartum care
    blood clotting disorders and, 537
    hemorrhoids during, 141
    multiple sclerosis and, 533
    preeclampsia during, 116, 508
Postpartum sterilization, 335t, 343–344, 344f
Postpartum Support International Helpline, 135, 279, 299, 465
Postpartum thyroiditis, 546
Postterm pregnancy
    defined, 172b, 220, 594b, 627b
    fetal well-being tests and, 583
    labor induction and, 219
    reasons for, 174–175
    TOLAC and, 262
Powdered formula, 326
Preeclampsia. See also High blood pressure; Hypertension
    another baby and, 672–673
    antiphospholipid syndrome and, 537–538
    asthma and, 530
    bed rest and, 457
    birth place choices and, 93
    calling ob-gyn about, 113b, 133b, 140b, 160b, 168b
    defined, 501
    delivery before 39 weeks and, 171
    diagnosis, 508–509
    eating disorders and, 496
    elective delivery and, 172
    exercise and, 375
    fetal well-being tests with, 582
    future risks, 297t
    gestational diabetes and, 515
    heart disease and, 543
    high protein levels and, 78
    hypertension and, 501, 506
    hyperthyroidism and, 546
    indicated preterm birth and, 600–601

INDEX • 751

Preeclampsia (continued)
    kidney disease and, 543
    labor induction and, 172, 220, 221b
    lupus and, 534
    multifetal pregnancy reduction and, 470b
    multiple pregnancy and, 476
    obesity and risks of, 490–491
    past pregnancies and, 6
    postpartum hemorrhage and, 639
    pregestational diabetes mellitus and, 521
    prevention, 510–511
    resources, 511
    risks, 507–508, 516
    with severe features, 509–510
    signs and symptoms, 117, 159, 160, 502b, 508
    sleep apnea and, 491
    TOLAC and, 263
    treatment, 509–510
    when it may occur, 116, 159
Preeclampsia Foundation, 118, 511
Preexisting health conditions, 3–4
Pre-exposure prophylaxis (PrEP), for HIV, 426
Pregestational diabetes mellitus
    blood sugar levels tracking, 522
    care after pregnancy, 526
    controlling, during pregnancy, 522
    exercise and, 524
    fetal well-being tests with, 525
    healthy eating and, 524
    labor and delivery, 525
    managing high and low blood sugar, 522–524
    medications, 524–525
    overview, 520–521
    prepregnancy care, 521–522
    risks to your pregnancy, 521
    special tests, 525
Pregnancy (pregnancies). *See also* Fetal well-being monitoring tests; Future pregnancies; Multiple pregnancy; Past pregnancies; specific months
    after miscarriage, 648
    after weight loss surgery, 494–495
    body changes during, 33–41f, 46–49
    CDC information on, 20
    choosing doctors for, 23–24
    choosing other practitioners for, 25–26, 25b
    confirmation, ultrasound exam for, 579
    depression screening during, 128–129b
    early loss. *See* Early pregnancy loss
    eating disorders and, 495–499
    foods to avoid or limit during, 364–366
    health problems during, 296, 298
    higher-order, 470b, 471
    how long? 456
    HPV vaccination and, 419
    involving your other children in, 118, 673–674
    late loss. *See* Stillbirth
    mental health during, 126–127, 128–129b
    news of, when to share, 64

Pregnancy (pregnancies) (continued)
    normal, 593
    obesity and, 489–494
    opioid use disorder and, 209
    prenatal care and, 62
    preventing Rh problems during, 610–612
    problems, TOLAC and, 262
    Rh factor in, 610–611f, 610–612
    signs and symptoms, 44
    spacing between, 132, 331, 669–670
    terms for length of, 172b, 594b, 627b
    tests, 47–49, 64, 221
    things to avoid during, 56–60
    travel and, 437
    vaccines and, 437
    weight gain during. *See* Weight gain during pregnancy
Pregnancy brain, 99
Pregnancy Discrimination Act, 441
Pregnant@Work website, 441, 449
Preimplantation genetic testing, 568, 574
Prelabor rupture of membranes (PROM). *See also* Preterm PROM
    bacterial vaginosis and, 428
    causes and risks, 597
    chlamydia or gonorrhea infections and, 424
    defined, 593
    delivery before 39 weeks and, 171
    diagnosis, 597–598
    exercise and, 376
    external cephalic version and, 250
    labor induction and, 220
    management, 598–599
    risk factors, 597
    as special concern, 145, 146
    trichomoniasis and, 427
Premenstrual dysphoric disorder (PMDD), 291
Premenstrual syndrome (PMS), 291
Prenatal care visits
    assisted vaginal delivery overview during, 462
    blood pressure checks at, 502
    blood type tests, 607
    childbirth (labor) partner and, 115, 184
    COVID-19 health crisis and, 29b
    depression screening, 127
    diagnostic testing, 568
    factors for, 26–27
    FMLA for, 442
    gestational diabetes and, 516–517
    group appointments, 26
    hepatitis B virus testing, 418
    how often? 28
    infection testing, 409
    making the most of, 27b
    multiple pregnancy and, 479
    multiple sclerosis and, 533
    obesity and, 490
    partners' role, 14b
    travel during pregnancy and, 444
    weeks 1 to 8, 52, 61–62
    weeks 9 to 12, 75–79

752 • INDEX

Prenatal care visits (continued)
    weeks 13 to 16, 92
    weeks 21 to 24, 115
    weeks 25 to 28, 130–131
    weeks 29 to 32, 145
    weeks 33 to 36, 155–156
    weeks 37 to 40, 170–171
    weight gain check, 364
    weight gain during pregnancy and, 488
    what happens during? 28
Prenatal vitamins. See Vitamins, prenatal
Prepregnancy care
    another baby and, 669, 670
    carrier screening, 8, 9t, 568
    checkup, 3–8, 9t
    family health history, 4–5
    getting pregnant, 15–20
    healthy lifestyle and, 9–15
    hypertension assessment and, 510
    importance, 3
    kidney disease and, 543
    medications and supplements, 5
    partners' role, 14b
    past pregnancies, 5–6
    preeclampsia and, 510–511
    preexisting health conditions, 4
    pregestational diabetes mellitus and, 520
    previous stillbirth and, 663
    protection against STIs, 7–8
    resources, 20
    vaccinations, 6–7
Prescription drugs. See also Illegal drugs;
    Medications
    acne treatment, 70, 337
    birth defect risks, 397–399
    breastfeeding and, 303–304, 313
    fetal growth restriction and, 626
    pregnancy complications and, 59
    prenatal care and, 62
    prepregnancy care and, 5, 13
    teratogenic, 396
Presentation, 231b, 254, 598. See also Breech
    presentation; Malpresentation
Preservatives, in vaccines, 410
Preterm babies
    breastfeeding, 302
    breech presentation and, 247
    CMV transmission through breast milk and,
        431, 604b
    delayed cord clamping and, 189, 463
    feeding expressed milk to, 319–320
    first few hours for, 269
    incision for cesarean delivery and, 258
    multiple, pumping milk for, 481
    multiple pregnancy and, 480
    preeclampsia and, 507–508
    resources, 604–605
    tocolytics and, 475
    umbilical cord prolapse and, 636
Preterm birth. See also Preterm delivery; Preterm
    labor
    after the baby is born, 241
    another baby and, 672

Preterm birth (continued)
    antiphospholipid syndrome and, 537–538
    asthma and, 530
    breech presentation and, 247
    caffeine and, 458
    CDC information on, 118
    chlamydia or gonorrhea infections and, 424
    chronic hypertension and, 504
    CMV and, 431
    defined, 593
    depression and, 127
    eating disorders and, 496
    extremely preterm, outcomes tool, 604
    first few hours for, 269
    future heart disease and, 297t
    incision for cesarean delivery and, 258
    indicated, 600–601
    kidney disease and, 543, 544
    labor induction and, 220
    lead exposure and, 105
    listeriosis and, 369, 433
    lupus and, 534
    marijuana and, 58
    medical evaluation of baby after, 241
    medications before, 601–602
    multiple pregnancy and, 473
    NICU stay for, 603
    obesity and, 491
    opioid use disorder and, 59
    outcomes-for-babies-born-before-26-weeks
        calculator, 603
    past pregnancies and, 6
    past preterm birth and, 604
    postpartum depression and, 291
    preventing another, 604
    prior, preterm PROM and, 597
    resources, 604–605
    risk factors, 595b
    risks, multifetal pregnancy reduction and,
        470b
    rubella and, 419
    seizure disorders and, 541
    smoking and, 56
    surfactant replacement therapy and,
        602–603
    survival, health problems and disabilities
        and, 602, 603
    syphilis and, 426
    terms describing, 172b, 594b, 627b
    thyroid disease and, 546
    time between pregnancies and, 331, 595b,
        669
    trichomoniasis and, 427
    unhealthy substances and, 13
    what to expect after, 603
Preterm delivery. See also Preterm birth
    fetal growth restriction and, 626
    placenta previa and, 616
Preterm labor. See also Preterm birth
    activity restriction and, 146
    bed rest and, 457
    calling ob-gyn about, 113b, 133, 133b,
        140b, 160b

Preterm labor (continued)
    cervical changes and, 593–594, 595
    defined, 593
    diagnosis, 595–596
    exercise and, 55, 376
    hydramnios and, 521
    hyperthyroidism and, 546
    management, 596
    multiple pregnancy and, 376, 474
    pregestational diabetes mellitus and, 521
    resources, 604–605
    risk factors, 55, 376, 594–595
    sexual activity and, 112
    signs of, 116–117, 133, 145–146, 159, 475*b*, 596*b*
    tocolytics and, 475
Preterm PROM, 146, 593, 597, 598, 599, 672. *See also* Prelabor rupture of membranes
Preventive care, health insurance, 443
Printing press operators, hazards for, 405*b*
Privacy, telehealth visits and, 29*b*
Private cord blood banks, 190, 191
Problems with baby's growth. *See* Growth problems for baby
Progesterone
    constipation and, 125
    menstrual cycle and, 16*f*
    pregnancy and, 15
    preventing another preterm birth and, 604
    reproduction, pregnancy, and birth and, 48
    sleepiness and, 46
Progestin, 333, 334, 337
Progestin-only birth control pills, 334–335*t*, 339, 347
PROM. *See* Prelabor rupture of membranes
Propylthiouracil, 546
Prostaglandins, 174, 224, 639
Protein
    breastfeeding and, 313
    maternal stores of, 55*b*
    urinary, preeclampsia and, 92, 117, 508–509
Protein C deficiency, 536–537
Protein foods
    in balanced diet, 351, 352
    five food groups and, 10, 361, 361*t*, 362
    nonmeat sources, 51
    vegetarian diets and, 367
Protein hydrolysate formulas, 326
Protein S deficiency, 536–537
Proteinuria, 508
Prothrombin G20210A mutation, 536–537
Pseudoephedrine, birth defects and, 454
Pubic symphysis, 124*f*, 125
Public cord blood banks, 190, 191
Pulmonary embolism (PE), 535, 535*b*
Pulse
    after cesarean delivery, 260
    after delivery, 275
    checking newborn's, 274
Pumped breast-milk feeding, 158, 188–189. *See also* Expressed milk
Pumping milk, blocked ducts and, 318

Pushing
    as stage 2 of childbirth, 232, 233*f*, 239–240, 633, 633*t*
    urge, active labor and, 238, 239
Pyelonephritis, 430

Q

Quad or quadruple screening tests, 92, 570*t*, 571
Quadruplets, 254, 469, 471, 474*t*, 480. *See also* Multiple pregnancy
Questions. *See also* Frequently asked questions
    after telehealth visits, 29*b*
    first prenatal care visit and, 26
Quickening, 85–86, 96. *See also* Baby's movement

R

Racket sports, 381
Radiation, 61, 76, 317, 403–404, 441, 446
Radioisotopes, 404
Radiological Society of North America, 589
Raising Multiples, 482
Rape, emergency contraception after, 346–347
Rash, 141, 427, 435. *See also* Measles infections; Rubella
Ready-to-use formulas, 326
Rear-facing car seats, 193–194, 194*f*
Recessive genes, 557–558
Recessive genetic disorders, 554*t*. *See also* Genetic disorders
Recovery
    after cesarean delivery, 259–261, 628
    after delivery, 273, 275–277
    after ectopic pregnancy, 652–653
    cesarean delivery on request and, 173, 255
    for cesarean versus vaginal delivery, 226, 244
    FMLA for, 442
    VBAC and, 263
Rectum
    bleeding from, IBD and, 540
    chlamydia or gonorrhea infections and, 424
    GBS in, 155, 431
    Kegel exercises and, 286*b*, 383
    muscles, tear involving, 287
    nerves, accidental bowel leakage and, 286–287
    pressure on, active labor and, 239
    uterus weight on, 125
    varicose veins near, 140
Red blood cells, 76, 78, 507. *See also* Anemia
    Rh antibodies and, 609, 610–611*f*
Reflexes, baby's, 271–272, 271*t*
Regional analgesia, 205–208, 343
Regional anesthesia, 144, 205–208
Relapse
    in multiple sclerosis, 533
    opioid use disorder and, 59
Relaxation techniques
    fear of needles and, 411*b*
    for pain relief during labor, 144, 184, 185, 235, 237
    stress of pregnancy and, 142

Relaxin, 96
Renting breast pumps, 322
Resident doctors, 237
Respiratory distress syndrome (RDS), 521
Respiratory illness, E. coli and, 369–370. See also Breathing
Respiratory system problems, placenta previa and, 616
Restrictive bariatric surgery, 494, 495
Retinoids, topical, 71
Reversible birth control. See also Birth control
    barrier methods, 339–342
    combined hormonal birth methods, 337–339, 338f
    forms, 332
    implant, 334–336, 334f
    injections, 336, 336f
    IUDs, 332–333, 333f
    progestin-only pills, 339
Rh antibodies
    problems caused by, 609, 610–611f
    RhIg and, 611
    screening, 130, 610
Rh factor
    blood type and, 78, 607
    in future pregnancy, 647
    in pregnancy, 610–611f, 610–612
RhIg. See Rh immunoglobulin
Rh immunoglobulin (RhIg), 130, 276, 610, 611–612, 647
Rh sensitization, 583
Rheumatoid arthritis (RA), 529, 532, 533
RhoGAM, 611
Ripening the cervix, 176, 223–224, 231b
Rooming in, 157–158, 189, 273
Root canals, 88
Rubella, 78, 403, 419, 624. See also Measles–mumps–rubella (MMR) vaccine
Rumination disorder, 498
Running, 381
Rupture of membranes. See also Prelabor rupture of membranes; Sweeping the membranes
    abnormal labor and, 634
    amniotomy for, 224–225
    endometritis and, 639
    labor and, 169, 232
    labor induction and, 176
    preterm labor and, 117, 133, 145, 475b, 596b
    umbilical cord prolapse and, 636
Rupture of uterus. See Uterine rupture

S

Saccharin (Sweet'n Low), 75, 366
Sacred hour, 270. See also Skin-to-skin care or contact
Sadness or depression? 456–457
Safe Kids Worldwide, 200
Salicylic acid, topical, 71
Salivation, excessive, 88
Salmonellosis, 369
Salt, during pregnancy, 365
Saltwater mouth rinse, 88
Sample Birth Plan, 182, 187, 708–710
Sashimi, 458
Saturated fats, 353, 354
Saunas, 405, 452
Schizophrenia, 544–545
Sciatica, 124–125, 124f
Screening panels, 568
Screening tests
    depression, 128–129b
    diagnostic tests compared with, 565t, 566
    genetic disorders, 8, 9t, 79, 81–82, 81t, 92, 553–555
    group B streptococcus, 155–156, 171
    lead, 104
    multiple pregnancy and, 479
    newborns, 274–275, 279
    Rh antibody, 130
    risk assessment using, 553
    sexually transmitted infections, 79, 156, 422, 425, 427
    showing increased risk, 572
Scrotum, 138, 273
Seasickness, 448
Seat belts, 447b, 448
Seated leg raises, 384, 384f
Seated overhead triceps extension, 384, 384f
Seated side stretch, 386, 386f
Second trimester
    Braxton Hicks contractions in, 671
    D&E in, 657
    defined, 49
    as honeymoon period, 86
    placenta previa and, 617
    preterm PROM and vaginal bleeding in, 597
    screening tests, 81t, 82, 570t, 571
    sexual desire during, 111
    surgery during, 453
    weeks 13 to 16 and, 85
    weight gain during, 54t, 101, 363t, 489t
Secondhand smoke, 13, 14b, 56, 313, 460. See also Smoking
Security, of telehealth visits, 29b
Sedatives, 204
Seizure disorders, 4, 396, 529, 541–542
Selective serotonin reuptake inhibitors (SSRIs), 127
Semen, 346, 425, 452
Sepsis, 632
Sequential screening for genetic disorders, 570t, 572
Sex (sexual activity). See also Birth control; Sexual intercourse; Sexually transmitted infections
    after childbirth, 293
    infection prevention and, 409
    lack of interest in, 294–295
    during pregnancy, 111–112, 164, 458
    STI transmission and, 422, 425
Sex, baby's, 116, 580
Sex chromosomes, 555, 556, 556f, 557f
    abnormalities, screening tests, 571

Sex toys, 7, 111, 458, 647
Sex-linked disorders, 558–559
Sexual abuse, 30–31
Sexual desire, 15, 111, 294
Sexual intercourse
    after childbirth, 294
    birth control after pregnancy and, 132, 331
    fertility and, 15, 17f
    genital warts and, 418
    methotrexate and, 651
    miscarriage and, 646
    during pregnancy, 111, 458
Sexually transmitted infections (STIs)
    birth control implant and, 336
    birth control injection and, 336
    CDC on, 437
    cervical cap and, 340
    chlamydia, 424–425
    circumcision and, 187
    combined hormonal birth control and, 339
    condoms and, 340
    diaphragms and, 340
    ectopic pregnancy and, 648
    genital herpes, 422–424
    gonorrhea, 424–425
    HIV and AIDS, 425–426
    IUDs and, 333
    partners' role, 14b
    prenatal care and, 75
    prepregnancy care and, 3–4
    progestin-only pills and, 339
    protection against, 7–8
    protection guidelines, 422
    resources, 437
    syphilis, 426–427
    trichomoniasis, 427
    Zika virus, 435–436
SHARE: Pregnancy and Infant Loss Support, 655, 664
Shellfish, 313, 365, 372, 407
Shingles, 421, 422
Ships, 437, 448
Shots. *See also* Vaccinations
    coping with fear of, 411b
Shoulder dystocia, 491, 515, 628, 634–635
Shoulder pain, 63–64, 502b
Shoulder presentation, 231b
Showers, 69, 185, 211, 234, 238, 318
Sick leave, 89, 443
Sickle cell disease
    as autosomal recessive disorder, 558
    carrier screening, 9t, 567t
    fetal growth restriction and, 624
    as genetic disorder, 554t, 563b
    neural tube defects and, 12b, 53b, 356
    placental abruption and, 618
    prenatal diagnostic tests for, 81t
Sickle Cell Disease Association of America, 578
Side sleeping, 69
Side-lying position, 288, 309b
SIDS. *See* Sudden infant death syndrome

Simple carbohydrates, 352, 517
Simple sugars, 74–75
Sitting issues, 100, 185, 210–211, 287
Sitz baths, 285, 287. *See also* Baths
Skin
    acne treatment, 70–71
    changes during pregnancy, 71, 82
    color of baby's, 271–272, 271t
    itchy, 141
    lupus and, 534
    TB tests on, 434
    treatments, pregnancy and, 60
Skin-to-skin care or contact, 189, 210, 270, 279, 306
SLE. *See* Lupus
Sleep
    after the baby is born, 273, 292–293
    exercise and, 55, 387
    mother, after delivery, 275
    pregnancy-related stress and, 89
    problems, 68–70, 99, 99f, 152
    safe, for babies, 195, 197f, 201
    snoring during, 167
    third trimester and, 138
Sleep apnea, 167, 491, 493
Small infant size, 297t. *See also* Baby's size; Fetal growth restriction; Growth problems for baby
Smartphone apps
    blood sugar levels tracking, 517
    fertility tracking, 17, 18b, 342
    fitness, 380, 381b
    frequently asked questions on, 455
Smells. *See also* Odors
    morning sickness and, 50
    vaginal discharge, 90, 91b
Smoking. *See also* Secondhand smoke
    blood pressure and, 502
    breastfeeding and, 313
    cessation aids, 399
    combined hormonal birth control and, 337
    ectopic pregnancy and, 649
    fetal growth restriction and, 624, 626
    gestational diabetes and, 520
    partners' role, 14b
    placenta previa and, 616
    placental abruption and, 618
    pneumococcal pneumonia vaccine and, 421
    preeclampsia and, 511
    pregnancy complications and, 56
    prepregnancy care and, 13
    preterm birth risk and, 595b
    preterm PROM and, 597
    quitting tips and tools, 21, 65
Smoothies, 101
Snacks, 12, 50, 61, 101, 362, 526
Snoring, 167
Social workers, 26, 284
Society for Maternal–Fetal Medicine, 31
Sodium, during pregnancy, 365
Solo practice ob-gyns, 25, 26

Solvents, as workplace hazards, 61, 441
Sophrology, 216
Soreness, vaginal area, 91b
Southeast Asian descent, carrier screening, 9t
Southern Iranian descent, carrier screening, 554t, 567t
Soy formulas, 326
Special Supplemental Nutrition Program for Women, Infants, and Children (WIC), 363
Sperm
 chromosomes in, 555–556, 646
 damage to, 14
 fertility and, 17, 17f
 IUDs preventing fertilization by, 333
 twins formation and, 470, 471f
 vasectomy and, 346
Spermicides, 334–335t, 341, 341f
Sphincter muscle, 287
Spices, imported, lead containing, 106
Spider veins, 86, 89, 147. *See also* Varicose veins
Spina bifida, 12b, 53b, 356. *See also* Neural tube defects
Spinal blocks
 for cesarean delivery, 256
 epidural block combined with, 208
 labor induction and, 226
 monitoring after delivery, 275
 observation after baby is born, 241
 as regional anesthesia, 144, 206f, 207–208
 side effects, 207b
 von Willebrand disease and, 538
Spinal muscular atrophy (SMA), 8, 9t, 558, 566, 567t
Splenda (sucralose), 75, 366
Sponge, birth control, 296, 334–335t, 340, 341f
Spoons hold, 321b
Spotting, 48, 63, 111, 167. *See also* Vaginal bleeding
Squatting, 185, 210–211, 215f, 240
Stairs, pain in walking up, 133b
Standard Days fertility awareness method, 342–343
Standing, 100, 185, 210–211, 440b, 441
Standing back bend, 387, 387f
State Children's Health Insurance Program (SCHIP), 444
State Health Insurance Exchanges, 443
States' opioid use laws and policies, 210
Station, during labor, 231b
Stem cells, 132, 189, 463
Sterile water, for powdered or condensed formulas, 326–327
Sterilization, 332, 334–335t, 343
 female, 343–345, 344f, 345f
 male, 345–346, 346f
Stevia (Truvia and SweetLeaf), 75, 366
Stillbirth
 another pregnancy after, 663–664
 chorioamnionitis and, 632
 diagnosis of, 657
 fetal well-being tests and, 581

Stillbirth (continued)
 the future after, 663
 genetic disorder risk and, 563b
 gestational diabetes and, 515
 grieving, 659–662, 660b
 hyperthyroidism and, 546
 listeriosis and, 369, 433
 lupus and, 534
 marijuana and, 58
 multiple pregnancy and, 480
 obesity and, 491
 opioid use disorder and, 59
 pregestational diabetes mellitus and, 521
 resources, 664
 rubella and, 419
 seeking support after, 662–663
 smoking and, 56
 subsequent pregnancies and, 6
 syphilis and, 426
 tests and evaluations after, 658–659
 thrombophilias and, 536
 unhealthy substances and, 13
 what went wrong? 658
 you and your partner after, 662
STIs. *See* Sexually transmitted infections
Stomach ache, 417
Stool, baby's, 311b
Stool softeners, 126, 286, 287, 288
Strength, activities or exercises for, 55, 381–382
Stress
 exercise and, 387
 lack of interest in sex and, 294
 multiple babies and, 481
 postpartum depression and, 291
 pregnancy-related, 89, 91b, 127, 133b
Stretch marks, 452–453, 453f
Stripping the membranes, 174, 176, 221b, 224, 225f, 238
Stroke
 blood clotting disorders and, 535
 chronic hypertension and, 504
 combined hormonal birth control and, 337
 eclampsia and, 507
 preeclampsia and, 491, 508
 risks, chronic high blood pressure and, 297t
Structural chromosomal disorders, 560, 561–562
Student nurses, 237
Substance Abuse and Mental Health Services Administration's Treatment Services Locator, 65
Substance use, 14b, 59, 595b, 624
Substance use disorders, 544–545
Sucralose (Splenda), 75, 366
Sudden infant death syndrome (SIDS)
 breastfeeding and, 302, 463
 pacifiers and, 195, 312
 resources, 201
 secondhand smoke and, 313
 smoking and, 13, 56
Sugar and sugar substitutes, 74–75, 366
Sun protection, 71, 652

Sunett (acesulfame-K), 75, 366
Supplemental Nutrition Assistance Program (SNAP), 363, 372
Supplements, 5, 29b, 60, 313, 460. *See also* Medications; Vitamins
Surfactant, 121, 602–603
Surgery
  breast, 158, 317
  ectopic pregnancy, 650, 652
  fetal, 555, 611
  fibroids, 222
  past, prenatal care and, 62
  during pregnancy, 453
  uterine, placenta previa and, 615
  weight-loss, 493, 494–495
Surma, 106
Sushi, 365, 370, 458
Swaddling, 210
Sweeping the membranes, 174, 176, 221b, 224, 225f, 238
Sweeteners, artificial, 74–75
SweetLeaf (stevia), 75, 366
Sweet'n Low (saccharin), 75, 366
Swelling, exercise and, 55
Swimming, 380, 388, 478
Symptothermal fertility awareness method, 342–343
Syphilis, 8, 79, 156, 403, 426–427, 658
Systemic analgesics, 204
Systemic lupus erythematosus (SLE). *See* Lupus
Systolic blood pressure, 502, 502b, 503

T

T-ACE test, 57b
Tai chi, 382
Talk therapy, 291
Tandem feeding, 319
Targeted carrier screening, 566
Taste alteration, epidural block or spinal block and, 207b
Tax credits, 444
Tay–Sachs disease
  carrier screening, 9t, 567t
  family history and, 563b
  as genetic disorder, 553, 554t, 558
  prenatal diagnostic tests, 81t
  resources, 578
Tdap vaccine. *See* Tetanus toxoid, reduced diphtheria toxoid, and acellular pertussis (Tdap) vaccine
Technology, for telehealth visits, 29b
Teeth, 86, 87–88, 93, 456. *See also* Dental care
Telehealth, ob-gyn visits and, 29b
Temperature
  core body, birth defects and, 405
  fertility awareness and, 342–343
  home monitoring, 29b
  mother's, after delivery, 275
  ovulation and, 19–20, 19f
Teratogens, 395–396
Testicles, 138, 273
Tetanus, 415–416

Tetanus toxoid, reduced diphtheria toxoid, and acellular pertussis (Tdap) vaccine
  postpartum, 276, 298
  prepregnancy, 6–7
  recommended during pregnancy, 130, 155, 412, 413t, 416
Tetracyclines, oral, 71
Thalassemias
  carrier screening, 9t, 567t
  family history of, 563b
  prenatal diagnostic tests, 81t
  types and risks, 554t
Third trimester
  antiphospholipid syndrome and, 538
  defined, 49
  fatigue during, 46
  fiber during, 460
  growth of baby monitoring in, 506
  hepatitis B infection testing, 418
  placenta previa and, 617
  preterm PROM and vaginal bleeding in, 597
  sexual desire during, 111
  stillbirth delivery in, 657
  vernix development during, 122
  weight gain during, 54t, 101, 363t, 489t
  39 weeks, delivery before, 171
    labor induction at, 221b
    problems for babies born before, 174, 222b, 255–256
    waiting to deliver until, 172, 173b, 176
3-in-1 car seats, 194
Three-dimensional (3D) ultrasound exam, 580
Throat cancer, 418
Thrombophilias, 535, 536–537, 639
Thyroid disease, 529, 532, 545–547, 548
Thyroid gland, 404, 454, 545, 547f
Thyroid hormone, 545
Tiredness, 138. *See also* Fatigue
Tobacco, 13, 56, 313, 502. *See also* Smoking
Tocolytics, 475, 599, 602
Toes, extra, 554t
TOLAC. *See* Trial of labor after cesarean delivery
Toxins, 56, 396, 401–403, 410. *See also* Environmental exposure history
Toxoplasmosis, 403, 434, 461
Trans fats, 353, 354
Transabdominal ultrasound exam, 77f, 580
Transducer, 62, 75, 77f, 580–581
Transfusion, blood
  ABO incompatibility and, 608
  cesarean delivery and, 259
  delayed cord clamping and, 190
  placenta accreta and, 621
  placenta previa and, 134, 616
  placental abruption and, 134, 619
  postpartum hemorrhage and, 639
  through umbilical cord, Rh antibodies and, 612
Translocation, chromosomal disorders and, 562
Transplants, 200

Transvaginal ultrasound exam, 62, 75–76, 77f, 580–581, 596, 600
Transverse incisions, 258, 258f, 262, 264
Transverse presentation, 254
Trauma, 291, 515, 609, 612. See also Birth injuries
Travel
  by air, 404, 446–447
  by car, 447b, 448
  deep vein thrombosis and, 445b
  international, 437, 446
  meningococcal meningitis and, 420
  overview, 444
  radiation exposure and, 404
  resources, 448–449
  safe, during pregnancy, 439
  by ship, 437, 448
  Zika virus and, 98b, 436
Travel insurance, 445
Travelers' Health website, CDC's, 446, 449
Tremors, early, genetic disorder risk and, 563b
Tretinoin, 71
Trial of labor after cesarean delivery (TOLAC), 253, 258, 261, 262–264, 638
Triceps exercise, 384, 384f
Trichomoniasis, 427
Triglycerides, 297t
Trimesters. See First trimester; Postpartum care; Second trimester; Third trimester
Triplets
  breastfeeding, 319
  cesarean delivery of, 480
  formation of, 471
  length of pregnancy, 474t
  NICU and, 474
  placenta previa and, 615
  placentas and amniotic sacs for, 472
Trisomy, 561, 564
Trisomy 13. See Patau syndrome
Trisomy 18. See Edwards syndrome
Trisomy 21. See Down syndrome
True labor, 150–152, 168–169. See also Labor
  differences between false labor and, 170t, 233t
Truvia (stevia), 75, 366
TTTS. See Twin–twin transfusion syndrome
Tuberculosis (TB), 79, 303, 434–435
Turkish descent, carrier screening, 9t, 554t, 567t
Turner syndrome, 561
Turning the baby
  attempts, RhIg after, 612
  breech presentation and, 160, 248, 249f, 250
  long second stage of labor and, 239
  Rh incompatibility and, 609
Twins. See also Multiple pregnancy
  breech presentation and, 247
  delivery, 480
  discordant, 477
  feeding, 319, 321b
  fraternal, 469–470
  getting ready for, 480–481
  identical, 469, 470–471

Twins (continued)
  length of pregnancy, 474t
  NICU and, 474
  placenta previa and, 615
  postpartum hemorrhage and, 639
  presenting, cesarean delivery and, 254
  resources, 482
  types, 472
  umbilical cord prolapse and, 636
  weight gain during pregnancy and, 363t, 478t
Twin–twin transfusion syndrome (TTTS), 476
Type A blood, 78, 607
Type AB blood, 607
Type B blood, 78, 607
Type O blood, 78, 607
Types 1 and 2 diabetes, 513. See also Diabetes mellitus

U

Ulcerative colitis, 540
Ulipristal pill, 347
Ultrasound exams. See also Biophysical profile
  of amniotic fluid amount, 134
  antiphospholipid syndrome and, 538
  baby's development, 44, 85, 95
  baby's growth and, 624–625
  of baby's position, 160
  of baby's size, 134
  biophysical profile and, 519, 585–587, 586f
  to confirm pregnancy, 62
  CVS and, 574
  Doppler, 237, 580, 584, 588, 625
  ectopic pregnancy and, 650
  elective labor induction and, 221
  estimated due date and, 48–49, 594b, 627b
  frequently asked questions, 582b
  genetic disorders and, 564, 570t
  hypertension and, 506
  keepsake, 457, 581
  macrosomia diagnosis, 628
  miscarriage diagnosis, 646
  modified biophysical profile and, 587
  molar pregnancy and, 653
  multiple pregnancy, 472, 479
  nuchal translucency screening, 81t, 569, 571
  obesity during pregnancy and, 491
  overview, 579
  parvovirus and, 433
  placenta percreta, 620
  placenta previa, 617
  prenatal care and, 75–76, 75f, 101–102
  preterm labor diagnosis and, 596
  PROM management and, 598
  resources, 589
  Rh incompatibility and, 612
  stillbirth, 657
  types and images, 75–76, 77f, 580–581
  uncertain results from, 457, 581
Umbilical artery, 588
Umbilical cord. See also Cord blood
  blood banking, 132, 187, 190–191, 240–241

Umbilical cord (continued)
    breech presentation and, 250
    compression, 635–636
    cutting, 240
    decreased amniotic fluid and, 220
    delayed clamping of, 189–190, 191, 463
    oxygen for baby through, 270
    postterm pregnancy and, 175
    pressure on, PROM and, 597
    problems, 254, 476, 583, 658
    prolapse, 222, 250, 636–637
2-Undecanone, Zika virus and, 436
Underweight, 54t, 490, 496
Unpasteurized milk, 370
Unsaturated fats, 353, 354
Upper body strength exercises, 382
Urethra, 257, 285, 286b, 383, 428–430, 429f
Urinalysis (urine tests), 62, 78, 92, 117, 155, 508–509
Urinary incontinence, 246, 285
Urinary tract infections (UTIs)
    of bladder, kidney, or urethra, 428–430, 429f
    calling ob-gyn about, 91b
    circumcision and, 187
    foodborne illness and, 369–370
    signs and symptoms, 90
    STI protection and, 7
    testing, 78
Urination
    active labor and, 238
    after delivery, 275
    frequent, 46, 150, 166
    postpartum problems, 285
    problems, 90, 282b
    trouble, epidural block or spinal block and, 207b
Urine
    baby's, 311b
    dark, hepatitis A infection and, 417
    leakage, 597
Urine cultures, 78
U.S. Department of Agriculture
    MyPlate food-planning guide, 10, 20, 293, 299, 359–360, 360f, 372
    Special Supplemental Nutrition Program for Women, Infants, and Children (WIC), 363
    Women, Infants, and Children (WIC) Breastfeeding Support Program, 305, 329, 372
U.S. Department of Health and Human Services, 147, 200, 372, 437
U.S. Department of Labor, 448
U.S. Environmental Protection Agency, 107, 372, 407
U.S. Equal Employment Opportunity Commission (EEOC), 441, 449
U.S. Food and Drug Administration (FDA), 365, 372, 397–398, 400, 410
U.S. National Library of Medicine
    on birth control, 347, 464
    on breech presentation, 251

U.S. National Library of Medicine (continued)
    on cesarean birth, 265
    on childbirth, 241
    on complications, 640
    on early pregnancy loss, 655
    on exercise and physical fitness, 393, 464
    on fetal growth restriction, 629
    on fetal well-being before labor, 589
    Genetics Home Reference, 576
    on hemolytic anemia, 612
    on hemorrhoids, 147
    on high blood pressure during pregnancy, 511
    on labor induction, 227
    on newborn screening tests, 279
    on placenta previa, 621
    on postpartum depression, 299
    on preterm babies, 604
    on Rh incompatibility, 613
    on skin and hair changes during pregnancy, 82
    on vasectomy, 347
Uterine artery embolization, 619, 639
Uterine atony, 637, 639
Uterine cancer, 337
Uterine contraction after delivery
    breastfeeding and, 302, 307f, 463–464
    exercise and, 289
    maternal blood vessels and, 241
    pain from, 276
    vaginal bleeding and, 284, 302
Uterine inversion, 638
Uterine rupture
    cesarean delivery and, 173, 244, 255, 259, 629, 633
    labor induction and, 225
    postpartum hemorrhage and, 638
    TOLAC and, 263–264
    trial of labor after cesarean delivery and, 261
    VBAC and, 80
Uterus. See also Contractions; Fundal height measurement; Uterine contraction after delivery; Uterine rupture
    abnormal labor and, 632
    abnormalities, breech presentation and, 247
    baby's development in, 32–41f, 121
    baby's position in, 155
    changes in size of, 102, 102f, 138
    core muscles and, 388
    eggs with aneuploidy and, 560
    fetal development of, 95
    fetal position in, 272
    infections, 171, 232, 259, 424
    IUD insertion into, 332
    Kegel exercises and, 286b, 383
    menstrual cycle and, 16f
    pelvic exam, 30f
    postpartum bleeding, 284
    pregnancy and, 15, 68
    scarring, 171
    sexual activity and, 111, 458

Uterus (continued)
　　size of, 86, 164, 472
　　surgery, placenta previa and, 615
　　tears, postpartum hemorrhage and, 638
　　tightening, preterm labor and, 117, 475b, 596b
　　ultrasound exam of, 76, 77f
　　weight gain during pregnancy and, 55b
UTIs. *See* Urinary tract infections

V

Vacation days, 89, 443
Vaccinations
　　after delivery, 276
　　another baby and, 670
　　CDC information on, 20
　　infection prevention and, 6–7, 410
　　international travel and, 446
　　postpartum period, 298
　　pregnancy and, 413–414t
　　prepregnancy care and, 3
Vaccines, 409, 410–411. *See also* specific diseases
Vacuum aspiration, 647
Vacuum device
　　abnormal labor and, 634
　　assisted vaginal delivery and, 239, 243, 245, 245f, 462
　　continuous labor support and, 213
Vagina. *See also* Pelvic exams
　　chorionic villus sampling and, 574, 574f
　　douching, 452
　　fetal development of, 95
　　forceps-assisted delivery and, 245, 245f
　　GBS in, 155, 431
　　genital warts in, 418
　　injuries, assisted vaginal delivery and, 246
　　Kegel exercises and, 383
　　local anesthesia injected into, 205
　　menstrual cycle and, 16f
　　mucus plug loss through, 169, 232
　　pelvic exams of, 30, 30f
　　perineum and, 276
　　tears, large babies and, 515
　　tears, postpartum hemorrhage and, 638
　　transvaginal ultrasound exam, 62, 77f, 580–581
　　umbilical cord prolapse and, 222
　　vacuum-assisted delivery and, 245, 245f
　　varicose veins near, 140
Vaginal birth. *See also* Assisted vaginal delivery
　　breech presentation and, 250
　　IUD insertion after, 333
　　labor induction and, 219
　　perineal pain and, 287–288
　　VBAC and, 262
Vaginal birth after cesarean (VBAC) delivery
　　benefits, 263
　　benefits and risks, 80–81
　　considerations, 262–263
　　defined, 253
　　discussions with your ob-gyn on, 157
　　trial of labor and, 261

Vaginal bleeding. *See also* Menstrual periods; Spotting
　　between 37 and 40 weeks, 167
　　abnormal, ectopic pregnancy and, 63, 649
　　after cesarean delivery, 259, 260, 261
　　amniocentesis and, 573
　　birth control implant and, 335
　　birth control injection and, 336
　　breakthrough, combined hormonal birth control and, 338
　　calling ob-gyn about, 113b, 133, 133b, 140b, 160b, 232, 282b
　　chorionic villus sampling and, 574
　　during early labor, 234
　　ectopic pregnancy and, 63
　　exercise and, 55, 376
　　heavy, cesarean delivery and, 173, 244, 255, 261b
　　heavy, IUD insertion after birth and, 333
　　heavy, placenta accreta and, 621
　　miscarriage and, 63
　　normal postpartum, 278b
　　placenta previa and, 617
　　placenta problems and, 134
　　placental abruption and, 618
　　postpartum, 284
　　during pregnancy, preterm birth risk and, 595b
　　during pregnancy, Rh incompatibility and, 609
　　during pregnancy, RhIg after, 611
　　PROM and, 597–598, 599
　　smoking and, 56
　　ultrasound exams for, 580
　　VBAC and, 263
Vaginal cancer, 418
Vaginal delivery. *See also* Vaginal birth
　　complications, obesity and, 492
　　going home after, 269
　　multiple pregnancy and, 480
Vaginal discharge. *See also* Cervical mucus
　　after cesarean delivery, 261
　　bad smelling, 282b
　　calling ob-gyn about, 91b, 113b, 133b, 140b, 160b, 168b
　　douching, 452
　　ovulation and, 15
　　postpartum, 285
　　pregnancy and, 90
　　preterm labor and, 117, 133, 145, 159, 475b, 596b
　　PROM and, 146, 597–598
　　as warning to stop exercises, 377b
Vaginal dryness, estrogen cream for, 294
Vaginal ring, for birth control, 337–339, 338f
Valproate (valproic acid), 53b, 356, 398
Vaping, 56
Variant of unknown significance, pregnancy and, 575
Varicella, 421–422, 624. *See also* Chickenpox; Shingles

Varicella vaccine
    after delivery, 276
    chickenpox exposure and, 461
    as live, attenuated vaccine, 411–412
    postpartum, 298
    pregnancy and, 6, 414t
Varicella zoster virus, 421
Varicose veins, 89, 140–141, 140f, 147, 287, 452, 452f
Vas deferens, 345–346
Vasectomy, 345–346, 346f
VBAC. See Vaginal birth after cesarean (VBAC) delivery
Vegetable shortening, sore nipples and, 314
Vegetables, 10, 101, 353, 361, 361t, 362
Vegetarians, 10, 367–368
Veins, 501
Ventilators, 602
Vernix, 38f, 122
Vertical incisions, 258, 258f, 264
Very preterm babies, 474, 599
Video chat, telehealth visits by, 29b
Vision problems. See also Eyes
    blood clotting disorders and, 535
    calling ob-gyn about, 168b
    delivery before 39 weeks and, 174, 256
    early preterm birth and, 116
    postpartum, 282b
    preeclampsia and, 117, 502b, 508
    pregestational diabetes mellitus and, 521
    prenatal care visits and, 27b
Visitors, postpartum period, 292
Vitamin A, 52, 353, 355t, 396, 460
Vitamin B$_1$, 358
Vitamin B$_2$, 358
Vitamin B$_6$, 51, 355t, 358
Vitamin B$_9$, 12b, 53b, 358
Vitamin B$_{12}$, 355t, 358, 494–495
Vitamin C, 52, 74b, 355t, 358–359
Vitamin D
    in balanced diet, 351
    celiac disease and, 539
    deficiency, 459, 494–495
    fats and, 353
    formula feeding and, 325
    recommendations and sources, 355t, 359
    supplements, 52, 310, 312
Vitamin E
    fats and, 353
Vitamin K shot, 274
    fats and, 353
    skin-to-skin contact and, 270
Vitamins. See also Supplements
    in balanced diet, 351
    deficiencies, weight-loss surgery and, 494–495
    as over-the-counter supplements, 399
Vitamins, prenatal
    another baby and, 670
    healthy eating and, 362
    morning sickness and, 50
    multiple pregnancy and, 477

Vitamins, prenatal (continued)
    nutrition and, 52
    recommendations and sources, 354, 355t, 356–359, 400
    smell of, 458
Vomiting
    baking soda mouth rinse after, 88
    calling ob-gyn about, 168b
    damaging effects on the body, 495
    epidural block or spinal block and, 207b
    foodborne illness and, 368b, 369
    managing, 50–51
    multiple pregnancy and, 477
    postpartum care for, 282b
    preeclampsia and, 117, 502b
    pregestational diabetes mellitus in, 523
    pregnancy and, 46, 456
    weight gain during pregnancy and, 489
Von Willebrand disease, 538–539, 639
Vulva
    cleaning, 452
    genital warts on, 418, 423f
    local anesthesia injected into, 205
    pushing too soon and, 238
    tears, learning care for, 276
    varicose veins in, 140, 287

W

Walking. See also Exercise
    during active labor, 237
    after childbirth, 388
    after delivery, 276
    constipation and, 286
    continuous labor support and, 213
    during early labor, 234
    epidural block and, 206
    multiple pregnancy and, 478
    pain relief during early labor and, 185, 210
    during pregnancy, 54–55, 380
    workplace accommodations for, 440b, 441
Walking epidural, 208
Warfarin, 396, 398, 537
Water. See also Baths; Fluids, drinking; Showers
    in balanced diet, 351, 359
    drinking during pregnancy, 459
    intake, constipation and, 73
    international travel and, 446
    labor in, 186, 211
    in vaccines, 410
    workouts, for exercise, 380
Water breaking. See also Rupture of membranes
    during active labor, 237
    calling ob-gyn about, 168b
    during early labor, 234
    labor and, 169, 232
    preterm labor and, 117, 133, 145
Weakness, 64, 204, 650
Weaning, 327
Weeks 1 to 8. See Months 1 and 2
Weeks 9 to 12. See Month 3
Weeks 13 to 16. See Month 4
Weeks 17 to 20. See Month 5

Weeks 21 to 24. *See* Month 6
Weeks 25 to 28. *See* Month 7
Weeks 29 to 32. *See* Month 8
Weeks 33 to 36. *See* Month 9
Weeks 37 to 40. *See* Month 10
Weight gain during pregnancy. *See also* Weight of mother
    components of, 55b
    excessive, future health risks, 297t
    excessive, macrosomia and, 627
    gestational diabetes and, 518
    guidelines on, 54t, 363t, 456
    hemorrhoids and, 141
    how much? 456
    multiple pregnancy and, 477–478, 478t
    prenatal care and, 62
    recommendations, 363–366, 363t, 489t
    sudden, calling ob-gyn about, 168b
    sudden, preeclampsia and, 117, 502b
    weeks 1 to 8, 53–54
    weeks 9 to 12, 73
    weeks 13 to 16, 91
    weeks 17 to 20, 101
    weeks 21 to 24, 112
    weeks 25 to 28, 122
    weeks 33 to 36, 155
Weight loss, 293, 493, 510, 521. *See also* Bariatric surgery
Weight of baby. *See also* Macrosomia
    alcohol and, 314
    breastfeeding and, 311b
    early preterm birth and, 116
    newborn, 272
    prenatal estimate of, 155
    TOLAC and, 262
    type of pregnancy and, 474t
    ultrasound exams and, 580
Weight of mother. *See also* Obesity; Overweight; Weight gain during pregnancy
    another baby and, 670
    dealing with comments about, 122, 488b
    healthy, reaching and maintaining, 11–13
    hyperemesis gravidarum and, 51
    importance of, 487–489
    low prepregnancy, 595b, 597
    obesity and pregnancy and, 489–493
    societal judgment on, 487
Weight training, 382
Well-woman health care, 298
West Indian descent, carrier screening, 9t, 567t
White coat hypertension, 503
Whooping cough (pertussis), 7, 415–416. *See also* Tetanus toxoid, reduced diphtheria toxoid, and acellular pertussis (Tdap) vaccine
WIC. *See* Women, Infants, and Children
Witch hazel, for hemorrhoids, 141, 287
Women, Infants, and Children (WIC)
    Breastfeeding Support Program, 304, 305, 322, 329, 372
    Special Supplemental Nutrition Program for, 363

Workplace and working
    breastfeeding at, 158, 328
    expressing milk at, 325
    hazards during pregnancy, 14, 60–61, 405–406, 405b
    health insurance, 443–444
    health risks, discussing with ob-gyn, 92
    pregnancy discrimination and, 64, 449
    pregnant workers' rights in, 439–443
    requesting accommodations, 440–441
    safety and health resources, 65, 407, 449
World Health Organization (WHO), 436
Wound healing, obesity and, 492

X
X chromosome, 556
X-linked genetic disorders, 555t, 558–559, 560f
X-rays, 76, 403–404, 454, 659

Y
Y chromosome, 556
Yeast infection, 90, 428
Yoga, 70, 216, 382, 478

Z
Zika virus
    birth defects and, 403, 435–436
    frequently asked questions on, 460–461
    pregnancy and, 437, 465
    travel and, 98b
Zinc, pica and, 91, 497
Zygotes, 43

618.24 You
Your pregnancy and childbirth